# 1,000,000 Books

are available to read at

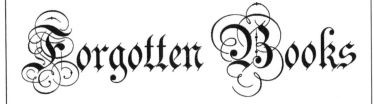

www.ForgottenBooks.com

Read online
Download PDF
Purchase in print

ISBN 978-1-334-71465-8
PIBN 10724911

This book is a reproduction of an important historical work. Forgotten Books uses state-of-the-art technology to digitally reconstruct the work, preserving the original format whilst repairing imperfections present in the aged copy. In rare cases, an imperfection in the original, such as a blemish or missing page, may be replicated in our edition. We do, however, repair the vast majority of imperfections successfully; any imperfections that remain are intentionally left to preserve the state of such historical works.

Forgotten Books is a registered trademark of FB &c Ltd.
Copyright © 2018 FB &c Ltd.
FB &c Ltd, Dalton House, 60 Windsor Avenue, London, SW19 2RR.
Company number 08720141. Registered in England and Wales.

For support please visit www.forgottenbooks.com

# 1 MONTH OF FREE READING

at

www.ForgottenBooks.com

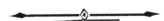

By purchasing this book you are eligible for one month membership to ForgottenBooks.com, giving you unlimited access to our entire collection of over 1,000,000 titles via our web site and mobile apps.

To claim your free month visit: www.forgottenbooks.com/free724911

\* Offer is valid for 45 days from date of purchase. Terms and conditions apply.

English
Français
Deutsche
Italiano
Español
Português

# www.forgottenbooks.com

**Mythology** Photography **Fiction** Fishing Christianity **Art** Cooking Essays Buddhism Freemasonry Medicine **Biology** Music **Ancient Egypt** Evolution Carpentry Physics Dance Geology **Mathematics** Fitness Shakespeare **Folklore** Yoga Marketing **Confidence** Immortality Biographies Poetry **Psychology** Witchcraft Electronics Chemistry History **Law** Accounting **Philosophy** Anthropology Alchemy Drama Quantum Mechanics Atheism Sexual Health **Ancient History** **Entrepreneurship** Languages Sport Paleontology Needlework Islam **Metaphysics** Investment Archaeology Parenting Statistics Criminology **Motivational**

# AN ENGLISH TRANSLATION

OF

# HE SUSHRUTA SAMHITA

## Vol. II.

NIDÁNA-STHÁNA TO KALPA-STHÁNA.

# AN ENGLISH TRANSLATION

OF

# THE SUSHRUTA SAMHITA

WITH

A FULL AND COMPREHENSIVE INTRODUCTION, ADDITIONAL TEXTS,
DIFFERENT READINGS, NOTES, COMPARATIVE VIEWS,
INDEX, GLOSSARY AND PLATES

IN THREE VOLUMES

EDITED BY

KAVIRAJ KUNJA LAL BHISHAGRATNA, M.R.A.S.

Vol. II.

NIDÁNA-STHÁNA, S'ÁRIRA-STHÁNA, CHIKITSITA-
STHÁNA AND KALAPA-STHÁNA.

———:·:———

CALCUTTA:
PUBLISHED BY THE AUTHOR,
NO. 10, KASHI GHOSE'S LANE

1911

*All Rights Reserved*

PRINTED BY M. BHATTACHARYYA, AT THE BHARAT MIHIR PRESS,
25, ROY BAGAN STREET, CALCUTTA.

# PREFACE.

It is with mingled feelings of pain and pleasure that we now place before the public the Second Volume of our English Translation of the Susruta Samhita. The arduous task of compiling a connected and succint history of any part whatever, of the ancient Hindu System of Medicine—requires greater leisure and more extensive reading than we can lay any pretension to. Years of patient study and constant discourse with our sainted preceptor the late lamented Mahamahopadhyaya Kaviraj Dwaraka Nath Sen, Kaviratna, that refulgent link of the golden chain of the Dhanvantaric succession, have enabled us, however, to grasp the leading facts, and during the last few years we have worked continuously, in moments snatched from the practice of an anxious profession that knows no respite, to arrange these facts in their present form. It breaks our heart to record the sad departure of our venerable Acharyya from this sublunary sphere to a land "from whose bourne no traveller e'er returns."

It is hardly necessary for us to reply to those critics who, through their ignorance of the original

Sanskrit works, persist in describing Ayurveda as an empirical system destitute of Anatomy, Physiology or Pathology in any scientific sense.

It behoves us, however, in this preface to meet some of the charges which have been brought against us.

Exception has been taken to our not including in the opening stanza the usual invocation to the Supreme Self (for a successful completion of the work) although it has found its way into almost all the printed editions of the work extant.

Now the stanza referred to finds no place in the various manuscript copies of the original work which are in our possession, or on which we have been able to lay our hands. The work was first put into print by the late Dr. Madhusudan Gupta and we believe that it was only in this printed edition that the benedictory address in question appeared for the first time, and that it has since crept, by the process of circulation, into subsequent printed editions.

In this opinion we are supported by the fact, that in none of the various commentaries and annotations on the Susruta Samhita is any mention made of the line in question, whereas, had it been the opening stanza of the original work, it would certainly have received at least a passing notice at the hands of the commentators, however easy or simple it might have been. Further, were it composed by Susruta himself, it would not have been in the form in which we find it in the printed editions. The ancient sages used invariably the auspicious expression "अथातः" or "ओम्" and the like, when commencing a work and never invoked any particular deity for a happy termination of their undertaking.* These are the reasons which have led us to omit the passage in our present translation.

Another objection raised by a certain section of the community is that we should not have at all undertaken to translate the work into the English language. Their contention is that the Ayurveda, being an integral portion of the Eternal Vedas, should, on no account, be rendered into a *Mlechchha Bhásha* and thus made accessible to the public at large, irrespective of caste or creed.

Such an objection, at this time of the day, is, to say the least, most puerile! Truth is truth, and latitudes and longitudes are not its boundary lines. The Vedas themselves have been translated into many European languages. To keep the truths promulgated by our ancient sages confined within the *coterie* of the privileged classes and thus to deprive the educated public of the

---

\* Thus :—

(a) "अथातो दीर्घञ्जीवितीयमध्यायं व्याख्यास्यामः"—Charaka Samhitá

(b) "अथातो धर्मं व्याख्यास्यामः"—Kanáda Vaiseshika Sutra

(c) "अथातो ब्रह्मजिज्ञासा"—Vedánta Sutra.

benefit of such truths would certainly be a sacrilege. In giving preference to English as the medium of translation we have been actuated by more reasons than one.

It cannot be gainsaid that English has now become almost the *lingua franca* of the world, and to disseminate the ancient wisdom of India throughout the world, we could not have selected a medium better than the English language.

Besides this, we have been actuated by the hope of drawing the direct attention of our benign Government to the scientific value of our system of Medicine by the adoption of such a procedure.

Here we must not stop without expressing our sincere and hearty thanks to our learned and valued friends Kaviraj Jogindranath Sen, M.A., Vidyabhusana, Kaviraj Jnanendranath Sen, B.A., Kaviratna and Professor Satyendranath Sen, M.A., Vidyávágisa, who have rendered us material help in the publication of this volume. We must freely admit that but for the active and continued co-operation of the above-named gentlemen we could not have brought out this volume so promptly and successfully. Our thanks are also due to Dr. S Sanyal, B.Sc., L.M.S. for his kind help, to Dr. S. N. Goswami, B.A., L.M.S. for his kindly supplying us with materials for writing the Introduction, and to our readers for their kind encouragement.

In conclusion, we implore our readers to excuse the errors of omission and commission which are inevitable in the execution of such a huge work, more especially when the author is encumbered with the responsible duties of his profession involving, as they do, the life and death of persons entrusted to his care.

10, Kashi Ghoshe's Lane,
    Calcutta.     } Kunja Lal Bhishagratna.
*November, 1911.*

# INTRODUCTION.

Ayurveda is not an Encyclopædia of ancient medical works, but a Treatise on Biology.

In the introduction of the first volume of our translation of the Susruta-Samhitá we have attempted to place before the public a correct interpretation of Váyu, Pitta and Kapha, the falsely so-called humours of the body* and it is a great pleasure to us, that our pronouncement has been very kindly accepted. In the introduction of the present volume we would draw the attention of the readers to the fact that Ayurveda is not at all an encyclopædic work,—an Encyclopædia of the Indian

---

\* Berdoe says :—"What is known as the Humoral Pathology formed the most essential part of the system of the Dogmatics. Humoral Pathology explains all diseases as caused by the mixture of the four cardinal humours, *viz.*, the blood, bile, mucus or phlegm and water. Hippocrates first leaned towards it, but it was Plato who devoloped it. The stomach is the common source of all these humours. When diseases deVelop, they attract humours. The source of the bile is the liVer, of the mucus the head, of the water the spleen. Bile causes catarrhs and rheumatism, dropsy depends on the spleen."

Be it observed that among the humours of Hippocrates there is no place for Váta although in point of fact both his Physiology and Pathology are to be traced to the "Tri-dhátu" of AyurVeda. The secret of this anomaly is that the theory of Váta was found to be a complicated one and Hipprocates, not being able to comprehend its original import, left it out and cautiously introduced, in its stead, his own theory of "water". So we find "Humoral Pathology is not of Indian origin ; neither it is the same which the Indian Rishis of Rigveda deVeloped under the name of Tri-dhátu." It is simply an imitation of Susruta who introduced blood ( शोणितचतुर्थं: ) as the fourth factor in the genesis of diseases. But the borrower, in his interpretation of Susruta, had made a mess of it. He retained blood, but substituted "water" in place of Váta, the most important of the three, for reasons best known to him.

ii INTRODUCTION.

system of Medicine in all its departments, but it is the Science of Life entire.

Though it is customary and convenient to group apart such phenomena as are termed mental and such of them as are exhibited by men in society, under the heads of Psychology and Sociology, yet it must be allowed that there are no absolute demarcations in Nature, corresponding to them, and so in the entire Science of Life, psychology and sociology are inseparably linked with Anatomy and Physiology, nay, more, with Pathology and Hygiene and above all with Treatment. In short the Biological Sciences must deal with whatever phenomena are manifested by living matter in whatever condition it is placed. Life in health ( सुखायुः ) as well as Life in disease ( दुःखायुः ), therefore, fall within the scope of Biology—even life exhibited by man in Society ( हिताहितं ) is not exempted from it.

हिताहितं सुखं दुःखमायुस्तस्य हिताहितम् ।
मानञ्च तत्र यचोक्तमायुर्वेदः स उच्यते ॥ चरक, श्रोकस्थान, १म अध्याय ।

**Ayurveda,—the entire Science of Life.**
In calling Ayurveda, therefore, the entire Science of Life, we are not guided by any prejudice of our own, but we rely solely on facts and figures, and these, when closely studied, will lead any one to arrive at the same conclusion, not unlike our own and to interpret Ayurveda as a collection of Biological Sciences in all departments. In the first place, for the guidance of our readers, we will mention that the name Ayurveda itself is a strong evidence in favour of its being called the **Science of Life**. Secondly, we will refer to the arrangement of the subject-matter in the Sárira-stháná which is popularly belived to be the anatomical portion of the book, as tending to the same conclusion. In this section, chapters on Midwifery and Management of Infants follow close to the heels of those on Anatomy and Physiology, and

**Negative Evidences thereof:—**
1. **The Name itself.**

**II. The arrangement of the subject-matters.**

these latter again are immediately preceded by chapters on Psychology. This intermixture is certainly an anomaly and can in no wise be satisfactorily explained unless we have to look upon these as general truths of Biology, elucidated by the Introduction of special truths exclusively collected from the science of medicine—भिषगादिषु संसार्थे सन्दर्शितानि । To call it Descriptive Anatomy or Physiology, in the modern sense of the term is simply ridiculous. The

**Want of Descriptive Anatomy and Physiology in the sections of Sarira-sthana itself :—**

absence of any reference to brain and spinal cord, to pancreas and heart, in a book of Anatomy and Physiology is unpardonable and in the Sárira-sthána we feel this absence almost to despondency. Moreover, in western medical science, Grey's Anatomy and Kirke's Physiology, for instance, in their bulk, exceeds, each, more than a thousand of pages and to present to the public, under the same name less than half a dozen of pages, as the result of Indian wisdom, is certainly a very miserable contrast—a contrast that is calculated to inspire no admiration, but, on the contrary, to generate in scientific minds an universal apathy, at least an apathy towards all that is connected with the system of Indian Medicine. In order to save our venerable Rishis from this disastrous plight, we announce here foremost of all, that our beloved Science of Ayurveda is by no means an Encyclopædic work, but

**Positive Evidences.**
**I The definition of Ayus.**
**Same as Life as defined by Mr. Herbert Spencer.**

distinctly possesses every characteristic that marks the Science of Biology. The very name Ayurvada indicates that it is actually a science of *Ayus* and the word *Ayus* is used here in the same sense as Mr. Herbert Spencer understands by his remarkable definition of Life.

In his masterly classification Mr. Herbert Spencer has, in his Biology, given, indeed, the first place to Anatomy and Physiology, but still it is divested of any elaborate chapters dealing with the subjects.

In the science of Life a short reference to the structures of the body or its functions is quite sufficient to illustrate its principles, and if we fail to find therein any discourse on the descriptive Anatomy and Physiology, we still consider that there is nothing amiss.

But unfortunately the fate of Ayurveda is otherwise. Though the very name indicates that it is Biology pure and simple, still it is denounced for its dificiencies in Anatomy and Physiology, and doomed for ever.

Sanskrit words are notorious for their confusion of meanings, but, as regards Ayurveda there exists no difference of opinion, at least, so far as the first word is concerned. *Ayus* is *Ayus* everywhere in Ayurveda and it is the only fault our venerable Rishis may be reasonably charged with, that they did not put themselves into any great trouble to explain *Ayus*, but, on the contrary, unlike scientific men, misspent their energy to ascertain the significance of the insignificant portion of Ayurveda, that is the meanings of the root *"Vida"* in the light of Grammar.

The scientific ear, ever unsatisfied with these grammatical eruditions, has ultimately thrust an Encyclopædic value upon what is properly speaking, a book of Biology. Of course, there is a marked difference between the two. An ordinary treatise on Biology deals with the general truths of life, and does not represent, by way of illustrations, all its special truths, nor their practical sides, but so far as Ayurveda is concerned, the general truths of Biology are thrown into the background and the special truths, gleaned exclusively from the science of medicine, are given great prominence (भिषगादिषु संसार्थं सन्दर्शितानि), so much so, that it is now regarded as a system of Medicine and Surgery which has neither Biology, nor Anatomy, nor Physiology, nor Pathology—but is a systematised Empiricism or Quackery. This is certainly a great misfortune. Apart from the name, the arrangement of the subject, to which we have just referred, at least, in the section of Sárira-sthána (the falsely so-called Anatomy of

## INTRODUCTION.

the Hindus),—is a direct contradiction to its bieng considered as an Encyclopædic work. The existence of the chapters on midwifery and management of infants in the same, following immediately the chapters on Anatomy, serves as a strong additional evidence thereof. It is an anomaly no doubt, that Midwifery has been offered a place in the section of Anatomy, but the confusion does not get at all confounded, if we are led to believe that the science of generation of a superior race (if we are at all permitted to use the term) forms, indeed, an important department of Practical Biology.

*Reasons for incorporating Midwifery into this Anatomical section.*

From whatever standpoint we look to the question, we find there are grounds to lead any one to pronounce in our favour and to come to the conclusion at which we now venture to arrive. Besides these two important facts, we now cite the following passage as a strong internal evidence in favour of our view. Maharshi Punarvasu, after giving us a short table of the principal structures of the human body, remarks that even this reference is considered by many as superfluous, on the ground, that an acquaintance with the molecular construction of an organism is quite sufficient to help us as a reliable guide to treatment.

*Internal evidence.*

*Reasons for omitting Descriptive Anatomy.*

The passage referred to is quoted below :—

"एके तदुभयमपि न विकल्पयन्ते प्रकृतिभावाच्छरीरस्य ।"

Now we ask the reader if this is not a sufficient evidence, proving to the hilt, that Ayurveda is nothing but Biology and that we run no risk of committing a grave omission if the chapter on Anatomy is wholesale dispensed with from Ayurveda. For the improvement of this awkward position—that in the section of Anatomy there should be no Anatomy—the entire credit is due to Susruta, as he has very wisely made the suggestion, that a knowledge of the anatomical structures of the body is of great value, at least so far as it

## INTRODUCTION.

helps the Surgeons and the Surgeons only in their operations.*
But so far as Biology is concerned with medicine, Susruta
does not forget to lay particular stress on the knowledge of
the molecular construction of the body. The following
memorable passages actually preached by this renowned
Surgeon, some three hundred centuries ago, still stands as a
model from which modern Science, even in its present advancement, can draw inspirations.

He says :—

1. न शक्यमचक्षुषा द्रष्टुं द्रेहि सूक्ष्मतमो विभुः ।
   दृश्यते ज्ञानचक्षुर्भिस्तपश्चक्षुर्भिरेव च ॥
   शरीरे चैव शास्त्रे च दृष्टार्थः स्याद्विशारदः ।
   दृष्टश्रुताभ्यां सन्देहमवापीद्याचरेत् क्रियाः ॥

2. तस्मान्निःसंशयं ज्ञानं हृत्वा शल्यस्य वाञ्छता ।
   शोधयित्वा मृतं सम्यग् द्रष्टव्योऽङ्गविनिश्चयः ॥
   प्रत्यचतो हि यद् दृष्टं शास्त्रदृष्टश्च यद्भवेत् ।
   समासतस्तदुभयं भूयो ज्ञानविवर्द्धनम् ॥

That is, the protean work of the protoplasm in which the
great Self resides cannot be detected by the body's eye ; to
know its work, mind's eye is necessary, along with the body's
eye. For acquiring efficiency in Surgery alone, the dissection

---

\* Susruta recommends dissection on dead human bodies and suggests
that it is only required of those who will practise surgery and that students
of medicine can do without it. Herophilus practised dissection on
living bodies and with the object of practising medicine successfully,
but it soon fell into disrepute and did not at all influence the art of
Medicine. He was condemmed even by his own pupil Philinus of cos
who declared that all the Anatomy his vivisecting master had taught him
had not helped him in the least in the cure of his patients. Such
indeed was the fate of vivisection for which Europe now takes pride.

But Susruta's, *Avagharshana* is now considered by many as the only
perfect mode of dissection ever known. It is with the help of this
method of dissection that the layers of epidermis and dermis could be
discovered and blood-vessels with their minute branches could be counted
to be as many as thirty millions. Not only this, but also in the opinion of
several European savants, Susruta still stands as a model of surgery and
European surgery has borrowed many things from Susruta and has yet
many things to learn.

of dead body (not of living body as proclaimed by Herophilus), nay, the *Avagharshana* which brings into view

**The knowledge of the Molecular Construction of the body is all that is wanted.**

the layers of the epidermis and the dermis, the number and branches of blood-vessels and nerves that lie embedded in muscles, etc., is only necessary. Professor Michael Foster's remarks in his article on Physiology in the Encyclopedia Britannica, to all appearnces, are just in the same line, if not identical with our extract, when he says "that the problem of Physiology, in the future, is largely concerned in arriving by experiment and inference, by the *mind's eye*, and not by the body's eye alone, assisted, as that may be, by lenses yet to be introduced at a knowledge of the molecular construction of the protean protoplasm ; of the laws according to which it is built up and the laws according to which it breaks down ; for these laws when ascertained will clear up the mysteries of the protean work which the protoplasm does."

In short the knowledge of the molecular construction of the body is just the thing with which Biology is concerned, and such is the unanimous verdict both in the East as well as in the West, in the most ancient and in the most modern Sciences of the world. Now, if the 'knowledge of the molecular construction of the protoplasm, of the laws according to which it is built up, and the laws according to which it breaks down,' is all that is necessary for an accurate knowledge of Anatomy and Physiology, our Ayurveda is pre-eminently the Science we want.

The following extracts, from Charaka Samhitá, are cited here to prove that we are quite justified in our contention.

1. शरीरावयवास्तु परमाणुभेदेनापरिसंख्येया भवन्ति—तेषां संयोगविभागे वायुः कारणम् । कर्म स्वभावश्चेति ।

2. शरीरसंख्यां यो वेद सर्वावयवशो भिषक् । तद्ज्ञानिमित्तेन स मोहेन न युज्यते ॥

That is, the body is composed of molecules and these are said to be numberless, because no body can count them up.

By their union, they build up the body, and this union is governed by three Laws, viz., the Laws of Váyu, Karma and Swabháva (which are almost equivalent to the three Biological Laws, *i e.*, the law of heredity, the law of external relations and the law of molecular motion caused by Ethereal vibrations compared with which nerve-impulses—akin to electric force,—are grosser and coarser shocks). So far we think we have proved that Ayurveda, as a Biology is not defective, if it contains no descriptive Anatomy and Physiology—descriptive in the same sense as Grey's Anatomy or Kirke's Physiology is. Its Histiology is molecular; its Pathology is molecular ; its Physiology is molecular. **Molecular in every sense is the Biology of the Hindus.** Virtually speaking, Ayurveda is our Science of Life, and we will presently shew that *Life* and *Ayus* are identical.

The continuous adjustment of molecules, their successive breaking down and building up within an organised living body, without destroying its identity, is the definition of *Ayus* as suggested by Maharshi Punarvasu.

He says :—

शरीरेन्द्रियसत्त्वात्मसंयोगो धारि जीवितम् ।
नित्यगश्चानुबन्धश्च पर्यायैरायुरुच्यते ॥

**The Definition of Ayu.** In another place the same definition is repeated with a slight modification and in this he enumerates चेतनानुवृत्ति:, (consciousness) as the most distinctive characteristic of *Ayus*. According to this definition, शरीरेन्द्रियसत्त्वात्मसंयोग: and चेतनानु-वृत्ति: re'er to an organised living body ; नित्यग: and अनुबन्ध: are identical with processes of breaking down and building up of the organism without destroying its identity. The idea of continuous adjustment is included also in these two words.

**The same as Life.** So we find, the definition of *Ayus*, as sugessted by Punarvasu, includes more than what is proposed in Mr. Herbert Spencer's definition of *Life*. The words धारि and जीवितम्, as explained by the great annotator Chakrapáni, represent two more distinct phases of Life, the first bearing upon the existence in the system of a preventive factor of putrefaction, the second pointing to the agent or agents that adjust the internal relations by delicate touches, which professor Michael Foster speaks of as "continuously passing from protoplasm to protoplasm and compared with which the nervous impulses (which are perhaps electrical in nature) are grosser and coarser shocks." Now this last epithet, *viz.*, "जीवितं," as explained by Chakrapáni—"जीवयति प्राणान् धारयति"—furnishes us with a clue to determine what *Ayus* ( आयु: ) actually means.

*More comprehensive than Life as defined by Mr. Herbert Spencer.*

*Prof. Michael Foster on the Theory of Sensation.*

*The Findings of the Upanishads.*

Our Sacred Upanishads now come forward to our relief and tell us, in the first place, "आयु: प्राण:," *i e*, Ayu and Prána are one and the same principle. In the second place, "य: प्राण: स वायु:", *i.e*, Prána and Váyu are identical. In the third place, "स एष एवायं वायुराकाशिनानन्य:", *i.e.*, Váyu is not unlike Ether. In the fourth place, "खं पुराणं वायुरं खं", *i e.*, the primitive fluid (according to Lord Kelvin) is divided into two parts, *viz.*, one without motion, another endued with motion. In the fifth place, "सर्वमित्याकाशे", *i.e.*, everything in this world are waves of this Ether endued with motion. In the sixth place, "वायुर्वाव संवर्ग:" "वायुरेव देवेषु, प्राण: प्राणेषु", *i e.*, Váyu is the universal store of energy; in the Physical world it is known by the name of Váyu; in the Living world it is called under a different name and that name is Prána (प्राण:)

From the above short table we come to know that the agent that adjusts the internal relations to external relations, is *Ayus* and that *Ayus* is Life, and that Life is a motion of the great etherial fluid which is known in Sanskrit as "खं" and that "वायुरं खं" is the sum of all the various energies—biological and abiological—which under the name of heat, light, electricity or consciousness, etc., manifest themselves both in the Physical as well as in the Metaphysical

*The same as primitive fluid as defined by Lord Kelvin.*

## INTRODUCTION.

world, and that Prána (प्राण:) is another name of the same force that, in acting on an aggregated living body, divides itself into five distinct forces, *viz.*, *Prána, Apána, Samána, Udána,* and *Vyána*, and subserves the functions of correlation ( वायु: ) and sustentation ( पित्तं ) and controls oxidation ( स्नेष्मा ). So Prána continuously helps to adjust, like the main-spring of a watch, the internal relations to the external relations. We are indebted to the master mind of Sankara for his able exposition of the functions of this main-spring,

**The Identity of Váyu and Ether.** that is, of the etherial vibrations (वायुप्राण:) as transformed into the *vital force* in an organised body. We quote below what he says about it in his celeberated commentary on the Vedánta Darsana.

**The five divisions of Váyu in its action on a living aggregate.** वायुरेवायमध्यात्ममापन्नः पञ्चव्यूहो विशेषात्मनाऽवतिष्ठ-मानः प्राणो नाम भण्यते न तत्त्वान्तरं नाऽपि वायु-मात्रम् । अतश्चोभे अपि भेदाभेदश्रुती न विरुध्येते ।
२।४।९ ।

That is, the primitive fluid that is endued with motion in its evolution of Life gets knotted into five divisions, viz , *Prána, Apána, Samána, Udána* and *Vyána*, and this acting on any aggregated living matter is called **Prana**. So what we call Prána is not the Váyu itself, but a particular mode of its motion. Hence the question of identity and non-identity is a matter of choice. Shortly speaking, this is the Biology of the Hindus. This too is the sum and substance into which (as a department of Biology), Physiology unfolds itself.

**Biology forms the basis —— Medical Science developed as so much collateral branches.** This too evidently serves as the line of demarcation between सुखायु: and दुःखायु:, हितायु: and अहितायु:. From this too Health and Disease, Hygiene and Treatment, Psychology and Sociology have all their origin and start. In fact, Biology forms the basis upon which the great edifice of the Indian Medical Science, as a collateral branch, has been developed.

**Conclusion.** The general truths of Biology a·e all there in the Ayurveda ; but the special truths from medicine have been given so great a prominence that the real character of the book has been over-shadowed and it has been transformed into a Science of Medicine.

\* \* \* \* \* \* \*

With a view to convey to the minds of our readers an idea of the different branches of the Medical Science which developed as a collateral branch of this great Science of Life, we would here touch upon a few of them in passing.

**Magnetism.** Magnetism had formed its way into the therapeutics of the ancient Hindus and animal magnetism was very extensively practised in India long before they were recognised by Mesmer in Germany and subsequently by John Elliotson in England.

**Hydropathy.** The Indian writers on Medical Science of the good old days have described in length the medicinal properties of the waters of the principal rivers, lakes, water-falls and mineral springs of the country that were known at the time and their respective curative powers as applied to various ailments that human flesh is heir to. This goes a long way to establish the fact that Hydropathy was known in India long before it was even dreamt of in the Western world.

**Massage.** The ancient Hindu sages from time immemorial had been cognizant of the benefits of massage and shampooing and taken to practising them. Whereas, it is but of late that the advantages of these methods have begun to be appreciated by the Western Medical School and it no longer hesitates to acknowledge them as efficacious therapeutic agents.

**Genesiology.** The Science of begetting healthy and beautiful children, which is just beginning to receive attention in other countries was not unknown to the ancient Hindus, and Manu in his *Mánava-dharma-Sástra* has laid down special injunctions which still form an integral part of the domestic life of the orthodox section of the community. As a matter of fact, they knew that mental impressions of the parents at the time of conception exercise a great influence over the future destiny of the child in embryo.

Thus we read in the Sástras :—"A woman, though at a distance, conceives a child of the shape of the person she loves ardently and thinks of at the time. Just as a tree that grows is not different from the parent tree whether we plant a branch or sow a seed, so the main features of the child partake of the features of its father, though there might be slight changes due to the soil."

The subtle soul co-operates with the Manas (the mind) ; the mind co-operates with the senses ; the senses perceive objects ; all this takes place in little or no time. The above is the connection between the soul and objects around us. What is there which the mind cannot comprehend ? Therefore, wherever the mind enters, the soul follows it.

"The soul being subtle, whenever it enters another soul, requires some time and an effort of the mind to know the latter. The soul, which intensely meditates on an object, assumes the shape of that object." etc, etc.

**Anæsthetics.**
In a book entitled Bhoja-Prabandha being a collection of the anecdotes realating to the reign of Bhoja Rája, by Pandita Ballala there is narrated the detail of an interesting surgical operation which had been performed on the Rájá, who was suffering from an excruciating pain in the head. All the medical aid obtaining at the same time was availed of, but in vain and his condition became quite critical when two brother physicians accidentally arrived in Dhar, who were duly called in. These physicians, after carefully examining the patient, held that unless surgically treated no relief could possibly be afforded to the Royal patient. Accordingly they administered an anæsthetic called **Sammohini** with

\* *Vide*—Baràha Mihir's Brihat Samhità Book, II. Chapter lxxv. Verses 1-3.

a view to render him insensible and, when completely under the influence of the drug, they trephined his skull, removed the malignant portion of the brain, the actual seat of the complaint, closed and stitched up the opening and applied a healing balm to the wound. Then they administered a restoration known as **Sanjivani** to the patient, who, thereupon, regained consciousness and felt quite at ease. This incident (as narrated by Thakur Saheb of Gondal in his Short History of Aryan Medical Science) goes to prove that the attendant physician of Buddha, is likewise recorded to have practised cranial surgery writh the greatest success. Instances of successful cases of abdominal section are also not rare. Thus it will appear that the ancient Indians knew and successfully practised surgical operations which are regarded now-a-days as the greatest triumphs of modern surgery. The purpose of chloroform in the palmy days of yore was used to be served by **Sammohini**, but there is hardly a drug known to modern Pharmacopæias, corresponding whith **Sanjivani** which certainly lessens the chances of deaths that at present sometimes occur under anæsthetics.

Let them, who allege that the Hiudu system of the healing Art is unscientific, now pause and reflect ere they make such an unwarranted and irresponsible assertion. How can a system which contains so accurate an account of the unions of bones and ligaments, anastomoses of nerves, veins and arteries, etc, and which assures the world of the existence of three crores and a half of veins and arteries in the human body giving facts and figures thereof with such mathematical precision, be regarded as being unscientific?

It is certainly an undeniable fact that one of the colossal achievements of modern Western Medical Science is its Anatomy; but the point at issue is whether the process of laying open the structures of the body with the lancets, is at all a satisfactory method. For, is it not a fact that the finest and the

**Dissection.**

minutest arteries of the skin are never disclosed, if the scalpel is used so recklessly to remove the skin all at once and not allowed to go deeper into the muscles to expose the minute branches of blood vessels and nerves that may happen to lie embedded therein ? But, on the contrary, look at the process promulgated by Susruta for demonstrating practical Anatomy ! Its originality and perfection beats hollow all the known methods, although it was discovered in almost the pre-historic age. The process prescribed by the Hindu system is as follows :—Cover a dead body with *Kusa* grass and place it at the edge of the water of a rivulet. After three days take it out carefully, and gradually take off the succsesive layers of the epidermis and dermis and of the muscles beneath by gently and lightly rubbing it over with a soft brush. Thus the smallest and the thinnest arteries, which have by this time swelled and obtained a distinct existence are made palpable everywhere even to the minutest.

The process is termed, as we have pointed before, **Avagharshana** by Susruta. The Western method might be an easier and a more off-hand one, but by no means precise.

**Avagharshana.** Though the merit of discovering this mode of dissection is due to Susruta, we are all blind to it and call Hippocrates the father of Medicine ! It is generally believed that with a view to further his researches and perfect his knowledge, it is Hippocrates who inaugurated the system of dissection of dead human bodies and he did the work secretly. Credulous people may lend a willing ear to such assertions but the fact is, that it was not till a century later that Hirophilus openly resorted to dissection of human bodies and thereby earned an undying fame in Europe, obliterating Susruta's name for ever, though, virtually speaking, he (Susruta) was the pioneer of dissection and figured in the world more than a millenium before the advent of Hippocrates and over eleven centuries prior to the age of Herophilus,

It would not, perhaps, be out of place here to mention that Dr. A. F. R. Hoernle, M. A , F. R. S , C. I. E., Ph. D., in his recent publication on Hindu Osteology, has proved it to the hilt, how systematic, scientific, unerring and exact were the researches of the ancient Hindus and what a mine of resplendent truths lay imbedded in them ! We, in our Introduction of the first volume of this work, have tried to prove how very superb, salutary and supremely happy was the theory of Váyu, Pitta, and Kapha promulgated by Susruta. There we have incidentally mentioned that the Science of Embryology was not unknown to the Hindu sages. In the present volume we mean to prove to a point that the main principles promulgated in the Anatomy, the Physiology and the Pathology of Susruta yield in no way to the principles on those subjects included by the modern Western Scientists and investigators. On the other hand, we boldly affirm that in the theories propounded by Susruta some two thousand years back there lies a fund of truths which might well throw a flood of light on the field of labour of the modern scientific men of the West. For is it not a fact that the theories of *Vamana* (causing to eject the contents of the stomach by mouth), *Virechana* (causing the evacuation of the intestines), *Nasya* (causing to inhale through the nose), *Anuvásana* and *Asthápana* which, in ancient India, had earned the appellation of Pancha-Karma, and had gained universal prevalence, and were extensively practised by oriental physicians from time immemorial, have, of late, been hailed by the medical authorities of the day as the most approved and commended mode of treatment.

Sceptics who care nor to examine and weigh solid facts, bluntly allege that the Ayurvedic system is not based upon experiment and observation—the key-stone of all true Science, and such being the case its Anatomy, Physiology, Pathology and Therapeutics are all erroneous. The suggestion, cruel and baseless as it is, originally emanated from an eminent Indian physician who has earned an unenviable reputation by writing a Treatise on Hindu Materia Medica. He says :—"It (the Ayurvedic system) is built not so much upon experiment and observation as upon an erroneous system of Pathology and Therapeutics." But such an expression would not stand the light of day. Indeed none but the ancient Hindu sages did set a high value on experiment and observation, and where they did not claim some occult knowledge or intuition, it is upon these two that they mainly based all their knowledge.

The Materia Medica of the Hindus is really a marvel. Its description of the properties of drugs belonging to the animal, vegetable and mineral kingdoms, and of the articles of food essential to the maintenance of health and strength, its selection of the specific dietaries and elimination of what are prohibited in particular ailments are every day being found correct. The European preparations of Indian drugs and diets are corroborative evidence thereof. The theory adopted by the ancient Hindus as the basis of their investigation is that every substance, whether vegitable or animal, possesses five properties namely,—Rasa, Guna, Viryya, Vipáka and Prabháva which lenses alone cannot reveal, nor the body's eye after observation and experiment made upon rats and rabbits. And those who have opportunities of studying and practising both the Eastern and Western Medical Science assert that the ancient Medical Science of the Hindus once reached the highest standard of excellence and perfection in Materia Medica, Therapeutics and Hygiene and was simply unrivalled and unapproachable, as it blended Philosophy with Science—the mind's eye with the body's eye.

A dispassionate examination of these facts (and such as can be multiplied to any extent), will convince an impartial reader that Ayurveda, as we find it described in Charaka Samhitá and Susruta Samhitá, if approached in a spirit of fairness and enquiry, might reveal the germs of not a few of the marvellous achievement of the present age in the domain of Medical Science and afford to the assiduous student a vast scope and varied materials for comparision between the Eastern and the Western systems, and render material help in improving upon the one with the aid of the other, and this to the benefit of the suffering humanity at large.

Lastly it is our prayer, that if Western Medical Science was ever anywise, directly or indirectly, benefited by the ancient Medical Science of the Hindus, it is but meet and fair that the former should come forward to render all possible aid to her parent Science, and that as it is almost dying now for want of aid and succour we look hopefully to our present benign Government in whose power lies the means of its complete regeneration.

PLATE No I.

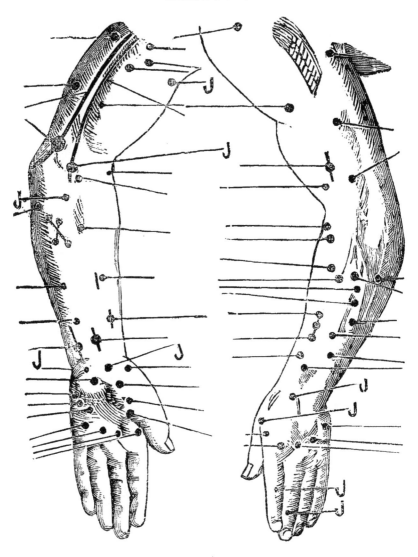

Vital points (Marmas) in the arm (inner side). | Vital points (Marmas) in the arm (outer side).

"J" indicates the points recognised in Juijutsu.

See Chapter VI, S'árira-S'thána.

PLATE No II.

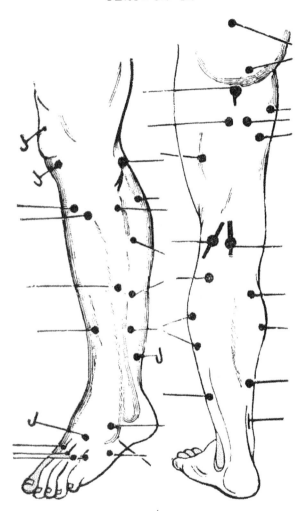

Vital points (Marmas) in the leg (outer side).  Vital points (Marmas) in the back of the thigh and the leg.

"J" indicates the points recognised in Juijutsu.

See Chapter **VI**, S'árira-Sthána.

# CONTENTS.

## NIDÁNA STHÁNA.
(SECTION ON PATHOLOGY).

### CHAPTER I.

**Diseases of the Nervous System, etc** :—The action of the Váyu in its normal state.—The Prána Váyu—The Udána Váyu—The Samána Váyu—The Vyána Váyu—The Apána Váyu.—Descriptions of the nature of the diseases—When they are localised in the different parts of the system.—Pathology of **Váta-rakta**—Its premonitory symptoms—Its prognosis.—Spasms—Convulsions—Epilepsy without Convulsions—Epilepsy with Convulsions.—Hemiplegia—Its Prognosis.—Wry-neck or Torticollis.—Facial Paralysis—Its Premonitory Symptoms—Its Prognosis.—Sciatica.—Erb's Paralysis.—Synovitis of the Knee-joints.—Lameness.—Váta-Kantaka.—Páda-Dáha—Páda-Harsha.—Ams'a-s'oshaka.—Ear-ache.—Deafness.—Nasal Voice.—Indistinct Speech.—Tuni.—Prati-tuni.—Tympanites.—Vátáshthilá.—Pratyashthilá. ... ... ... Pages 1—17.

### CHAPTER II.

**Hæmorrhoids** :—Classifications—Pathology—Premonitory Symptoms.—Vátaja Type—Pittaja Type—Kaphaja Type—Raktaja Type—Sannipátaja Type—Congenital Type.—Figwarts or condylomatous growths about the genitals.—Prognosis. ... ... ... ... 18—24.

### CHAPTER III.

**Urinary Calculii** :—General Ætiology.—Premonitory Symptoms.—Leading Indications.—S'leshmaja As'mari—Pittaja As'mari—Vátaja As'mari.—Seminal Concretions.—Supervening Symptoms.—Situation of the Bladder.—How stones are formed in the Bladder. ... ... 25—30.

## CHAPTER IV.

**Fistula-in-ano** and **Fistular Ulcers** :—Classifications—Premonitory Symptoms.—Derivation of the term Bhagandara.—Vátaja Type—Pittaja Type—Kaphaja Type—Sánnipátika Type—Traumatic Type—S'ata-ponaka Type—Ushtra-griva Type—Parisrávi Type—S'ambukávarta Tppe—Unmárgi Type.—Fistulous Pustules.—Prognosis.   ...   ...  31—34.

## CHAPTER V.

**Cutaneous Affections in general** :—Premonitory Symptoms—Ætiology—Classifications.—Aruna-Kushtha—Audumbara—Rishya-jihva—Kapála Kushtha (Macula).—Kákanaka—Pundarika—Dadru (ring-worm)—Sthulárushka—Eka-Kushtha (Ichthyósis)—Charma-dala (Hypertrophy of the skin)—Visarpa-Kushtha—Parisarpa-Kushtha—Sidhma—Vicharchiká (Psoriasis)—Vipádiká—Kitima (Keloid)—Pámá (Eczema)—Kachchhu—Rakasá (Dry Erythema)—Kilása.—Congenital cause of Kushtha.—Prognosis.—How Kushtha becomes contageous.—Some other contagious diseases enumerated.   ...   ...   ...   ...  35—42.

## CHAPTER VI.

**Diseases of the Urinary tracts** :—Pathology—Premonitory Symptoms.—General characteristics.—Kaphaja Type—Pittaja Type—Vátaja Type.—Names and Symptoms of **Kaphaja** Meha—Surá-meha—Lavana-meha—Pishta-meha—Sándra-meha—S'ukra-meha.—Names and Symptoms of **Pittaja** Meha—Nila-Meha—Haridrá-meha—Amla-meha—Kshára-Meha—Manjishthá-meha—Rakta-meha.—Names and Symptoms of **Vátaja** Meha—Sarpir-meha—Vasá-meha—Kshaudra-meha—Hasti-meha.—Supervening Symptoms.—Kaphaja Types—Pittaja Types—Vátaja Types.—Abscesses.—Carbuncles.—Pimples.—Pustules, etc., due to Prameha.—Prognosis.—Symptoms of Madhu-Meha. ...   ...   ...   ...  43—49.

## CHAPTER VII.

**Dropsy** with an abnormal condition of the abdomen:—Classifications.—Predisposing causes.—Premonitory Symptoms.—Vátaja, Pittaja and Kaphaja Types—Tridoshaja Type.—Enlargement of the Spleen and the Liver with dropsy of the Abdomen.—Vaddha-gudodara—Parisrávi-Udara.—Jalodara (Ascites).—General Characterstics of Dropsy.—Prognosis. 50—54.

## CHAPTER VIII.

**False Presentations and Difficult Labour** :—Causes.—Definition.—Classifications and Symptoms.—Abortion.—Miscarriage.—Prognosis. **Cæsarian Section.** ... ... ... ... 55—60.

## CHAPTER IX

**Vidradhi** (Abscess, etc.) :—Definition and Classification—Vátaja, Pittaja and Kaphaja Types—Sánnipátika Type—Traumatic Type—Raktaja Type—Incurable type of **External** Abscess.—**Internal** Abscesses—Their localities.—Differentiating diagnosis of Gulma and Vidradhi.—Incurable Type . ... ... ... ... ... 61—66.

## CHAPTER X.

**Erysipelas, Sinus** and **Diseases affecting the mammary glands of women** :—Definition of Erysipelas —Vátaja, Pittaja and Kaphaja Types —Sánnipátika Type—Kshataja Type.—Prognosis.—**Nádi-Vrana** (Sinus).—Classification—Vátaja, Kaphaja and Pittaja Types—Dvandvaja and Tri-doshaja Types—S'alyaja Type.—**Stana-roga.**—Breast-milk—Its character—Its normal and abnormal traits.—Stana-Vidradhi (Inflammation of mammary glands). ... ... ... ... 67—71.

## CHAPTER XI.

**Glands, Scrofula, Tumours** and **Goitre** :—Dosha-origened Glands —Sirája gland (aneurysm or Varicose Veins).—Apachi (**Scrofula, etc.**)—Its symptoms.—Tumour—Its symptoms—Blood-origined Tumour.—Mámsa-Arvuda.—Prognosis.—Adhyarvuda.—Dvirarvuda.—Cause of its not being suppurated.—Definition of **Goitre**—Its specific Symptoms—Vátaja Goitre—Kaphaja Goitre—Medoja Goitre.—Prognosis.—General shape of Goitre.— ... ... ... ... ... 73—78.

## CHAPTER XII.

**Hydrocele, Hernia, Scrotal Tumours, Upadamśa** (disease of the genital organ) and **Elephantiasis:**—Classification of Vriddhi—Definition and Premonitory Symptoms of Vriddhi.—Symptoms of Dosha-origined Vriddhi.—Medoja Vriddhi—Raktaja Vriddhi—Hydrocele.—Inguinal

Hernia.—**Upadams'a**—Symptoms of different Dosha-origined types of Upadams'a.—Raktaja Upadams'a.—Definition of Elephantiasis.—Causes and Symptoms of different kinds of Elephantiasis.—Prognosis of Elephantiasis.—Localisation of Elephantiasis. ... ... ... 79—84.

## CHAPTER XIII.

**Diseases known by the general name of Kshudra-Roga** (minor ailments):—The Names and Symptoms of the diseases included therein.—Ajagalliká—Yava-prakhyá—Andháláji—Vivritá—Kachchhapiká—Valmika—Indra-vriddhá—Panasiká—Páshána-Gardabha—Jála-Gaiddabha—Kakshá—Vishphota—Agni-Rohini—Chippa—Kunakha—Anus'ayi—Vidáriká—S'arkarárbuda—Pámá—Vicharchiká—Rakasá—Páda-dáriká—Kadara—Alasa—Indra-lupta (Alopecia)—Dárunaka—Arumshiká—Palita—Masuriká etc.—Tila-kálaka—Nyachchha—Charma-kila—Vyanga—Parivartiká—Avapátiká—Niruddha-Prakas'a—Niruddha-guda—Ahi-putana—Vrishana-kachchhu—Guda-Bhrams'a. ... ... ... 85—93.

## CHAPTER XIV.

**Śuka-dosha:**—Its classification.—Symptoms of different Types.—Progonsis. ... ... ... ... ... 94—96.

## CHAPTER XV.

**Fracture and Dislocation, etc :**—Their Causes.—General features of Sandhi-mukta (Dislocation).—Diagnostic Symptons of Dislocation.—Different kinds of Kánda-bhagna (Fracture)—General symptoms of Kánda-bhagna.—Curable and incurable Types. ... ... ... 97—100.

## CHAPTER XVI.

**Mukha-Roga** (Diseases which affect the cavity of the mouth in general):—General Classification and Localisation.—Diseases of the **lips**.—Dosha-origined Types.—Raktaja Type—Mángsaja Type—Medoja Type—Diseases of the **roots of the teeth.**—Their Names and specific Symptoms.—**Danta-Nádi** (Sinus at the root of a tooth).—Diseases of the **tooth proper.**—Their Names and specific Symptoms.—Diseases of the **tongue**—Their Names and specific Symptoms.—Diseases of the **Palate**—Their Names and specific Symptoms.—Diseases of the **Throat and Larnyx**

—Their Names and specific Symptoms —The different Kinds and Symptoms of Rohini.—Diseases in the entire cavity. ... ... 101—111.

**End of the contents of Sutra-sthána.**

---

# SÁRIRA STHÁNA.

(SECTION ON ANATOMY).

## CHAPTER I.

**The Science of Being in General :**—The Twenty-four Tattwas or first Principles.—The Purusha or the Primordial Being or the Self-conscious Reality.—The Prakriti or the External Nature personified or the non-conscious Eternity—Traits of Commonalty and Diversity.—Comparison of the Philosophy of A'yurveda with that of Sámkhya as well as with the other branches of Philosophy.—Prakriti and Purusha how understood in the A'yurveda—Different kinds of *Manas* (mind).—The five Primary Elements of Creation—Their specific function—Their mutual co-operation in creation. ... ... ... ... ... 113—121.

## CHAPTER II.

**Purification of Semen and Cataminal fluid etc.** :—Derangement of Semen.—Specific treatment.—Derangement of Cataminal fluid.—Specific treatment.—Traits of pure and healthy Semen and Cataminal fluid. —Menorrhœa.—Amenorrhœa.—Their treatment.—Regimen to be observed during Menses.—Conduct of husband during the period.—Prohibited period.—Conception—Subsequent Conduct.—Causes of different Colours in the child.—About twins—Causes of the child being of Defective Organ —Fecundation without sexual intercourse—Causes of Deformity in the child —State of the Fœtus—Its activity while in the womb. ... 122—133.

## CHAPTER III.

**Pregnancy, etc.** :—Combination of Self with the Impregnated Matter.—Factors which determine Sex.—Period and Signs of Menstruation. —Signs of Pregnancy.—Prohibited conducts during Gestation.—Development of the Fœtus.—Longings and its effects during pregnancy.—Development of the Fœtus from the Sixth to the Eighth month.—Time of Delivery. —Different opinions on the formation of the Fœtal body.—The solution— Factors respectively supplied by the Paternal and Maternal Elements, etc.— External Signs of Male, Female and Twin conception. ... 134—143.

## CHAPTER IV.

**The development of Factors in the womb** as well as the **Factors** which contribute to the growths of its different bodily organs and principles :—Different folds of skin over the fœtus.—The definition of Kalás and their Varieties.—Seat of the semen.—Why and how semen is discharged.—Placenta.—Formation of different limbs and organs of the Fœtal body.—Sleep and its effect.—Heart and its action.—Effects of daysleep.—Somnolence.—Effect of Sleep on an Enciente woman —Gnawing. —The temperaments.—Symptoms of Vátaja, Pittaja and Kafaja temperaments - Symptoms of Dvandvaja and Sánnnipátika temperaments.—Sáttvika, Rájasika and Támasika features. ... ... ... 144—158.

## CHAPTER V.

**The Anatomy of the Human body** :—Definition of fœtus.— Enumeration of the different Limbs and Members of body.—Their Numbers— The Cavities or Viscera.—Channels.—Kandará.—Jála or Plexuses.—Kurcha or Cluster.—Sevani or Sutures.—Asthi-Sangháta.—-Simanta.—Bones of the four Extremeties.—Bones of the Trunk.—Bones above the Cavicles— Different kinds of Bones and their situation—Sandhi or Joints.— Joints of the four Extremities.—Sandhis of the Koshtha and Clavicles.— Their forms, distinctions and locations,—The Snáyu or Ligaments.— Their Number and Situations.—Muscles.—Muscles in the extremities in the Koshtha—Of the Head and Neck.—Extra Muscles in Women.—The Vaginal Canal—The Uterus—The Womb.—Superiority of Surgery — Preparations of dead body—Mode of dissection. ... ... 156—172.

## CHAPTER VI.

**The Marmas or Vital parts of the body:**—Classifications of Marmas—Their different Numbers.—Their Locations.—Their Names and Distributions.—The different Heads of Marmas.—Qualitative Classes.— Different opinions on Marmas.—Marmas of the Extremities.—Marmas of the Thorax, etc.—Marmas in the Back.—Marmas in the Clavicular region. —Their specific Symptoms when injured. ... ... 173—190.

## CHAPTER VII.

**The Description and Classification of Sirá or the Vascular System:**—Their Numbers and action.—Names and Classification of the principal Sirás.—Their specific Locations.—The Pitta, Kapha, Váyu and Rakta-carrying Sirás.—Specific Colours of Sirás.—The specific Sirás not to be punctured.—Sirás of the four Extremeties, Trunk and the region above the Clavicles and their roots. ... ... ... 191—197.

## CHAPTER VIII.

**The method of Venesection :**—Persons unfit for Venesection :—Preliminary Rules.—The Jantra-Vidhi or how the patient should be placed in cases of Venesection.—Venesection in the Extremeties.—Venesection on the different parts of the body.—Proper and Defective Venesection—Classification and definition of Defective Venesection. ... ... 198—208.

## CHAPTER IX.

**The Description of the Arteries, Nerves and Ducts :**—Region and Number of Dhamanis.—Functions of the up-coursing Dhamanis.—Functions of the down-coursing Dhamanis. - Functions of the lateral coursing Dhamanis.—The Situation of the Srotas and the specific Symptoms when pierced at the roots. ... ... ... 209—215.

## CHAPTER X.

**Nursing and Management, etc. of Pregnant Women** from the day of conception till parturition :—General rules.—Especial Regimen during the period of Gestation.—Sign of imminent Parturition—Effects of premature Urging—Preliminary Measures.—Post-parturient Measures.—Natal Rites.—Diet for Children.—Treatment of the Mother—Makkalla pain and its treatment.—Management of the Child.—Lactation.—Selection of Wet-nurses.—Examination, etc. of Breast-milk.—Treatment of Wet-nurses.—Infantile Diseases and their Diagonosis.—Treatment of Infants.—Infantile Elixirs.—Nursing of child.—Symptoms when malignant stars, etc. strike the child.—Eductation and Marriage.—Defective Pregnancy—Its Symptoms and Medical treatment.—Miscarriage—Its treatment.—Management of Pregnancy and special Recipe for Pregnant Women according to e months of Gestation. ... ... ... ... 216—238.

**End of the contents of Śárira Sthána.**

# CHIKITSITA STHÁNA.

(Section on Therapeutics).

## CHAPTER I.

**The two kinds of inflamed Ulcers**:—The Causes, Symptoms and Classification of Ulcers.—Idiopathic and Traumatic ulcers.—General and specific Symptoms—Symptoms of different Dosha-origined ulcers.—Symptoms of Blood-origined ulcers.—Symptoms of **Suddha** Vrana.—Therapeutics.—The sixty different Factors of medical treatment of ulcers.—Upadrava or the Supervening Symptoms of ulcers. ... ... 269—264.

## CHAPTER II.

**The medical treatment of Traumatic Wounds or Sores** :— Different Shapes and Classifications of Sores.—Their definitions—Their specific Symptoms—Their treatment.—Treatment of Cuts or Incised Wounds.—Treatment of Excised Wounds—Treatment of Viscera when perforated.—Subsequent treatment.—Treatment of Diabetic Ulcers.— Treatment of Ulcers due to Kushtha or malignant Ulcers. ... 265—278.

## CHAPTER III.

**The medical treatment of Fractures and Dislocations** :— Symptoms of incurable fractures.—Bandage.—Diet.—Defective Bandaging —Washing.—Prrgnosis.—Treatment of fractures in particular limbs.— Gandha-Taila.—Suppuration of fractured Bones—Symptoms of Complete union of fractured Joints. ... ... ... 279—288.

## CHAPTER IV.

**The medical treatment of Váta-Vyádhi or Nervous disorders :** —Nervous affection of the A'más'aya—Nervous affections of the Pakvás'áya —S'álvana-upanáha.—General Measures beneficial to Váta-Vyádhi.—The Tilvaka-Ghrita.—The Anu-Taila.—The S'ata-páka and Sahasra-páka Taila. —The Patra-lavana.—The Kánda or Sneha-lavana.—The Kalyánaka-lavana. ... ... ... ... ... 289—296.

## CHAPTER V.

**The medical treatment of Mahá-Váta-Vyádhi :**—Causes of Váta-Rakta.—Its definition—Premonitory symptoms—Specific features of Váta-Rakta—Prognosis.—Preliminary remedial measures.—Plasters etc.—Treatment of Váta-Rakta with a preponderance of different Doshas.—The five Pradehas—Guda-Haritaki and Pippali-Vardhamána Yogas.—Diet.—Regimen of conduct.—The Medical Treatment of Apatánaka.—Traivrita Ghrita.—Treatment of Pakshágháta.—Treatment of Manyá-stambha.—Treatment of Apatantraka.—Treatment of Ardita.—Kshira-Taila—Tympanites etc.—Hingvádi-Vati.—Symptoms and Treatment of Uru-stambha.—Therapeutic properties of Guggulu ... ... 297—315.

## CHAPTER VI.

**The medical treatment of Arśas (Hæmorrhoids) :**—General remedial measures.—Application of Kshára (Alkali).—Symptoms of satisfactory, excessive and defective Cauterisation.—Diet—Rectal Speculum.—Plasters.—Treatment of Internal piles.—Dantyarishta.—Abhayárishta.—Bhallátaka-yoga.—Other forms of Bhallátaka-yoga.—Regimen of diet and conduct. ... ... ... ... .. 316-328.

## CHAPTER VII.

**The medical treatment of Aśmari (Urinary Calculus, etc) :**—Different modes of treatment in As'mari.—Treatment of Vátaja, Pittaja and Kaphaja As'mari.—Alkaline treatments.—Modes of Surgical operations.—Prognosis.—Lithotomic operations.—Post-surgical measures.—Surgical treatment in Seminal Concretions.—Diet.—Parts to be guarded in Litho-tomic operations. ... ... ... ... 329-337.

## CHAPTER VIII.

**The medical treatment of Bhagandara (Fistula-in-ano, etc) :**—Classification.—General treatment.—Specific measures.—Different Forms and Names of incision.—Treatment of Ushtra-griva.—Treatment of Parisrávi.—Bhagandara in infants—Treatment.—Treatment of traumatic type.—Treatment of Tri-doshaja type.—Syandana Taila.—Description of instrument.—Regimen of diet. ... ... ... 338-345.

B

## CHAPTER IX.

**The medical treatment of Kushtha (Cutaneous Affections in general)**:—Pathology.—Conduct of diet and regimen.—Regulation of diet and conduct.—Preliminary treatment.—Treatment of Doshaja types.—Mahá-tikta Ghrita.—Tikta-Sarpih.—Medicinal plasters.—Alkaline treatment.—Treatment of S'vitra.—Nila-Ghrita.—Mahá-nila Ghrita.—Treatment by Bleeding, Emetics and Purgatives.—Vajraka Taila.—Mahá-Vajraka Taila.—Treatment by Khadira.—Diet. ... ... ... 346-361.

## CHAPTER X.

**The medical treatment of Mahá-Kushtha (Major Cutaneous Affections).**—Mantha-Kalpas.—Diet.—Medicated Arishtas, Ásavas, Surás (Wine) and Powders.—Medicinal Ayas-kriti.—Aushadha Ayas-kriti.—Mahaushadha Ayas-kriti.—Khadira preparations....Khadira-Sára preparations. ... ... ... ... .. 362-371.

## CHAPTER XI.

**The medical treatment of Prameha** (Diseases of the Urinary tracts):—Two-fold Classifications, Causes and Symptoms.—Forbidden articles of food and drink.—Articles of diet.—Preliminary treatment.—The five medicinal remedies.—Specific treatment of Kaphaja Meha—Specific treatment of Pittaja Meha.—Specific treatment of Vátaja Meha.—Palliative measures—Medicinal Arishtas, Ásavas, Yavágus, etc.—Mode of treating a poor Prameha-patient.... ... ... ... 372-378.

## CHAPTER XII.

**The medical treatment of Prameha-Pidaká** (the Abscesses or Eruptions which mark the sequel of a case of Prameha):—Curable cases of Prameha-Pidaká.—Treatment.—Dhánvantara-Ghrita.—Fomentations forbidden in cases of Madhu-meha.—S'ála-sárádi Avaleha.—Naváyasa Churna.—Lohárishta.—Traits of cure. ... ... .. 379-385.

## CHAPTER XIII.

**The medical treatment of Madhu-meha**:—S'ilá-jatu—Its origin, properties and use.—The Mákshika-Kalpa.—The Tuvaraka-Kalpa. 286-391.

## CHAPTER XIV.

**The medical treatment of Udara (Dropsy** with an abnormal condition of the Abdomen) :—Symptoms of curable and incurable types.—Diet of articles forbidden.—Treatment of Vátaja, Pittaja and Kaphaja types.—Treatment of Dushyodara.—General treatment of Udara.—Haritaki Ghrita.—Mahá-vriksha Ghritá.—Chavya Ghrita.—Ánáha-Vartis.—Treatment of Plihodara.—Shat-palaka Ghrita.—Treatment by Venesection.—Treatment of Baddha-Gudodara.—Treatment of Parisrávi Udara.—Treatment of Udakodara.—Treatment by tapping.—Diet. ... 392-403.

## CHAPTER XV.

**The medical treatment of Mudha-Garbha** (Difficult and mal-presentation of the Fœtus and Difficult Labour) :—Varieties of Mudha-Garbha.—Incantations.—Postures of the Fœtus.—Operations involving destruction of the Fœtus.—Craniotomy.—After-measures.—Diet and regimen of conduct.—The Balá Taila.—The Balá-Kalpa. ... 404-411.

## CHAPTER XVI.

**The medical treatment of Vidradhi** (Abscesses) and **Tumours:**—Classifications.—Treatment of Vátaja, Pittaja and Kaphaja Vidradhi.—Karanjádya Ghrita.—Treatment of traumatic and blood-origined types.—Treatment of internal Vidradhi.—Treatment of Vidradhi.—Treatment of Majja-játa Vidradhi. ... ... ... ... 412-417.

## CHAPTER XVII.

**The medical treatment of Erysipelas** etc., **Sinus and Diseases of the Mammary Glands** :—Classifications of curable and incurable types of **Visarpa** (Erysipelas)—Treatment of Vátaja and Pittaja Visarpa.—Gauryádi Ghrita.—Treatment of Kaphaja Visarpa.—Treatment of **Nádi-Vrana** (Sinus).—Treatment of Vátaja, Pittaja, Kaphaja and S'alyaja Nádi (Sinus).—Alkaline treatment—Treatment by Plug-stick—Bballatakádya Taila—Treatment of **Stana-Roga**—Purification of breast-milk—Surgical treatment of Stana-Roga. ... ... ... ... 418-426.

## CHAPTER XVIII.

**The medical treatment of Granthi** (Glandular Swellings), **Apachi** (Scarvi), **Arvuda** (Tumour) and **Gala-ganda** (Goitre) :—General treatment of **Granthi**—Treatment of Vátaja, Pittaja, Kaphaja and Medoja Granthi.—Medical treatment of **Apachi**.—Surgical treatment of Apachi.—**Arvuda**—Treatment of Vátaja, Pittaja, Kaphaja and Medoja types of Arvuda (Tumour).—**Gala-ganda**—Treatment of Vátaja, Kaphaja and Medoja types of **Gala-ganda** (Goitre). . ... . 427-438.

## CHAPTER XIX.

The medical treatment of **Vriddhi** (Hernia, Hydrocele, Scrotal Tumour, etc.), **Upadamśa** (Diseases of the Genital Organ) and **S'lipada** (Elephantiasis):—Treatment of Vátaja, Pittaja, Raktaja, Kaphaja, Medoja and Mutraja **Vriddhi**.—Treatment of Antra-Vriddhi.—Treatment of **Upadamśa**—General treatment—Treatment of Vátaja, Pittaja, Kaphaja, Tridoshaja and Raktaja types of Upadams'a.—Treatment of **Slipada**—General treatment—Treatment of Vátaja, Pittaja and Kaphaja types of S'lipada—Alkaline remedies. ... ... .. 439—449.

## CHAPTER XX

The medical treatment of **Kshudra-Roga** (Minor Ailments):— Treatment of Aja-gallıká and Yava-prakhyá.—Treatment of Vivritá, etc.— Treatment of S'arkarárvuda, etc.—Treatment of Páda-dári, etc.—Treatment of Alasa and Kadara.—Treatment of Baldness and Alopecia, etc.— Treatment of Dárunaka, etc.—Treatment of Jatu-mani, etc—Treatment of Yuvána-pidaká—Treatment of the Retroflexion of the Prepuce.—Treatment of the Constriction or Stricture of the Urethra—Its surgical treatment.— Treatment of the Stricture of the Anus, etc.—Treatment of Valmika, Ahiputana and the Prolapsus of the Anus. ... . 450-458.

## CHAPTER XXI.

The **medical treatment of the Sores on the Penis produced by the Śuka** :—The specific treatment of the different types of S'ukadosha—General treatment —Prognosis. ... ... .. 459-461.

## CHAPTER XXII.

The **medical treatment of the Affections of the Mouth** :— Treatment of Vátaja, Pittaja, Kaphaja and Medoja types of **Oshtha-**

kopa—Treatment of the diseases of the **Danta-mula.**—Treatment of **Danta-Veshta** etc.—Paridara—S'aushira—Upakus'a—Danta-Vaidarbha—Adhimámsa.—Treatment of Danta-nádi.—Treatment of the diseases of the different types of **Tooth** proper.—Treatment of **Tongue-diseases**—Treatment of Vátaja, Pittaja and Kaphaja types of tongue-diseases—Treatment of the different types of **Tálu-gata** diseases—Treatment of **Throat**-diseases.—Treatment of Vátaja, Pittaja, Kaphaja and Raktaja types of Rohini.—Treatment of the different types of the Sarva-sara Mukha-Roga.—Incurable types of Mukha-Roga. ... ... 462-474.

## CHAPTER XXIII.

**The medical treatment of Śopha** (Swellings).—Classifications of general S'opha—Its causes.—The specific symptoms of Dosha-origined types of S'opha.—Symptom of Vishaja S'opha—Complications—Prognosis.—The Special treatment of the different types of S'opha.—General remedies.—Diet. ... ... ... ... ... 475-477.

## CHAPTER XXIV.

**The Rules of Hygiene and the Prophilactic Measures :**—Tooth-brushing—Cases where tooth-brushing is forbidden.—Eye and Mouth-washing —Collyrium.—S'iro'bhyanga.—Combing —Anointing.—Parisheka. —Affusion.—Effusion.—Anointments.—Prohibitions of Anointments, etc.—Physical Exercise.—Rubbing and Friction.—Massage.—Bathing.—Prohibition of Bathing.—Anulepana.—A'lepa.—Food.—Pravata and Niváta.—Sleep—General Rules of Conduct.—Rules for Drinking Water, etc.—Curd (Dadhi)—When and How to be taken.—Women unfit to visit.—Evil Effects of the foregoing Abuses. — ... ... 480-502.

## CHAPTER XXV.

**The medical treatment of a Variety of Diseases :**—Diseases of the Ear-lobes—Classification—Causes and Symptoms—General treatment—Specific treatment.—Treatment of Palita.—Treatment of Vyanga, etc.
503-504.

## CHAPTER XXVI.

**The medical treatment for increasing the Strength and the Virile Power of weak persons :**—Definition of Váji-Karana—Means of Váji-karana.—Causes and Symptoms of the six Forms of Sexual incapacity.—Incurable types.—Remedies—Utkáriká—Pupaliká.—Cakes etc. 510-514.

## CHAPTER XXVII.

**The Recipes and Modes of using Elixirs and Rejuvenators :—** The Human Organism—Which will make it invulnerable to the inroads of any Disease and Decay.—Time of using Rasâyana.—Rasâyana for Mental and Physical maladies—Vidanga-Rasâyana—Vidanga-kalpa —Kâs'marya-kalpa.—Balâ-kalpa.—Ati-balâ, Nâga-balâ, Vidâri and S'atâvari-kalpa.—Várâhi-kalpa —Use of S'ana (-seeds)... ... ... 515-521.

## CHAPTER XXVIII.

**The Elixirs and Remedial Agents** which tend to improve the Memory and invigorate the Mental Faculties as well as to increase the Duration of Human Life :—S'vetâvalguja Rasâyana—Krishnâvalguja-Rasâyana—Manduka-parni-Rasâyana— Bráhmi-Rasâyana — Bráhmi-Ghrita —Vachâ-Rásayana—S'ata-páka-Vachâ-Ghrita.—Measures for prolonging life.—Uses of Gold. ... ... ... ... 522-523.

## CHAPTER XXIX.

**The Restorative and the Constructive Agents** which arrest innate morbific tendencies and decays :—Classifications of Soma.—Mode of using the Soma.—Regimen of Diet and Conduct after taking Soma.—Its Therapeutic effects.—Distinctive features of the Soma-plants—Their descriptions—Their Habitats. ... ... ... ... 530-538.

## CHAPTER XXX.

**The Tonic Remedies which remove Mental and Physical Distress :**—Persons unfit for the use of Rasâyna —Names of the healing drugs.—The Mode of their use.—Regimen of Diet and Conduct—Dosage—Therapeutic effects.—Differentiating traits.—Mode of Culling the above drugs.—Their Habitats.—The common Habitat of all the Oshadhis.

539-545.

## CHAPTER XXXI.

**The medicinal uses of Sneha, etc,** :—Classifications of Sneha—Description of Sneha—The specific uses.—Measures of drugs.—The Kasháya-páka-Kalpa —The Sneha-páka-Kalpa.—Alternative methods.—Application of Sneha according to specific Dosha and Season.—Degrees of Cooking a Sneha—Distinctive traits of the complete cooking of a Sneha.—Process of Internal Use of Sneha —The Specific Uses of Clarified butter—The Dosage.—Evil Effects of over-dosage—Sadyah-Sneha.—Forbidden cases of Sneha-pána —Good Effects of Sneha-pána. .. .. 546-557.

## CHAPTER XXXII.

**The medical treatment by measures of Sveda** (Fomentations, Diaphoretic measures etc.).—Classifications of Sveda.—Its Specific Applications.—Effects of Sveda —Prohibited cases of Sveda.—Symptoms of perfect and imperfect Sveda.—Measures to be followed after Sveda. 558-564.

## CHAPTER XXXIII.

**The Distresses which prove amenable to the use of Purgatives and Emetics** :—Importance of Purgatives and Emetics.—Mode of application of Emetics.—Symptoms of excessive, satisfactory and deficient Emetics.—Effects of satisfactory Emetics.—Cases where Emesis is forbidden.—Cases where Emesis is recommended.—Mode of administering Purgatives.—Classifications of Koshtha.—Diet.—Benefits of proper Purgation.—Persons who should not be purged.—Persons who should be purged.—Necessity of applying Sneha before the administration of Purgative or Emetic. ... ... ... ... ... 565-589.

## CHAPTER XXXIV.

**The treatment of the Disorders resulting from an Injudicious Use of Emetics or Purgatives** :—Their Classes.—Causes and treatment.—Evils of an Unpurged Residue of a Purgative or Emetic.—Evils of a Digested Purgative, etc.—Evils of insufficient or excessive expulsion of the Doshas.—Flatulent Colic.—Partial and Deficient Medication (Ayoga).—Over-drugging with purgatives, etc. (Ati-yoga).—Hæmorrhage due to excessive Vomiting or excessive Purging (Jivádána).—Jiva-s'onita, how to be known.—Flatulent distention of the Abdomen (Ádhmána).—Cutting pain in the Anus, etc.—Dysenteric stools (Parisrâva).—Diarrhœa (Pravâhikâ).—Overwhelming the heart.—Retention (Vibandha) of flatus, stool and urine.   ...   ...   ...   ..  577—589.

## CHAPTER XXXV.

**The Dimensions and Classifications of a Netra and a Vasti with their therapentic applications :**—The importance of Vasti-Karma.—The application of Vasti in different diseases.—Dimensions of the Pipe.—Materials of the Pipe.—Construction of the Vasti.—Classifications of the Vasti.—Nomenclature of the Vasti.—Application of Niruha-Vasti and Ásthápana-Vasti.—Their therapeutic Effects—The different Defects of a Vasti.   ...   ...   ...   ...   ..  590—598

## CHAPTER XXXVI.

**The medical treatment of the mishaps which are consequent on the Injudicious Application of the Pipe and the Vasti :**—Remedies for the injudicious application of the Pipe.—Disorders resulting from a defective Vasti (bladder) and its contents.—Disorders resulting from the defective Position of the Patient.—Remedies for the Complications of the defective position of Niruha-Vasti and Sneha-Vasti.—Intervals for the application of Purgative, Emetic, Ásthápana-Vasti and Anuvásana-Vasti.   ...   ...   ...   ...   ...  599—607.

## CHAPTER XXXVII.

**The treatment with Anuvásana-Vasti and Uttara-Vasti :**—The Process of Anuvásana-Vasti—The process of preparing several medicated Oils and Snehas.—Proper time for the application of Sneha-Vasti.—The mode of applying a Sneha-Vasti.—Symptoms of insufficient, excessive, and satisfactory application of Anuvásana-Vasti.—Diet after the application of a Vasti.—The Successive Actions of a Vasti.—Distresses from Injudicious Application of Sneha-Vasti.—Specific Symptoms —Their remedies.— **Uttara-Vastis**—Dimensions of the Pipe of the Vasti for a Male and for a Female patient.—Mode of application.—Vaginal Uttara-Vasti.—Diseases amenable to Uttara-Vasti. ...   ...   ...   ...  608—626.

## CHAPTER XXXVIII.

**The mode of applying, as well as the treatment with a Nirudha-Vasti** :—The mode of Preparing a Vasti.—The mode of Applying a Vasti.—Symptoms of a satisfactory application of a Vasti.—Subsequent treatment and Diet —Drugs to be used in a Niruha-Vasti.—The Formula of a Niruha-Vasti.—The process of preparation.—The Dvádasa-Prasriti — Classifications of Vastis according to the range of their therapeutic applications.—Corrective Vastis.—Lekhana-Vasti.—Váji-Karana-Vasti.— Vrimhana-Vasti.— Pichchhila-Vasti.— Gráhi-Vasti.— Sneha-Vasti.— Utkles'ana-Vasti.—Dosha-hara-Vasti.— Soothing Vasti.—Yukta-ratha-Vasti.—Siddha-Vasti.—Mustádika-Vasti.—Variations in the composition of Vastis in cases of persons of different Temperaments.—Nomenclature of different Vastis and their Specific Uses.                    ...   ...   ...   637—646.

## CHAPTER XXXIX.

**The treatment of distressing Symptoms which are manifested in a patient** :—The quantity of diet to be taken after the exhibition of a Niruha-Vasti.—Internal application of Sneha after Blood-letting.—Preparations of different diets.—Diet to be taken according to the Dosha and to the Strength of the patient.—Regimen of conduct.—Articles of diet.
647—652.

## CHAPTER XL.

**The treatment which consists in employing the Dhuma** (Fumes), **Nasya** (Snuffs) and **Kavala** (Gargles) ;—Classifications of Dhuma—Materials of different Dhuma-Varti.—Formation of the Pipe used in Dhuma-Pána—Mode of inhalation of different Dhumas—Prohibitive cases —Time of Dhuma-pána (Smoking)—The therapeutic effects of Dhuma-Pána—Mode of Smoking.—**Snuffs** and **Errhines** (Nasya)—The Nomenclature of the term "Nasya"—Classifications of Nasya—S'iro-Virechana—Its application—Dosage of Sneha-Nasya—Effects of proper, excessive and deficient application of a Sneha-Nasya—Avapida-Nasya—Forbidden cases.—Prati-marsha Nasya when to be used— Its effects.—Specific use of Sneha-Nasya —**Kavala-graha** (Gargles)—Classification—Mode of application—Their uses—Kavala and Gandusha distinguished—How long Kavala should be retained—Symptoms of satisfactory, deficient and excessive Gargling.—Prati-sárana—Its classification and effects.    ...  653—671.

**End of the Contents of the Chikitsita Sthána.**

# KALPASTHÁNA.

(SECTION ON TOXICOLOGY).

—:o:—

## CHAPTER I.

**The mode of Preserving Food and Drink from the effects of Poison** :—The necessary qualifications of a Superintendent of the Royal Kitchen—The necessary features of a Royal Kitchen.—Characteristic features of a Poisoner.—Indications of poisoned food and drink, etc.—General treatment.—The mode of preparing Soup, etc. ... ... 673—684.

## CHAPTER II.

**The Indications** (Effects, Nature and Operations) **of Sthávara Poisons** :—Sthávara Poison—Its source.—Names of the different Vegetable and Mineral poisons.—Effects of poison on the Human organism.— Effects of Bulb-poisons—Specific properties and actions of Bulb-poisons—Definition of Dushi-visha—Symptoms of weak and slow poisoning—Derivative meaning of Dushi-visha.—Symptoms of the different stages of Sthávara Poisoning—The medical treatment.—Keshátakyádi-Yavágu—Ajeya-Ghrita —Vishári Agada.—Treatment of the supervening Symptoms of Poisoning.— Prognosis. ... ... ... ... ... 685—694.

## CHAPTER III.

**The Subject of** (the nature, virtue, etc. of) **Animal Poisons** :— Different locations—Characteristic features and purifications of poisoned Water.—Poisons in the Atmosphere and its purification.—Mythological origin of Poison.—Properties of Poison—Nature and Location of Snake-poison—General treatment of poisoning—Symptoms of taking poison internally.—Fatal bites.—Prognosis. .. ... .. 695—702.

## CHAPTER IV.

**The Specific Features of the Poison of a Snake-bite** :—Clasifications of Snakes—Classifications of Snake-bites—Their specific Symptoms— Characteristic features of the different species of Snakes.—Features of the different Castes amongst Snakes.—Particular Habits of the different kinds of Snakes.—Names of the different species of Darvi-kara Snakes—Names of the different species of Mandali Snakes—Names of the different species of Rájimán Snakes—Names of the different species of Nirvisha Snakes—Names and Origin of the different species of Vaikaranja Snakes—Sub-families of the Vaikaranja Snakes.—Characteristic features of Male and Female Snakes—Features of their bites—General and specific symptoms of a bite by a Darvikara Snake—Specific symptoms of a bite by a Mandali Snake—Specific symptoms of a bite by a Rájimán Snake—Specific symptoms of bites by Snakes of different Sexes and Ages, etc.—Symptoms of the different stages of poisoning from the bites of a Darvi-kara Snake—Different stages of poisoning from the bite of a Mandali Snake—Different stages of poisoning from the bites of a Rájimán Snake.—The *Vegántara* (or the intervening) Stages.—Different Stages of poisoning in cases of Lower Animals.—Different stages of poisoning in cases of Birds. ... ... 703—714.

## CHAPTER V.

**The medical treatment of Snake-bites** :—General treatment of Snake-bites.—Mantras (Incantations)—Blood-letting in Snake-bites—Specific treatement of the bite by a Hooded (Darvi-kara) Snake, a Mandail Snake and a Rájimán Snake.—Contra-indication to blood-letting in cases of Snake-bites.—Dosage of Collyrium, etc., to be resorted to in cases of different Beasts and Birds.—General dosage of medicines in cases of Snake-bites—Specific treatment of poisoning according to the Physical Symp'oms—Specific treatment of the different Supervening Symptoms —Remedy for the aggravated Doshas due to Poison—Medical treatment of persons made unconscious from the effects of a Fall or Suspended Animation.—Symptoms of wounds from Poisoned Darts, etc.—Treatment of a Poisoned Wound—Recipe of different Agadas—Mahágada—Ajitágada—Tárkshyágada—Rishabhágada — Sanjivana Agada—Darvi-kara-Rájila-visha-hara-Agada —Mandali-Visha-hara Agada—Vams'a-tvagádi Agada—Pancha-s'irisha Agada—Sarva-Kámika Agada—Ekasara Agada. ... ... 715—727.

## CHAPTER VI.

**Cases of Rat-poisoning** :—Different Varieties of Rats—General Symptoms of Rat-poisoning—Specific symptoms and treatment of Rat-poisoning—General treatment.—Causes of **Rabies**—Symptoms of Hydrophobia—Prognosis.—Symptoms of Jala-trása—Its treatment—Treatment of bites by rabid-dogs—Treatment of teeth and nail-scratching. 728—736.

## CHAPTER VII.

**Treatment with the Sounds of a** (medicated) **Drum, etc., possessed of Anti-venomous Virtues** : —Ksháragada—Its Uses and Therapeutic Effects—Kalyánaka-Ghrita—Amrita-Ghrita -- Mahá-sugandhi Agada—Rules of Diet and Conduct.—Symptoms of Elimination of Poison. 737—741.

## CHAPTER VIII.

**On insects, i.e., the measures, etc. to be adopted in cases of Insect-bites, etc.** :—The Germination and Classification of Insects — Insects of Vátaja, Pittaja, Kaphaja and Sánnipátika temperaments.— Symptoms of their Bites—The Kanabha class of Insects—The Gaudheyaka class of Insects—S'ata-padi—Manduka (Frogs)—Pipiliká (Ants)—Makshiká (Stinging Flies)—Mas'akas (Mosquitoes).—Incurable classes—Treatment of a bite by strong and acute-poisoned Insects—Recipes of Remedies in different cases.—Origin and Classification of Scorpions—Specific traits and characteristics of Mild-poisoned Scorpions, Madhya-visha Scorpions and Tikshna-visha Scorpions—Treatment of Scorpion-bites.—Spider-bites.— Development of Lutá-poison—Its Potency—Location.— Characteristics of Poison according to its seat in the body of a Spider—Mythological Account of the Origin of **Lutá**.—The different names of Spiders and the general Symptoms of their Bodies— Specific Symptoms of Spider-bites and their Treatment—General Remedies—Specific symptoms of the Incurable cases of Spider-bites—Their treatment.—Surgical Treatment—Treatment of Ulcers incidental to the Bites by Insects or Snakes. ... ... 742—762.

**End of the Contents of the Kalpa Sthána.**

# THE SUSHRUTA SAMHITÁ
## NIDÁNA STHÁNAM.

---

### CHAPTER I.

Now we shall discourse on the **Vátavyádhi-** (diseases of the nervous system) **Nidánam**.*

**Metrical text:**—Having clasped the feet of the holy Dhanvantari, who had arisen out of the primordial ocean with the pitcher of ambrosia on his head, and who was the foremost of all knowers of truth, Sus'hruta interrogated him as follows :—"Tell me, O thou, the foremost of discoursers, all about the different locations and functions of the bodily Váyu (nerve force), both in its normal and agitated conditions, (as well as when it changes its natural seat through a concourse of disturbing or aggravating causes) Instruct me on the nature of distempers, which result from its deranged condition." 2.

The holy Dhanvantari, the greatest of all healers, having listened to the foregoing words of Sus'hruta, replied as follows·—This vital Váyu (nerve force), which courses through the body, is self-begotten in its origin, and

---

\* The term Nidánam, usually translated as Pathology, is meant to include factors, which fall within the respective provinces of Pathology, Etiology, Symptomology and Pathognomy as well. For the meaning and functions of Vàyu see Introduction vol. I. pp xli.—xlii.

is regarded as identical with the divine energy of eternal life (God), inasmuch as it is unconditional and absolute in its actions and effects, eternal and self-origined, and is subtile and all-pervading (like the sky and the atoms). It is the primary factor, which determines the principle of cause and effect in all forms of created things, whether mobile or immobile. It is so called (Váyu) from the fact of its coursing (skr. Vá—to move) throughout the universe. It determines the growth, origin and disintegration of all animated organisms, and as such, it receives the homage of all created beings. Although invisible in itself, yet its works are patent or manifest. It is cold, light, mobile, dry and piercing, and follows a transverse course. It is characterised by the two attributes (proper-sensibles or Gunas) of sound and touch. It abounds in the fundamental quality of Rajas (principle of cohesion and action), is of inconceivable prowess, propels all the deranged or obstructing prinicples (Doshas) in the organism, (or in other words, is primarily concerned with the deranged principles of the body which are pathogenic in their actions) It is instantaneous in its action, and radiates or courses through the organism in constant currents. It has its primary field of action in the intestinal tract (Pakvádhána) and the rectum (Guda). In its deranged state, it is the principal factor, which, (in combination with the deranged Pittam and Kapham), lies at the root of all diseases, and is accordingly termed the king of diseases (Rogarát). 3.

**The action of Váyu in its normal State :**—Now, hear me describe the symptoms, which mark the Váyu, as it courses through the organism. The Váyu, in its normal or undisturbed condition, maintains a state of equilibrium between the different Doshas and the root principles of the body (Dhátu) ; it further tends to maintain uniform state in the metabolism of the body, (protoplasmic, Agni\*) and helps the organs of sense-perception in discharging their specific functions. The bodily Váyu, like the Pittam in the organism, is grouped under five different subheads according to the difference in its functions and locations, and is classified as the Prána, Udána, Samána, Vyána and Apána.† These five classes of Váyu, located in their specific regions, contribute towards the integration and maintenance of the body.  4—6

**The Prána Váyu :**—The Váyu, that courses in (governs) the cavity of the mouth,‡ is called the Prána, its function being to force down the food into the cavity of the stomach, and to assist the different vitalising principles of the body (such as the internal heat or fire etc ) in discharging their functions in life, and to contribute to the general sustenance of the body. A deranged condition of this particular kind of Váyu (Prána) is usually followed by hic-cough, dyspnœa and other kindred distempers  7.

**The Udána Váyu :**—The most important of the vital Váyus, which courses (sends its vibrations) upward, is called the Udána. It produces speech, song, etc. In its deranged state it brings on diseases which are specifically confined to regions lying above the clavicles  8.

**The Samána Váyu :**—The Samána Váyu courses in (governs) the stomach (Ámáshaya) and in the

---

\* See Introduction Vol I. p.p XLVIII—XLIX Mahâmahopâdhyâya Dvárká Nátha Kaviratna interprets this Agni as digestive heat (*Jatharágni*).

† The Prána Váyu is identical with the energy of the nerve centre in the medulla ; the Udána with that of the one which is situated in the speech centre. The Samána is same as the energy of the epigastric plexus, the Udána is same as the energy of the Motor-Sensory Nerves, and the Apána is identical with the force of the Hypogastric plexus

‡ The field of its action includes the regions of the heart, throat, head and the nose.

region of intestines (Pakvàshaya). Its functions consist in digesting the chyme brought down into the intestines in unison with the digestive ferment (Agni), and especially in disintegrating its essence from its refuse or excreted matter. A deranged or aggravated condition of the Samána Váyu causes dysentery, Gulma, and impaired digestion, etc. 9

**The Vyána Váyu :**—The Váyu known as the Vyána courses (acts) through the whole organism, and its functions consist in sending the lymph chyle etc. all through the body and in helping the out-flow of blood (Asrik) and perspiration Five kinds of muscular move-ments\* are ascribed to the action of the Vyána Váyu, a deranged condition of which is generally attended with diseases which are not confined to any particular region, member, or organ of the body, but are found to affect the whole organism (such as, fever, etc). 10.

**The Apána Váyu :**—The Váyu known as the Apána acts in the lower region of the intestines (Pakvádhána). Its functions consist in bearing down the fœtus and the fæces and in evacuating the urine, semen and catamenial blood. An enraged condition of this Váyu tends to bring on serious diseases, which are peculiar to the urinary bladder and the distal portion of the large intestine (Guda). An aggravated condition of both the Vyána and Apána Váyus may produce Prameha and disorders of the seminal fluid, while a simultaneous excitement of the five vital Váyus leads to a sure and speedy termination of life. 11-12.

Now we shall describe the nature of diseases, brought about by the localization of the variously aggravated Váyus in the different parts of the body.—In the cavity

---

\* Such as expansion, flexion, lowering down and lifting up or lateral thrusting of any part of the body.

of the stomach (Ámáshaya) the deranged or aggravated Váyu gives rise to vomiting, vertigo, epileptic fits, thirst and pain at the sides (Párs'va Śula) and about the region of the heart (Hridgraha) In the intestines (Pakváshaya) the enraged or disturbed Váyu gives rise to a rumbling in the intestines a piercing pain about the region of the umbilicus, scanty and painful urination and stool, or their entire suppression (Anáha), and pain about the region of the coccyx (Trika) 13—15. Similarly, incarcerated in the sense-organs, such as the ears, etc. it tends to deprive them of their respective faculties. In the skin (lymph chyle) it produces a discolouring of the complexion, parchedness and twitching in the skin, and causes a complete local anæsthesia, giving rise to a tingling, piercing pain in the skin, which spontaneously bursts, or becomes marked with cracks and fissures. Similarly, the aggravated Váyu interfering with the principle of blood gives rise to ulcers. In the flesh, it produces painful nodes and tumours (Granthi), while in the principle of fat it brings on almost painless tumours (Granthi) unattended with any kind of ulcer. Incarcerated in the veins &c. (Sirá) it produces a stiffening or painful contraction, or a varicose or neuralgic condition; in a ligament (Snáyu), it produces numbness (anæsthesia), palsy, aching pain and convulsive jerks; in a long joint, it tends to deprive it of its contractibility and produces a painful inflammatory swelling (about the affected part). In the bones it produces a wasting (atrophy) of the bones which crack and begin to spontaneously burst, attended with the characteristic bone-ache Again in that important principle of life, the marrow, it tends to dry it up and produces a sort of pain, extending all over the body which knows no respite or abatement. Similarly, in the principle of semen it tends to produce a scanty, defective, or excessive emission of that vital fluid, or a complete stoppage thereof. 16—23.

The Váyu, thus disturbed and agitated, affects in succession the lower and the upper extremities of the body, and the head, or extends all over the body and deranges all its root-principles (Dhátu) The symptoms, which mark such conditions of the body, are numbness (paralysis), convulsive contortions of the limbs (Ákshepa), anæsthesia, and various kinds of pain (Śula), and swelling (Śopha) of the body. The deranged Váyu, having entered the natural seats of the Pittam or Kapham, develops symptoms, which are peculiar to either of them, and gives rise to numerous diseases. 24—25.

The symptoms, which characterise the union of the deranged Váyu with the Pittam (in its particular seat) are a burning sensation, heat, thirst, and loss of consciousness, in addition to the symptoms of the Vátaja disease so generated in that particular part of the body, while a similar unison with the Kapham develops coldness, swelling and heaviness (of the affected part). The disturbed or agitated Vàyu in unison with the principle of blood gives rise to a sort of pricking pain (pins and needles in the affected locality), which can not bear the least touch, or is marked by complete anæsthesia, and symptoms, peculiar to the deranged Pittam, follow in its train. 26—28.

Vomiting, and a burning sensation, etc. in the body, mark the instance when the Prâna Váyu is surcharged (Ávrita) with the Pittam ; while weakness, lassitude, somnolence and a general discolouring of the complexion ( D. R.,—loss of taste ) characterise a case when it is surcharged with the deranged Kapham A burning sensation in the body, loss of consciousness or epileptic fits, and a sense of giddiness (vertigo) and physical languor are the indications, which distinguish a case of the Udàna Vàyu being surcharged with the Pittam ; while a stoppage or absence of perspiration, appearance of goose-flesh on the skin, impaired digestion, coldness and numbness of the affected part characterise a case of the same being surcharged with the Kapham. 29—32.

Copious flow of perspiration, heat with a burning sensation in the body, and epileptic fits indicate a case when the Samána Váyu has become united with the Pittam ; while a copious flow of stool and urine, and an excess of mucous secretion (Kapham) from the nose (fluent coryza) etc. and horripilation mark a case, where it has become saturated with the Kapham. 33—34.

Heat and a burning sensation in the affected part and a profuse menorrhagia mark a case when the Apána Váyu becomes surcharged with the Pittam, whereas a sense of heaviness in the lower limbs characterises a case when it becomes overcharged with the Kapham. 35—36.

[Symptoms such as,] burning and jerking in the limbs, and a sense of physical languor become manifest in the event of the Vyána Váyu being surcharged with the Pittam, while a general heaviness of the limbs, stiffness or numbness of the bone-joints, and an incapability of locomotion indicate the fact of its being surcharged with the Kapham. 37—38.

### The Nidánam of Váta Raktam :—

An over-indulgence in grief, excessive sexual intercourse, inordinate physical exercise, drinking large quantities of wine, observance of a regimen of diet and conduct in a particular season of the year which is improper to it, use of articles of food which are not congenial to one's own temperament and an improper or baneful use of such oleaginous substances (as oil, clarified butter etc.) are the factors, which vitiate in common the blood and Pittam of a person. The foregoing causes especially tend to vitiate or agitate the Váyu and blood in persons of delicate constitutions, or in corpulent persons, or in those who observe a form of perfect continence. 39

The vital Váyu becomes enraged or agitated by excessive riding on horses, camels or elephants or through the lifting or carrying of great weights, etc., or by an inordinate indulgence in things which are possessed of the specific virtue of enraging or aggravating that vital principle. On the other hand, an over-indulgence in such articles of food as are heat-making in their potency, or a surfeit of edibles largely composed of sharp, acid or alkaline substances, as well as a large consumption of potherbs etc., or an exposure to heat tends to vitiate the blood of the organism, and which on account of such contamination, tends to speedily obstruct the passage of the fleet-coursing Váyu. The Váyu, thus impeded in its course, becomes more and more agitated each moment, and is prone to speedily agitate the blood in a similar way. The antecedence of the term "Váta" or "Váyu" in the nomenclature of the disease (Váta-Rakta) is owing to the precedence accorded to the action of the deranged Váyu in bringing about the malady, although it effects this in concert with the vitiated blood of the organism 40.

Similarly, the disease brought about by the agitated Pittam, in conjunction with the vitiated or agitated blood, is called the **Pitta-Raktam**, while the one incidental to the combination of the deranged Kapham with the vitiated blood is called **Kapha-Raktam**. In a case of **Váta-Raktam**, the legs, or the lower extremities can not bear the least touch (Hyperæsthesia) and a sort of pricking, piercing pain (pins and needles) is experienced in those regions. The legs become withered or atrophied and lose all sensibility to touch. In a case of **Pitta-Raktam**, the legs become extremely red, hot, soft and swollen, characterised by a sort of indescribable burning sensation. In a case of **Kapha-Raktam**, the legs become swollen and numbed. The swelling assumes a whitish hue and feels cold to the touch, and is accompanied by excessive itching. In the Sánnipátika or Tridoshaja form of **Dushta-Raktam**, the legs exhibit symptoms, which are respectively peculiar to all the three preceding types  41—43.

**Premonitory Symptoms:**—In the incubative stage of the disease the legs perspire and become cold and flabby, or (on the contrary), the local perspiration is stopped and the legs become hot and hard. Moreover, a pricking pain is experienced in the affected parts which are marked by complete anæsthesia, heaviness, or heat, and discolouring of the skin. The disease creeps in either from the lower extremities, or in some cases, first affects the upper ones and gradually extends all over the body like an enraged rat-poison.

**Prognosis:**—The form of the disease in which the skin of the part lying between the instep and the knee-joint becomes abraded or spontaneously bursts open, exuding pus and blood, attended with loss of strength (Prána) and flesh, curvature of the fingers, and eruptions of nodules, should be regarded as incurable; while a case of one year's standing admits only of palliative measures.  44.

The enraged or agitated Váyu, while coursing swiftly through the Dhamanis (nerves) of the body, shakes it in quick succession, and a disease, (exhibiting such symptoms as shaking or convulsive jerks), is originated which is called Ákshepaka* (spasms, convulsions). The form of the disease, in which the patient falls to the ground, at intervals, is called **Apatánaka** (Epilepsy without convulsions) The aggravated or agitated Váyu, charged with an abnormal quantity of Kapham, sometimes affects and stuffs the entire nervous system, and gives rise to a form of disease, which is called **Dandápatánakam**† (Epilepsy with convulsions), inasmuch as it deprives the body of its power of movement and flexibility, making it stiff and rigid like a rod (Danda). 45—46.

The disease but rarely yields to medicine and, is cured in rare instances only with the greatest difficulty ; its characteristic symptom being a paralysis of the jaw-bone, which makes deglutition extremely difficult. The disease in which the enraged Váyu bends the body like a bow is called **Dhanushtambha** (Tetanus). The disease admits of being divided into two distinct types accordingly as the body of the patient is curved internally (**Antaráyáma**, lit :—inwardly or forwardly extended, emprosthotonos), or externally (**Vahiráyáma**, lit :—extended or bent on the back, resting on his heels and occiput—Opisthotonos). When the extremely enraged and powerful bodily Váyu (nerve-force), accumulated in

---

\* The patient suffers from Vanishings (*támyaté*) and loss of consciousness through the instrumentality of the enraged and aggravated Váyu, hence the disease is so named—*Gayadása*.

† Jejjada holds that the enraged Váyu, in unison with the deranged Kapham, gives rise to another kind of convulsions (Ákshepaka) which he has denominated as Dandá-patánakh which, exhibits such symptoms as coldness, swelling and heaviness of the body on account of its being brought about by a concerted action of the deranged Pittam and Kapham. Several authorities aver that there are four distinct types of Ákshepakah, such as Dandá-patánakh, Antaráyámah, Vahiráyámah, and Ákshepakh of traumatic (Abhighátaja) origin.

the regions of the fingers, insteps, abdomen, chest, heart and throat, forcibly draws in the local ligaments (Snáyu), the body becomes contracted and bent forward, bringing about a curvature of the inner trunk. The disease in this form is called **Antaráyáma Dhanushtambha**. The movements of the eyes become impossible, which become fixed in their sockets; the jaw-bones become paralysed, the sides are broken, and the patient ejects (at intervals quantities of) slimy mucous (Kapham). These are the features which mark the first type (Antaráyàma Dhanushtambha). On the contrary, when the same enraged Váyu, centred or lodged in ligaments which traverse the posterior side of the body, attracts them violently, the body is naturally bent backward. The patient experiences a sort of breaking pain at the chest, waist and thighs, (which are ultimately broken). The disease is called **Vahiráyáma**, and should be looked upon as beyond the pale of all medicinal treatment. 47—50.

Four types of Ákshepaka are usually recognised in practice such as, the (1) one incidental to the concerted action of the enraged bodily Váyu and Kapham (2), the one brought about through the union of the enraged Váyu with the deranged Pittam, (3), the one due to the single action of the agitated Váyu (4) and the one due to any external injury or blow (Abhighátaja).* An attack of *Apatànkah* due to excessive hæmorrhage, or following closely upon an abortion or miscarriage at pregnancy (difficult labour), or which is incidental to an external blow or injury (traumatic), should be regarded as incurable. 51—52.

* Brahma Deva designated the four types of the disease, as Apatânakah, Samsrishta Ákshepakab, simple Ákshepakah and the Abhighâtaja (traumatic).

The disease, in which the extremely agitated Váyu affects the nerve chains (Dhamanis) which spread either in the left or in the right side of the body, whether in the upward, downward, or lateral direction, making them lax and vigourless, and in which the joints of the other side of the body become useless and inoperative, is called **Pakshághata** (Hemiplegia) by eminent physicians. The patient, the whole or half of whose body has become (almost) inoperative and lost all sensibility, but who retains his consciousness so long as there remains the least vestige of vitality in the affected part, suddenly falls down and expires. 53—54.

**Prognosis:**—A case of Pakshághata (Hemiplegia), brought about through the single action of the enraged or agitated Váyu of the body, can be cured only with the greatest care and difficulty. A case of the same disease, engendered by the aggravated Váyu in conjunction with the deranged Pittam or Kapham, proves amenable to medicine (Sádhya). It becomes incurable when caused through the waste of the root principles (Dhátu) of the body. 55.

**Apatantrakah** (Convulsions) :—The Váyu, aggravated (by its specifically exciting factors and principles) and dislodged from its natural seat or receptacle in the body in consequence thereof, courses upwards and finds lodgment in the regions of the head, heart and temples. It presses upon those parts and gives rise to convulsive movements of hands and legs, or at times bends them down.

**Symptoms :**—The patient lies with his eyes closely shut, or stares with a sort of fixed or vacant gaze, the eyes remaining fixed or immovable. The patient loses all perception, and groans. Respiration becomes difficult, or symptoms of temporary asphyxia and unconsciousness set in. Consciousness and a normal condition of the organism return with the passage of the enraged Váyu from the heart, while on the other hand the patient relapses into unconsciousness simultaneously with the envelopment of the heart with that enraged and Kapha-saturated Váyu. This disease is called Apatantrakah and is ascribed to the action of the enraged Váyu surcharged with the deranged Kapham. 56.

**Manyástambha:**—The local Váyu, agitated through such causes as sleep in the day time, reclining with the neck on an uneven place or pillow, gazing upward for a considerable length of time, or looking aside in a contorted way, and enveloped in the deranged Kapham, gives rise to the disease known as Manyástambha (wry neck or torticollis) 57.

**Arditam** (Facial Paralysis):—*Pregnant women, mothers immediately after parturition (Sutiká), infants, old and enfeebled persons are most prone to fall victims to this disease*. It has been also known to result from excessive hæmorrhage or loss of blood The local Váyu, extremely enraged or aggravated by continuous talking in an extremely loud voice, chewing of hard substances, loud laughter, yawning, carrying extremely heavy loads, and lying down in an uneven position on the ground, finds lodgment in the regions of the head, nose, upper lip, chin, forehead and the joints (inner cornea) of the eye, and produces the disease called *Arditam* by distorting the face.

**Symptoms:**—The neck and half of the face longitudinally suffer distortion and are bent. The head shakes; the power of articulating speech is lost, and the

---

\* The portion of the text included within asterisks has been rejected by Jejjaḋicháryya as spurious.

eyes are distorted into a variety of shapes. The portions of the neck and the chin, as well as the teeth on the affected side become painful.

**Premonitory Symptoms :**—The disease generally commences with shivering, horripilation, cloudiness of vision, upcoursing of the bodily Váyu and anæsthesia, a pricking pain in the affected locality, numbness or paralysis of the jaw-bone, or of the cervical muscles of the neck. Physicians, conversant with the Ætiology of diseases, call it Arditam (Facial paralysis). **Prognosis** :—A case of Arditam, appearing in an extremely enfeebled or emaciated patient, or exhibiting such symptoms as a winkless vision, inarticulate speech which hardly seems to come out of the throat, excessive palsy of the face, as well as the one of more than three years' standing, should be deemed as incurable. 58.

**Gridhras'i** (Sciatica).—The disease in which the two great nerve-trunks (Kandarà), which emanating from below the lower extremity of the thigh reach down to the bottom of the insteps and toes, and become stuffed or pressed with the enraged Váyu, thus depriving the lower extremities of their power of locomotion, is called Gridhras'i. 59.

**Vis'vachi** (Erbe's paralysis or Bracial neuralgia):— The disease in which the enraged Váyu affecting the nerve-trunks (Kandará) which run to the tips of fingers from behind the roots of the upper arms, making them incapable of movement and depriving them of their power of flexion or expansion is called Vis'vachi.* 60.

**Kroshtukas'irsha** (Synovitis of the knee-joints):—An extremely painful swelling in the knee-

---

* When the aforesaid nerve of a single arm is affectd the disease is restricted to it alone, while it attacks the both when both their nerves are affected.

joints, which is originated through the concerted action of the deranged Váyu and the vitiated blood is called Kroshtukas'irsha from the fact of its resembling the head of a jackal (Kroshtuka) in shape. 61.

**Khanja** (Lameness)—The disease proceeds from the drawing up of the nerve trunks (Kandará) of a leg by the deranged Váyu lying about the region of the waist. When both the legs are similarly affected, the patient is called a **Pangu**. He, whose legs tremble before starting for a walk and who afterwards manages to go on limping is called a **Kaláya Khanja** one in whom the bone-joints become loose. 62—63.

**Váta Kantaka :**—The local Váyu, enraged by making a false step on an uneven ground, finds lodgment in the region of the ankle (Khudaka, instep according to others), thus giving rise to a disease which is called Váta Kantaka. The burning sensation in the soles of the feet caused by the enraged local Váyu, in conjunction with the deranged Pittam and blood, is called **Páda-dáha**, which is generally seen to afflict persons of pedestrian habits. When the legs are deprived of all sensibility of touch, and a sort of tingling pain is experienced in them it is termed **Pádaharsha**, which is due to the deranged action of the Váyu and Kapham. The disease in which the enraged local Váyu dries up the normal Kapham lying about the shoulder-joints is called **Ansa-shoshaka**. The form in which the aggravated local Váyu contracts the nerves of the arms is called **Avavahuka**\*. 64—67.

**Vádhiryayam** (deafness) :—The disease occurs only when the deranged Váyu, either singly or sur-

---

\* The Ansa-shosha is due to the single action of the enraged Vâyu, while Ava-vâhuka is due to the concerted action of the deranged Vâyu and Kapham.

charged with the Kapham, stuffs the sound-carrying channels (Srota) of the ears. 68.

**Karna s'ulam :**—The disease in which the deranged Váyu causing a piercing pain in the regions of the cheekbones, head, temples and neck, gives rise to a sort of aching pain in the tympanum, is called Karna-s'ulam (otitis). The local Váyu, deranged and saturated with the Kapham stuffing the nerves (Dhamani) which conduct of the sound of speech, produces complete (in some cases partial) loss of the power of speech—*e g.* **Muka** (dumbness), **Minmina** (nasal voice) and **Gad-gada** (indistinct speech) 69—70

A sort of pain, which (rising from the bowels or the urinary bladder and ranging downward) gives rise to a bursting sensation in the regions of the anus and the genitals, is called **Tuni**, whereas the one, rising upward from the preceding parts and extending up to the region of the intestines, is called **Prati-tuni**. A distension of the abdomen (Udara), attended with the incarceration of flatus (Váyu) and an intense pain and rumbling in its inside, is called **Ádhmánam** (Tympanites). When it first affects the stomach (Ámasáya) and is unattended with an oppressive feeling about the heart and pain at the sides it is called **Pratyádhmánam** The Váyu saturated with the deranged Kapham causes the preceding type of distemper. 71—74.

A knotty stone-like tumour (Granthi) of considerable density, whether fixed or mobile, and appearing below the umbilicus, and having an elevated shape which is always found to be extended in an upward direction, is called a **Vátásthilá**, (which) as its name implies, is due to the action of the local deranged Váyu. The tumour, thus formed, obstructs the emission of flatus and impedes the evacuation of fæces. A tumour of similar shape, appearing laterally or across the region of the abdomen (Jathara) and obstructing the passage of stool, urine and flatus (Váta) is called a **Pratyashthilá**. 75—76.

Thus ends the first Chapter of the Nidâna Sthânam in the Sushruta Samhitâ, which treats of the Nidânam of the diseases of the nervous system.

## CHAPTER II.

Now we shall discourse on the **Nidánam** of **Ars'as** (Hæmorrhoids). 1.

Hæmorrhoids may be divided into six classes viz — (i) *Vátaja* (due to the action of the deranged Váyu), (ii) *Pittaja* (due to the action of deranged Pittam), (iii) *Kaphaja* (due to the action of deranged Kapham), (iv) *Raktaja* (due to the action of the vitiated blood), (v) *Sannipátaja* (due to the concerted action of the deranged Váyu, Pittam and Kapham) and (vi) *Sahaja* (congenital).

**Pathology :**—The deranged Váyu, Pittam, etc. enraged by their specific aggravating causes, or by such acts or conduct as partaking of food composed of incompatible substances, eating before the previous meal has been digested, inordinate sexual intercourse, sitting on the haunches, excessive riding, and the voluntary suppression of any natural urging of the body, either severally or in combination of two or three Doshas, or vitiating the blood of a person, who observes no moderation in food and drink &c , become dislodged from their natural seats in the body [according to the law of Prasáranam (expansion and change of place by a deranged organic principle)] and are carried down through the large intestine (Pradhána Dhamani) into the descending colon and getting lodged therein, give rise to growths of polypi or fleshy condylomata, which are known as **piles**. These growths chiefly appear in persons suffering from impaired digestion (Agni), and gain in size through friction with the wearing apparel, weeds, wood, lumps of clay or stone, or by contact with cold water. 3.

The lower end of the large intestine, which passes into the flexure of the rectum and measures four and a half fingers in length, is called the Gudam (lit—the channel of fecal matter), the interior of which is provided with three spiral grooves. Each of these grooves or ring-like muscles lie a finger and a half apart, and are respectively known as Pravábini, Visarjani and Samvarani, or the grooves of out-flow, defecation and closure of the anus (sphincter ani), covering a space of four fingers and having laterally an elevation of one finger's width. 4.

**Metrical Texts :**—These grooves are like the involuted indentures of a conch shell, situated one above the other, coloured like the palate of an elephant. A part of the channel, half a finger's width in length as it is usually measured from the outer hairy orifice of the rectum, is called the anus (Gudoushtha). 5—6.

The first of the aforesaid grooves or rings lies about a finger's width apart from the orifice of the anus.

**Premonitory Symptoms :**—A non-relish for food, a tardy and difficult digestion of food (brought into the stomach), acid eructations, a sense of weakness in the thighs, a rumbling sound in the intestines, emaciation of the body, frequent eructations, swellings around the eyes, a croaking sound in the intestines, cutting pain in the rectum (Guda), apparent indications of an attack of phthisis, jaundice, dysentery, cough, dyspnœa, vertigo, somnolence, excessive sleep, weakness of the organs (Indriya), are indications which predict the advent of this disease, and which become more marked with its progress. 7.

**The Vátaja Type :**—Piles, due to the action of the aggravated Váyu, are non-exuding, rose-coloured, and uneven in their surface. They resemble the Kadamba flowers in structure and are either tubular or sharp-pointed like a needle, sometimes assuming the shape of the wild Tundikeri flower. The stool of a hæmorrhoid patient of this type becomes excessively hard, and can be evacuated only in a sitting posture, with the greatest pain and difficulty. An excruciating pain is experienced in the regions of the waist, back, sides, anus, umbilicus and the genitals. Symptoms peculiar to Gulma, Ashthilá, enlarged spleen and abdominal dropsy add to the distress of the patient, whose skin, nails, eyes, teeth, face, urine and stool also assume a dark black colour. 8.

**The Pittaja Type:**—Piles, brought on through the action of the deranged Pittam, are slender, blue-topped, shifting in their nature, yellowish in their hue, or are coloured like shreds of liver, resembling in shape the tongue of the Śuka bird. They are thick at middle, like barley grains, or resemble the mouth of leeches and secrete a sort of slimy exudation. The stool is marked with blood, and the patient complains of a painful, burning sensation (in the rectum) at the time of defecation. Fever, with a burning sensation and thirst, and epileptic fits, supervene. The skin, nails, eyes, face, teeth, stool, and urine of the patient assume a yellow hue. 9.

**The Kaphaja Type:**—Piles, due to the action of the deranged Kapham, become white, are sunk about their roots, and are hard, round and glossy. They assume a greyish hue and resemble the teats of a cow or the stones of the Karira, or of a Panasa fruit. These piles do not burst, nor do they exude any sort of secretion. The patient feels an irresistible tendency to scratch the excrescences. The stools become copious in quantity and are charged with mucous (Śleshmá), resembling the washings of meat. Indigestion, fever with shivering (Śita-jvara), and heaviness of the head and œdema with a non-relish for food are the symptoms which become manifest with the progress of the disease. The skin, finger nails, eyes, teeth, face, stool and urine of the patient also assume a white colour. 10.

**The Raktaja Type :**—Piles (hæmorrhoids), having their origin in the vitiated condition of the blood resemble the sprouts of the Vata tree in shape and are of the colour of red coral, or the seeds (dark red) of Gunja berry. They exhibit all the symptoms, which are peculiar to the Pittaja type of this disease. Pressed hard by the constricted fæces in their passage through the anus, they suddenly give rise to a hæmorrhage of vitiated (venous) blood, and symptoms characteristic of excessive bleeding are found to supervene. 11.

**The Sannipáta Type :**—In a case of hæmorrhoids due to the concerted action of the deranged Váyu, Pittam and Kapham, symptoms characteristic of each of these *types* manifest themselves in unison. 12.

**The Congenital Type :**—Congenital hæmorrhoids (**Sahaja Arśas**) are usually ascribed to defects in the semen and ovum of one's parents and should be medicinally treated with an eye to the special deranged Doshas involved in the case. The polypi (in this type) are hardly visible and are rough and yellowish, with their faces turned inward. They are extremely painful. A person suffering from this type of piles gets thinner and thinner every day and eats but very little. Large veins (Sirá) appear on the surface of the body. The patient becomes irritable, the semen decreases in quantity, making the procreation of a small number of children possible only by him. The voice becomes feeble, the digestion is impaired, and disorders affecting the head nose, ears and eyes follow. A croaking sound is heard in the intestines, attended with a rumbling in the abdomen. All relish for food vanishes and the region of the heart seems to be smeared with a kind of sticky paste (of mucous), etc. 13.

**Auhoritative verse on the subject :—** A qualified physician should undertake the medical treatment of hæmorrhoids which occur either about the outer or the middle groove of the rectum, (in as much as they prove amenable to medicine). A polypus, appearing about the innermost ring or groove of the rectum, should be treated without holding out any definite hope of cure to the patient. 14.

**Lingárs'as** (Fig warts or condylomatous growths about the genitals) **:**—The deranged and aggravated Váyu etc., finding lodgment in the genitals, vitiate the local flesh and blood, giving rise to an itching sensation in the affected localities. The parts become ulcerated (through constant scratching) and the ulcers become studded with sprout-like vegetations of flesh(warts),which exude a kind of slimy, bloody discharge. These growths, or excrescences generally appear on the inner margin, or on the surface of the glans penis, in the form of soft, slender vegetations of skin, resembling the hairs of a small brush (Kurchaka). These vegetations ultimately tend to destroy the penis and the reproductive faculty of the patient.

**Bhagárs'as :**—The deranged Váyu etc. of the body, lodged in the vaginal region of a woman, gives rise to similar crops of soft polypi in the passage. They may crop up isolated at the outset, and (by coalescing) may assume the shape of a mushroom or an umbrella, secreting a flow of slimy, foul-smelling blood.

The deranged Váyu, etc. may further take an

upward course, and finding a lodgment in the ears, nose, mouth and eyes may produce similar warts in those localities. Warts, which crop up inside the cavities of the ears, may bring on earache, dumbness, and a foul discharge from those organs, while those (cysts) cropping up in the eyes will obstruct the movement of the eye-lids, giving rise to pain and a local secretion and ultimately destroy the eye-sight. Similarly, such growths in the nostrils produce catarrh, excessive sneezing, shortness of breath, headache, nasal speech and the complaint known as Putinasya. Such vegetations cropping up in and about the lips, palate or the larynx, tend to make the speech confused and indistinct. When appearing in the mouth, they impair the faculty of taste, and diseases which affect the cavity of the mouth follow. The excited Vyána Váyu, united with the aggravated Kapham, produces a kind of hard papillomatous growths on the skin (about the anus) which are called the Charmakilas (papillomata).* 15.

**Authoritative verses on the subject:**
—These Charmakilas may be attended with a kind of pricking pain through an excess of the deranged Váyu, whereas those which have their origin in the deranged Kapham (lymphatics) assume a knotty shape and become of the same colour as the surrounding skin. On the other hand, they become dry, black or white, and extremely hard through an exuberance of the deranged local blood and Pittam. 16.

The symptoms of polypi, appearing in the neighbourhood of the anus, have been described in full, while the general characteristics of those, which are found to crop up around the genitals, have been briefly discoursed

---

* According to others, Charmakilas may crop up on the skin of any part of the body.

upon. An intelligent physician should ponder over the two groups of symptoms while engaged in treating a case of piles. A case of piles exhibiting symptoms peculiar to the two deranged Doshas is called the **Samsargajam.** Six distinct types of bio-Doshaja piles are known in practice.* 17.

**Prognosis :**—A case of piles due to the concerted action of the three deranged Doshas of the body, (with its characteristic symptoms) but partially developed, may be temporarily checked (Yápya). Cases, which are of more than a year's standing, as well as those in which the hæmorrhoids are due to the concerted action of the two Doshas (Samsargaja), or are situated in the middle groove of the rectum, may be cured but with the greatest difficulty. Cases of the Sánnipátika or congenital (Sahaja) types should be given up as incurable. The Apána Váyu, in a person whose rectum is overrun with such polypus growths, tries to pass out through the anus, but is driven back upward, being obstructed in its passage by the vegetations, and then mixes with his Vyána Váyu, thus imparing (the five-functioned) fire (Pittam) in his body. 18-19.

* Such as (1) the one due to the concerted action of the deranged Pittam and Kapham, (2) the one incidental to the simultaneous derangement of the Vàyu and the Kapham, (3) the one brought about through the disordered condition of the Váyu and blood, (4) the one due to the combination of the deranged Pittam and Kapham, (5) the one produced by the concerted action of the deranged Pittam and blood, (6) the one which results from the combined action of the deranged Kapham and blood.

Thus ends the second Chapter of the Nidánasthánam in the Sus'ruta Samhitá which deals with the Nidánam of piles.

## CHAPTER III.

Now we shall discourse on the **Nidánam** of **As'-mari** (urinary calculi). 1.

The disease admits of being divided into four several types, such as the Vátaja, the Pittaja, the Kaphaja and the S'ukraja (Seminal) concretions. An exuberance or preponderance of the deranged Kapham should be understood as the underlying cause of all invasions of this disease. 2.

**General ætiology :**—The Kaphah of a man, who neglects to cleanse (Sams'odhana) the internal channels of his organism, or is in the habit of taking unwholesome food, enraged and aggravated by its own exciting causes, is carried into the urinary bladder. Here it becomes saturated with the urine, and gives rise to the formation of concretions or gravels in its cavity. 3.

**Premonitory Symptoms :**—An aching pain in the bladder, with a non-relish for food, difficulty in urination, an excruciating pain in the scrotum, penis, and the neck of the bladder, febrile symptoms, physical lassitude, and a goat-like smell in the urine are the symptoms, which indicate the formation of gravel in the bladder. 4.

**Metrical Text :**—The deranged Doshas involved in a particular case respectively impart their specific colour to the urine, and determine the character of the accompanying pain. The urine becomes thick, turbid, and vitiated with the action of the aggravated Doshas, and micturition becomes extremely painful. 5.

**Leading Indications :**—A sort of exciuciating pain is experienced either about the umbilicus, or in the bladder, or at the median rape of the perineum, or about the penis, during micturition when gravel is forming in the bladder. The urine is stopped at intervals in its out-flow, or becomes charged with blood, or flows out twisted and scattered like spray, leaving a sediment of clear, sandy, red or yellow particles of stone, which resembles a Gomedha gem in colour. Moreover a pain is experienced in the bladder at the time of running or jumping or in swimming, or while riding on horseback, or after a long journey. 6.

**The Śleshmas'mari :**—Stone or gravel, originated through the action of the deranged Kapham, saturated with an excessive quantity of that Dosha by the constant ingestion of phlegm-generating (Sleshmala) substances, increases in size at the lower orifice of the bladder and ultimately obstructs the passage of the urine. The pressure and recoil of that incarcerated fluid on the walls of the urinary badder gives rise to a kind of crushing, bursting, pricking pain in that organ, which becomes cold and heavy. A Kapha-origined stone or gravel is white and glossy, attains to a large size, to that of a hen's egg, and has the colour of the Madhuka flower. This type is called S'leshmás'mari. 7.

**The Pittaja As'mari :**—The Kapham charged (dried) with the deranged Pittam becomes hard (condensed) and large in the aforesaid way, and lying at the mouth of the bladder obstructs the passage of the urine. The bladder, on account of the flowing back of the obstructed urine into its cavity, seems as if it has been exposed to the heat of an adjacent fire, boiling with the energy of an alkaline solution. A kind of sucking, drawing and burning pain is experienced in the organ. This type of Aśmari is further marked by symptoms which characterise Ushna-váta (stricture). The concretion is found to be of a reddish, yellowish black colour like the stone of the Bhallátaka fruit, or it is coloured like honey. This type is called Pittaja Aśmari. 8.

**The Vátáśmari :**—The deranged Kapham (mucus) inordinately saturated with the bodily Váyu, acquires hardness and gains in dimensions, and these lying at the mouth of the bladder obstructs the passage of the urine. The incarcerated fluid causes extreme pain in the organ. The patient constantly under severe pain gnashes his teeth or presses his umbilical region, or rubs his penis, or fingers his rectum (Páyu) and loudly screams. A burning sensation is experienced in the penis, and urination, belching and defecation become difficult and painful.* The concretions in this type of Aśmari are found to be of a dusky colour, rough, uneven in shape, hard, facetted and nodular like a Kadamva flower. This type is called Vátáśmari. 9.

Infants are more susceptible to an attack of any of the three preceding types of Aśmari, inasmuch as they are fond of day sleep or of food composed of both wholesome and unwholesome ingredients, and are in the habit of eating before the digestion of a previous meal, or of taking heavy, sweet, emollient and demulcent food: In children the bladder is of diminished size and poor in muscular structure. These facts contribute to the easy possibility of the organ being grappled (with a surgical instrument) and of the stone being extracted with the greatest ease in cases of infantile Aśmari. 10.

**The Śukráśmari :**—Śukráśmaris or seminal concretions are usually formed in adults owing to the germination of semen in their organisms. A sudden or abrupt stoppage of a sexual act, or excessive coition tends to dislodge the semen from its natural receptacle

---
* Stool and urine can be voided only with the greatest straining.

in the body. The fluid thus dislodged, but not emitted, finds a wrong passage. The Váyu gathers up the fluid (semen), thus led astray, and deposits it (in a round or oval shape) at a place lying about the junction of the penis and the scrotum and dries up the humidity with which it is charged. The matter, thus formed, condensed, and hardened, is called the seminal stone (Śukráśmari), which then obstructs the passage of the urine, giving rise to pain in the bladder, painful micturition, and swelling of the scrotum. The stone vanishes under pressure in its seat*. 11—12.

**Authoritative verses on the subject :**—Concretions, sands and sediments found to be deposited in the urine in a case of Bhashma-meha are but the modifications, or attendant symptoms of a case of stone in the bladder (Aśmari). The same group of symptoms and the same kind of pain are exhibited and experienced in a case of gravel (*S'arkarâ*) as in a case of stone (Aśmari) in the bladder. The local Váyu coursing in its natural direction helps the discharge of calculi (Aśmari) with the urine in the event of they being extremely attenuated in structure. Particles of a stone broken by the Váyu are called urinary calculi (*S'arkarâ*). A pain about the cardiac region, a sense of weakness and lassitude in the thighs, a griping pain in the regions of the spleen and liver (Kukshi-śula), a shivering sensation, thirst, hiccough or eructations, darkness or sallowness of complexion, weakness, emaciation with a non-relish for food and

---

\* We can not but contemplate with admiration the fact that Sushruta was aware of the formation of seminal or spermatic concretions in the seminal vesicles through degenerative changes of spermatozoa and other secretions and their subsequent calcification as lately discovered by the savants of the West.—*Translator*

impaired digestion are the symptoms which are manifest in a gravel-patient. A gravel (S'arkará) obstructed at the mouth of the urinary channel is detected by the following indications :—*viz.*, weakness, lassitude, emaciation, cachectic condition of the body, pain over the hepatic region (Kukshi-s'ula), a non-relish for food, sallowness of complexion, hot and high coloured urine, thirst, pressing pain at the cardiac region and vomiting. 13.

The bladder is situated in the pelvic cavity, surrounded on its different sides by the back, loin (Kati), umbilicus, scrotum, rectum (Guda), groins and penis. This organ is provided with a single aperture or opening and lies with its mouth downward, covered with nets of nerves (Sirá) and ligaments (Snáyu), in the shape of a gourd. The organ is extremely thin in structure; and thus situated within the pelvic cavity, it is connected, through its mouth or external orifice, with the rectum, the penis, and the testes. It is also known by the name of Maládhára (the receptacle of impure matter) and forms (one of) the primary seats of vital energy (Prána)*. The urinary ducts (ureters) pass close by the large intestines (Pakvás'aya) and constantly replenish the bladder and keep it moist with that waste product of the system in the same manner as rivers carry their contributions of water into the ocean. These passages or ducts (which are two) are found to take their origin from hundreds of branches (or mouths *tubuli uriniferi*), which are not visible to the naked eyes, on account of their extremely attenuated structures and carry, whether in a state of sleep or wakening, the urine from below the region of the

---

* The text has *Pránáyatanam*, which means that an injury to the urinary bladder may be attended with fatal result.

stomach† (Amásaya) into the bladder keeping it filled with this important fluid of the body, just as a new pitcher, immersed up to its neck in a vessel full of water, is filled by transudation through its lateral pores. 14.

In the same way the Váyu, Kapham and Pittam are carried into the bladder (through their respective ducts or channels), and in unison with the retained urine, give rise to the formation of stone, on account of the slimy character of the deposit produced. Stone is formed in the same way in the bladder as sediments are ultimately deposited from clear and transparent water at the bottom of a new pitcher which contains it. As the wind and lightning jointly condense the rainwater into hailstones, so the bodily Váyu and Pittam (heat) jointly contribute to the condensation of the Kapham in the bladder and transform it into stone.

The Váyu in the bladder, coursing in its natural downward direction, helps the full and complete emission of urine ; while coursing in a contrary direction, it gives rise to various forms of maladies such as, Prameha, strangury, as well as seminal disorders ; in short, it produces any urinary trouble to which the bladder may be subjected. 15.

† From the kidneys.

Thus ends the third Chapter of the Nidâna Sthânam in the Sushruta Samhitâ which treats of the Nidânam of urinary calculi.

# CHAPTER IV.

Now we shall discourse on the **Nidánam** of **Bhagandaram** (fistula in ano and fistular ulcers). 1.

The deranged Váyu, Pittam, Kaphah and Sannipátah (a simultaneous derangement of the three bodily Doshas) and extraneous causes (such as a blow etc.) give rise to the types of Bhagandaram known as Sátaponaka, Ushtragriva, Parisrávi, Samvukávarta and Unmargi. The disease is so named from the fact that it bursts the rectum, the perineum, the bladder and the place adjoining to them (thus setting up a mutual communication between them). The pustules, which appear in this regions are called as Pidakás in their unsuppurated stage, while they are called Bhagandaram when they are in a stage of suppuration. A pain about the sacral bone and an itching about the anus, accompanied by a swelling and burning sensation, are the premonitory symptoms of this disease. 2.

**The Sátaponakah Type :**—The Váyu, excited, condensed, and rendered motionless by a course of unwholesome food, gives rise to a pustule within one or two fingers' length from the rectum (anal region, —Guda), by vitiating the flesh (areolar tissue) and blood (of the locality). It assumes a vermilion colour and is characterised by a variety of pricking, piercing pain. If neglected at the outset, the pustule runs into suppuration. Owing to its vicinity to the bladder, the abscess or the suppurated pustule exudes a kind of slimy secretion and becomes covered with hundreds of small sieve-like holes, through which a constant frothy discharge is secreted in large quantities. The ulcer, thus formed, seems as if it is being thrashed with a rod, pierced with a sharp instrument, cut with a knife, and pricked by needles. The region of the anus cracks and bursts, and jets of urine, fecal matter, flatus (Váta) and semen are emitted through these sieve-like holes. This type of fistula is called Sátaponakah (Sieve-like fistula in ano). 3.

**The Ushtra-grivah Type:**—The enraged Pittam, carried down by the Váyu (into the rectum) finds lodgment therein, and there gives rise to a small, raised, red pustule, which resembles the neck of a camel in shape, and is characterised by a varied kind of pain, such as sucking etc. The pustule, not medicinally treated at the beginning, runs into suppuration. The incidental ulcer seems as if it is being burnt with fire or alkali, and emits a hot, fetid discharge. Jets of urine, flatus (Váta), fecal matter and semen flow out of the ulcer in the event of it not being healed up with proper medicinal remedies. This type is called Ushtragrivah 4.

**The Parisrávi Type:**—The enraged Kaphah, carried down by the Váyu (into the rectum) and lodged therein, gives rise to a white, hard, itching pustule in that locality, characterised by a variety of itching pains, etc. If neglected at the outset, it soon runs into suppuration. The incidental ulcer becomes hard and swollen, marked by excessive itching and a constant secretion of slimy fluid. Jets of urine, fecal matter, flatus and semen are emitted through the ulcer in the event of it not being well cared for at the outset. This type is called Parisrávi. 5.

**The Śamvukávartah Type:**—The enraged Váyu, in conjunction with the aggravated Pittam and Kapham, is carried down, and finds lodgment (in the region of the rectum), giving rise to a pustule of the size of the first toe, and characterised by a piercing pain, and burning, itching sensations etc. Such a pustule, neglected at the outset, speedily suppurates, and the incidental ulcer exudes secretions of diverse colours, characterised by a kind of whirling pain, which revolves about, in the direction of the involuted indentures (within the grooves of the rectum) such as are found within the body of a river or fresh water mollusc. This is called Śamvukávartah. 6.

**The Unmárgi Type :**—Particles of bones, eaten with (cooked) meat by an imprudent, greedy, gluttonous person, may be carried down with the hard and constipated stool by the Apána Váyu (into the rectum), thus scratching or abrading the margin of the anus, or burrowing into the rectum in the event of their being evacuated in improper directions through (transverse or horizontal postures). The scratch or abrasion is soon transformed into a fetid and putrid ulcer, infested with worms and parasites, as a plot of miry ground will soon swarm with a spontaneous germination of similar parasites. These worms and parasites eat away the sides of, or largely burrow into, the region of the anus, and jets of urine, fecal matter, and flatus (Váyu) are found to gush out of these holes. This type of Bhagandaram is called Unmárgi. 7.

**Authoritative verses on the subject :**—A pustule, appearing about the region of the anus and characterised by a slight pain and swelling, and spontaneously subsiding, should be regarded as a simple pustule, which is of a quite different nature from a fistula in ano, which has contrary features (*i.e.*, invariably found to be attended with a violent pain and swelling etc., and takes a long time to heal). A Fistula-pustule crops up within a space of two fingers' width of the *Páyu* proper (distal end of the rectum), is sunk at its root, and attended with pain and febrile symptoms. Pain, itching and burning sensations are experienced about the anus after a ride in a carriage, or after defecation. The anus becomes swollen, and the waist painful in the premonitory stages of Bhagandaram. 8—9.

**Prognosis :**—Almost all the types of this disease (Fistula in ano) yield to medicine after a prolonged course of treatment, and are hard to cure, except the Sannipàtah and traumatic ones, which are incurable. 10.

Thus ends the fourth Chapter of the Nidâna Sthânam in the Sushruta Samhitâ, which treats of the Nidânam of Fistula in ano (Bhagandaram).

# CHAPTER V.

Now we shall discourse on the **Nidánam** of **Kushtham** (cutaneous affections in general). 1.

Improper diet or conduct; especially ingestion of improper, unwholesome, indigestible, or incongenial food; physical exercise or sexual intercourse immediately after partaking of any oleaginous substance, or after vomiting; constant use of milk in combination with the meat of any domestic, aquatic or amphibious animal; a cold water bath after an exposure to heat; and repression of any natural urging for vomiting etc. are the factors which tend to derange and aggravate the fundamental principle of Váyu in a person. The enraged or aggravated Váyu, in combination with the agitated Pittam and Kapham, enters into the vessels or ducts (Sirá), which transversely spread over the surface of the body. Thus the enraged Váyu deposits the Pittam and Kapham on the skin through the medium of their channels and spreads them over the entire surface of the body. The regions of the skin in which the aforesaid morbific diatheses are deposited become marked with circular rings or patches. The morbific diatheses (Doshas), thus lodged in the skin, continue to aggravate, and having been neglected at the outset, tend to enter into the deeper tissues and thus contaminate the fundamental principles (Dhátus) of the body. 2.

**Premonitory Symptoms :**—A roughness of the skin, sudden horripilation, an itching sensation in the surface of the body, excess or absence of perspiration, anæthesia of the parts, a black colour of the blood, and a rapid growth and expansion of any ulcer (appearing on the body) are the symptoms which mark the premonitory stages of Kushtham. 3.

**Classification :**—[Diseases, falling under the group of Kushtham, may be divided into two broad subdivisions], viz.,—*Mahákushthas* (major) and *Kshudra (minor) Kushthas*, the first consisting of seven, and the second of eleven different types, aggregating eighteen in all. The Mahákushthas are classified as, Aruna, Audumvara, Rishya-Jihva, Kapála, Kákanaka, Pundarika, and Dadru. The minor or Kshudra-kushthas (Lichen and Dermatitis) are Sthulárushkam, Mahàkushtham, Eka-kushtham, Charmadalam, Visarpah, Parisarpah, Sidhma, Vicharchiká, Kitima, Pámá, and Rakasá. All the types of Kushtham, whether major or minor, involve the action of the deranged Váyu, Pittam or Kapham, and are connected with the presence of parasites in those localities.* The preponderance of any particular morbific diathesis (Dosha) in any case of Kushtham should be looked upon as its originating cause. The type, known as Aruna Kushtha, is due to the action of the preponderant Váyu; Audumvara, together with Rishya-Jihva, Kapála and Kákanaka, to a preponderance of the deranged Pittam; while Pundarika and Dadru owe their origin to an excess of the deranged Kapham. These types of major or minor Kushthas are successively more extensive in their action and more incurable on account of their respectively invading a greater number of the bodily elements (Dhátus). 4—6.

**Mahákushthas :**—Aruna-kushtha owes its origin to an exuberance of the deranged Váyu. It is slightly vermilion-coloured, thin and spreading in its

---

\* Certain authorities hold that, all types of Kushtham (cutaneous affections) to be of parasitic origin. The *Garuda Puranam* avers that, the parasites, which infest the external principles of the body, are the primary causes of cutaneous affections—*Kushthaika-hetavontarjáh shlemshajá váhya sambhaváh.* Ch. CLXIXV. 4.

nature. A sort of pricking, piercing pain (is experienced in the affected locality) which loses all sensibility to the touch. The type known as **Audumbara** is coloured and shaped like a ripe or mature *Audumbara* fruit and has its origin in the deranged Pittam. The type called **Rishyajihva** is rough and resembles the tongue of a Rishya (Deer) in shape and colour. The type known as **Kapála** (Macula cærulæ) resembles a black (deep blue) Kharpara ( baked clay ). The **Kákanaka** type is characterised by a dark red and black colour like the seed of the *Gunja* berry. A sort of sucking and burning pain is experienced in the affected locality in all the four preceding types of the disease which are the outcome of the deranged Pittam. The whole diseased surface seems as if burning with fire, and emitting hot fumes They are speedy in their origin and rapidly suppurate and break. All these types soon become infested with parasites These are the general features of these forms of Kushthas. 7.

**Pundarika:**—The patches resemble the petals of a (full blown) lotus flower in colour, and **Dadru** (Ringworm) assumes the colour (faint blue) of an Atasi flower, or of copper. They are spreading in their nature and are found to be overspread with pustules. Both the Dadru and Pundarika types are raised, circular, and characterised by itching and take a considerable time to be fully patent. These are the general characteristics of Dadru and Pundarika. 8.

**Kshudra Kushthas :**—We shall now describe (the features of the diseases known as) **Kshudrakushthas** (M. Text):—The type known as **Sthulárushka** appears about the joints. It is extremely thick at its base, is cured with the greatest difficulty, and is strewn over with hard pustules (Arungshi). In the type known as of **Mahákushtham** the skin contracts, and with the bursting of the skin (a piercing pain is felt in the affected part), which loses all sensibility to the touch, accompanied by a general sense of lassitude in the limbs. In the **Ekakushtham** (Ichthyosis) type the skin assumes a reddish black colour. It is incurable. In the form known as **Charmadalam** (Hypertrophy of the skin) a burning, sucking, drawing pain is experienced in the palms of the hands and in the soles of the feet which become characterised with an itching sensation. The disease, which affects in succession the (organic principles of) skin, blood and flesh, and speedily extends all over the body, like Erysipelas, and is attended with a burning sensation (Vidáha), restlessness, suppuration and a piercing pain and loss of consciousness (epileptic fits), is called **Visarpa Kushtham**. The form in which a number of exuding pustules gradually extend over the surface of the body is called **Parisarpa** Kushtham. The type of the disease which is white and thin, and is characterised by itching and does not create any disturbance (in the patient), is called **Sidhma** (Maculæ atrophicæ). This form is generally found to restrict itself to the upper part of the body. **Vicharchiká** (Psoriasis) is characterised by excessive pain and itching and gives rise to extremely dry crack-like marks on the body [hands and feet]. The same form of malady attended with pain, burning and itching, and restricting itself solely to the lower extremities, is called **Vipádiká**. The type in which the eruptions exude (a kind of slimy secretion) and which are circular, thick, excessively itching, glossy and black-coloured is called **Kitima** (Keloid tumours). Small pustules or pimples characterised by an itching, burning secretion and appearing on the surface of the body are called **Pámá** (Eczema). The preceding kinds of pimples attended with burning vesicles, are called **Kachchus** and are found to be chiefly confined to the legs, hands and buttocks. A sort of dry and non-exuding pimples characterised by excessive itching and appearing all over the body, is called **Rakasá** (dry Erythema). 9-10.

The forms known as Sthulárushka, Sidhma, Rakasá, Mahákushtham and Ekakushtham should be considered as offspring of the deranged Kapham. Parisarpa-kushtham alone is due to the action of the deranged Váyu, while the remaining types (of minor Kushtham) owe their origin to the action of the deranged Pittam. 11.

**Kilásam :**—The disease known as Kilásam is but another form of Kushtham. It may be divided into three types according as it is brought about through the action of the deranged Váyu, Pittam or Kapham. The difference between Kilásam and Kushtham is that the former confines itself only to the Tvaka (the skin) and is marked by the absence of any secretion.\* A case of Kilásam caused by the action of the deranged Váyu is circular, vermilion-coloured and rough to the touch. The affected part when rubbed peals off scales of morbid skin. A case of Kilásam, due to the action of the deranged Pittam, is marked by eruptions, resembling the petals of a lotus flower (in shape and colour), and are attended with an extremely burning sensation. In the type originated through the action of the deranged Kapham, the affected part (skin) assumes a glossy, white colour, becomes thick and is marked by an itching sensation. The form in which the eruptions or patches extend and become confluent, invading even the soles of the feet,

---

\* A case of Kushtham has its primary seat in the blood and skin (of the patient), in which it lies confined during the period of incubation, after which it attacks the skin and secretes the characteristic secretion of the deranged Dosha involved in it.

the palms of the hands and the region of the anus, and in which the local hairs assume a red colour should be regarded as incurable. A case of Kilásham, which is the outcome of a burn (cicatrix) should be likewise considered as incurable. 12.

A preponderance of the deranged Váyu in a case of Kushtham (leprosy) is indicated by a contraction of the skin, local anæsthesia, a copious flow of perspiration, swelling, and piercing or cutting pain in the affected part, together with a deformity of the limbs and hoarseness. Similarly, an excess of the deranged Pittam in a case of Kushtham, should be presumed from the suppuration of the affected part, from the breaking of the local skin, from the falling off of the fingers, from the sinking of the nose and ears, from the redness of the eyes and from the germination of parasites in the incidental ulcer. An excessive action of the deranged Kapham, in a case of Kushtham, gives rise to itching, discolouring and swelling of the affected part which becomes heavy and exudes the characteristic secretion. The types, Pundarika and Kákanam, which are due to the germinal defect of the patient, are incurable, inasmuch as they involve (according to Dallana) the concerted action of the three simultaneously deranged Doshas from the very outset. 13.

**Memorial verses** :— As a tree, full grown in the course of time, has driven its roots, which derive their nourishment from the rain water, deeper and deeper into the successive strata of the soil, so this disease (Kushtham), first affecting and confining itself to the upper layers of the skin, will invade the deeper tissues and organs etc. of the patient, if unchecked until almost all the fundamental principles or elements Dhátus are attacked by its virus in the course of time. 14.

The symptoms of a case of Kushtham confined only to the serous (Tvaka) fluid of the skin are the loss of the perception of touch, a scanty perspiration, itching and discoloration and roughness of the affected part. The symptoms which manifest themselves when the disease is confined to the blood are complete anæsthesia, horripilation, absence of perspiration, itching and excessive accumulation of pus in the affected parts. The symptoms of Kushtham affecting only the flesh are thickness of the patches, dryness of the mouth, roughness and hardness of the patches which become covered with pustular eruptions and vesicles, and an excruciating pricking pain in, and numbness of, the affected part. The symptoms of (Kushtham) invading the principle of fat only are a fetid smell and an excessive accumulation of pus in the affected part and a breaking of the skin, exposing deep gashing wounds which soon become infested with parasites. The body seems as if covered with a plaster. Symptoms of (Kushtham) affecting only the bones and the marrow are a sinking (lit: breaking) of the nose, a redness of the eyes, loss of voice and the germination of parasites in the incidental ulcers. Symptoms of the disease restricting itself only to the principle of semen are a crippled state of the hands and distortion of the limbs, loss of the power of locomotion, spreading of ulcers and all the other symptoms peculiar to the preceding types of the disease. 15—20.

A child, which is the offspring of the contaminated semen and ovum of its parents afflicted with Kushtham, should be likewise regarded as a Kushthi. 21.

**Prognosis:**—A case of Kushtham appearing in a person of prudence and discretion and confined only to the serum (Tvaka), flesh and blood of his organism should be regarded as curable. A palliative treatment is the only remedy in cases where the disease is found to invade the principle of fat ; whereas a case where the poison is found to have penetrated into any of the remaining organic principles should be given up as incurable. 22.

Wise men hold that, for killing a Bráhmana, or a woman, or one of his own relations, for theft, as well as for doing acts of impiety, a man is sometimes cursed with this foul disease by way of divine retribution. The disease reattacks a man even in his next rebirth in the event of his dying with it. Uncured Kushtham (leprosy) is the most painful, and most troublesome of all diseases. 23—24.

A Kushthi (leper), getting rid of this foul malady by observing the proper regimen of diet and conduct and by practising expiatory penances and by resorting to proper medicinal measures, gets an elevated status after death. 25.

Kushtham (Leprosy) is a highly contagious disease ; the contagion being usually communicated through sexual intercourse with a leper (Kushthi), or by his touch or breath, or through partaking of the same bed, and eating and drinking out of the same vessel with him, or through using the wearing apparel, unguents and garlands of flowers previously used by a person afflicted with this dreadful disease. Kushtham (Leprosy), fever, pulmonary consumption, ophthalmia and other Aupasargika disease (incidental to the influences of malignant planets or due to the effects of impious deeds) are communicated from one person to another. 26.

Thus ends the fifth Chapter of the Nidànasthànam in the Sushruta Samhitá which treats of the Nidánam of cutaneous affections (Kushtham).

# CHAPTER VI.

Now we shall discourse on the Nidánam of **Prameha** (diseases of the urinary tracts). 1.

It may be prognosticated that an idle man, who indulges in day sleep, or follows sedentary pursuits or is in the habit of taking sweet liquids, or cold and fat-making or emollient food, will ere long fall an easy victim to this disease. 2.

**Pathology:**—The bodily principles of Váyu, Pittam and Kaphah of such a person get mixed with improperly formed chyle of the organism. Thus deranged, they carry down through the urinary ducts the deranged fat, etc.* of the body and find lodgment at the mouth (neck) of the bladder, whence they are emitted through the urethra†, causing diseases, known by the (generic) name of **Prameha.** 3

**Premonitory symptoms:**—A burning sensation in the palms of the hands and of the soles of the feet, a heaviness of the body, coldness or sliminess of the skin and limbs, sweetness and whiteness of the urine, somnolence, lassitude, thirst, a bad-smelling breath, a shortness of breath, slimy mucous deposit on the tongue, palate, pharyx and teeth, clotted hair and an inordinate growth of the finger and toe nails are the indications which mark the advent of the disease. 4.

**General Characteristics:**—A copious flow of cloudy or turbid urine characterises all the types of the disease, which, together with the abscesses and eruptions (Pidaká) which mark its sequel, should be

---

* The particle "cha" in the text denotes other Virus or morbific matter. Dallana.

† Remain incarcerated therein according to others.

regarded as involving the concerted action of the deranged Doshas (Váyu, Pittam and Kaphah). 5.

**The Kaphaja Types :**—Cases of Prameha, which are caused by an exuberance of the deranged Kapham, may be grouped under ten subheads such as, *Udaka-meha, Ikshu-meha, Surà-meha, Sikatà-meha, S'anai-meha, Lavana-meha, Pishta-meha, Sàndra-meha, S'ukra-meha* and *Phena-meha*. The ten aforesaid types are curable, inasmuch as the medicines which tend to remedy the deranged Kapham (Dosha), the cause of the disease, prove also remedial to the other principles of the body (flesh, marrow, blood, semen etc) deranged (Dushya) from the same causes. 6.

**The Pittaja Types :**—The types, which are brought about through an exuberance of the deranged Pittam, are named as *Nila-meha, Haridrá-meha, Amla-meha, Kshàrá-meha, Manjishthà-meha*, and *S'onita-meha*. Palliation is all that can be effected in these types, inasmuch as the medicines which tend to correct the deranged Pittam, which has brought on the disease, fail to exert similar virtues on the organic principles (Dushyas) deranged by it. 7.

**The Vátaja Types :**—The types of Prameha which are produced by an aggravated condition of the bodily Váyu are divided into four subgroups, such as *Sarpi-meha, Vasà-meha, Kshoudra-meha* and *Hasti-meha*. These should be regarded as most incurable inasmuch as no kind of medicine can restore the fleet-coursing, deep diving (*i e.* invading the bones and the marrow) Váyu, which at the same time also augments the Pittam, to its normal state and thus advances (unchecked) in its work of disintegration. 8.

The deranged Kaphah, in conjunction with the (morbid) Pittam, Váyu and fat, gives rise to all Kaphaja types of Prameha. The deranged Pittam, in conjunction with the deranged Váyu, blood, fat and Kapham, produces the Pittaja ones; while the deranged Váyu, in unison with the deranged Kapham, Pittam, fat, marrow and Vasá (myosin), engenders the types of Vátaja Prameha. 9.

**Symptoms of Kaphaja-Mehas :**—The urine* of a person suffering from an attack of **Udakameha** becomes white and water-like and is passed without the least pain. In a case of **Ikshumeha** the urine resembles the expressed juice of sugarcane. It has the colour of wine in a case of **Surámeha.** The urine in a case of **Sikatámeha** is passed with pain and is found to leave a sediment of extremely fine and sand-like concretions (*Sikata's*). In a case of **Sanaimeha** the urine gushes out at intervals in jets and is charged with a slimy mucous (kaphah). The urine in a case of **Lavauameha** becomes limpid (non-viscid) and acquires a saline taste There is horripilation at the time of micturition in a case of **Pishtameha** (Chyluria), the urine resembling a stream of water, charged with a solution of pasted rice (Pishtam).

In a case of **Sándrameha**, the urine becomes thick and turbid, while in a case of **Sukrameha** the urine resembles semen (or the urine is found to be charged with semen :—Mádhaba). In a case of

---

\* The Sanskrit term Meha literally means to micturate. The verbal noun Mehanam signifies urination as well as the act of passing any morbid urethral secretion. Hence the urine in most of these cases denotes the fact of its being charged with pus or any other morbid secretion of the urinary organs such as Ojah (albumen), marrow, etc., which imparts their characteristic colours to the fluid,—a fact which determines the nomenclature of the disease and forms the keynote of its diagnosis in the Ayurveda.—Ed.

**Phenameha** the patient passes frothy urine in broken jets. 10.

**Symptoms of Pittaja Mehas :**—Now we shall describe the characteristic features of the types of Prameha, which are due to the action of the deranged Pittam. The urine in a case of **Nilameha** becomes frothy, transparent and bluish. The urine in a case of **Haridrámeha** becomes deep yellow like turmeric (Haridrá) and is passed with a burning pain. The urine in a case of **Amlameha** acquires an acid taste and smell. The urine in a case of **Ksháramċha**\* resembles an alkaline solution filtered (through a piece of linen). The urine in a case of **Manjisthámeha** resembles the washing of the Manjisthá, while in a case of **Raktameha**, the urine is found to be of blood-colour (or charged with blood – Mádhava). 11.

**Symptoms of Vátaja-Mehas :**—Now we shall describe the characteristics of the different types of Prameha, which are due to an exuberance of the deranged Váyu. In a case of **Sarpimeha**, the urine looks like a stream of clarified butter, while in one of **Vasámeha** it resembles the washings of Vasá. In a case of **Kshaudrameha,** the urine looks like honey and acquires a sweet taste. In one of **Hastimeha**, the patient passes a copious quantity of urine, like an excited elephant, at a time, and in one unbroken stream, (the organ becoming steady immediately after the act of micturition). 12.

**Supervening symptoms :**—The fact of the urine being assailed by a swarm of flies, lassitude, growth of flesh (obesity), catarrh, looseness of the limbs, a

---

\* The urine acquires a distinct alkaline taste, smell, colour and touch. (Mádhaba Nidánam).

† Charaka has included it within Kshaudra Meha and Madhu Me a.

non-relish for food, indigestion, expectoration of mucous, vomiting, excessive sleep, cough and laboured breathing (Svása) are the supervening traits (Upadrava) of the **Kaphaja Prameha.** A piercing pain in the testes, a pricking (veda) pain in the bladder, a shooting pain (Tuda) in the penis, a griping pain at the heart, acid eructations, fever, dysentery, a non-relish for food, vomiting, a sensation as if the entire body is emitting fumes, a burning sensation in the skin, thirst, epileptic fits, insomnia, jaundice (Pándu) and a yellow colour of the stool and urine are the supervening symptoms which mark the **Pittaja types** of Prameha. An oppressive feeling at the heart (Hridgraha), eager longings for foods of all tastes, insomnia, numbness of the body, fits of shivering, colic pain and constipation of the bowels are the supervening symptoms, which specifically mark the **Vátaja types.** Thus we have described the nature of the twenty different types of Meha with their supervening evils as well. 13-16.

The ten different types of Pidaká (abscess, carbuncles, pimples, pustules etc ) are found to crop up on the bodies of patients, suffering from Prameha, and abounding in fat and Vasá, and whose fundamental principles have been affected by the simultaneous derangement of the Váyu, Pittam and Kapham. They are named as **Sarávika, Sarshapiká, Kachchapiká, Jálini, Vinatá, Putrini, Masuriká, Alaji, Vidáriká** and **Vidradhiká** 17.

**Metrical Texts :—**An abscess which is raised at the margin and dipped in its centre, so as to resemble an Indian saucer in its shape is called **Sarávika.** Pimples or pustules of the shape and size of white mustard seeds are called **Sarshápiká.** An abscess, resembling (the back of) a tortoise in shape and attended with a burning sensation, is called **Kachchapiká** by the wise.

An abscess studded with slender vegetations of flesh and attended with an intolerable burning sensation is called **Jálini.** A large blue-coloured abscess (carbuncle) appearing on the back or the abdomen, and exuding a slimy secretion and attended with a deep-seated pain is called **Vinatá** A thin and extensive abscess (studded with slender pustules—D.R.) is called **Putrini.** Pimples to the size of lentil seeds are called **Masuriká.** A dreadful abscess which is of a red and white colour, studded over with blisters or exuding vesicles is called **Alaji. A** hard and round abscess as large as a (full-grown) gourd is called **Vidárika.** An abscess of the Vidradhi type is called **Vidradhiká** (carbuncle) by the wise. An incidental abscess in a case of Prameha should be regarded as having its origin in the same morbific principle (Dosha) as that which has produced the disease (Prameha) 18-28.

**Prognosis :**—A Pidaká, or an abscess, appearing about the region of the heart, anus, head, shoulder, back or at any of the vital joints (Marma) of the body, and attended with other supervening symptoms producing extreme prostration [impaired digestion—D. R.] in the patient should be abandoned as incurable. In a case of Vátaja meha, the deranged Váyu presses all the fundamental principles out of the body through the urethra and rages rampant in the lower part of the body, united with the deranged fat, marrow and Vasà. Hence a case of Vátaja meha, (or its accompanying abscess), is held as incurable. 29-30.

A person in whom the premonitory symptoms (Purvarupam of Prameha) have appeared and who passes a little larger quantity of urine than usual, should be considered as already afflicted with it. A person afflicted with all or half of the premonitory symptoms of the disease and passing a copious quantity of urine should be considered as one suffering from an attack of Prameha. 31—32.

A Prameha patient afflicted with deep-seated abscesses and other distressing symptoms, which are usually found to supervene in the disease, should be pronounced as suffering from Madhumeha and adjudged incurable. A Madhumeha patient seeks a halting place while walking, wants a place to sit on while halting, lies down if he finds a sitting place, and sleeps if he lies down. 33—34.

As five mixed colours such as grey, brown, Kapila (bluish yellow), Kapota (blackish grey), Mechaka (light-green) may be produced by combination of the five primary colours in definite proportions (such as white, green, black, yellow and red), so a diversity of causes, through the relative preponderance of the particular kinds of food, and of the deranged Doshas, root principles (Dhátu) and excretions of the body (Mala), may be attributed to the origin of Prameha. 35.

**Memorial verses :**—All types of Prameha, not properly treated and attended to at the outset, may ultimately develop into those of **Madhumeha** types, which are incurable. 36

For English equivalents of the different types of Prameha compare :—
Cystitis (Acute Infective)—Frequent, painful micturition, small quantity of urine voided with pain and urgency. Urine—slightly acid or alkaline in reaction, cloudy, containing blood corpuscles. Cystitis (Chronic Infective) —Great and frequent pain, in the lumbar region, rigor. Urine—thick, offensive and alkaline, containing ropy mucous and blood. Cystitis (Non-Infective)—Symptoms like those of acute inflammatory type. Urine— acid and cloudy with mucous. Blood is generally present in considerable quantity. Neuralgia of the bladder, compare Albuminuria, Albumosuria, Hœmoglobinuria, Hœmaturia, Peptonuria, Pyuria, Spermatorrhœa and Diabetes, Proteuria and Polyuria.

Thus ends the sixth Chapter of the Nidâna Sthânam in the Sushruta Samhitâ, which treats of the Nidânam of Prameha.

## CHAPTER VII.

Now we shall discourse on the **Nidánam of Udara** (dropsy with an abnormal condition of the abdomen). 1.

**Metrical Text :**—The royal sage Dhanvantari, the foremost of all pious men who equalled in splendour and glory the lord of the celestials, thus blissfully discoursed on the Nidánam of Udara to Susruta, the son of the holy Visvámitra, who devoutly approached him for that purpose. 2.

**Classification :**—This disease may be divided into eight different types, of which four are produced by the several actions of the three deranged **Doshas** of the body and their concerted action as well. Of the remaining types, two being known as Plihodara (including Yakritodara), and Vaddha-Gudodara (tympanites due to the constriction of the anus), the seventh Ágantuka (traumatic or of extraneous origin), and the eighth Dakodara (Ascites proper). 3.

**Predisposing Causes :**—The deranged Doshas of a person of extremely impaired digestion, addicted to the habit of taking unwholesome food, or of eating dry, putrid food, or of violating the rules of conduct to be observed in connection with oleaginous measures etc.,* are aggravated and find lodgment in the abdomen. Thus appearing in the shape of an abdominal tumour (Gulma), they give rise to this dreadful disease, attended with all its characteristic symptoms. The lymph chyle formed out of the assimilated food gets vitiated, and, impelled by the aggravated Váyu, it percolates

---

* These include purgative, emitic, A'sthá'panam and Anuva'sanam measures.

through the peritoneum in the same manner as a quantity of oil or clarified butter kept in a new earthen pot will transude through the pores of its sides. It thus gradually distends the skin (Tvak) of the abdomen. The process becomes general all through the abdominal region and the disease (Udara) is produced in consequence. 4—5.

**Premonitory sypmtoms :**—The precursory symptoms of the disease are loss of strength, complexion and appetite, emaciation of the muscles of the abdomen, appearance of veins on its surface, acid reaction of food closely following upon its digestion (Vidáha), pain in the bladder, and swelling of the lower extremities. The patient cannot ascertain whether his meal has been digested or not. 6.

**The Vátaja, Pittaja, and Kaphaja Types:**—A case of Udara in which the abdomen enlarges on its sides and posterior part, and is overspread with nets of black veins should be ascribed to the action of the deranged Váyu. A pain (Śula), suppression of the stool and urine (Anába) and a cutting and piercing pain and flatulent rumbling in the intestines are the symptoms which likewise characterise this **Vátaja** form of Udara. A sucking pain in the abdomen, thirst, fever with a burning sensation, yellow colour of the swollen skin of the abdomen, on the surface of which yellow veins appear, yellow colour of the eyes, nails, face, stool and urine and the rapid increase of the dropsical swelling, are the characteristics of the **Pittaja Udara.** In a case of **Kaphaja** type the dropsical swelling is cold to the touch and becomes overspread with white-coloured veins. The abdomen seems heavy, hard, glossy and is extremely distended. The swelling slowly increases, and the finger-nails and face of the patient become white, and he complains of a general lassitude. 7—9.

**The Tridoshaja Type :**—Evil-natured women (with a view to win the affections of their husbands or lovers sometimes) mix with their food and drink such refuse matters of their bodies as nails, hair, fæces, urine, catamenial blood etc. (which are supposed to be possessed of talismanic virtues). The three **Doshas** of the body, vitiated by such food or drink, or through imbibing any sort of chemical poison (Gara) administered by one's enemy, or by taking poisonous waters, or Dushi-Visha (slow poison whose active properties have been destroyed by fire or any antipoisonous medicine), will vitiate the blood and give rise to a kind of dreadful dropsical swelling of the abdomen, marked by the specific symptoms of each of them  The disease is aggravated in cold and cloudy days and a burning sensation is felt (in the inside of the abdomen). The patient becomes pale, yellow and emaciated, and is afflicted with thirst and dryness in the mouth, and loses consciousness at short intervals. This disease is also known as the dreadful **Dushyodaram.** 10.

**Plihodaram.**—(Spleen with dropsy of the abdomen) :—Now hear me describe the symptoms of Plihodaram. The blood and the Kapham of a person, deranged and aggravated through the ingestion of phlegmagogic food, or of those which is followed by an acid digestionary reaction (Vidáha), often enlarge the spleen, (which gives rise to a swelling of the abdomen). This disease is called **Plihodara** by the experts. Plihodaram protrudes on the left side of the abdomen, its characteristic symptoms being lassitude, low fever, impaired digestion, loss of strength, jaundice, weakness, and other distressing symptoms peculiar to the deranged Pittam and Kapham. A similar enlargement of the liver through similar causes on the right side of the abdomen is called **Jakriddályudaram.** 11—12.

**Vaddha-gudodaram***:—The fecal matter, mixed with the deranged Váyu, Pittam etc. of the body, lies stuffed in the rectum of a person whose intestines have been stuffed with slimy food (as pot herbs) or with stones and hair (enteritis). They give rise to a sort of abdominal dropsy by swelling the part between the heart and the umbilicus which is called Vaddha Gudodaram. Scanty stools are evacuated with the greatest pain and difficulty and the patient vomits a peculiar kind of matter with a distinctly fecal smell (scyabalous?). 13.

**Parisrávi-Udaram :**—Now hear me describe the causes and symptoms of the type of Udaram which is called **Parisrávi-udaram**. Thorny or sharp-pointed substances (such as fish-bones etc.), carried down with the food in a slanting way from the stomach into the abdomen, sometimes scratch or burrow into the intestines. Causes other than the preceding ones, (such as a long yawn or over-eating etc.) may contribute to the perforation of the intestines, giving rise to a copious flow of a watery exudation which constantly oozes out of the anus and to a distension of the lower part of the abdomen situated below the umbilicus. This is called Parisrávyudaram which is marked by a cutting pain and a burning sensation. 14.

**Dakodaram :**—Now hear me describe the causes and symptoms of the type known as **Dakodaram** (ascites). The drinking of cold water immediately after the application of an Aunvásanam or Ásthápanam enema, or closely following upon the exhibition of any purgative or emetic medicine, or just after the taking of a medicated oil or clarified butter, etc. tends to derange

---

* Dropsical swelling of the abdomen with tympanites due to the constriction of the rectum known as intestinal obstruction.

the water-carrying channels of the body. The same result may be produced by the drinking of oil, etc. in inordinate quantities The water, by percolating or transuding through the walls of these channels, as before described, inordinately enlarges the abdomen, which becomes glossy on the surface and is full of water, being rounded about the umbilicus and raised like a full-bloated water-drum. The simile is complete as it fluctuates under pressure, oscillates, and makes a peculiar sound like a water-drum under percussion. 15

Distension of the stomach, incapacity of locomotion, weakness, impaired digestion, œdematous swelling of the limbs, a general sense of lassitude and looseness in the limbs, suppression of flatus and stool, and a burning sensation and thirst are among the general characteristics of the disease in its various forms. 16.

**Prognosis :**—All cases of Udaram after the lapse of considerable time develop into those of ascites, and a case arriving at such a stage should be given up as incurable. 16—17.

Thus ends the seventh Chapter of the Nidàna Sthànam in the Sus'ruta Samhitá which treats of the Nidánam of Udaram.

# CHAPTER VIII.

Now we shall discourse on the Nidănam of **Mudhagarbham** (false presentations and difficult labour). 1.

**Causes of Mudha-garbham** :—Sexual intercourse during pregnancy, riding on horseback, etc., or in any sort of conveyance, a long walk, a false step, a fall, pressure on the womb, running, a blow, sitting or lying down on an uneven ground, or in an uneven posture, fasting, voluntary repression of any natural urging of the body, partaking of extremely bitter, pungent, parchifying articles, eating in inordinate quantities of Sákas and alkaline substances, dysentery (Atisára), use of emetics or purgatives, swinging in a swing or hammock, indigestion, and use of medicines which induce the labour pain or bring about abortions, and such like causes tend to expel the fœtus from its fixture. These causes tend to sever the child from the uterine wall with its placental attachment owing to a kind of Abhighátam (uterine contraction) just as a blow tends to sever a fruit from its pedicel. 2.

**Definition**:—The fœtus, thus severed and dislodged from its seat, excites peristalsis not only in the uterus, but induces a sort of constant, spasmodic contraction of the intestinal cavities (Koshthas), producing pain in the liver, spleen, etc. The Apána Váyu, thus obstructed through the spasmodic contraction of her abdomen, produces any of the following symptoms, viz. a sort of spasmodic pain in the sides, or in the neck of the bladder, or in the pelvic cavity, or in the abdomen, or in the vagina, or Anába (tympanites with obstruction, etc.) or retention of urine, and destroys the fœtus, if immature, attended with bleeding. In case the fœtus continues to develop and is brought in an inverted posture at the entrance to the vaginal canal, and is impacted at that place, or if the Apána Váyu gets disordered and consequently cannot help the expulsion of the same, such an obstructed fœtus is called **Mudha-garbhah.** 3.

**Classification and Symptoms:**—Cases of Mudha-garbha may be roughly divided into four different classes such as, the *Kilah*, the *Pratikhurah*, the *Vijakah* and the *Parighah*. The sort of false presentation in which the child comes with its hands, legs and head turned upward and with its back firmly obstructed at the entrance to the vagina, like a stake or a kila, is called **Kilah.** The sort of presentation, in which the hands, feet and head of the child come out, with its body impacted at the entrance to the vagina, is called **Prathikhurah.** The type in which only a single hand and the head of the child come out (with the rest of its body obstructed at the same place), is called the **Vijakah.** The type in which the child remains obstructing the head of the passage in a horizontal position, like a bolt, is called the **Parighah.** Certain authorities aver that, these are the only four kinds of Mudhagarbha. But we can not subscribe to the opinion (which recognises only four kinds of false presentations), inasmuch as the deranged Váyu (Apána) can present the fœtus in various different postures at the head of the vaginal canal. Sometimes, the two thighs of the child are first presented, and sometimes it comes with a single leg flexed up. Sometimes the child comes with its body, bent double, and thighs drawn up, so that only breech is obliquely presented. Sometimes the child is presented, impacted at the head of the passage with its chest, or sides, or back. Sometimes the child is presented with its arm around its head, resting on the side, and the hand coming out first. Sometimes only the two hands are first presented, the head leaning on one side; sometimes the two hands, legs and the head of the child, the rest of the body being impacted at the exit in a doubled up posture. Sometimes one leg is presented, the other thigh being impacted at the passage (Páyu). I have briefly described these eight sorts of presentation of which the last two are irremediable. The rest should be given up as hopeless if these are attended with the following complications *viz.*, deranged sense-perception of the mother, convulsions, displacement or contraction of the reproductive organ (yoni) a peculiar pain like the after-pain of child birth, cough, difficult respiration, or vertigo. 4.

**Memorial verses :**—As a fruit, fully matured, is naturally severed from its pedicel and falls to the ground and not otherwise, so the cord, which binds the fœtus to its maternal part, is severed in course of time, and the child comes out of the uterus ( into this world of action ). On the other hand, as a fruit, worm-eaten or shaken by the wind or a blow, untimely falls to the ground, so will a fœtus be expelled out of its mother's womb, before its time. For four months after the date of fecundation, the fœtus remains in a liquid state, and hence its destruction or coming out of the womb goes by the name of **abortion.** In the course of the fifth and sixth months the limbs of the fœtus gain in firmness and density, and hence, its coming out at such a time is called **miscarriage.** 5-7.

**Prognosis :**—The enceinte who violently tosses her head in agony (at the time of parturition) and the surface of whose body becomes cold, compelling her to forego all natural modesty, and whose sides and abdomen are covered with nets of large blue-coloured veins, invariably dies with the dead child locked in her womb. The death of the fœtus in the womb may be ascertained by the absence of movements of the fœtus (in the womb) or of any pain of child-birth, by a brown or yellow complexion of the *enceinta*, cadeverous smell in her breath, and colic pain in the abdomen and its distension owing to the continuance of the swollen and decomposed child in the womb. 8-9.

The death of a child in the womb may result from some emotional disturbance of its mother, (such as caused by bereavement or by loss of fortune during pregnancy); while an external blow or injury (to the womb) or any serious disease of the mother may also produce the like result. A child, moving in the womb of a dead mother, who had just expired (from convulsions etc) during parturition at term, like a goat (Vastámára) should be removed immediately by the Surgeon from the womb (by Cæsarean Section);* as a delay in extracting the child may leads to its death. 10-11.

---

* Cæcsarean Section means incision of the uterus through the abdominal walls and extrication of the fœtus therefrom. Operation like this upon a dead subject requires no skill of a surgeon. Any one can do it without the help of any anatomical knowledge. In modern times, when the mother's life is in peril, and the expulsion of the fœtus becomes nearly impossible, by the natural passage, owing to an existence of deformity either in the parturient canal or in the forms and structures of the fœtus, to save both mother and child this operation is principally undertaken.

The evidence of similar attempts, in ancient India, is found recorded in passages like what we have just translated and that the operation was practised on living subjects, there is not the least doubt about it. This custom is still preserved in Central Africa, and it is possible that the Egyptians like Hindu philosophy and religion learnt this also from the Hindus. "Felkin," says "Baas in his History of Medicine p. 70 "saw a case of the Cæsarean operation in Central Africa performed by a man. At one stroke

**Additional Text:**—The bladder is ruptured, the dead child lies like a weight upon the placenta and is pressed upward on the spleen, liver and gall bladder. The mother shivers and is oppressed with tremor, dryness of the tongue, dyspnœa and perspiration. She complains of a cadaverous smell in her breath and stands in danger of imminent death. By these symptoms a physician shall know the death of the child in the womb. This portion is partly recognised by Brahmadeva and is totally rejected by Jejjadáchárya as spurious.

an incision was made through both the abdominal walls and the uterus. The opening in the latter organ was then enlarged, the hæmorrhage checked by the actual cautery, and the child removed. While an assistant compressed the abdomen, the operator then removed the placenta. The bleeding from the abdominal walls was then checked. No sutures were placed on the walls of the uterus but the abdominal parietes were fastened together by seven figure-of-eight sutures, formed with polished iron needles and threads of bark. The wound was then dressed with a paste prepared from various roots, the woman placed quietly upon her abdomen, in order to favour perfect drainage, and the task of the African Spencer Wells was finished. It appears that the patient was first rendered half unconscious with banana wine. One hour after the operation the patient was doing well. And her temperature never rose above 101 F. nor her pulse above 108. On the eleventh day the wound was completely healed, and the woman apparently as well as usual."

When we read this evidence of Felkin, we are reminded of the operative steps as described in our own ancient book of Surgery from which modern surgeons have been able to borrow the operation of rhinoplasty. It is a great pity that while in Africa the same practice is still retained intact, we in India by spurious attempts and disgraceful contortions, subs. titutions of false readings and dismal knowledge of grammar and rhetoric try to prove in the face of strong evidence that in ancient India Cæsarean Section was attempted only on cases where one "might not perspire"

If we take विपन्नायाः in the sense of "a woman whose life is in great danger" and not exactly in the sense of "a woman who is dead" as recommended by Dallan and Arundutta (and which might have been the meaning if instead of विपन्न a word like आपन्न had been used in the text), we find at once that Weber's remark in his History of Indian Literature p. 270 "that in Surgery they (the Hindus) attained to high proficiency" is not based on the solitary evidence of rhinoplasty alone.

In performing obstetric operations with success examples like this are not rare. If the two different readings वक्षमार and वक्षिहार be taken conjointly into consideration we are impressed with the idea that in ancient

India Cæsarean operations were very frequently undertaken in cases of puerperal eclampsia, where the mother had been in the deplorable condition of a goat suffering from cramps and convulsions as well as in cases of an accidental death not unlike that which fell to the lot of the poor mother of him in whose name the operation is called. वस्त=goat मार= destroyer (See Monier William's Dictionary) hence a goat-destroyer=a tiger or wolf) or in cases where the presence of deformity in the parturient canal or of malformation of the fœtus prevented the natural delivery of a living child. The incision is not to be made anywhere else but exactly in the place where Felkin saw the illiterate Negro successfully apply his knife, the selection of वस्ति' द्वारा as suggested by some commentators being a tempest on a tea pot especially when the subject is beyond the grave. In a living subject the selection of a proper site for the operation is of course very commendable. Hence we venture to suggest that extraction of the living fœtus from the womb by making incision through this part of the pelvis was also attempted later on. We extract here the two different readings and leave our readers to judge whether we are correct to draw the above inferences.—Ed.

वस्तिद्वारे विपन्नायाः कुचि: प्रस्यन्दते यदि जन्मकाले ततः शीघ्रं पाटयित्वोदरे-च्छिद्युम् । Bágabhata S'árira S:hánam. ch. II. slo. 53.

वस्तमार विपन्नायाः कुचि: प्रस्यन्दते यदि सत्यचणाज्जन्मकाले तं पाटयित्वोदरे-द्विषक् ।

Thus ends the eighth Chapter of the Nidána Sthánam in the Sus'ruta Samhitá, which treats of Nidánam of difficult labour and false presentations.

# CHAPTER IX.

Now we shall discourse on the Nidánam of **Vidradhi** (abscess etc.). 1.

The blessed Dhanvantari, the honoured of the gods, who for the promulgation of the knowledge of the Áyurveda and for administering proper medicines (to the sick), took his birth at Kási, (Benares) as a king, thus fully discoursed on the symptoms of Vidradhi (abscess etc.) to his disciple, Sus'ruta. 2

**Definition and classification :—**The extremely deranged and aggravated Váyu, Pittam and Kapham, resorting to the bone and vitiating the Tvaka (skin), blood, flesh, and fat of a person (with their own specific properties), gradually give rise to a deep-seated, painful, round or extended swelling which is called **Vidradhi** by the wise. The disease admits of being divided into six types such as the *Vátaja* type, the *Pittaja* type, the *Kaphaja* type, the *Sànnipàtika* type, the *Kshataja* type (traumatic), and the *Asrija* (which has its seat in the vitiated blood). Now we shall describe their specific symptoms. 3-4.

**The Vátaja Type :—**This abscess assumes a black or vermilion colour, is felt rough to the touch and is characterised by a sort of excruciating pain. The growth and suppuration of the abscess are brought about in a variety of forms (owing to the variable and irregular action of the deranged Váyu inolved in these cases). 5.

**The Pittaja Type :—**This abscess assumes a blackish yellow colour or one like that of a ripe Audumvara fruit. It is attended with fever and a burning sensation, and is of rapid growth and suppuration. 6.

**The Kaphaja Type:**—This abscess is shaped like an Indian saucer (s'aráva) and seems cold to the touch. It assumes a light yellow colour and is characterised by numbness, itching and little pain. The growth and suppuration of this abscess is very slow. The secretions from a Vátaja abscess are thin, those from a Pittaja type are yellow, while the exudations from a Kaphaja abscess are white. 7.

**The Sánnipátika Type:**—An abscess of the Sánnipátika type is of varied colour, and is attended with a varied sort of pain (sucking, drawing, turning etc.) and exudes secretions of various colours (white, yellow, etc.). It is little raised or elevated at its top, large and irregular in its shape and does not uniformly suppurate in all its parts. 8.

**Ágantuja** or **Kshataja Type:**—The local or inherent heat of an ulcer, (caused by a blow or a dirt) in a person, addicted to unwholesome regimen, is augmented and conducted by the deranged Váyu and vitiates the blood and Pittam, thus giving rise to a kind of abscess which is known as the Ágantuja Vidradhi (traumatic abscess). Symptoms of the Pittaja type likewise mark this type of abscess and fever, thirst and a burning sensation attend it from the very beginning. 9.

**The Raktaja Type:**—This abscess assumes a black or tawny colour, covered with a large number of black vesicles, and fever and an intolerable burning and pain attended with all the symptoms peculiar to the Pittaja type, mark the present form of the disease. It is called Raktaja Vidradhi. Of external Vidradhis or abscesses, those of the Sánnipátika type should be regarded as incurable. 10—11.

**Antara-Vidradhi :**—Now we shall describe the characteristic features of internal abscesses (Antara-

Vidradhi). The Váyu, Pittam and Kaphah of the body, deranged through eating heavy, incompatible and incongenial (to the physical temperament of the eater) articles of food or of dry, putrid and decomposed substances, or by excessive coition and fatiguing physical exercise, or by voluntary repression of any natural urging of the body or through the eating of food which is followed by an acid reaction, either severally or collectively give rise to a tumour-like (Gulma), raised, or elevated abscess in the interior of the organism, which is often felt to be shaped like an ant-hill. 12-13.

**Localities :**— They are generally found to be seated at the mouth (neck) of the bladder, or about the umbilicus, or in the sides, or in the Kukshi (inguinal regions), or on the Vrikkas, or on the liver, or in the heart, or on the Kloma, or on the spleen, or in the rectum. Their general characteristics are identical with those of the several types of external abscess. The symptoms of their suppurated or unsuppurated stages should be determined in the light of the chapter on Ámapakvaishanyiam (Ch XVII Sutra.). 14-15.

**Their specific symptoms :**—Now hear me describe the symptoms which specifically mark these internal abscesses according to their seats in the different regions of the organism. An abscess appearing in the **rectum** (Guda) is marked by the suppression of the flatus (Váta). Seated in the **bladder,** it gives rise to difficulty of urination and scantiness of urine. Appearing about the **umbilicus** it produces a distressing hic-cough and a rumbling sound (Átopa) in the intestines. Seated in either of the sides (**Kukshi**) it tends to aggravate inordinately the váyu of the body. Appearing in the **inguinal region** it gives rise to an extreme catching pain at the back and waist. Seated in either of the **Vrikkas** it brings about a contraction of the sides. Appearing on the **spleen,** it produces symptoms of difficult and obstructed respiration. Seated on the **heart** it gives rise to an excruciating and piercing pain within its cavity and a drawing pain (Graha) extending all over the body (D R.—cough). Seated in the **Liver** its characteristic indications are thirst and difficult breathing (D. R.—hic-cough) whereas a sort of unquenchable thirst is the symptom which marks its seat on the **Kloma.** 16-17.

**Prognosis :**—An abscess appearing on any vital part (Marma) of the organism, whether large or small in size, suppurated or unsuppurated, should be deemed' as extremely hard to cure. Discharge from an abscess formed in the region of the organism above the umbilicus and (spontaneously bursting), will flow out through the mouth whereas similar secretions from down the umbilical region of (the abdomen), naturally find an outlet through the fissure of the anus. The case in which the secretions (pus etc.) find a downward channel and outlet may end in recovery of the patient, whereas the one in which the secretions take an upward course invariably proves fatal. An incision made by surgeon from the outside into an internal abscess, other than the one situated on the heart, or on the bladder or on the umbilicus may occasionally, prove successful, but the one, seated on any of the preceding vulnerable visceras (heart, bladder etc.) of the body and surgically opened invariably ends in death. 18-19.

A woman, who has miscarried or has been even safely delivered of a child at term, may be afflicted with a dreadful abscess in the event of her taking injudicious and unhwholesome food after parturition The abscess in such a case, which is attended with extreme hyper-pyrexia (Dáhajvara) should be considered as having had its origin to the vitiated blood (Raktaja Vidradhi) accumulated in the organism. The abscess, which appears in the Kukshi (in the iliac region) of a safely delivered woman owing to the presence of the unexpelled blood-clots in those regions after childbirth, should be also diagnosed as a case of Raktaja abscess. The unexpelled blood is called Makkalla. Such an abscess, if not absorbed in the course of a week. is sure to suppurate. 20 - 21.

**Differentiating diagnosis of Gulma and Vidradhi\*:**—Now I shall discuss the features which distinguish a Gulma (internal tumour) from a Vidradhi (internal abscess). It may be asked, how is it that Gulma, (internal tumour) though caused by, and involving the co-operation of the same deranged Doshas as an internal abscess, does not suppurate, while the latter (Vidradhi) does run to suppuration ? 22— 23.

The answer is that a Gulma (internal tumour), though caused by the same deranged Doshas as a Vidradhi (internal abscess), does not resort to any deranged organic matter, such as flesh, blood, etc., while, on the contrary, in a case of Vidradhi, the diseased flesh and blood of a locality are in themselves transformed into an abscess. An internal tumour (Gulma) is like a water bubble floating and moving about within a cavity

---

\* A Gulma according to Sus'ruta does not suppurate, but the term "Api" (also) contemplates instances in which a Gulma may suppurate as in the case where it has got its basis in the deranged flesh etc. of the locality. Charaka asserts that retarded digestion of the ingested food followed by digestionary acid reaction, colic pain, insomnia with fever and a non-relish for food and a sense of oppression, etc. are the symptoms which indicate that suppuration has set in a Gulma, and he advises that it (Gulma) should be treated with poultices, etc.

of the body etc. without any fixed root of its own. Hence, it is that a Gulma (internal tumour) does not suppurate at all. Suppuration sets in in an abscess only because it largely contains flesh and blood unlike a Gulma (internal tumour) which is not formed of any such organic matter, and depends only on the aggravated Doshas giving birth to it. Hence, a Gulma does not suppurate at all. 24.

**Incurable Types :**—A case of an internal abscess suppurating about the heart, bladder or umbilicus as well as one of the Tridosha type (appearing in any part of the organism) should be given up as incurable. The abscess in which the marrow suppurates (generally) becomes fatal. The suppurating process in an internal abscess, which generally affects the underlying bone, is sometimes found to affect the marrow. The suppurated marrow, failing to find an outlet on account of the compactness of the local flesh and bone, produces a sort of burning sensation in the locality which consumes the body like a blazing fire. The disease confined to the bone, like a piercing dirt, torments the patient for a considerable length of time. An incision (made into the affected bone) is followed by the secretion of a fat-like, glossy, white, cold and thick pus. Men, learned in the knowledge of the Medicinal Sástras, designate such an abscess as an Asthigháta-Vidradhi (abscess of the bone) which involves all the three kinds of deranged Doshas, and is attended with various kinds of pain which mark them respectively. 25-26.

Thus ends the ninth Chapter of the Nidánasthánam in the Sus'ruta Samhitá which treats of the ætiology of abscess.

# CHAPTER X.

Now we shall discourse on the Nidánam of **Visarpa** (erysipelas), **Nádi** (sinus) and **Stana-roga** (diseases affecting the mammæ of a woman). 1.

**Definition of Visarpa :**—The deranged and aggravated Doshas, (Váyu, Pittam and Kapham) having recourse to, and affecting the Tvaka (Skin), flesh and blood, speedily give rise to a sort of shifting, elevated swelling (Sotha) marked by the characteristic symptoms of any of them involved in the case. This swelling tends to extend all over the body. The disease is called **Visarpa** from the fact of its extending or swiftly shifting character (Skr. srip —to go, to extend). 2.

**The Vátaja Type :**—The swelling (Sotha) is soft and rough and assumes a black colour attended with an aching pain in the limbs and a cutting or piercing pain (in the affected locality). It is further marked by (all the usual) symptoms of the Vátika fever. A case of this type in which uneven flame coloured vesicles or bulbs appear on the affected part through the extreme vitiation (of the Váyu and Pittam) should be given up as incurable. 3.

**The Pittaja and Kaphaja Types :**— The Pittaja Visarpa (erysipelas) rapidly extends (over the body), attended with severe fever, a burning sensation, suppuration and cracking (of the skin. A large number of vesicles appears on the spot which assume a blood-red colour. A case of this type, characterised by the destruction of the local flesh and veins owing to the excessively aggravated condition of the deranged Doshas (Kaphha and Pittam) and a collyrium-like black colour (of the swelling), should be regarded as incurable. The **Kaphaja Visarpa** extends slowly and the process of suppuration is tardy. The affected part becomes white, glossy and swollen, and is marked by a slight pain and excessive itching. 4-5.

**The Sánnipátika Type :**—The Visarpa of the Tridoshaja type is deep-seated and the affected part assumes all colours and is attended with all sorts of pain which are peculiar to the three aforesaid types The local flesh and veins are destroyed in the suppurating stage of this disease and hence, it shouldbe looked upon as incurable 6.

**The Kshataja Type** (Erysipelas due to a wound or an ulcer):—The Pittam of a person with a temperament marked by the extreme aggravation of all the three Doshas, in conjunction with the blood, resorts to a wound* in his body and immediately gives rise to Erysipelas (Sopha—lit rash) which assumes a reddish-brown colour, with high fever with a burning sensation, and suppuration in its train, and it is found to be covered with black vesicles to the size of *Kulattha* pulse. 7.

**Prognosis :**—The Vátaja, Pittaja and Kaphaja Visarpas are curable ; the Sánnipátika and Khataja ones being incurable. The symptoms, which indicate an unfavourable prognosis in a case of Vátaja or Pittaja Erysipelas. have been described before Those, which attack the vital parts (Marmas) of the body, can be cured only with the greatest difficulty.† 8.

---

\* Or through the extreme augmentation of all the three doshas in the ulcer (Sadyah kshata-Vrana) according to others.

† Golden coloured (yellow) Erysipelas due to the action of the (deranged) Pittam is incurable (*Pittátmá Kànchana-vapuscha ta há na sydhyet.*).—D. R.

**The Nádi-Vrana :**—The pus of an abscess or swelling burrows into the affected part if a person neglects it in its fully suppurated stage, dubious of its being so conditioned, or not, or even neglects to open a fully suppurated abscess. An abscess or swelling is called a Gati Vrana owing to an excessive infiltration of pus, and it is also called a Nádi-vrana owing to the presence of a large number of recesses or cavities in its inside There are five different types of *Nádi-vrana* (sinuses) such as the Vátaja, Pittaja Kaphaja, Tridoshaja and Salyaja. 9—10

**The Vátaja, Kaphaja and Pittaja Types :**—The **Vátaja** Sinus is rough and short-mouthed, characterised by an aching pain (in its inside) It exudes a sort of frothy secretion which becomes greater at night and is attended with an aching pain. Thirst, lassitude, heat and a piercing pain (in the affected locality) are the usual accompaniments of the **Pittaja types**. Fever is present from the beginning and the Sinus exudes a large quantity of hot and yellow coloured secretion which is more by day than by night. The **Kaphaja Sinus** becomes hard and is characterised by itching and a slight pain (numbed?). It is found to secrete a copious quantity of thick, shiny, white-coloured pus which becomes greater at night 11-13.

**Dvandaja and Tridoshaja Types :**— A case of Nádi-Vrana involving the concerted action of any two of the deranged Doshas (Váyu, Pittam and Kapham) and exhibiting symptoms peculiar to both, is called a **Dvandaja*** one. There are three

---

* Gáyadása does not read the symptoms of *Dvi-doshaja* (*i e.*, due to two morbific principles) types of sinus a given in the text which he has rejected as spurious

types of this class of disease, (such as the *Vàta-pittaja, Vàta-kaphaja* and *Pitta-kaphaja*) A case of **Nádi-vrana**, exhibiting symptoms of the three aforesaid types, and attended with fever and a burning sensation, difficult breathing, dryness of the mouth and syncope, is called Tridoshaja. An attack of this type should be regarded as dreadful and fatal, casting around the gloom of death. 14-15.

**The Śalyaja Nádi-Vrana :**—A foreign matter (such as dirt, bone, splinter etc.), lodged within the body and invisible to the eye, tends to burst open the skin, etc. of the locality along its channel of insertion and gives rise to a type of Sinus. It is characterised by a constant pain, and suddenly and rapidly exudes a sort of hot, blood-tinged, agitated, frothy secretion. This type is called *Śalyaja*. 16.

**The Stana-Roga:**—These may be divided into as many types as the aforesaid Nádi-Vrana and are caused by the same exciting factors as the last named malady. The milk-carrying ducts remain closed in the breast of a nullipera thus barring the possibility of the descent of the Doshas through them and of an attack of any disease at that part of the body. On the contrary, such ducts in the breast of a primipara open and expand of their own accord, thus making the advent of diseases possible that are peculiar to the mamma. 17-19

**The breast-milk :** -The sweet essence of the Rasa (lymph chyle) drawn from the digested food courses through the whole body and is ultimately concentrated in the breast of a mother or a woman (big with child) which is called milk. 20.

**Its character :**—The breast-milk, like semen, lies hidden and invisible in the organism, though permeating it in a subtle or essential form. The characteristic features of the breast-milk bear analogy to those of semen  The breast milk is secreted, and flows out at the touch, sight or thought of the child in the same manner as the semen is dislodged and emitted at the sight, touch or recollection etc. of a beloved woman  As the strong and unclouded affections of a man are the cause of the emission of semen, so the fondest love of a mother for her children brings about the secretion of her breast-milk  Both semen and breast-milk are the product of the essence of digested food, this essence being converted into milk in women. 21—22.

**Its abnormal and normal Traits:—** The milk of a mother vitiated by the deranged Vàyu of her system has an astringent taste and floats on water  The milk of a mother vitiated by the deranged Pittam has an acid and pungent taste and becomes marked with a yellow hue,* if left to float on water. The milk of a mother vitiated by the deranged Kapham is thick and slimy and sinks in water. The milk of a mother vitiated by the concerted and simultaneous derangement of the three Doshas of the body is marked by the combination of all the preceding symptoms. An external blow or hurt too (Abhighàta) sometimes produces vitiation of the mother's milk. 23.

The milk (of a mother), which instantly mixes with water, tastes sweet and retains its natural greyish tint, should be regarded as pure  24.

The bodily Doshas having recourse to the breasts of a woman whether filled with milk or not and vitiating the local flesh and blood give rise to mammary diseases,

---

* The particle 'Cha" in the text indicates that the colour may turn blue or pink in some cases

(Stana-roga). All the types of abscess (Vidradhi) excepting the one called the Raktaja out of the six types described before are found to attack the mammæ, and their symptoms should be understood as identical with those of external abscesses. 25.

Thus ends the tenth Chapter of the Nidánam Sthánam in the Sus'ruta Samhitá wich treats of the œtiology and symptoms of Erysipelas, Sinus and mammary abscesses.

# CHAPTER XI.

Now we shall discourse on the Nidànam of **Granthi** (Glands etc.), **Apachi** (Scrofula etc.), **Arvuda** (Tumours) and **Galaganda** (Goitre). 1.

The deranged and unusually aggravated Váyu etc. (Pittam and Kapham), by vitiating the flesh, blood and fat mixed with the Kapham (of any part of the organism), give rise to the formation of round, knotty, elevated swellings which are called **Granthi** (Glandular inflammation). 2.

**The Dosha-Origined Types :**—The swelling (Sopha) of the **Vátája type** seems as if it were drawn into and elevated or as if severed or pricked with a needle, cleft in two or drawn asunder or as if cut in two or pierced. The knotty growth assumes a black colour, and is rough and elongated like a bladder. On bursting a granthi of this type exudes clear bright red blood. The **Pittaja Granthi** is characterised by heat and an excessive burning sensation (in its inside). A pain, like that of being boiled by an alkali or by fire, is felt in the inside. The knotty formation assumes a red or yellowish colour and exudes a flow of extremely hot blood on bursting. The **Kaphaja Granthi** is slightly discoloured and cold to the touch. It is characterised by a slight pain and excessive itching, and feels hard and compact as a stone It is slow or tardy in its growth and exudes a secretion of thick white-coloured pus when it bursts. 3-5.

**The Medaja Type :**—The fat origined Granthi is large and glossy and gains or loses in size with the gain or loss of flesh by the patient. It is marked by a little pain and an excessive itching sensation and exudes a secretion of fat resembling clarified butter or a gruel, in colour and consistency, made of the levigated paste of sesamum on bursting. 6.

**Sirá-Granthi**—(aneurism or varicose veins) :— The bodily Vàyu in weak and enfeebled persons, deranged by over-fatiguing physical exercises, straining or exertion or by pressure, presses on, contracts, dries or draws up the ramifications of veins (Sirà) or arteries (of the affected locality), and speedily gives rise to a raised knotty formation which is called a Sirá-Granthi. In the event of its being shifting and slightly painful, it can be cured only with the greatest difficulty. Whereas a case in which the knotty formation is painless, fixed, large and situated at any of the vital parts of the body (Marmas), should be deemed incurable.* 7.

**Apachi**—(Scrofula etc.) :—The augmented and accumulated fat and Kapham give rise to string of hard glossy, painless, nodular, or elongated granthi (swellings) about the joints of the jawbones, at the waist, joint, about the tendons of the neck, about the throat or about the region of the arm-pits. These glands (Granthis) resembling the stones of the Ámalaka fruit or the spawn of fish in shape or like some other shape, are of the same colour as the surrounding skin ; and a string or a large crop of such glandular knots, gradually growing is called Apachi† on account of the extensive nature of their growth. 8-9.

---

\* In several editions an additional line is to be found running as men well conversant with symptoms (of *Granthis*) recognise a type of Granthi due to the action of the deranged flesh and blood, which exhibits symptoms identical with those of a tumour (*Mansjra'srayam chárvuda laskhanena tulyam hi drishtamath lakshanajanih*). But Jejjata has rejected it as of questionable authority.

† These glandular formations appear about the root of the penis, about the sides, in the arm-pits and about the throat and the tendons of the neck.

These knotty formations are characterised by itching and a slight pain. Some of them spontaneously burst exuding secretions while others are observed to vanish and re-appear (in succession). Such vanishings, re-appearances, or fresh formations continue for a considerable time. The disease undoubtedly owes its origin to the deranged fat and Kapham, and may only be made amenable (to medicine) with the greatest difficulty lasting for years at a time. 10.

**Arvuda**—(tumour etc.) :—The large vegetation of flesh which appears at any part of the body, becomes slightly painful, rounded, immovable and deep-seated, and has its root sunk considerably deep in the affected part, and which is due to the vitiation of the flesh and blood by the deranged and aggravated Doshas (Váyu, Pittam and Kapham) is called an Arvuda (tumour) by the learned physicians*. The growth of an Arvuda is often found to be slow, and it seldom suppurates. The characteristic symptoms of an Arvuda which owes its origin to the deranged condition of the Vàyu, Pittam, Kapham, flesh or fat, are respectively identical with those, which mark the cases of Granthis, brought about by the same deranged principles of the body. 11.

**Raktaja–Arvuda :**—The deranged Doshas (Vàyu, Pittam and Kapham) contracting, compressing

---

They resemble spawns of fish in shape and size and are due to the action of the deranged Váyu, Pittam and Kapham. The appearance of such glands in the upper part of the body should be attributed to the action of the deranged and aggravated Váyu. They are extremely hard to cure in as much as their growth (formation) involves the concerted action of the morbific principles (Doshas) of the body.—**Bhoja.**

Charaka, who designates this disease as *Gandamálá*, describes its location in regions about the jawbones alone.

*That they having recourse to the flesh, produce deep-seated vegetations (of flesh) is the reading adopted by Gayádása and others.

and drawing the vessels (Sirá) and blood (of the affected part), raise a slightly suppurated and exuding tumour which is covered with small warts and fleshy tubercles and is called a **Raktárvuda**. This tumour is rapid in its growth and exudes a constant flow of (vitiated) blood. The complexion of the patient owing to depletive actions and other concomitant evils of hæmorrhage becomes pale and yellow. The type should be considered incurable on account of its having its origin in the blood.* 12—13.

**Mánsárvuda :**—The flesh of any part of the body hurt by an external blow etc. (hurting it with a log of wood—D.R.) and vitiated in consequence, gives rise to a sort of swelling (tumour) which is called Mánsárvuda, which originates through the action of the deranged Váyu. It is glossy, painless, non-suppurating, hard as a stone, immobile, and of the same colour as the surrounding skin. Such a tumour appearing in a person addicted to meat diet becomes deep seated owing to the consequent vitiation of the bodily flesh and soon lapses into one of an incurable type. 14.

**Prognosis :**—Even of the aforesaid curable types (such as the Vátaja, etc.), the following types of Arvudam (tumours) should be likewise regarded as incurable, those which appear in the cavity of a Srota channel or an artery, or any vulnerable joint of the body and are characterised by any sort of secretion and also immovable, should be deemed incurable. An Arvudam (tumour) cropping up on one existing from before is

---

* Although all types of Arvuda have their origin in the deranged flesh and blood, preponderant action of the deranged blood is found in *Raktá. arvuda*, while a dominant action of the deranged flesh marks the *Mánsárvuda* type.

called **Adhyarvudam,** which should be likewise deemed as incurable. A couple of contiguous Arvudam (tumours) cropping up simultaneously or one after another is called **Dviarvudam,** which should be held as equally incurable (with one of the foregoing types). An Arvuda (tumour) of whatsoever type, never suppurates owing to the exuberance of the deranged Kapham and fat as well as in consequence of the immobility, condensation and compactness of the deranged Doshas (Váyu, Pittam and Kapham involved in the case, or out of a specific trait of its own nature. 15-16.

**Definition of Galaganda** (Goitre):—The deranged and aggravated Vàyu in combination with the deranged and augmented Kapham and fat of the locality affects the two tendons of the neck (Manyás) and gradually gives rise to a swelling about that part of the neck characterised by the specific symptoms of the deranged Doshas (Vàyu or Kapham) and principles involved in the case. The swelling is called Galganda (Goitre). 17.

**Symptoms of the Dosha-origined Types :**—The swelling or tumour in the **Vátajá** goitre is characterised by a pricking pain (in its inside) marked by the appearance of blue or dark coloured veins Sirá) on its surface. It assumes a vermilion or tawny brown hue. The goitre becomes united with the local fat in course of time, and gains in size, giving rise to a sense of burning in the throat, or is characterised by the absence of any pain at all. A Vátaja goitre is rough to the touch, slow in its growth, and never or but rarely suppurates. A sense of dryness in the throat and the palate as well as a bad taste in the mouth likewise marks this type. The swelling in the **Kaphaja Type** assumes a large shape and becomes hard, firm, cold and of the same colour (white). There is but slight pain and the patient feels an irresistible inclination to scratch the part. It is slow in its progress and suppuration is rare and tardy. A sweet taste is felt in the mouth and the throat and the palate seem as if smeared with a sort of sticky mucous. 18-20.

**Symptoms of the Medaja Type:—** The swelling is glossy, soft (heavy—D.R) and pale-coloured. It emits a fetid smell and is characterised by excessive itching and an absence of pain. It is short at its root and hangs down from the neck in the shape of a pumpkin (Alávu), gradually gaining its full rotundity at the top. The size of the goitre is proportionate to the growth or loss of flesh of the body. The face of the patient looks as if it has been anointed with oil and a peculiar rumbling sound is constantly heard in the throat. 21.

**Prognosis :** - A case of goitre attended with difficult respiration, a softening of the whole body, weakness, a nonrelish for food, loss of voice as well as the one which is more than of a year's standing should be abandoned by the physician as incurable. 22.

**Metrical Text :—** A pendent swelling whether large or small and occurring about the region of the throat and resembling the scrotum in shape is called a Gala-Ganda. 23.

Thus ends the eleventh Chapter of the Nidána Sthánam in the Susrutá Samhitá which treats of the Nidánam of Granthi, Scrofula, etc.

# CHAPTER XII

Now we shall discourse on the Nidánam of **Vriddhi** (hydrocele, hernia, scrotal tumours etc), **Upadansa** (disease of the genital organ, and **Slipada** (elephantiasis). 1.

**Classes :** -There are seven different types of **Vriddhi** such as the Vátaja, Pittaja, Kaphaja, Raktaja, Medaja, Mutraja and the Antra-vriddhi. Of these both the Mutraja-vriddhi (hydrocele or extravagation of the urine), and Antra-vriddhi types, though owing their origin to the deranged condition of the bodily Vàyu, have been so named after the organic matters or anatomical parts (urine, iliac colon etc.) involved in them. 2.

**Definition and Premonitory symptoms :**—Any of the deranged Doshas (Vàyu, Pittam, etc) lying in the nether regions of the body may resort to the spermatic cords (Dhamani) and give rise to a swelling and inflammation of Phalacosha (scrotal sac) which is called **Vriddhi** (scrotal tumour etc.). A pain in the bladder, scrotum, penis and the waist (Kati) incarceration of the Vàyu and the swelling of the scrotum, are the premonitory symptoms of the disease. 3—4.

**The Dosha-origined Types :**—The type in which the scrotum becomes distended with Vàyu like an inflated air-drum, marked by roughness of (its surface) and the presence of a varied sort of Vàtaja pain (in its interior) without any apparent cause is called **Vataja Vriddhi**. The swollen scrotum, of the **Pittaja Vriddhi**, assumes the colour of a ripe

*Audumvara* fruit and is attended with fever, a burning sensation and heat in the affected part. It is of a marked rapid growth and speedy suppuration (of the scrotum). The swollen organ in the **Kaphaja Vriddhi** becomes hard and cold to the touch accompanied by little pain, and itching (in the affected part). In the **Raktaja** type the swollen scrotum is covered over with black vesicles, all other symptoms of the type being identical with those of the Pittaja one. In the **Medaja** type the swollen scrotum looks llke a ripe *Tàla* fruit and becomes soft, glossy and slightly painful. The patient feels a constant inclination to scratch the part. The **Mutraja-vriddhi** (hydrocele) owes its origin to a habit of voluntary retention of urine, its characteristic symptoms being softness and fluctuation on the surface of the swollen scrotum like a skin-bladder filled with water, painful urination, pain in the testes and swelling of the scrotum. 5.

**Antra-vriddhi** (Inguinal hernia):—The local Vàyu enraged and unusually aggravated by lifting a great load, wrestling with a stronger person, violent physical strain or a fall from a tree and such like physical labour doubles up a part of the small intestine and presses it down into the inguinal regions lying there strangulated in the form of a knot (Granthi) which is known as **Antra-vriddhi** (inguinal hernia). The part not properly attended to at the outset descends into the scrotum which becomes ultimately elongated and intensely swollen and looks like an inflated air-bladder. It (hernia) ascends upwards under pressure, making a peculiar sound, (gurgling); while let free it comes down and again gives rise to the swelling of the scrotum. This disease is called Antra-vriddhi and is incurable. 6.

**The Upadansam:**—An inflammatory swelling of the genital, whether ulcerated or not is called **Upadansa**.* The disease owes its origin to the action of the local Doshas, aggravated by promiscuous and excessive sexual intercourse, or by entire abstinence in sexual matter; or by visiting a woman, who had observed a vow of lifelong continence or one who has not long known a man, or one in her menses or one with an extremely narrow or spacious vulva, or with rough or harsh or large pubic hairs; or by going unto a woman whose partturient canal is studded with hairs along its entire length; or by visiting a woman not amorously disposed towards the visitor and vice versa; or by knowing a woman who washes her private parts with foul water or neglects the cleanliness of those parts, or suffers from any of the vaginal diseases, or one whose vagina is naturally foul; or by going unto a woman in any of the natural fissures of her body other than the organ of copulation (Vi yoni); or by pricking the genital with finger nails, or biting it with the teeth, or through poisonous contact, or through practice of getting the (penis abnormally elongated by pricking the) bristles of a water parasite (*Suka*) into its body; or by practising

---

* Upadans'a is not syphilis whole to whole. Certain types of Upadans'a such as the Raktaja and Sànnipátika types which entail the destruction of the organs concerned exhibit certain symptoms which are common to syphilis as well. The secondary eruptions and tertiary symptoms of syphilis are not mentioned by the A'yurvedic Rishis who used to treat it only with vegetable medicines and this fact intimates the probability that the secondary and tertiary symptoms of syphilis might not arise by their efficient and able treatment from the very beginning, preventing the absorption of the poison into the system. The practice of ablution, so common among the Hindus, might be taken into consideration as one of the important preventive factors. Maharshi Charaka has comprised it within the chapter on 'Senile Impotency'.—Ed.

masturbation, or any unnatural offence with female quadrupeds; or by washing the genitals with filthy or poisonous water; or through neglect to wash the parts after coition, or voluntary suppression of a natural flow of semen or urine or through any hurt or pressure on the organ etc. The inflammation of the genital thus engendered is called Upadansa. The disease admits of being divided into five distinct types, such as, the Vàtaja, Pittaja, Kaphaja, Tridoshaja and the Raktaja. 7—8.

**The symptoms of different Types :—** The roughness of the genitals, the bursting or cracking of the integuments of the penis and prepuce etc., numbness and swelling of the affected part which is perceived rough to the touch and the presence of a varied sort of pain peculiar to the deranged Vàyu are the characteristic indications of the **Vátaja type.** In the **Pittaja** type fever sets in (from the very beginning), the penis becomes swollen and assumes the colour of a ripe Indian fig (reddish-yellow), attended with a sort of intolerable burning sensation The process of suppuration is rapid and a variety of pain peculiar to the deranged Pittam, (distinguishes it from the other forms of the disease). The penis becomes swollen, hard and glossy in the **Kaphaja type** marked by itching and a variety of pain characteristic of the deranged Kapham. In the blood-origined type (**Raktaja**) the organ bleeds heavily and is covered with the eruptions of large black vesicles. Fever, thirst, (Sosha), burning sensations and other characteristic symptoms of the deranged Pittam are also present. Palliation is all that can be occasionally effected in these cases. Symptoms specifically betraying to each of the Vátaja, Pittaja and Kaphaja types concurrently manifest themselves in the **Sánnipátika** type of Upadansá. The organ cracks, the ulcers or cancers become infested with parasites and death comes in to put a stop to the suffering of its wretched victim. 9—13.

**Slipadam** (Elephantiasis) :—The disease in which the deranged Vàyu, Pittam and Kapham, taking a downward course, are lodged in the thighs, knee-joints, legs and the inguinal regions and spread to the feet in course of time and gradually give rise to a swelling therein, is called **Slipadam**. There are three types of Slipada severally due to the actions of the deranged Váyu, Pittam and Kapham. 14—15.

**The symptoms of the different Types:**—The swollen parts assume a black colour in the **Vátaja** type and are felt rough and uneven to the touch. A sort of spasmodic pain without any apparent reason is felt (at intervals in the seat of the disease), which largely begins to crack or burst. The **Pittaja** type is characterised by a little softness and yellowish hue (of the diseased localities) and often attended with fever, and a burning sensation. In the **Kaphaja** type the affected localities become white, glossy, slightly painful, heavy, contain large nodules (Granthis) and are studded over with crops of papillæ. 16

**Prognosis :**—A case of elephantiasis of a year's growth as well as the one which is characterised by excessive swelling (of the affected parts), exudation and vegetation of knotty excrescences resembling the summits of an ant-hill should be given up as incurable. 17.

**Memorable Verses :**—A preponderance of the deranged Kapham marks the three types of the disease, in as much as, the heaviness and largeness (of the swelling) can not be brought about by any other factor than Kapham. The disease is peculiar to countries in which large quantities of old rain-water remain stagnant during the greater part (lit.- all seasons) of the year making them damp and humid in all seasons. 18-91

The disease is usually found to be confined to the legs and hands of men but cases are on record in which it has extended to the ear, nose, lips and the regions of the eyes. (Penis—Mádhaba-Nidánam). 20.

Thus ends the twelfth Chapter of the Nidánastbánam in the Sus'ruta Samhitá which treats of the Nidánam of scrotal tumours, hernia, Upadans'am and elephantiasis.

# CHAPTER XIII.

Now we shall discourse on the Nidánam of **Kshudrarogam** (diseases which are known by the general name of minor ailments). 1.

These diseases are generally divided into forty-four distinct varieties or types such as :—Ajagalliká, Yavaprakshyá, Andhálaji, Vivritá, Kachchapiká, Valmika, Indravriddhá, Panasiká, Páshána-garddabha, Jála-garddabha, Kakshá, Vishphota, Agni-rohini, Chippam, Kunakha, Anus'aye, Vidáriká, Sarkará-Arbudam, Pámá, Vicharchiká, Rakasá, Pádadáriká, Kadara, Alasa, Indralupta, Dárunaka, Arunshiká, Palitam, Mas'uriká, Yauvana-pidaká, Padmini-kantaka, Yatumani, Mas'aka, Charmakila, Tilakálaka, Nyachchya, Vyanga, Parivartiká, Avapátiká, Niruddha-prakás'a, Niruddha-guda, Ahiputanam, Vrishana-kachchu, and Guda-bhrans'a * 2.

**Metrical Texts :**—The species of pimples or eruptions which are shaped like the *Mudga* pulse and are glossy, knotty and painless is called **Ajagalliká**. They are of the same colour (as the surrounding skin) and their origin is usually ascribed to the action of the deranged Kapham and Váyu. The disease is peculiar to infants.† **Yáváprakshyá** :—The eruptions

---

* Brahmadeva comprising *Garddavika, Irvellika, Gandhapidiká* and *Tilakálaka* in the list reads it as consisting of thirty-four different species. Jejjata does not hold the four forms of disease commencing with *Garddavika, etc.* as included within the list. Gayádása, finding them included in all the recensions reads *Garddabhiká,* etc. as included within the list of *Kshudra Roga,* and Pámá etc. as included within the list of Kshudra Kushtham.

† They afflict certain infants—Dallana.

which are shaped like the barley-corns, extremely hard, thick at the middle, knotty and affect (lit.—confined to) the flesh are called Yavaprakshyá. They are due to the action of the deranged Váyu and Kapham. **Andhálaji**:—The dense, raised, slender-topped eruptions which appear in circular patches and exude a slight pus are called Andhálaji. They are due to the action of the deranged Váyu and Kapham. **Vivritá**:—Pustules or eruptions, which are coloured like a ripe fig. fruit and are flat-topped and appear in circular patches with an intolerable burning sensation, are called Vivrita They are due to the action of the deranged Pittam. 3 - 6.

**Kachchapiká :**—A group of five or six hard, elevated, nodular eruptions (Granthis), arranged in the shape of a tortoise (which may appear on the surface of any part of the body), are called Kachchapiká. They are due to the action of the deranged Kapham and Váyu. **Valmika :**—The knotty undurated eruptions (Granthis) which gradually appear on the soles, palms, joints, neck and on the regions above clavicles and resemble an ant-hill in shape, slowly gaining in size are called **Valmika** Ulcers attended with pricking pain, burning, itching sensations and exuding mucopurulent discharges appear around the aforesaid eruptions (Granthis). The disease is due to the action of the deranged Kapham, Pittam and Váyu. 7—8.

**Indravriddhá :**—Pimples or eruptions (Pidaká) arising (on the surface of the body), arranged in the same circular array as marks the distribution of the seed (sacks) in a lotus flower are called **Indravriddhá** by the physicians. The disease is caused by the action of the deranged Váyu and Pittam. **Panasika :**—Eruptions (Pidaká) of a sort of extremely painful pustules all over the back or the ears which resemble the

Kumuda bulb in shape, are called **Panasiká**. They are due to the action of the deranged Kapham and Váyu. **Páshána-Garddabha** :—A slightly painful and non-shifting hard swelling, which appears on the joint of the jawbones, (Hanu-sandhi, is called Páshána-Garddabha. The disease is the effect of the deranged Kapham and Váyu. **Jála-Garddabha** :—A thin and superficial swelling, which like erysipelas is of a shifting or progressive character and is further attended with fever and a burning sensation and which is but rarely found to suppurate, is called Jála-Garddabha.* The disease results from the deranged Pittam **Kakshá** :—The disease characterised by the eruptions of black and painful vesicles (Shphota) on the back, sides, and on the region about the arm-pits, is called Kakshá. The disease is likewise attributed to the action of the aggravated Pittam. **Vishphotaka** :—The disease in which eruptions of burnlike vesicles (Shphota) crop up on the whole surface of the body, or on that of any particular locality, attended with fever, is called Vishphotaka. The disease is the effect of vitiated blood and Pittam. 9—14.

**Agni-Rohini†** :—Vesicles (Shphota) having the appearance of burns and cropping up about the waist

---

* The circular raised spots studded with Vesicles are called Garddabhá. They are reddish and painful and produced by the action of Váyu and Pittam. Gayádása reads it so.

† Dallana quotes from another Tantram that the morbific principles in men, aggravated through the action of the enraged and augmented Pittam and blood, give rise to vesicles (blisters) like red-hot charcoal by breaking open the flesh at the waist, attended with extreme pain, high fever and an insufferable burning sensation which, if not properly remedied, bring on death within a fortnight, or ten days of their first appearance. These (Vesicles) are called *Vahni-Rohini*. And again from another work. he cites that a case of *Vahni-Rohini* due to the action of the deranged.

(Kakshá) by bursting the local flesh, and which is attended with fever and a sensation as if a blazing fire is burning in the inside (of the affected part), are called Agni-Rohini. The disease is caused by the concerted action of the three deranged Doshas (Váyu, Pittam and Kapham). It is incurable and ends in the death of the patient either on the seventh\*, tenth or fifteenth day (of its first appearance). 15.

**Chippam :**—The deranged Váyu and Pittam vitiating the flesh of the finger-nails, give rise to a disease which is characterised by pain, burning and suppuration. The disease called Chippam, is also denominated *Upanakha* and *Kshataroga*. **Kunakham** —The nails of fingers becoming rough, dry, black, and injured through the action of the Doshas enraged through the effect of a blow, are called Kunakha (bad nails). It is also called *Kulinam*. **Anusayi :**— A small swelling (on the surface of the body) which is of the same colour (as the surrounding skin), but is deep-seated, and suppurates in its deeper strata, is called *Anusayi* by the physicians. The disease is the effect of the deranged Kapham. **Vidáriká :**—A round reddish swelling rising either on the auxiliary or inguinal regions in the shape of a gourd (*Vidárikanda*) is known as Vidáriká. The disease is due to the concerted action of the deranged Váyu, Pittam and Kapham and is characterised by symptoms peculiar to each of them. 16--19,

---

Kapham proves fatal within a fortnight, that due to the deranged Pittam, within ten days, and that due to the deranged Váyu, within a week.

\* The patient dies on the seventh day in a case of disease marked by the dominant Váyu, on the tenth day in a case marked by the dominant Pittam and on the fifteenth day in a case of dominant deranged Kapham.

**Sarkarárbudam :**—The deranged Váyu and Kapham having recourse to and affecting the flesh, veins (Sirá), ligaments (Snáyu) and fat give rise to a sort of cyst (Granthi) which when it bursts exudes a copious secretion in its nature somewhat like honey, clarified butter or Vasá. The aforesaid Váyu, when aggravated through excessive secretion, dries and gathers the flesh up again in the shape of (a large number of) gravel-like concretions (Sarkará) known accordingly as Sarkarárbudam. A fetid secretion of varied colour is secreted from the veins (Sirá) in these Granthis which are sometimes found to bleed suddenly. The three varieties of the skin disease called **Pámá** (Eczema), **Vicharchiká** (Psoriasis) and **Rakasá** have already been discussed under the head of Kushtham (Chapter. V.). 20—21.

**Pádadáriká :**—The soles and feet of a person of extremely pedestrian habits become dry (and lose their natural serous moisture). The local Váyu thus aggravated gives rise to peculiar painful cracks (Dári in the affected parts) which are called Pádadàriká. **Kadara** :—The knotty (Granthi), a painful, hard growth raised at the middle or sunk at the sides, which exudes a secretion and resembles an Indian plum (Kola—in shape), and appearing at the soles (palms according to—Bhoja) of a person as an outcome of the vitiated condition of the local blood and fat produced by the deranged Doshas incidental to the pricking of a thorn etc. or of gravel is called a Kadara (corns). **Alasa** :—An affection, caused by contact of poisonous mire and appearing between the toes, which is characterised by pains, burning, itching and exudation, is called Alasa. 22—25.

**Indralupta :**—The deranged Váyu and Pittam having recourse to the roots of the hairs bring about their gradual falling off, while the deranged blood and Kapham of the locality fill up those pores or holes, thus barring their fresh growth and recrudescence. The disease is called **Indralupta,*** **Rujya or Khálitya** (Alopecia). **Dárunaka:**—The disease in which the hairy parts of the body (roots of hairs) become hard, dry and characterised by an itching sensation is called Dárunaka The disease is due to the action of the deranged Kapham and Váyu. **Arunshiká :**—Ulcers (Arunshi) attended with mucopurulent discharges and furnished with a number of mouths or outlets and appearing on the scalps of men as the result of the action of local parasites and of the deranged blood and Kapham (of the locality) are called Arunshiká. **Palitam :**—The heat and Pittam of the body having recourse to the region of the head owing to overwork, fatigue, and excessive grief or anger, tend to make the hair prematurely grey, and such silvering of the hair (before the natural period of senile decay) is called Palitam. **Masuriká** (variola) :—The yellow or copper-coloured pustules or eruptions attended with pain, fever and burning and appearing all over the body, on (the skin of) the face and inside the cavity of the mouth, are called Masuriká. **Yauvana-pidaká**—**(Mukhadushiká)** :— The pimples like the thorns of a Sálmali tree, which arefound on the face of young men through the deranged condition of the blood, Váyu and Kapham, are called Yauvana-pidaká or pimples of youth. **Padmini-Kantaka :** —The circular, greyish patches or rash-like eruptions

---

* Women are generally proof against this disease owing to their delicate constitution and to their being subjected to the monthly discharge of vitiated blood and at the same time to their undergoing no physical exercise, and hence there is little chance of the bodily Pittam being deranged and bringing on this disease.

studded over with thorny papilla of the skin resembling the thorns on the stem of the lotus marked by itching are called Padmini-kantaka. The disease is due to the deranged condition of the Váyu and Kapham. **Yatu-mani (mole)** :—The reddish, glossy, circular, and painless, congenital marks (Sahajam) or moles on the body not more elevated (than the surrounding skin) are called Yatumani. The disease is due to the deranged condition of the blood and Pittam. 26—33.

**Maśaka (Lichen) :** —The hard, painless, black and elevated eruptions on the body (skin) resembling the Másha pulse in shape, caused by the aggravated condition of the bodily Vàyu are called Maśaka **Tilakálaka**:—The black painless spots on the skin about the size of a sesamum seed and level with the skin are called Tilakálaka. This disease is caused through the aggravated condition of the Váyu, Pittam and Kapham.† **Nyachcham**:—The congenital, painless, circular, white or brown (Śyáva) patches on the skin, which are found to be restricted to a small or comparatively diffused area of the skin, are called Nyachcham. **Charmakila** (hypertrophy of the skin) :—The causes and symptoms of the disease known as Charmakila have been already described (under the head of the Arśa-Nidànam). **Vyanga** :— The Váyu being aggravated through wrath and over-fatiguing physical exercise, and surcharged with Pittam, and suddenly appearing on the face of a person, causes thin, circular, painless and brown-coloured patches or stains. They are known by the name of Vyanga * 34-38.

\* According to certain authorities it is due to the absorption of blood by Váyu and Pittam.

† According to others the spot goes by the name of *Nilikam*, if it is black-coloured and appears anywhere other than on the face.

**The Parivartiká :**—The vital Váyu (Vyána) aggravated by such causes as excessive massage (masturbation), pressure, or local trauma, attacks the integuments of the penis (prepuce) which being thus affected by the deranged Váyu forms into a knot-like structure and hangs down from the glans penis. The disease known as Parivartiká or Phymosis is due to the action of the deranged Váyu aggravated by any extraneous factor. It is marked by pain and burning sensation; and sometimes suppurates. When the knotty growth becomes hard and is accompanied by itching, then it is caused by the aggravated Kapham. 39.

**Avapátiká :**—When the integuments of the prepuce is abnormally and forcibly turned back by such causes as coition under excitement, with a girl (before menstruation and before the rupture of the hymen and consequently with a narrow external orifice of the vagina) or masturbation or pressure or a blow on the penis, or a voluntary retention of a flow of semen or forcible opening of the prepuce, the disease is called Avapátiká or paraphymosis. **Niruddha-prakás'a :**—The prepuce affected by the deranged Váyu entirely covers up the glans penis and thus obstructs and covers up the orifice of the urethra. In cases of partial obstruction a thin jet of urine is emitted with a slight pain. In cases of complete closing the emission of urine is stopped without causing any crack or fissure in the glans penis in consequence. The disease is called Niruddha-prakás'a which is due to the deranged Váyu and is marked by pain (in the glans penis). 39-41.

**Niruddhaguda :**—The Váyu (Apána) obstructed by the repression of a natural urging towards defecation stuffs the rectum, thus producing constriction of its passage and consequent difficulty of defecation. This dreadful disease is known as Niruddha-gudam (stricture of the rectum) which is extremely difficult to cure. **Ahiputana** :—A sort of itch-like eruptions appearing about the anus of a child owing to a deposit of urine, perspiration, feces etc consequent on the neglect in cleansing that part. The eruptions which are the effects of the deranged blood and Kapham soon assume an Eczematous character and exude a purulent discharge on account of constant scratching. The Eczema (Vrana) soon spreads, and coalesces and proves very obstinate in the end. The disease is called Ahiputana. **Vrishana-kachchu** :—When the filthy matter, deposited in the scrotal integuments of a person who is negligent in washing the parts or in the habit of taking daily ablutions, is moistend by the local perspiration, it gives rise to an itching sensation in the skin of the scrotum, which is speedily turned into running Eczema by constant scratching of the parts. The disease is called Vrishana-kachchu and is due to the aggravated condition of the Kapham and blood. **Guda-Bhransa** :—A prolapse or falling out of the anus (due to the Váyu) in a weak and lean patient through straining, urging or flow of stool as in dysentery is called Guda-Bhransa or prolapsus ani. 42—45.

Thus ends the thirteenth Chapter of the Nidána Sthánam in the Sus'ruta Samhitá which treats of the Nidánam of minor ailments.

# CHAPTER XIV.

Now we shall discourse on the Nidánam of the disease known as **Śukadosha.** 1.

Any of the eighteen different types of the disease may affect the genital (penis) of a man who foolishly resorts to the practice of getting it abnormally elongated and swollen by plastering it with **Śuka** (a kind of irritating water insect) and not in the usual officinal way.

**Classification :**—Diseases, which result from such malpractices, are knonwn as,—Sarshapiká, Ashthiliká, Grathitam, Kumbhiká, Alaji, Mriditam, Sammudhapidaká, Avamantha, Pushkariká, Sparśaháni, Uttamá, Śatoponaka, Tvakapáka, Śonitárvudam, Mánsárvudam, Mánsapáka, Vidradhi and Tilakálak. 2.

**Metrical Texts :**—The tiny herpetic eruptions (Pidaká) which resemble the seeds of white mustard in shape and size, (and are found to crop up on the male organ of generation) on account of a deranged condition of the blood and Kapham, as the result of an injudicious application of Śuka plasters are called **Sarshapiká** by the wise. Eruptions of hard stone-like pimples, (Pidaká) irregular at their sides or edges and which are caused by the aggravation of the local Váyu by the use of a plaster of the poisonous Śuka, are called **Ashthiliká**. The knotty Granthis (nodules) on the penis owing to its being frequently stuffed with the bristles of a Śuka insect are called **Grathitam**. This type is caused by the deranged action of the Kapham. A black wart resembling the stone or seed of a jambolin fruit in shape is called **Kumbhiká**. This type is due to the deranged condition of the blood and Pittam. 3—5.

An **Alaji** (incidental to an injudicious application of Śuka on the penis) exhibits symptoms, which are identical with those manifested by a case of Alaji in Prameha (Ch. vi). A wart (papilloma) attended with swelling of the part and caused by the aggravated Váyu on the hard and inflamed penis causing pressure (on the urethra) is called **Mriditam**. The pustule or eruption appearing on the penis on account of its being extremely pressed by the hand (for the insertion of the hairs of the Śuka) in its dorsum is called **Sammudhapidaká**. (It is the outcome of the aggravated Váyu*). A large number of elongated pustules on the penis (incidental to an application of Śuka to the part) which burst at the middle, causing pain and shivering, is called **Avamantha** (epithelioma). 6—10.

The **Pushkariká** type of the disease is marked by the eruptions of small pimples around the principal one. The type has its origin in the deranged condition of the blood and Pittam, and is so called from the part of the excrescenses being arranged in rings or circles like the petals of a lotus flower in shape. A complete anesthesia (of the affected organ) owing to the vitiated blood by the injudicious application of a Śuka is called **Sparśaháni**. Pustules appearing on the penis through the vitiation of the local blood and Pittam by such constant applications are called **Uttamá**. A suppuration of the prepuce under the circumstance is called **Tvakapákh**. There is fever with a burning sensation in the affected organ. The disease is due to the vitiated condition of the blood and Pittam. 11—15.

The type of the disease in which the penis is marked by the eruption of black vesicles and is covered over with a large number of red pimples or pustules with

---

\* According to Dallana it is due to the action of Váyu and blood.

an excruciating pain in the ulcerated region of the organ is called **Śonitárvudam**. The vegetation of a fleshy tumour on the penis (incidental to a blow on the organ to alleviate the pain of inserting the hairs of the Śuka insect into its body), is called **Mánsárvudam**. A suppuration as well as sloughing of the penis attended with different kinds of pain which severally mark the deranged Váyu, Pittam and Kapham is called **Mánsapáka**. This type is caused by the concerted action of the deranged Váyu, Pittam and Kapham. 15-18.

The specific symptoms of a Tridoshaja Vidradhi as described before (Chap. ix.) mark the one which affects the penis (owing to an injudicious application of the highly poisonous irritant Śuka to the organs) The disease is called **Vidradhi**. A process of general suppuration and sloughing of the organ marks the type which is produced by the application of a black Śuka or one of a variegated coloured insect of the same species. The type is called **Tilakálaka**, and should be regarded as Tridoshaja one. 19 – 21.

**Prognosis :**—Of the above enumerated malignant diseases of the penis, those known as Mánsárvuda, Mánsapáka, Vidradhi and Tilakálak shoulda be deemed as incurable. 22.

<small>Thus ends the fourteenth Chapter of the Nidána Sthánam in the Sus'ruta Samhitá which treats of Nidánam of different types of S'ukadohsa.</small>

# CHAPTER XV.

Now we shall discourse on the Nidánam of **Bhagnam** (fractures and dislocations etc. of bones). 1

Various kinds of fracture may be caused from a variety of causes, such as by a fall, pressure, blow, violent jerking or by the bites of ferocious beasts etc. These cases may be grouped under the two main sub-divisions such as **Sandhi-Muktam** (dislocation) and **Kánda-Bhagnam** (fracture of a kánda). 2.

Cases of Sandhi-muktam (dislocation) may be divided into six different types, such as the *Utplishtam, Vis'lishtam, Vivartitam, Adhah-Kshiptam, Ati-kshiptam* and *Tiryak-kshiptam.* 3

**General features of a dislocation :—** Incapability of extension, flexion, movement, circumduction and rotation (immobility, considered in respect of the natural movements of the joint), of the dislocated limb, which becomes extremely painful and cannot bear the least touch. These are said to be the general symptoms of a dislocation. 4.

**Diagnostic symptoms of a dislocation :—**In case of a friction of a joint by two articular extremeties (**Utplishtam**) a swelling is found to appear on either side of the articulation attended with a variety of pain at night. A little swelling accompanied by a constant pain and disordered function of the dislocated joint, marks the case of simple-looseness (**Vislishtam**) of the articulation ; while pain and unevenness of the joint owing to the displacement of the connected bones distinguish a case of **Vivartitam** (lateral displacement). An excruciating pain, and looseness of the dislocated bone are the symptoms which characterise a case in which a dislodged bone is seen to drop or hang down from its joint (**Adhah-kshiptam**). In a case of abnormal projection (**Ati-kshiptam**), the dislocated bone is removed away from its joint which becomes extremely painful. A case of oblique dislocation (**Tiryak-kshiptam**) is marked by the projection or displacement of the bone on one side accompanied by a sort of intolerable pain. 5.

**Different kinds of Kánda Bhagnam :**—Now we shall describe the Kánda-Bhagnam (fracture etc.). Fractures may be divided into twelve different kinds which are known as, Karkatakam, Aśvakarnam, Churnitam, Pichchitam, Asthi-chchalitam, Kándabhagnam, Majjágatam, Atipátitam, Vakram, Chchinnam, Pátitam and Sphutitam. 6.

**General symptoms of Kánda-bhagnam :**—A violent swelling (about the seat of fracture) with throbbings or pulsations, abnormality in the position (of the fractured limb), which cannot bear the least touch, crepitus under pressure, a looseness or dropping of the limb, the presence of a variety of pain and a sense of discomfort in all positions are the indications which generally mark all kinds of fracture (Kánda-bhagnam). 7.

**Diagnostic symptoms:**—The case where a fractured bone, pressed or bent down at its two articular extremities, bulges out at the middle so as to resemble the shape of a knot (Granthi), is called **Karkatam**. The case where the fractured bone projects upward like the ear of a horse is called **Aśvakarnam**. The fractured bone is found to be shattered into fragments in a case of the **Churnitam** or comminuted kind which can be detected both by palpation and crepitation. A smashed condition of the fractured bone marks a case of the **Pichchitam** kind which is often found to be marked by a great swelling. The case where the covering or skin of the bone (periosteum) is cast or splintered off is called the **Asthi-chchallitam**. The case where the completely broken or severed bones are found to project through the local skin, is called **Kánda-bhagnam** (compound). The case where a fragment of the fractured or broken bone is found to pierce into the bone and dig out the marrow, is called **Majjánugatam**, (Impacted fracture). The case where the fractured bone droops or hangs down is called **Ati-pátitam**. The case where the unloosened bone (from its position) is bent down in the form of an arch is called **Vakram** The case where only one articular extremity of the bone is severed is called **Chhinnam**. The case where the bone is slightly fractured and pierced with a large number of holes, is called **Pátitam**, an excruciating pain being the leading indication. The case where the bone largely cracked and swollen becomes painful as if stuffed with the bristles of a Śuka insect is called **Sphutitam** (Green-stick fracture). Of the several kinds of fracture, cures are effected with extreme difficulty in a case of the Churnitam, Chhinnam, Ati-pátitam or Majjánugatam kind. A case of displacement or laxation occurring in a child or in an old or weak patient or in one suffering from asthma (Śvasa) or from any cutaneous affection (Kushtha) or Kshata-Kshina disease is difficult to cure. 8.

**Memorable verses :**—The following cases are to be given up as hopeless —*viz* fracture of the pelvic bone (or of bones that are of this description, wherever they may be situated); dislocation of the pelvic joints ; compound fracture of the thigh bone or of the flat bones) ; fracture into small pieces of the frontal bone or its dislocation ; simple fracture of the breast-bones, back-bone and temporal and cranial bones. If the dislocations and fractures be improperly set from the outset (Ádito)* or if the union be anyhow disturbed there is no hope for recovery. 9—11.

If fractures happen at any time of the first three stages of **adult life** which has been described before (vide Sutrasthána Chap. XXXV.) and if they are set up by an able surgeon they have a great chance of being united. 12.

A bending of a gristle or cartilage (**Taruna**) is called its fracture. A **Nalaka** (long bone) bone is usually found to be severed. A **Kapála** bone is found to be cracked, while a **Ruchaka**† (tooth) is found to be splintered off. 13.

* The word *Ádito* may be taken into the sense of congenital malformation which is beyond remedy.

† The presence of the particle 'cha' denotes **Valya-asthi**.

Thus ends the fifteenth Chapter of the Nidána Sthánam in the Sus'ruta amhitá which treats of the Nidánam of dislocations and fractures.

# CHAPTER XVI.

Now we shall discourse on the Nidánam of **Mukharogam** (diseases which affect the cavity of the mouth in general). 1.

**General Classifications:**—Sixty five* different forms of mouth disease are known in practice. They are found to attack seven different localities viz. the lips, the gums of the teeth, tongue, palate, throat and the entire cavity; of these eight are peculiar to the lips; fifteen, to the roots of the teeth; eight to the teeth; five to the tongue; nine to the palate; seventeen to the throat; and three to the entire cavity. 2—3.

**Diseases of the lips:**—The eight forms which affect the lips, are either Vátaja, Pittaja, Kaphaja, Sánnipátika, Raktaja, Mánsaja, Medaja or Abhighátaja (Traumatic). 4.

**The Vátaja Type:**—The lips become dry, rough, numbed, black, extremely painful and the affected part seems as if it were smashed and pulled out or cracked by the action of the aggravated **Váyu**. In the **Pittaja type**—the lips become blue or yellow-coloured and studded with (a large number of small) mustard-seed-like eruptions, which suppurate and exude a purulent discharge attended with a burning sensation (in the locality). In the **Kaphaja type**—the affected lips are covered with small eruptions, which are of the same colour as the surrounding part, and become slimy, heavy or thick, cold and swollen. Pain is absent in this type and the patient feels an irresistible inclination to scratch the parts. In the **Sánnipátaja type**, the lips change

---

* According to others sixty-seven—but Dallan does not support this.

colour, becoming black, yellow, or ash-coloured (white) at intervals and are found to be studded with various sorts of eruptions. 5—8.

**The Raktaja type:**—(Produced by the vitiated condition of the blood) the affected lips look as red as blood and profusely bleed and crops of date coloured (chocolate-coloured) eruptions appear on their surface. In the **Mánsaja type** (due to the vitiated condition of the local flesh), the lips become heavy, thick and gathered up in the form of a lump of flesh. The angles of the mouth become infested with parasites which germinate and spread themselves in the affected parts. In the **Medaja** (fat-origined) **type** the lips become numbed, soft, heavy and marked by an itching sensation. The skin of the inflamed surface becomes glossy and looks like the surface layer of clarified butter exuding a thin crystal-like (transparent) watery discharge. In the **Abhigátaja** (Traumatic) **type**, the lips become red, knotty and marked by an itching sensation and seem as if pierced into or cut open with an axe and (become cracked and fissured). 9—12.

**Disease of the roots of the teeth :**—Diseases which are peculiar to the roots of the teeth, are known as Sitáda, Danta-pupputaka, Danta-veshtaka, Saushira, Máha-Saushira, Paridara, Upakusa, Danta-vaidarbha, Vardhana, Adhimánsa and the five sorts of Nádi (sinus). 13.

**Sitáda** (Scurvy);—The gums of the teeth suddenly bleed and become putrified, black, slimy and emit a fetid smell. They become soft and gradually slough off. The disease has its origin in the deranged condition of the local blood and Kapham. **Danta-pupputaka** (gum boil):—The disease in which the roots of two or three teeth at a time is marked by a violent swelling and pain is called Danta-pupputaka. The disease is due to the vitiated condition of the blood and Kapham. **Danta-veshtaka :**—The teeth become loose in the gums, which exude a discharge of blood and pus. This disease is due to the vitiated blood of the locality. **Saushira :**— The disease in which an itching painful swelling appears about the gums attended with copious flow of saliva is called S'aushira (Alveolar abscess). It is caused by the deranged blood and Kapham of the locality. **Mahá-S'aushira :**—The disease in which the teeth become loose, the palate marked by sinuses or fissures, the gums putrified, and the whole cavity of the mouth inflamed, is called Mahás'aushira, the outcome of the concerted action of the deranged Doshas of the body. 14—18.

**Paridara :**—The disease in which the gums become putrified, wear off and bleed is called Paridara (bleeding gums). The disease has its origin in the deranged condition of the blood, Kapham and Pittam. **Upakus'a :**—The disease in which the gums become marked by a burning sensation and suppuration and the teeth become loose and shaky (in their gums) in consequence and bleed at the least shaking, is called Upakus'a. There is a slight pain, and the entire cavity of the mouth becomes swollen and emits a fetid smell ; this disease is due to the vitiated condition of the blood and Pittam   19.

**Danta-Vaidarbha :**—The disease which is consequent upon the friction of the gums marked by the appearance of a violent swelling about the portion (so rubbed and in which) the teeth become loose and can be moved about, is called Danta-vaidarbha which is due to an extraneous cause such as a blow etc  **Vardhana :**— the disease which is marked by the advent of an additional tooth (the last molar) through the action of the deranged Vâyu with a specific excruciating pain of its own, is called Vardhana or eruption of the Wisdom tooth. The pain subsides with the cutting of the tooth. **Adhimánsa :**—The disease in which a violent and extremely painful tumour appears about the root of the tooth, and is situated in the farthest end of the cavity of the cheek-bone accompanied by a copious flow of saliva is called Adhimánsa or Epulis. It is due to the deranged Kapham. The five sorts of **Nádi** (sinus) which affect the roots of the teeth (are either Vátaja, Pittaja, Kaphaja, Sánnipátaja or Abhighàtaja), their symptoms being respectively identical with those of the types of Nádi-vrana. 20 - 24.

**Diseases to the teeth proper :**—Diseases which are restricted to the teeth proper are named as, Dálana, Krimi-dantaka, Danta-harsha, Bhanjaka, Sarkará, Kapálika, Syáva-dantaka and Hanu-moksha. 25.

**Dálana :**—The disease in which the teeth seem as if being cleft asunder with a violent pain is called Dálana or toothache, the origin of which is ascribed to the action of the aggravated state of the bodily Vàyu. **Krimi-dantaka :**—The disease in which the teeth are eaten into by worms, is called Krimi-dantaka (caries). The teeth become loose and perforated by black holes accompanied by a copious flow of saliva. The appearance of an extremely diffused swelling (about the roots of decayed teeth) with a sudden aggravation of the accompanying pain without any apparent cause is also one of its specific features. **Danta-harsha :**—The disease in which the teeth cannot bear the heat, cold or touch is called Danta-harsha. It is due to the deranged condition of Váyu. **Bhanjaka :**—The disease in which the face is distorted, the teeth break, and the accompanying pain is severe, is called Bhanjaka (degeneration of the teeth). The disease is due to the deranged condition of the Váyu and Kapham. **Śarkará** :—The disease, in which sordes, formed on the teeth and hardened (by the action of the deranged Váyu), lie in a crystallised form at the roots of the teeth, is called Śarkará (Tartar). Such deposits tend to destroy the healthy growth and functions of the teeth. **Kapaliká** :—The disease in which the preceding crystallised deposits get cemented together and afterwards separate from the teeth taking away a part of their coating (enamel) is called Kapáliká (calcareous deposit) which naturally makes an erosion into and destroys the teeth **Syáva-dantaka** :—The disease, in which the teeth variously scorched by the action of the deranged Pittam assumes a blackish or blue colour, is named as Syáva-dantaka (black teeth). **Hanu-moksha** :— The disease in which the Váyu aggravated (by such causes, as by loud talking, chewing of hard substances, or immoderate yawning) produces the dislocation of the jawbones is called Hanu-moksha It is identical with Ardditam as regards its symptoms. 26 – 33.

**Diseases of the tongue :**—The five kinds of diseases which affect the organ of taste are the three sorts of Kantakas due to the three deranged Doshas (Vátaja Pittaja and Kaphaja), Alása and Upa-jihviká. 34.

**The three Kantaks :**—In the **Vátaja Kantaka** type the tongue becomes cracked, loses the sense of taste and becomes rough like a teak leaf (giving the organ a warty appearance). In the **Pittaja Kantaka** form the tongue is coloured yellow and studded over with furred blood-coloured papillæ with the burning sensation (of the Pittam in them). In the **Kaphaja Kantaka** type the tongue becomes heavy, thick and grown over with vegetation of slender fleshy warts in the shape of *S'álmali* thorns    **Alása** :—The severe inflammatory swelling about the under surface of the tongue is called Alása, which if allowed to grow on unchecked gives rise to numbness and immobility of the organ and tends to a process of rapid suppuration at its base. The disease is caused by the deranged blood and Kapham   The **Upa-jihvá** :—The disease in which a (cystic) swelling shaped like the tip of the tongue appears about the under-surface of that organ by raising it a little is called Upa-jihviká (Ranula). The accompanying symptoms are salivation, burning and itching sensations in the affected organ; these are due to the deranged Kapham and blood (of the locality).  35—37.

**Disease of the palate :**—Diseases which are peculiar to the part of the palate are named Gala-s'undiká, Tundikeri, Adhrusha, Mànsa-kachchapa, Arvuda, Mànsa-sanghàta, Tálu-s'osha and Tálu-páka.  38.

**Gala-sundiká :**—The diffused and elongated swelling, caused by the deranged blood and Kapham, which first appears about the root of the palate and goes on extending till it looks like an inflated skin-bladder is called Gala-s'undiká (tonsilitis) by physicians. Thirst, cough, difficult breathing are the indications of the disease. **Tundikeri** :—A thick swelling resembling the fruit of the *Tundikeri* plant in shape and appearing about the root of the palate attended with a burning, piercing or pricking pain and suppuration is called Tundikeri (abscess of the tonsil). **Adhrusha** :—A red, numbed swelling appearing about the same region, as the effect of the vitiated blood of the locality, attended with severe fever and pain, is known by the name of Adhrusha. **Mánsa-kachchapa** :—A brownish and slightly painful swelling somewhat shaped like the back of a tortoise (and appearing about the region of the soft palate) is called Mánsa-kachchhapa. The disease is slow in its growth or development and is due to the deranged Kapham. **Arvuda :**—A swelling shaped like the petal of the lotus lily and appearing in the region of the soft palate as an outcome of the aggravated condition of the local blood is called Arvudam. The swelling is identical with the Raktárvuda described before **Mánsa-Sangháta** :—A vegetation of morbid flesh at the edge or extremity of the soft palate through the action of the deranged Kapham is called Mánsa-Sangháta. It is painless. **Tálu-pupputa :**—A painless permanent swelling to the shape of the *Kola* fruit (plum) caused by the deranged fat and Kapham at the region of the soft palate is called Tálu-pupputa. **Tálu-sosha :**—The disease of the soft palate in which the patient feels a sort of parched sensation with dyspnœa and a severe piercing pain in the affected part is called Tálu-sosha, which has its origin in the aggravated condition of the bodily Váyu acting in concert with the deranged Pittam. **Tálu-páka** —The disease in which the deranged Pittam sets up a very severe suppurative process in the soft palate is called Tálu-páka. 39-47.

**The diseases of the throat and larynx :**—The diseases peculiar to the throat and the larynx are seventeen in number and are known as the five types of Rohini, Kantha-Sáluka, Adhijihva, Valaya, Valása, Eka-vrinda, Vrinda, Sataghni, Giláyu, Gala-vidradhi, Galaugha, Svaraghna, Mánsatána, and Vidári. 48.

**General features of Rohinis :**—The aggravated Váyu, Pittam, Kapham, either severally or in combination, or blood may affect the mucous of the throat and give rise to vegetations of fleshy papillæ, which gradually obstruct the channel of the throat and bring on death. The disease is called Rohini (Diphtheria). 49

**The Vátaja Rohini :**—A vegetation of extremely painful fleshy Ankuras (nodules), crops up all over the tongue which tend to obstruct the passage of the throat and are usually accompanied by other distressing symptoms characteristic of the deranged Váyu. **Pittaja-Rohini** :—The Ankuras (nodules) in the present type are marked by speedy growth and suppuration, and are accompanied by a burning sensation and high fever. **Kaphaja Rohini** :—The Ankuras (nodules) become heavy, hard and characterised by slow suppuration gradually obstructing the passage of the throat. 50-52.

**The Sánnipátika Type :**—Suppuration takes place in the deeper strata of the membrane accompanied by all the dangerous symptoms peculiar to the three aforesaid types of the disease. It is rarely amenable to treatment **Raktaja Type** :—Symptoms characteristic of the Pittaja type of the disease are present and the fleshy outgrowth formed in the throat, is found to be covered with small vesicles. This type is incurable.* 53—54

**Kantha-Sálukam :**—The disease in which a hard rough nodular growth (Granthi) in the shape of a plum-stone crops up in the throat, which seems as if it has been stuffed with the bristle of a *S'uka* insect or been pricked by thorns is called Kantha-Sálukam. The disease is due to the action of the deranged Kapham. It is amenable to surgical treatment only. **Adhijihva :**— A small swelling like the tip of the tongue caused by the

---

\* The reading Sádhya (curable) which is to be met with in the several printed editions of Mádhab's Nidánam in lieu of the reading Asádhya (incurable) is not to our mind correct.

deranged blood and Kapham over the root of the tongue is called Adhijihva, which should be given up as soon as suppuration sets in. **Valaya** :—A circular or ring-shaped raised swelling obstructing or closing up the upper end of the œsophagus (structure of œsophagus) is called Valaya. It cannot be cured and hence should be given up. It is due to the deranged action of the Kapham in the locality. **Valása** :—The disease in which the unusually aggravated Váyu and Kapham give rise to a swelling in the throat, which is extremely painful and causes a difficulty of respiration, ultimately producing symptoms of complete asphyxia is called Valása by learned physicians and is very difficult to cure. 55—58.

**Eka-vrinda and Vrinda\***:—The disease in which a circular, raised, heavy and slightly soft swelling appears in the throat attended with itching, a slightly burning sensation and a slight suppuration is called **Eka-vrinda**. The disease is due to the effect of vitiated blood and Kapham. The disease in which a round elevated swelling attended with high fever and a slightly burning sensation is formed in the throat through the aggravated condition of the blood and Pittam is called **Vrinda**. A piercing pain in the swelling points to its Vátaja origin. 59—60.

**Śataghni :**—The disease in which, through the concerted action of the deranged Váyu, Pittam and Kapham, a hard throat obstructing Varti (jagged membrane) edged like a Śataghni† and densely beset with fleshy excrescences is formed along the inner lining of

---

\* The diseases of the throat are 17 in number. Taking Vrinda as a separate disease they amount to 18 ; but Vrinda, affecting similar place and being similar in appearance with but a slight distinction of symptoms, is only a particular state of Eka-vrinda, and not a separate disease.

† Sataghni is a kind of weapon used in ancient warfare.

that pipe is denominated as Śataghni. Various kinds of pains, (characteristics of each of the deranged Váyu, Pittam and Kapham) are present in this type which should be necessarily considered as irremediable. 61.

**Giláyu :**—The disease in which the aggravated Kapham and blood give rise to a hard and slightly painful (D. R extremely painful) glandular swelling in the throat to the size of the stone of the *Ámalaka* fruit is called Giláyu. A sensation as if a morsel or bolus of food is stuck in the throat is experienced which by its very nature is a surgical case. 62.

**Gala-vidradhi:**—The disease in which an extensive swelling occurs along the whole inner lining of the throat, owing to the concerted action of the deranged Váyu, Pittam and Kapham is called Gala-vidradhi which exhibits all the features present in a Vidradhi of the Sánipátika type. **Galaugha**—The disease in which a large swelling occurs in the throat so as to completely obstruct the passage of any solid or liquid food and also that of Udána-váyu (choking the pharynx, larynx and the mouth of the esophagus), attended with a high fever is called Galaugha, the origin of which should be ascribed to the action of the deranged blood and Kapham. **Svaraghna:**—The disease in which the patient faints owing to the choking of the larynx by the deranged Kapham which is marked by stertorous breathing, hoarseness, dryness and paralysed condition of the throat is called Svaraghna which has its origin in the deranged Váyu. 63—65

**Mánsatána :**—The disease in which a pendent, spreading and extremely painful swelling appears in the throat which gradually obstructs the pipe is called Mánsatána. It invariably proves fatal and is caused by the deranged Váyu, Pittam and Kapham . 66

**Vidári :**—The disease in which a copper-coloured swelling occurs in the throat, marked by a pricking and burning sensation, and the flesh of the throat gets putrefied and sloughs off (and emits a fetid smell) is called Vidári. The disease is of a Pittaja origin and is found to attack that side of the throat on which the patient is in the habit of lying. 67.

**The disease in the entire cavity :**—Cases which are found to invade the entire cavity of the mouth (without being restricted to any particular part thereof) may be either due to Vátaja, Pittaja, Kaphaja or Raktaja type and are known by the general name—**Savra-Sara.** 68.

In the **Vátaja type** the entire cavity of the mouth is studded with vesicles attended with a pricking sensation in their inside. In the **Pittaja type** a large number of small yellow or red-coloured vesicles attended with a burning sensation crops up on the entire (mucous membrane lining the cavity of the mouth. In the **Kaphaja** variety a similar crop of slightly painful, itching vesicles of the same colour as the skin (is found on the entire inner surface of the mouth.) The blood-origined **Raktaja** type is nothing but a modification of the Pittaja one (giving rise to similar symptoms); it is also by others called **Mukha-páka.** 69-72.

Thus ends the sixteenth Chapter of the Nidána Sthánam in the Sus'ruta Samhitá which treats of the Nidánam of the diseases of the mouth.

## Here ends the Nidána Sthánam.

# THE SUŚRUTA SAMHITA

## ŚÁRIRA STHÁNAM.

(SECTION ON ANATOMY).

——:*o*:——

## CHAPTER I.

Now we shall discourse on the Śáriram which treats of the science of Being in general **(Sarva-Bhuta Chintá Śáriram).** 1.

The latent (lit : unmanifest) supreme nature (**Prakriti**) is the progenitor of all created things She is self-begotten and connotes the three fundamental or primary virtues of Sattva, Rajas and Tamas. She is imaged or embodied in the eightfold categories of **Avyakta** (unmanifest), Mahán (intellection), Ahamkára (Egoism) and the five Tanmátras or elementals (proper sensibles) and is the sole and primary factor in working out the evolution of the universe. The one absolute and original nature is the fundamental stone house of materials out of which the bodies of all self-conscious (Karma-Purusha) working agents (agents who come into being through the dynamical energy of their acts or Karmas) have been evolved in the same manner as all water, whether confined in a tank or a reservoir, or coursing free through the channels of streams and of mighty rivers, have been welled up from the one and shoreless primordial ocean. 2.

Out of that latent unmanifest (Avyakta) or original nature (impregnated by the atoms or elemental units of consciousness or Purushas) Intellection or Mahán has been evolved, and out of Mahán egoism. This Mahán or intellection should be likewise considered as partaking of the three fundamental attributes (Sattva, Rajas, and Tamas) of the latent (Avyakta) or original nature.* Ahamkára or egoism in its turn may be grouped under three subheads as the Vaikárika Taijasa (operative) or Rájasika, and Bhutádi (illusive or Tàmasika). 3.

The eleven organs of cognition, communication or sense perception have emanated from the co-operation of the aforesaid Vaikárika Ahamkára with the Taijasa or Rajasa. They are the ears, skin, eyes, tongue, nose, speech, hands, genitals, anus, feet and the mind (Manah). Of these foregoing organs the first five are intellectual or sense organs (Vuddhi-Indriya); the next five being operative (Karma-Indriya). The mind (Manah) partakes of the character of both the intellectual and operative organs alike. 4-5.

The five Tanmátras or elementals (or the five proper sensibles of hearing, touch, sight, taste, and smell) characterised by the Nescience, etc. have been evolved out of the Bhutádi etc. (or Támasa Ahamkára) concerted with the Taijasa Ahamkára through the instrumentality of the Vaikárikam. The gross or perceptible modifications of these five Tanmátras are sound, touch, taste, sight and smell. From the combination of the aforesaid five Tanmátras (Bhutádi) taken one at a time, have successively emanated the five gross matters of space such as

---

* Sattva, Rajas and Tamas:—Adhesion, cohesion and disintegration in the Physical plane ; affection, love and hate in the moral ; emancipation, spiritual affinity and sin in the Psychic.

Simply phenomenal or the simple outcome of the phenomenal evolution without being by other specific attributes of matter and hence Sàttvika or illuminating or quasi-spiritual,

ether, air, heat, (fire,) fluid (water), and earth (solid). These twenty four categories combinedly form what is technically known as the twenty four elements (**Tattvas**). Thus we have discoursed on the twenty four fundamental principles (Chaturvins'ati-tattvam). 6.

Hearing, touch, sight, taste and smell respectively form the subjects of the five intellectual (Vuddhi) organs of man, whereas the faculty of speech, handling, pleasure, ejections or evacutation, locomotion successively belong to the (remaining) five operative (Karma-Indriya) ones. The original nature (Avyakta), Mahán* (intellection), Egoism (Ahamkára), the five sensibles (Tanmátras), and the five gross material principles in their nascent stage in evolution form what is included within the eight categories of Nature (Prakriti), the remaining sixteen categories being her modifications (Vikára). The objects of intellection (Mahán) and Egoism (Ahamkárá) as well as of the sense organs of knowledge and actions are the material principles (Ádibhautika) though they are spiritual in themselves and in their nature.

The tutelary god of intellection (Buddhi) is Brahmá. The god Is'vara is the presiding deity of the sense of egoism (Ahamkára) ; the moon god is that of the mind (Manah); the quarters of the heaven, of the ears ; the wind god is that of the skin ; the sun is that of the eyes; the water is that of the taste ; the earth is that of the smell ; the fire is that of the speech ; Indra is that of the hands ; Vishnu is that of the legs ; Mitra is that of the anus and Prajápati is that of the organs of generations  7.

* Mahán, Ahamkára and the five Tanmátras, though but modifications of the original Nature in themselves, have been included within the category of Nature (Prakriti) in asmuch as they form the immediately prior or antecedent conditions of the evolution of the phenomenal universe.

All the aforesaid (twenty-four) categories or elementals (Chaturvinsati-Tanmátras) are devoid of consciousness. Similarly the modifications of the primal cause of Prakriti such as the Mahat etc. are all bereft of consciousness in as much as the cause itself, the Avyakta or the original nature is devoid of it The Purusha or the self-conscious subjectivity, enters into the primal cause (Mula-Prakriti or original Nature) and its necessary effect (the evolved out phenomena) and makes them endued with his own essence or self-consciousness. The preceptors and holy sages explain the proposition by an analogy that as the milk in the breast of a mother, though unconscious in itself, originates and flows out for the growth and sustenance of her child ; (as the semen in the organism of an adult male though devoid of consciousness, flows out during an act of sexual intercourse) ; so these twenty-four primary material principles (elementals), though unconscious in themselves, tend to contribute towards the making of the self-conscious self or the universal individual (the aggregate of limited or conditional selves) for the purpose of working out his final liberation or emancipation *i.e.*, attainment of the stage of pure consciousness or perfect knowledge. 8.

Now we shall describe the tracts which the Purusha (subjective or self-conscious reality) and Prakriti or nature (passive non-conscious eternity) pass in common as well as those wherein they differ from each other. 9.

**Traits of commonalty :**—Both the Purusha and Prakriti are eternal realities, both of them are unmanifest, disembodied, without a beginning or origin, eternal, without a second, all—pervading and omnipresent.

**Traits of diversity :**—Of the Purusha and the Prakriti, only the latter is non-conscious and possesses the three fundamental qualities of Sattva, Rajas and Tamas. Prakriti performs the function of the seed or in otherwords she lies inherent as the seed or the primary cause in the latter phenomenal evolution of the Mahat etc. and contributes the maternal element in the conception, development and birth of the primordial cosmic matter (phenomenal universe), fecundated by the Purusha (self-conscious subjectivity) in its different stages of evolution. These stages are called Mahat, Ahamkára etc. ; and Prakriti is not indifferent, as the Purusha is to the pleasures and misery of life. But the Purusha (units or atoms of consciousness), devoid of the threefold virtues of Sattva etc. are non-concerning hence non-producing and bereft of the seed-attributes of lying inherent in all as the primary cause of evolution. They are mere witnesses to the joys and miseries of life, and do not participate in their enjoyment though imprisoned in the human organism. 10

Since an effect is uniform in virtue to its producing cause, the evolutionised effects or products of the Prakriti such as the Mahat, Ahamkára etc. must needs partake of the three fundamental qualities (Sattva, Rajas and Tamas) which are predicated of the Prakriti. In other words, these Mahat, Ahamkára, etc, are but the modifications of the three fundamental qualities of Sattva, Rajas and Tamas. Moreover, certain authorities hold that the Purushas are units of self-consciousness, possessed of the three aforesaid qualities owing to their antecedent conditions or causes (the gross material universe) being permeated with and characterised by them. 11.

**Metrical Text** (Vaidyake) :—It is asserted in the Áyurveda that it is only the gross-sighted ones and men capable of observing only the superficial appearances, who confound eternal order or sequence of things and events (Svabhába), God (Isvara).* Time (Kála), sudden and unlooked for appearances of the phenomena (Yadrichchhá), Necessity (Niyati) and transformation (Parináma) with the original Nature (Prakriti). The five different forms of matter (such as Ether etc) are nothing but the modifications or transformed states of the original nature and are characterised by the three universal qualities of Sattva, Rajas and Tamas, and all created things, whether mobile or immobile, should be considered as alike exponented by the same. In the Science of medicine the cause of a disease is the one sole aim to be achieved by means of administering proper medicinal remedies (matter), and hence the properties of matter are the only fit subject to be dealt with in a book on pharmacy. And further, because the immediately prior cause of the human organism is a proper and congenial admixture of the sperm and ovum (matter), the sense organs are the resultants of phenomenal—evolution of matter, and the objects of sense perception are equally material or phenomenal in their nature. 12 –14.

**Memorable verse :** –A man by a particular organ of his body perceives the same matter which forms the proper object of that sense organ in as much as the perceiving sense organ and the perceived sensible are produced by the same material cause. The matter,

---

* The second factor according to Sánkhya, in the order of cosmic evolution, which as the seed of the universe, was hid in the burning disc of the central, primordial Sun, out of which the different solar systems have come into being.

which specifically forms the object of a particular sense organ, cannot be perceived by the other. We see a flower with the eyes and not with the nose. 15.

The Science of medicine does not lay down that the self-conscious **Selves** (Kshetrajna) are all pervading, but on the contrary it asserts that they are real and eternal and are born in the planes of divine, human or animal existence according to their good or evil deeds in life. The existence of these self-conscious entities can be ascertained duly by inference inasmuch as they are extremely subtle in their essence. The self-conscious self is possessed of infinite consciousness, is real and eternally subject to the process of being evolved out into a finite, organic individual through the dynamics of the combined sperm and ovum. The view is further corroborated by a dictum of the Sŕuti which holds that **Purusha** (individual) is nothing but a combination of a self-conscious self and the five kinds of matter (Mahábhutas) formed into an organic body. This Purusha or individual, which is called Individual of action (**Karma-Purusha**), falls within the scope of the science and art of medicine.\* 16—17.

\* Here lies the difference between Sànkhya and Áyurveda. While the former discourses on in material character of the soul, the latter commences to discuss on the questions how the material environment in which the soul is said to inhabit is evolved, and how the inclusion of the spiritual within the material organism is effected.

Hence Sus'ruta's Physiology, like that of Charaka, is in the strictest sense of the word molecular and his science of life is an attempt at explanation of consciousness from the materialistic standpoint, which agrees with the views of modern western science. Intellect according to Sus'ruta is material and belongs to the same category which the Sánkhya system of philosophy in its explanation of evolution enumerates originally as seven. The soul, according to Sus'ruta, is an independent existence and is often associated with what is called life. Where there is life, there is a soul, and it is not everywhere the same. The soul in Sus'ruta is individual

**The attributes of an organic individual :**—Longing for pleasure, shunning of pain, enemity, energetic undertaking of work, respiration (Prána), emission of flatus (Apána), closing and opening of the eyelids, intellect (Vuddhi), sentiment (Manah), deliberation, discretion, memory, knowledge of art, perseverance, sensation and perception, are the attributes of an organic individual. 18.

**Distinctive features of the different classes of mental temperaments :**—An absence of all killing or hostile propensities, a judicious regimen of diet, forbearance, truthfulness, piety, a belief in God, spiritual knowledge, intellect, a good retentive memory, comprehension, and the doing of good deeds irrespective of consequences, are the qualities which grace the mind of a person of a **Sáttvika temperament.** Feeling of much pain and misery, a roving spirit, non-comprehension, vanity, untruthfulness, nonclemency, pride, an over winning confidence in one's own excellence, lust, anger and hilarity are the attributes which mark a mind of the **Rájashika cast.** Despondency, stupidity, disbelief in the existence of God, impiety, stupification, and perversity of intellect, lethargy in action and, sleepiness are the qualities which mark a mind of a **Támashika stamp.** 19,

**The distinctive traits of the five material of Elements of the world :**—The properties of **Ákáśa** (ether) are sound, the sense of hearing, porosity and differentia evolution of the veins, ligaments etc. into their characterised species (Viviktatá.)

---

राशिज्ञ पुरुष: and takes cognisance of sorrow, disease and death by its union with the body .( वर् महाभूते शरीरि समवाय: पुरुष इत्युच्यते ). Hence the living frame together with the soul that is said to inhabit it forms the subject-matter of Ayurvedic medical treatment. Ed.

The properties **Váyu** (etherin) are touch, the skin, all functional activities of the organism, throbbing of the whole body (Spandana) and lightness. The properties of **Teja** (fire or heat) are form, the eyes, colours, heat, illumination, digestion, anger, generation of instantaneous energy and valour. The properties of **Ápa** (water or liquid) are taste, the tongue, fluidity, heaviness, coldness, olioginousness and semen. The properties or modifications of **Prithivi** (the earth matter or solid) are smell, the nose, embodiment and heaviness. 20.

Of these the ether or Akása abounds in attributes of the Sáttvika stamp, the Váyu or etherin in Rájashika, the Teja in Sáttvika and Rájashika, the water in Sáttvika and Támashika and the earth in Támasha attributes. 21.

**There are Memorable Verses :** —These qualities are found to characterise and enter into the successive elements in the order of their enumeration. The specific attributes of these elements are manifest in the substances which are respectively originated from them. The term Prakriti or original nature connotes the eight categories (of Avyakta, Mahán, Ahamkára, and the five Tanmátras) and the rest of the twenty four fundamental principles are its modifications. The Purusha forms the twentyfifth principle. These twentyfive fundamental principles of cosmogony have been dealt with in the present treatise (Salya-Tantram) as well as in the other treatise (Sálaky-Tantram and Sánkhya Philosophy). 22—23.

Thus ends the first Chapter of the S'árira Sthánan in the Sus'ruta Samhitā which deals with the science of Being in general.

# CHAPTER II.

Now we shall discourse on the Sáriram which treats of the purification of semen and cataminal fluid etc. **(Śukra-Śonita-Śuddhirnáma Śáriram).** 1.

A man is incapable of begetting children, whose seminal fluid, affected by the aggravated Váyu, Pittam or Kapham, emits a cadaverous smell, or has acquired a clotted or shreddy character or which looks like putrid pus, or has become thin, or smells like urine or stool. 2.

**Deranged Semen :**—Semen vitiated by the deranged Váyu acquires a (reddish-black) colour and gives rise to a pain (piercing and cutting etc.) which characterises the Váyu (at the time of being emitted). Similarly semen deranged by the Pittam gets a (yellowish or bluish etc.) colour and produces the specific pain (burning and sucking etc.) of the deranged Pittam (at the time of emission). Semen vitiated by the action of the deranged Kapham has a (white) colour and produces the pain (itching sensation etc.) peculiar to the deranged Kapham (at the time of its outflow). The semen vitiated by blood is tinged with a bloody hue, produces all kinds of pain peculiar to the deranged Sonita (Pittam). The semen smells like a putrid corpse and is emitted in large quantities. The shreddy or clotted character of the fluid (**Granthila**) should be ascribed to the action of the deranged Váyu and Kapham. If vitiated by the action of the deranged Pittam and Kapham it looks like putrid pus (Putipuya). Thin semen is caused by the deranged Váyu and

Pittam as described before. A concerted action of the deranged Váyu, Pittam, and Kapham causes the semen to smell like urine or fecal matter. Of these, the cadaverously smelling, shreddy and clotted, putrid pus-like and thinned semen can be remedied and corrected only with the greatest difficulty ; while the one, having the smell of stool or urine, should be regarded as beyond cure. The remaining kinds are curable. 3.

**Deranged Ártavam :**—The catamenial fluid (Ártavam) of a woman vitiated by the deranged Váyu, Pittam, Kapham, or blood, either severally or in combination of two or more Doshas should be likewise considered as unfit for the purpose of fecundation. Vitiated catamenial fluid exhibits the characteristic colour and pain of the deranged Doshas or blood (underlying at its roots). Of the several kinds (of vitiated catamenial fluids) those which smell like a putrid corpse or fetid pus, or which is clotted, or is thin, or emits the smell of urine or fecal matter, should be deemed as being beyond remedy, the rest being amenable. 4.

**Memorable Verses :**—The first three types of seminal derangements or defects should be corrected by an intelligent physican with an application of medicated oil etc. (Sneha-karma), diaphoric measures etc* or uretheral injections (Uttara-vasti). A medi-cated Ghrita prepared with a (decoction and Kalka of) *Dhátaki* flowers, *Khadira, Dádima* and *Arjuna* barks should be given to drink to a man whose semen emits a cadaverous smell (Kunapa). As an alter-native, a medicated Ghrita prepared with (a decoction and levigated paste or Kalka of) the drugs forming the *S'álasárádi* group should be given to him. In a case of

---

* The word "Ádi" in the text includes emetics, purgatives, Anuvá-sánam and Ásthápanam measures according to their specific Doshas.

clotted and shreddy semen (Granthi), the patient should be made to drink a medicated Ghrita prepared with a (decoction and Kalka of) *S'athi,* or with an alcaline solution prepared from the ashes of the burnt *Palás'ha* wood. In the case of a pus-like appearance of the fluid the patient should be treated with the medicated Ghrita prepared with (a decoction and Kalka of) the drugs included within the groups of *Parushakádi* and *Vatádi* (Nyágrodhádi) Ganas. In a case of thin semen, measures laid down under the same head before, as well as those to be hereafter described should be resorted to. Similarly a medicated Ghrita, prepared with (a decoction and Kalka of) *Chitrakk* roots, *Ushira* roots and Hingu, should be drunk in a case of the semen smelling like urine or fecal matter. In all cases of seminal disorders as well as in menstrual anomalies, Uttara-Vssti (uretheral or vaginal injection) should be made after having recourse to the application of medicated oil etc. (Sneha-karma, purgatives, emetics, Ásthápana and Anuvásana measures. 5—12

**Treatment of deranged Ártava:—**In all the four cases when the catamenial blood would be found to be vitiated (by the deranged Váyu, Pittam, Kaphah or Śonita), the preliminary remedial measures of the application of oil etc. purgatives etc. (Pancha-karma) should be first employed and then the following measures should be undertaken *viz.* application of **Kalka**, (levigated paste of drugs), **Pichu** (medicated plugs—pecharies etc), **Pathya** (diet) and **Áchamana** (washes with decoctions) as described under the treatment of Gynœcological cases etc. Appearance of clots of blood (Granthi) in place of the healthy menstrual fluid would indicate, decoction or a pulverised compound of Páthá, Trushuna and Vrikshaka (Kutaja).

A decoction of *Bhadras'riyam*\* and *Chandanam* is indicated in the case when the menstrual fluid would smell like fetid pus, or contain marrow. The remedies described under the head of seminal disorders, should be likewise prescribed in cases of menstrual anomalies caused by the action of the deranged Váyu, Pittam and Kaphah according to the requirements of each individual case under treatment. Sáli-rice, barley, wine and meat with cholagogue properties should be deemed as a wholesome diet in these cases. 13—16.

**Traits of pure and healthy semen and menstrual blood :**—Semen which is transparent like crystal, fluid, glossy, sweet and emits the smell of honey ; or like oil or honey in appearance according to others, should be considered as healthy. The catamenial blood (Ártava) which is red like the blood of a hare, or the washings of shellac and leaves no stains on cloths (which may be washed off by simply soaking them in water) should be considered as healthy. 17—18.

**Asrigdara** (Menorrhagia) :—An abnormal or excessive discharge of the menstrual blood (Ártava), or its long persistence even after the wonted time, or its appearance at a premature or unnatural period (as well as contrarity in its colour or properties) is called **Asrigdara**. All types of the disease (Asrigdara) are attended with an aching in the limbs and a painful flow (of the catamenial fluid). In case of excessive hœmorrhage (from the uterus), symptoms such as weakness, vertigo, loss of consciousness, darkness of vision, or difficult breathing, thirst, burning (sensation of the body), delirium, palour, somnolence and other Vátaja

---

\* Bhadras'riyam is S'richandanam according to Dallana or white Sandal wood according Gayádása.

troubles (convulsion, hysteria etc.) may set in. A physician should treat a case of Asrigdara with measures and remedies as laid down under the head of **Rakta-pittam** (hœmorrhage) in a case when the patient is young (of sixteen years), careful in her diet, and the disease unattended with severe complications. 19—21.

**Amenorrhœ :**—In a case of suppression of menstruation (**Amenorrhœ**) caused by the obstruction of the deranged Doshas (Váyu and Kapham) in the passage, the patient should be advised to take fish, *Kulattha* pulse, *Màsha* pulse, *Kànjikam* (fermented sour gruel etc.), *Tila*, wine (Surá), cow's urine, whey, half diluted *Takra*, curd and *S'uktam* for her diet. The symptoms and treatment of thin and scanty menstruation have been described before. Still in such a case measures laid down for the treatment of **Nashta-Rakta** (amenorrhœ) may be adopted. Under a course of treatment described as before, the semen or the catamenial blood of a person would be resorted to their healthy and normal condition. 22—23.

A woman with (healthy) catamenial flow should forego the bed of her husband during the first three days of her uncleanness, as well as day sleep and collyrium. She shall not shed tears nor bathe, nor smear her person (with sandal paste etc.), nor anoint her body, nor pare her nail, nor run, nor indulge in loud and excessive laughter and talk, nor should she hear loud noise, nor comb her hair, nor expose herself to droughts, nor do any fatiguing work at all ; because if a woman sleeps in the day time (during the first three days of her period) her child of subsequent conception becomes sleepy or somnolent. The woman who applies collyrium along her eyelids (during those days), gives birth to a blind child ; by shedding tears (during her period) a woman gives birth to a child of defective eyesight ; by bathing or smearing her body (with sandal paste etc ) a miserable one ; by anointing her body a leper (Kushthi) ; by paring her nails a child with bad nails ; by running a restless one ; by indulging in excessive laughter, a child with brown (Syàva) teeth or palate or tongue ; by excessive talking a garrulous child or one of incoherent speech ; by hearing loud sounds, a deaf child ; by combing her hair, a bald one ; whereas by exposure to the wind or by doing fatiguing work (during the first three days of her period) she gives birth to an insane child (conceived immediately after it). Hence these acts (day sleep etc ) are to be avoided. 24.

**Regimen to be observed in her menses :**—A woman in her menses should lie down on a matress made of *Kus'a* blades (during the first three days of her uncleanness), should take her food from her own blended palms or from earthen sauces, or from trays made of leaves. She should live on a course of Habishya diet and forswear during the time, even the sight of her husband. After this period, on the fourth day she should take a ceremonial ablution, put on a new (untorn) garment and ornaments and then visit her husband after having uttered the words of necessary benediction  25.

**Metrical Text :**—A child conceived after the period resembles the man whom she first sees after ablution on the fourth day of her menses ; hence she should see none but her husband* at that time (so that the child may resemble his father). After that the priest shall perform the rites (Garbhàdhàna ceremony),

---

* In the case of the husband being absen· at the time, she should look at the sun.

to help the conception of a male child and after the ceremony a wise husband should observe the following rules of conduct. 26—27.

**Conduct of Husband :**—A husbaud wishing to beget a son by his wife, should not visit her bed for a month (before the day of the next flow) Then on the fourth day of her uncleanness, he should anoint or lubricate his body with Ghrita, should partake of a food in the afternoon or evening composed of boiled *S'áli* rice, milk and clarified butter, and then visit the bed of his wife The wife also, in her tern, should observe a similar vow of sexual abstinence (Brahma-chárini) for a month before that day on which she should anoint or lubricate her body with oil, partake of food largely composed of oil and *Màsha* pulse, and then meet her husband at night. The husband then having uttered the appropriate Veda Mantras and having awakened confidence in the wife, should go unto her on the fourth, sixth, eighth, tenth or on the twelfth night of her menses for the progenation of a male child. 28.

**Metrical Text :**—A visit to the wife on any of these nights leads to the continual increase of the wealth, progeny, and the duration of the husband's life. On the other hand, a visit to one's wife on the fifth, seventh, ninth, or eleventh day of her flow leads to the conception of a female child The thirteenth and the remaining days (till the next course) are condemned as regards intercourse. 29 —30

**Prohibited Period etc. :**—A going unto one's wife on the first day of her monthly course tends to shorten one's life and a child born of the act dies immediately after its delivery. The same result is produced by a visit on the second day, or the child dies lying-in room *i.e.* ten days of its birth ; A visit on the third day leads to the child's being deformed and short-lived. A child which is the fruit of a visit on the fourth day lives long, will be well developed and remain in the full vigour of health. The semen cast in the womb of a woman during the continuance of her monthly flow does not become fruitful because it is carried back and flows out in the same manner as a thing thrown into a stream does not go against but is carried away with the current. Hence a husband should foreswear the company of his wife during the first three days of her uncleanness, when she also should observe a vow of sexual abstinence ; the husband should not visit his wife within the month (after the twelfth day of her menses). 31.

After the impregnation on any of these nights, three or four drops (of the expressed juice) of any of the following drugs such as *Lakshanà*, *Vata-S'unga'*, *S'ahadevá* or *Vis'vadevá*, mixed with milk should be poured into the right nostril of the enceinte for the conception of a male child and care should be taken that she does not spit it away. 32.

**Metrical Text :**—A co-ordination of the four factors of menstrual period (**Ritu**), healthy womb (**Kshetra**), nutrient liquid *i.e.* chyle of digested food (**Ambu**), healthy semen (**Vija**) and the proper observance of the rules is necessary for the conception and development of a healthy child just as the proper season (Ritu), good soil (Kshetra), water (containing nutrient matter) and vigorous seeds (Vija) together with proper care, help the germination of strong and undiseased sprouts. A child which is the fruit of such conception is destined to be beautiful, of vigorous health, generous, long-lived, virtuous, attached to the good of its parents and capable of discharging its parental obligations. 33.

**Causes of different colours of the Child:**—The fiery principle (Teja-dhátu) of the organism, which is the originator of all colours of the skin (complexion), happening to mix largely with the watery principle of the body at the time of conception, serves to make the child a fair complexioned one (Gaura-varna); mixed with a large quantity of the earth principle (Kshiti) of the body, it makes the chiid a dark complexioned one (Krishna-varna). In combination with a large quantity of earth and ethereal principles of the organism, it imparts a dusky (Krishna-s'yáma) complexion (to the full developed fœtus). A similar combination of watery and ethereal principles serves to make the child dusky yellow (Gaura-s'yáma). Others on the contrary aver that the complexion of the child is determined by the colours of the food taken by its mother during the period of gestation. 34.

A child is born blind in the failure of the fiery principle (Teja-dhátu) of the organism in reaching the region of its still undeveloped eyes (part—where the eyes would be); so also a penetration by the same (Teja-dhátu) into its blood accounts for the blood-shot eyes of the child. Entered into the Pittam it makes the child a yellow-pupiled one (Pingaláksha). Entered into its bodily Kapham it makes it a white-eyed body and mixed with its bodily Vàyu, a child of defective eyesight. 35.

**Memorable verses:**—As a lump of condensed clarified butter melts and expands if placed by the side of a fire, so the ovum (Ártava) of a woman is dislodged and glides away in contact with an adult male*.

---

* Sus'rutá's theory is that ovulation occurs about the same time as menstruation and rather initiates the latter, and the shed ova are washed out with the menstrual flow, hence there is a possibility of conception on

A seed divided into two by the deranged Váyu within the (cavity of the) uterus (Kukshi) gives rise to the birth of **twins**, conditioned by the good or evil deeds of their prior existence * A child born of scanty paternal sperm becomes **an Ásekya** and feels no sexual desire (erection) without previously (sucking the genitals and) drinking the semen of another man. A child begotten in a sordid vagina is called a **Sougandhika**, whose organ does not respond to the sexual desire without smelling the genitals of others. The man who first becomes a passive member of an act of sodomy and then again commits sodomy with the woman (he visits) is called a **Kumbhika** (or Guda-yoni and is included within the category of a Kliva). 36—40.

The man who cannot copulate with a woman without previously seeing the sexual intercourse of another couple is called **Irshaka**. A child born of an act of fecundation foolishly or ignorantly effected during the menses of its mother by its progenitor by holding her on his bosom during the act is called a **Shanda** and invariably exhibits effeminate traits in his character. A daughter born of a woman riding on her husband during the act of sexual intercourse will develop masculine traits in her character. 41—43.

connexion during the period of flow. But when the menstruation stops of itself by the end of the third day, it also indicates that ovulation has ceased and no ovum is left to be fertilized, hence the question arises how can there be conception then on connexion on the fourth day and thereafter? The explanation (as in the following verse) is that the ovulating organ though quiescent at the time is again stimulated to activity by intercourse with a male and new ova are shed which are ready to be fertilized by the semen.—Ed.

* Gayi interprets the term "Dharmetara" to mean evil deeds (other than good) and quotes verses from S'rutis, S'mritis and Tantras on expiations of sin in support of his view.

Semen is developed in the four types of Kliva known as Ásekya, Sougandhika, Kumbhika and Irshaka, whereas a Shanda is devoid of that fluid (Sukra). The semen carrying ducts of an Ásekya etc. are expanded by the drinking of the semen as above described which helps the erection of his reproductive organ. 44-45

The conduct and character of a child and its inclination to particular dietary are determined by those of its parents during the act of fecundation. A boneless (*i. e.* with cartilaginous bones) monstrosity is the outcome of the sexual act in which both the parties are female and their Sukra (sexual secretion) unite some how or other in the womb of one of them. Fecundation may take place in the womb of a woman, dreaming of sexual intercourse in the night of her menstrual ablution The local Váyu carries the dislodged ovum into the uterus and exhibits symptoms of pregnancy, which develop month after month till the full period of gestation. The offspring of such a conception is a **Kalala** (a thin boneless jelly-like mass) on account of the absence of the paternal elements\* in its development. Such monstrosities as serpents, scorpions, or gourd shaped fœtus delivered from the womb of a woman should be ascribed as the effects of deadly sins. 46-49.

The child of a mother whose wishes are not honoured and gratified during pregnancy stands in danger of being born palmless, hunchbacked, lame, dumb or nasal voiced through the deranged condition of the Váyu of its mother's body. The malformation of a child in the womb should be ascribed to the atheism of its parents, or to the effects of their misdeeds in a prior existence, or

---

\* Hair, beard, nails, teeth, arteries, veins, ligaments and semen are called paternal elements inasmuch as these are said to be inherited by the child from its father

to the aggravated condition of the Váyu, Pittam and Kapham. 50—51.

A fœtus in uterus does not excrete fæces or urine, owing to the scantiness of the fecal matter, etc , in its intestines and also to the obstruction and consequently lessened admission of the Vàyu into its lower bowels. A child in the womb does not cry inasmuch as its mouth remains covered with the sheath of the *placenta i.e. fœtal membranes* (Yaráu) and its throat is stuffed with Kapham. The processes of respiration, sleeping and movement of the fœtus in the womb are effected through those of its mother. 52—53.

The adjustment of the different limbs and organs of the body of a child in the womb at their proper places, the non-development of hair on its palms and soles and the subsequent cutting and falling off of its teeth are spontaneously effected according to the laws of nature after the model of its own species. An honest, pious, erudite man, who has acquired a vast knowledge of the Sástras in his prior existence, becomes largely possessed of mental traits of the Sáttvika stamp in this life too and also remembers his prior births (**Játismara**). Acts similar to those, which a man performs in a prior existence, overtake him also in the next. Similarly the traits and the temperament which he had developed in a previous existence are likewise sure to be patent in the next. 54—55.

Thus ends the second Chapter of the S'árira Sthánam in the Sus'ruta Samhitá which treats of the purification of sperm and ovum.

# CHAPTER III.

Now we shall discourse on the Sáriram which treats of pregnancy, etc. (**Garbhá Vakránti Śáriram**). 1.

The male reproductive element (Śukra) is endowed with Soma-guna (i.e , thermolytic properties) the female element Ártava) presents the opposite property and is therefore Agni-guna (i e , thermogenetic properties). The principles of earth, water, fire, air and ether are also present in men in their subtle forms and contribute to the formation of the material parts by their molecular adjustment in the way of supplying nutrition and in way of the adding to their bulk. 2.

**Combination of Self with the impregnated matter :**—The local Váyu (nerve-force) heightens or aggravates the heat generated by the friction of the sexual organs in an act of copulation. The Váyu and heat thus aggravated tend to dislodge the semen from its sac or receptacle in a man which enters into the uterus of a woman through the vaginal canal and there it mixes with the ovum (Ártavam) dislodged and secreted by similar causes. The combined ovum and semen are subsequently confined in the uterus (Garbháśaya). After that, He who is known by the epithets of **Self-conscious**, impressioner (creator of sensations and perceptions), toucher, smeller, seer, hearer, taster, Self or Ego, creator, wanderer, witness, ordainer, speaker, though eternal, unmanifested and incomprehensible in his real nature, takes hold of the five subtle or essential material principles contributed by the united impregnating matter, assumes a subtle shape throughout, marked by the three fundamental qualities of Sattva, Rajas and Tamas, and led away by the Váyu, lies confined in the uterus to be subsequently evolved out in the shape of a god, animal, or monster, as determined by his acts in the former existence. 3.

**Factors which determine sex :**—The birth of a male-child marks the preponderance of semen over the ovum (in its conception); the birth of a daughter shows the preponderance of the maternal element. A child of no-sex (hermaphrodite) is the product when ovum and sperm are equal (in their quality and quantity). The first **twelve nights** after the cessation of the flow should be deemed as the proper period for conception, as being the time during which the ova are secreted. Certain authorities hold that there are women who never menstruate to all appearances  4—5.

**Memorable verses :**—The face of a woman (lit: a woman of undetected menstruation) becomes full and lively. A moist and clumsy deposit is found on the body, face, teeth and gums. She feels a desire for sexual intercourse and speaks sweet words Her eyes, hair, and belly droop down. A sort of distinct throbbing is felt in her aims, thighs, mammæ, umbilicus, perineum and buttocks. Her sexual desire grows intense and prominent, and its gratification gives her utmost joy and pleasure. These symptoms will at once indicate that a woman has menstruated (internally). 6.

Just as the petals of a full blown lotus flower are gathered up during the night, so the uterus (Yoni) of a woman is folded up (*i. e.*, os of the uterus is closed) after the lapse of the menstrual period (*i e.* fifteen days from the date of the flow). The menstrual flow, accumulated in the course of a month, is led in time by the local Váyu through its specific duct (Dhamani) into the mouth of the uterus (Yoni) whence it flows out odourless and blackish. 7.

**Period of Menstruation :**—The process (menstruation) commences at the twelfth year, flowing once in every month, and continues till the fiftieth* year when it disappears with the sensible decay of the body. 8

A visit† to one's wife on even days during the catamenial period (twelve days in all from the cessation of the flow) leads to the conception of a male child while an intercourse on odd days results in the birth of a daughter. Hence a man, seeking a male-issue, should approach his wife for the purpose in a clean body and with a quiet and calm spirit on an even date. 9.

A sense of fatigue and physical languor, thirst, lassitude and weariness in the thighs, suppression of the flow of semen and menstrual secretion (Sukra and Sonita) out of the uterus (Yoni), and throbbing in the organ (after coition) are symptoms of a recent fecundation. 10.

**Signs of Pregnancy**—(M. T.' :—A black rash (areola) around the nipples of the mammæ, the rising appearance of a row of hair (as far as the umbilicus), contractions of the eye-wings, sudden vomitings, nausea which does not abate even on smelling perfumes, water-

---

\* Some are of opinion that the menstruation continues up to the sixtieth year.

† According to Videha, menstrual secretion flows less on even days, hence a son is born if the sexual intercourse be made on those days ; whereas menstrual secretion becomes more on odd days, so a daughter is born if the intercourse be made on odd days.

According to Bhoja, a son is born from intercourse on even days and a daughter is born from that on odd days. The birth of a male issue is due to the preponderance of semen Virile and that of a female sex is due to the preponderance of menstrual secretion. If both the secretions be equal (in quality and quantity) a hermaphrodite is issued.

brash, and a sense of general lassitude are the indications of pregnancy. 11.

**Prohibited conducts during gestation :**—Immediately on the ascertainment of her pregnancy, a woman should avoid all kinds of physical labour, sexual intercourse, fasting, causes of emaciation of the body, day-sleep, keeping of late hours, indulgence in grief, fright, journey by carriage or in any kind of conveyance, sitting on her haunches, excessive application of Sneha-karmas etc., and venesection at an improper time (*i.e*, after the eighth month of gestation), and voluntary retention of any natural urging of the body. 12.

**Metrical Text :**—The child in the womb feels pain in the same part of its body as the one in which its mother feels any ; whether this (pain) may be from an injury or through the effect of any deranged morbific principle (Dosha) of her organism. 13.

**Development of the Fœtus:**—In the **first month** of gestation a gelatinous substance is only formed (in the womb) ; the molecules of the primary elements (Mahábhuta—air, fire, earth, water, and ether) being acted upon by cold (Kapham), heat (Pittam) and air (Váyu or nerve-force) are condensed in the **second month**. A lump-like appearance (of that confused matter) indicates the male-sex (of the embryo). An elongated-like shape of the matter denotes that the fœtus belong to the opposite sex ; whereas its tumour-like shape (like a Sálmali-bud) predicts the absence of any sex (*i e.* a hermaphrodite). In the **third month**, five lump-like protuberances appear at the places where the five organs —namely the two hands, two legs and the head—would be and the minor limbs and members of the body are formed in the shape of extremely small papillæ. In the **fourth month** all the limbs and organs (of the body of the embryo) become more potent and the fœtus is endowed with consciousness owing to the formation of viscus of the heart. As heart is the seat of consciousness, so as the heart becomes potent, it is endowed with consciousness and hence it expresses its desire for things of taste, smell etc. (through the longings of its mother). The enciente is called double-hearted (**Dauhrida**) at the time, whose wishes and desires—not being honoured and gratified—lead to the birth of a paralysed, hump-backed, crooked-armed, lame, dwarfed, defect-eyed, and a blind child. Hence the desires of the enciente should be gratified, which would ensure the birth of a strong, vigorous and long-lived son. 14.

**Memorable Verses :**—A physician should cause the longings of a pregnant woman (**Dauhrida**) to be gratified inasmuch as such gratifications would alleviate the discomforts of gestation ; her desires being fulfilled ensure the birth of a strong, long-lived, and virtuous son. A non-fulfilment of her desires during pregnancy, proves injurious both to her child and her ownself. A non-gratification of any sensual enjoyment by its mother (Dauhrida) during gestation tends to painfully affect the particular sense-organ of the child.

**Longings and its effects during pregnancy :**—An enciente longing for a royal interview during her gestation (fourth month) gives birth of a child, who is sure to be rich and to hold a high position in life Her longing for fine silks, clothes, ornaments etc. indicates the birth of a beautiful child of æsthetic taste. The birth of a pious and self-controlled child is indicated by its mother's longing for a visit to a hermitage. The desire of a pregnant woman to see a divine image or an idol, predicts the birth of a child in her womb who would grace the council of an august assembly in life. Similarly, a desire to see a savage animal on the part of a pregnant woman signifies the presence of a child of savage and cruel temperament in her womb. A desire for the flesh of a Godhà indicates the presence of a sleepy, drowsy person in her womb who would be tenaciously fond of good things in life. Similarly a longing for beef on the part of the mother (during gestation) indicates the birth of a strong and vigorous child capable of sustaining any amount of fatigue and physical pain A longing for buffalo-meat of the mother indicates the birth of a hairy, valiant and red-eyed child (in her womb); a longing for boar-flesh indicates the birth of a drowsy child though valiant ; a longing for venison indicates that of an energetic, determined and sylvan-habited child ; a longing for Srimàra-meat indicates that of a distracted person ; a longing for the flesh of Tittira bird indicates that of a child of timid disposition ; whereas a desire on the part of an enciente for the flesh of any particular animal indicates that the child in the womb would be of such stature and would develop such traits of character in life as are peculiar to that animal. The desires of a woman during her pregnancy are determined by ordained fate and effects of the acts of the child in its prior existence (that are to be happened during the present life). 15.

**Development of the Fœtus :**—In the **fifth month** the fœtus is endowed with mind (Manah) and wakes up from the sleep of its sub-conscious existence. In the **sixth month** cognition (Buddhi) comes in. In the **seventh month** all the limbs and members of its body are more markedly developed. The Ojo-dhátu (in the heart of the fœtus) does not remain silent in the **eighth month** \* A child born at that time (eighth month) dies for want of Ojo-dhátu soon after its birth, a fact which may be equally ascribed to the agency of the malignant monsters   Hence (in the eighth month of gestation) offerings of meat should be made to the demons and monsters (for the safe continuance of the child). The parturition takes place either in the ninth, tenth, eleventh or twelfth month of conception, otherwise something wrong with the fœtus should be apprehended. 16.

The umbilical chord (Nádi) of the fœtus is found to be attached to the cavity of the vein or artery of its maternal part through which the essence of lymph-chyle (Rasa) produced from the assimilated food of the mother, enters into its organism and fastens its growth and development, (a fact which may be understood from the analogy of percolation or transudation of blood). Immediately after the completion of the process of fecundation, the vessels (Dhamani) of its maternal body which carry the lymph-chyle (Rasa) and run laterally and longitudinally in all directions through it, tend to foster the fœtus with their own transudation all through its continuance in the womb. 17.

**Different opinions on the formation of the fœtal body :**—Śaunaka says that probably the head of the fœtus is first developed since head is the only organ that makes the functions of all other organs possible. **Kritaviryya** says, it is the heart that is first developed since heart is the seat of Manah and Buddhi (mind and intellect). The son of

---

\* Sometimes it passes from the body of the child to that of the mother and *vice versa*.

**Paraśara** says that the developmeut of the umbilical region of fœtus must necessarily precede (that of any other part of its body) inasmuch as it is through umbilical chord that an embryo draws its substance from mother's body. **Márkandeya** says that the hands and feet of a fœtus are first te be developed since they are the only means of movements in the womb. **Śubhuti Gautama** says that the development of the trunk is the earliest in point of time since all other limbs and organs lie soldered to and imbedded in that part of the body. But all these are not really the fact. **Dhanvantari** holds that the development of all the parts of the body of an embryo goes on simultaneously ; and they can not be perceived or detected in their earlier stages of development in the womb owing to their extremely attenuated size like a mango fruit or sprouts of bamboo. As the stone, marrow, pith etc of a ripe and matured mango-fruit or the sprouts of bamboo, cannot be separately perceived in the earlier stage of their growth but are quite distinguishable in the course of their development, likewise in the early stage of pregnancy the limbs and organs of the body (fœtus) are not perceptible for their extremely attenuated stage but become potent (and therefore they are distinctly perceived) in the course of time for their development. 18.

**Factors respectively supplied by the paternal and maternal elements :**—Now we shall describe the parts and principles of the body of a fœtus which are respectively contributed by the paternal element, maternal factor, the serum (Rasaja), the soul (Átmaja), the natural (Sattvaja) and the innate physiological conditions (Sátmyaja). The hairs of the head and body, beard and moustaches, bones, nails, teeth, veins (Śira), nerves, arteries (Dhamani), semen and all the steady and hard substances (in the organism of a child) are contributed by the **paternal element** in the conception Pitraja ; whereas flesh, blood, fat, marrow, heart, umbilicus, liver, spleen, intestines, anus (Guda) and all other soft matters in the body owe their origin to the **maternal element** (Mátrija) ; strength, complexion, growth, rotundity and decay of the body are due to the **serum** (Rasaja). The sensual organs, conciousness, knowledge, wisdom, duration of life (longivity), pleasure and pain etc. are the outcome of the spiritual element in man (Átmaja). We shall describe the **Sattvaja** features of the body in the next chapter. Valour, healthfulness, strength, glow and memory are the products of a child naturally born with physiological conditions of the parents (Sátmyaja). 19.

**Signs of male and female conception :**—An enciente, in whose right mammæ the milk is first detected, who first lifts up her right leg at the time of locomotion, whose right eye looks larger, or who evinces a longing largely for things of masculine names, dreams of having received lotus flowers (red and white), Utpala, Kumuda, Ámrataka, or flowers of such masculine denomination in her sleep, or the glow of whose face becomes brighter during pregnancy, may be expected to give birth to a male child; whereas the birth of a daughter or a female child should be pre-assumed from the contriety of the foregoing indications. An enciente whose sides become raised and the forepart of whose abdomen is found to bulge out will give birth to a sex-less (hermaphrodite) child. An enciente, the middle part of whose abdomen becomes sunk or divided in the middle like a leather-bag, will give birth to a twin. 20.

**Memorable verses :**—Those women who are devout in their worship of the gods and the Bráhmins and cherish a clean soul in a clean body during pregnancy are sure to be blest with good, virtuous and generous children ; whereas a contrary conduct during the period is sure to be attended with contrary fruits. The development of the limbs and the members etc. of a fœtus in the womb is natural and spontaneous, and the qualities and conditions which mark these organs are determined by the acts of the child which are anterior to its genesis and were done in its prior existence. 21-22.

Thus ends the third Chapter of the S'árira Sthánam in the Su'ruta Samhitá which treats of the generation and pregnancy.

# CHAPTER IV.

Now we shall discourse on the S'áriram which treats of the development of a fœtus in the womb, as well as of the factors which contribute to the growth of its different bodily organs and principles (**Garbha-Vyakáranam-S'áriram**). 1.

The Pittam (fiery or thermogenic) and S'leshma (lunar principles of the body, the bodily Váyu, the three primary qualities of Sattva, Rajas, and Tamas (adhesion, cohesion and disintegration), the five sense organs, and the Self (Karma-Purusha) are the preserver of the life (Pránáh) of the Fœtus. 2

**Folds of Skin :**—Seven folds or layers of covering (Tvaka—skin) are formed and deposited on the rapidly transforming product of the combination of (semen) S'ukra and S'onita (fertilized ovum) which have been thus charged with the individual **Soul** or Self in the same manner as layers (of cream) are formed and deposited on the surface of (boiling) milk. Of these the first fold or layer is called **Avabhásini** (reflecting) as it serves to reflect all colours and is capable of being tinged with the hues of all the five material principles of the body. The thickness of this fold measures eighteen-twentieth of a *Vrihi** (rice grain) and it is the seat of skin diseases, such as Sidhma, Padma-

---

\* The complexion of a person is due to this first layer ; and as the colour of an opaque body is due to the rays that are reflected from its surface, this layer is rightly named Avabhás'ini or reflecting layer.

\*\* The text runs "Vriherashtadashabhága," which means eighteen (or so many) parts of a Vrihi ; and Dallan comments that "Vrihi" stands for a measure equal to the twentieth division of a Vrihi or rice grain.

kantaka etc. The second fold (from the surface) is called **Lohita**; it measures a sixteen-twentieth of a *Vrihi* and is the seat of such (cutaneous affections) as Tilakálaka, Nyachcha and Vyanga etc. The third fold or layer is called **Sveta**, which measures in thickness, a twelve-twentieth of a *Vrihi*, and forms the seat of such diseases as Ajagalli, Charmadala, and Masaka etc. The fourth fold or layer is called **Támrá** measuring an eight-twentieth of a *Vrihi* and forms the seat of such diseases as the various kinds of Kilása and Kushtha etc. The fifth fold or layer is called **Vedini**, measuring in thickness a five-twentieth of a *Vrihi* and forms the seat of Kushtha, Visarpa, etc. The sixth fold or layer is called **Rohini**, which is of equal thickness as a *Vrihi* (grain), and is the seat of Granthi, Apachi, Arvuda, Slipada and Gala-ganda etc. The seventh fold or layer is called **Mánsa-dhará** twice a *Vrihi* in thickness and is the seat of Bhagandara, Vidradhi, and Arsa etc. These dimensions should be understood to hold good of the skin of the fleshy parts of the body, and not of the skin on the forehead, or about the tips of the fingers, inasmuch as there is a surgical dictum to the effect that an incision as deep as the thickness of the thumb may be made into the region of the abdomen with the help of a Vrihi-mukha (instrument). 3

The **Kalás** too number seven in all and are situated at the extreme borders (forming encasement and support) of the different fundamental principles (Dhátus) of the organism. 4.

**Memorable Verses :**—As the duramen or core of a piece of wood or stem becomes exposed to view by cutting into it, so the root principles (**Dhátus**) of the body may be seen by removing the successive layers or tissues of its flesh. These Kalás are extensively supplied with Snáyus (fibrous tissues), bathed in mucous, and encased in a membranous covering. 5-6

**Mánsadhará-Kalá:**—Of these Kalás, the first is named **Mánsadhará** (fascia), in the contained flesh (bodily substance of the Kalá) of the Sirá (veins), Snáyu (fibrous tissues), Dhamani (arteries) and other Srotas (channels) are found to spread and branch out. 7.

**Memorable Verse :**—As the roots and stems of a lotus plant respectively situated in the ooze and water (of a tank), do simultaneously grow and expand, so the veins etc. situated in the flesh, grow and ramify. 8.

**Raktadhará-Kalá :**—The second Kalá is called **Raktá-dhará** (Vascular tissue of the blood vessels etc.). The blood is contained in these inside the flesh and specially in the veins (Sirá) and in such viscera of the body as the liver and spleen. 9.

**Memorable Verse :**—As a plant containing latex in its tissues, when injured or pricked, exudes milky juice, so blood oozes out instantaneously on the flesh of the body (supplied with the Raktádhará-kalá) being injured. 10.

**Medadhará-Kalá :**—The third Kalá is called **Medadhará** (adipose tissue). Meda (fat) is present (chiefly) in the abdomen of all animals, as well as in the cartilages (small bones). The fatty substance present in large bones is called **Majjá** (marrow). 11.

**Memorable Verse :**—Marrow is found inside large bones, whereas a substance similar in appearance and found inside other bony structures (cartilages) should be considered as **Meda**, mixed with blood. The fats, present in purely muscular structures, go by the name of **Vasá** (muscle-fat). 12-13.

**Śleshmádhará-Kalá :**—The fourth Kalá is called **Śleshmádhará** (Synovial tissues) and is present about all the bone-joints of animals. 14.

**Memorable Verse :**—As a wheel easily turns upon a well greased axle, so the joints moistened by the mucous (Śleshmá) contained in these sacs admit of easy movements. 15.

**Purishadhará-Kalá :**—The fifth kalá is called **Purishadhará** and being situated in the Kostha (abdomen) serves to separate the fæcal refuse in the (Pakváśaya) lower gut (from other ingested matters). 16.

**Memorable Verse :**—This Kalá extends about the liver, upper and lower intestines and other abdominal viscera and keeps the fœces in the lower intestines (Undukam) separate and hence is called Maladhará-kalá 17.

**Pittadhará-Kalá :**—The sixth Kalá is called **Pittaphará-kalá**; it holds (the chyme derived from) the four kinds of solid and liquid foods (in the Pitta-sthánam or biliary region) propelled from the stomach (Ámáśaya or Grahani-Nádi) and on its way to the (Pakáśaya) intestines (for the proper action of the digestive juices upon it) 18.

**Memorable Verse :**—The four kinds of food, viz. those that are chewed, swallowed, drunk, or licked, and brought into the intestines (Kostha) of a man, are digested in proper time through the heating agency (action) of the Pittam 19.

**Śukradhará-Kalá :**—The seventh Kalá is called **Śukradhará** (semen-bearing), which extends throughout the entire body of all living creatures. 20.

**Memorable Verse :**—The physician should know that like fat (Sarpi) in the milk, or sugar in the expressed juice of sugar-cane, the (seat of) semen is co-extensive with the whole organism of a man (or animal).

The semen passes through the ducts situated about two fingers' breadth on either side (vas deferens) and just below the neck of the bladder and finally flows out through the canal. The semen of a man during an act of sexual intercourse with a female under exhilaration comes down from all parts of his body owing to the extreme excitement (engendered by the act). 21-33.

The orifices of the Ártava—carrying channels (vessels of the uterine mucosa) of a pregnant woman are obstructed by the fœtus during pregnancy and hence there is no show of menses (during gestation). The menstrual blood thus obstructed in its downward course ascends upwards; a part of it accumulates and goes to the formation of placenta (**Apará**), while the rest ascends higher up and reaches the breasts; this is the reason why the breasts of a pregnant woman become full and plump. 24.

The spleen and liver of the fœtus are formed out of blood; the lungs are made of the froth of the blood; and the Unduka or fæcal receptacle, of the refuge matter (Mala) of the blood. 25,

**Metrical Texts :**—The intestines (Antra), the bladder (Vasti), and the anus (Guda) of the fœtus are formed out of the essence of the blood and Kapham, baked by the Pittam into which Váyu enters as well. As fire fed by draughts of air refines the dregs of golden ore and transforms it into pure metal, so blood and Kapham acted upon by the heat of the Pittam are transformed into the shape of the intestines etc. in the abdomen. The tongue is made of the essence of the flesh, blood and Kapham. The Váyu, combined with heat (Pittam) in adequate proportion, rends through the internal channels into the flesh and transforms them into muscles (**Peśi**). The Váyu, by taking off the oily principles of fat (Meda), transforms them into (Sirá and (fibrous tissues) Snáyu, the underbaked (Mridu) ones being converted into the Sirá and the overbaked (Kshara) ones into the Snáyu. The internal cavities (Aśayas) of the body mark the spots or regions where the Váyu had constantly stayed in its embryo stage. 26-29.

The kidneys (Vrikkas) are made out of the essence of the blood and fat. The **testes** are formed out of the essence of the blood, flesh, Kapham and fat. The **heart** is formed out of the essence of blood and Kapham; and the vessels (Dhamanis) carrying the vital principles of the body are attached to it (heart). The spleen and the lungs are situated below and beneath the heart on the left side, and the liver and Kloma (Pancreas ?) below and beneath it (heart) on the right. The heart is the special seat of consciousness (**Chetaná**) in all creatures. Sleep sets in when this viscus (heart) of a person becomes enveloped by the effects of the Tamas (principles of illusion or nescience). 30-31.

**Memorable Verse :**—The heart which is of the shape of a lotus bud hangs with its apex downward, folding itself up during sleep and expanding with the return of wakening or consciousness. 32.

**Sleep and its virtues :**—Sleep is the illusive energy of God (lit.—the all-pervading deity) and naturally has its sway over all created beings. The kind of sleep which sets in when the sensation-carrying channels (Snáyu) of the body are choked by Sleshmá, which abounds in the quality of Tamas, is known as **Támasi-nidrá.** It is this sleep which produces unconsciousness at the time of dissolution or death. A man of **Támasika-temperament** sleeps both in the day and night; one of the **Rájasika-temperament** sleeps either in the day or in the night; while sleep never visits the eyelids of a man of **Sáttvika-temperament** before midnight. Persons with enfeebled Kapham and aggravated Váyu, or suffering from bodily and mental troubles, get little sleep, and if at all, their sleep is of the Vaikárika or delirious type (*i e.* much disturbed)*. 33-34.

**Memorable Verses** :—O Suśruta ! the heart is said to be the primary seat of consciousness (**Chetaná**) in the animated beings. Sleep overcomes a man whenever the heart is enveloped in the illusive effects of Tamas. Sleep is the offspring of Tamas and it is the quality of Sattvam that brings on awakening. This is the fundamental law of Nature. The self-conscious individuality (**Self**), ensconced in the material frame of man which is composed of the five material elements, recollects through the agency of the mind (Manah), which abounds in the quality of Rajas, the renaissance of his by-gone existences, and wakens up in his psychic plane the pictures of good or evil deeds done by him therein. Dreams are but the embodiment of these recollections. The self or **Jivatmá**, though he sleeps not himself, is said to be sleeping, whenever the sense organs are overpowered by the illusive energy of Tamas. 35.

Day sleep is forbidden in all seasons of the year, except in summer and in the case of infants, old men, and persons enfeebled by sexual excesses, or in Kshatakshina diseases and in case of habitual tipplers. A sleep in the day may be enjoyed after the fatigue of a long journey, riding, or physical labour, or on an empty stomach. It may be allowed as well to men suffering from the loss of fat, Kapham or blood, to those of

---

\* Such persons may get sleep only, when being tired and exhausted they cease to think of their affairs.

*C f.* Charaka :—When the active self of a person, tired in body and mind, loses touch with his worldly affairs, sleep comes to him.

scanty perspiration, or of dry or parched constitution; and also to those who have been suffering from indigestion and who may sleep for a Muhurta (48 minutes) in the day time. Those who have kept late hours in the night may sleep in the day for half the time they have watched in the night (and no more). Day sleep is the outcome of perverted nature and all the Doshas of the body are aggravated by a sleep in the day, bringing on many a troublesome complaints such as cough, asthma, catarrh, heaviness of the body, aching or lassitude in the limbs, fever, loss of appetite etc. On the other hand, the keeping of late hours in the night develops symptoms (Upadrava) which are peculiar to the deranged Váyu and Pittam. 36.

**Memorable Verses:**—Hence, one should not sleep in the day, nor keep late hours. Having known both these acts to be injurious, the wise should observe moderation in sleep. A conformity to the preceding rule of conduct is rewarded with health, good humour, strength, healthful complexion, virility and beauty, a frame which is neither too fat nor too thin, and a long life of a hundred years). A day sleep may not prove injurious to those who are habituated to it and conversely keeping late hours at night may not tell upon the health of those to whom it is customary. 37-39.

An aggravated condition of the bodily Váyu or Pittam, an aggrieved state of the mind, loss of vital fluid, and a hurt or an injury may bring on insomnia, the remedy being the adoption of measures antagonistic to those which destroy sleep. The following measures are useful in cases of sleeplessness—such as anointing the body, rubbing of oil on the head, soft massages of the body (with cleansing paste) and shampooing; a diet consisting of cakes and pastry made up of Sáli-rice and wheat prepared with sugar or other derivatives of sugar-cane, sweet or soothing articles with milk or meat juice or flesh of animals of the Biskira or Vileśaya class, and eating of grapes, sugar and sugar-cane at night, are beneficial (in such cases); so also a soft and pleasant bed, and easy and convenient seats and means of loco-motion. Hence, a wise physician should advise those and similar other measures to allay insomnia. 40-41.

Excessive sleep should be remedied by emetics, Sanśodhana measures, fastings, bleeding, and works which tend to disturb the mental equanimity of man. Keeping up at night is beneficial to persons afflicted with obesity, poison or the deranged Kapham; so also a nap in the day is beneficial to people troubled with hiccough, colic pain, dysentery, indigestion, or thirst. 42-43.

**Somnolence or Drowsiness etc. :**—In this kind of light sleep, or in the preliminary stage of sleep, the sense organs are overpowered and remain only partially cognisant of their respective objects and all (subjective and objective) symptoms of a sleepy person such as, yawning, sense of fatigue and heaviness of the limbs, present themselves in succession; these are the special features of **Tandrá**. One (prolonged) inhaling of the air through a widely open mouth and subsequent exhaling with the contraction of the limbs and tearful eyes are (all together) called **Jrimbhá** or yawning.

A sense of fatigue without any physical labour which comes upon a person unaccompanied by hurried respiration is called **Klama**. It obstructs the proper functions of the senses as also the workings of the active organs.* An inordinate love of pleasure and a great aversion to pain, attended with an apathy to all sorts of

---

* Hand, leg, anus, and generative organ etc.

work even with the capacity of carrying them through is called **Álasyam** (laziness) Nausea, without vomiting of ingested food, attended with salivation and formation of sputum, and cardiac distress are the symptoms of **Utklesham**. A sweet taste in the mouth, drowsiness, a beating pain in the heart, dizziness, and non-relish for food are the signs of **Glâni** (languor). A feeling as if the whole body were wrapped in a wet sheet, accompanied by an extreme heaviness of the heart, is called **Gauravam**. 44-50.

Loss of consciousness (**Murchchá**) is due to an excess of the deranged Pittam and to the quality of the Tamas; vertigo (**Bhrama**) is due to an aggravated state of the Váyu, Pittam, and to the quality of the Rajas; drowsiness (**Tandrá**) is due to a similar condition of the Váyu, Kapham and to the quality of the Tamas; while sleep (**Nidrá**) is produced by the predominance of Kapham and to the quality of the Tamas in the organism. 51.

The growth of a fœtus in the womb is effected by the serum (Rasa) prepared out of the food (assimilated by its mother) incarcerated by the Váyu in the internal passage of its body. 52.

**Memorable Verses :**—Be it clearly understood that there exists fire or heat (Jyoti) in the umbilical region of the fœtus which is fanned by its bodily Váyu and thus contributes to the growth of its body. The same Váyu in combination with the heat (thus generated), expands the upward, downward, and lateral channels (in the body of the embryo) and thus leads to the growth of the fœtus. The eyes (**Dristi**—aperture of sight) and the hair-follicles of a man do not

---

\* In the text we find the word "Indriya" which refers to both Jnánendriya (sensory functions) and Karmendriya (motor functions) of the body.

participate at all (in the general expansion of the body). This is a law of nature, and is the opinion of Dhanvantari. On the other hand the growth of hair and finger nails continue even when the body enters the stage of decay. This also is a law of nature. 53-56.

**The Temperaments :**—The temperaments (**Prakriti**) of persons may be of seven different types, according as the deranged Doshas of the body are involved therein, either severally, or in combination of two or of all the three together. The temperament (Prakriti) of a man is determined by the preponderance of the particular Doshas at the time of his generation (actual combination of the semen and ovum) and is marked by that preponderant Dosha. The characteristics of the different Prakritis are now described. 57-58.

**Vátaja-Temperament :**—A man of *Vátika-temparament* is wakeful, averse to bathing and cold contact, unshapely, thievish, vain, dishonest and fond of music; the soles of his feet, and the palms of his hands are much fissured ; has often a rough and grisly beard and moustache, finger nails and hairs in him ; he is hot-tempered and is given to biting his finger nails and grinding his teeth (when asleep). Morally he is impulsive, unsteady in his friendship, ungrateful, lean, and rough ; his body is marked with a large number of prominent veins (Dhamani); he is incoherent in his habit and vacillating in his temper. He is a fast walker and dreams of scaling the skies in his sleep. His eyes are always moving. His mind is never steady. He makes few friends, is capable of accumulating very little money and talks incoherently. The traits of his character etc. seem to resemble those of a goat, jackal, hare, mouse, camel, dog, vulture, crow, and of an ass. 59-60.

**Pittvaja-Temperament :**—A man of *Pittvaja temperament* perspires copiously emitting a fetid smell. His limbs are loosely shaped and yellowish in colour. The finger nails, eyes, palate, tongue, lips, soles and palms of such a person are copper-coloured. He looks ugly with wrinkles, baldness and grey hair; he eats much, is averse to warmth and irritable in temper, though he cools down very soon. He is a man of middling strength and lives up to middle age. He is intelligent and possesses a good retentive memory and loves to monopolise the conversation (by pulling down any speaker that may be present). He is vigorous and is simply irresistible in battle. He dreams in his sleep of such things as meteors, lightning-flashes, fire, Nágeshvara, Palas'a or Karnikára plants. He is never overpowered with fear nor bends before a powerful antagonist; he protects the suppliant and is very often afflicted with suppuration in the cavity of the mouth. The traits of his character resemble those of a serpent, an owl, a Gandharba (heavenly musician), Yaksha, cat, monkey, tiger, bear, and of a mongoose. 61-64.

**Kaphaja-Temperament :**—The complexion of a man of *S'leshmá* temperament resembles either the colour of a blade of grass, blue lotus, polished sword, wet Arishta, or that of the stem of the Sara grass. He is comely in appearance, fond of sweet tastes, grateful, self-controlled, forbearing, unselfish and strong; he does not hastily form any opinion, and is fast in his enmity. His eyes are white; his hair curly and raven black. He is prosperous in life. His voice resembles the rumblings of a rain-cloud, the roar of a lion, or the sound of a Mridanga. He dreams in his sleep of large lakes or pools decked with myriads of full blown lotus flowers, swans and Chakravákas. His eyes are slightly red towards the corners, the limbs are proportionate and symmetrically developed with a cool effulgence radiating from them He is possessed of the qualities of the Sáttvika stamp, capable of sustaining pain and fatigue and respectful towards his superiors He possesses faith in the Śástras and is unflinching and unchanging in his friendship; he suffers no vicissitudes of fortune, makes large gifts after long deliberation, is true to his word and always obedient to his preceptors. The traits of his character resemble those of Brahma, Rudra, Indra, Varuna, a lion, horse, an elephant, cow, bull, an eagle, swan and of the lower animals. 65-68.

A combination of two different temperaments should be called a double temperament or a **Dvandaja** one; and one of all the three temperaments in a person should be stated as a **Sánnipátika** one. 69.

The temperament of a man is never altered, nor does it suffer any deterioration or abatement. A change, abatement or deterioration in any particular case should be regarded as the harbinger of death. As a worm, bred in poison, is not troubled with it, so the temperament of a person however painful to others does no inconvenience to himself. Several authorities hold that the temperaments of persons have their origin in the material elements of the body and accordingly they classify them as the **Vátika Prakriti**, the **Taijasa Prakriti**, and the **Ápya** (watery) **Prakriti**, the characteristic traits of which respectively correspond to the first three temperaments described above. 70—71.

A man of the **Párthiva** temperament is large in his stature, and is firm, strong and muscular in his limbs. A man of the **Nabhasa** temperament is pious and long-lived, has large aural cavities. The mental temperaments are classified according to their qualities. 72.

**Sáttvika Features :**—The features of a **Brahma-káya** person are cleanliness of person and conduct, belief in the existence of God, a constant reader of the Vedas, a worship and reverence of elders and preceptors, hospitality and celebration of religious sacrifices. Those of a **Mahendra-káya** person are valour, command, constant discussion of the Sástras, maintenance of servants and dependents and magnanimity. The features of a **Karuna-káya** person are a liking for exposure to cold, forbearance, a brown hue of the pupils, golden colour of the hair and sweet speech. The features of a **Kouvera-káya** person are, arbitration of disputes, capacity of bearing hardships, earning and accumulation of wealth, and capacity of propagation or fertility. The features of a **Gandharva-káya** person are love of garlands and perfumes, fondness of songs and music, and love making. The features of a **Yamya-Sattva** person are sense of duty, promptness, firmness of action, courage, memory, purity, and absence of anger, illusion, fear and malice. The features of a **Rishi-Sattva** man are divine contemplation, observance of vows, complete sexual abstinence, performance of Homas, celebration of religious sacrifices, knowledge, wisdom and cultivation of divine or spiritual science. These seven types of men should be considered as belonging to the Sáttvika group (of Sáttvika mental temperament). Now hear me describe the features of men of Rájasika stamp (of mind). 73.

**Rájasika Features :**—Asura-Sattva men are affluent in circumstances, dreadful, valorous, irascible, jealous of other men's excellence, gluttonous and fond of eating alone without sharing with any one else. A **Sarpa-Sattva** man is irritable, laborious, cowardly, angry, double-dealing, and hasty in eating and sexual intercourse. A **Sakuna-Sattva** man is gluttonous, intemperate in sexual matters, irritable and fickle. A **Rákshasa-Sattva** man is solitary in his habits, fierce, jealous of others excellence, externally pious, extremely vain and ignorant. The characteristics of a **Paisácha-Sattva** man are eating food partaken of by another, irritability of temper, rashness, shamelessness, and covetousness of female possessions. Those of **Preta-Sattva** man are utter want of knowledge as regards duty, laziness, miserableness, envy, covetousness, niggardliness. These six belong to the Rájasika cast of mind. Now hear me describe the characteristic traits of men of the Támasika temperaments. 74.

**Támasika Features:**—The features of a **Pásava-Sattva** man are perverseness of intellect, parsimoniousness, frequent sexual dreams and incapacity of ascertaining or discerning anything. The features of **Matsya-Sattva** man are unsteadiness, stupidity, cowardice, fond of intermissive quarrel and oppression and a longing for water. The features of a **Vanaspati-Sattva** man are fondness of staying at the same place, constant eating and absence of truthfulness, piety, riches and enjoyment. Thus the three types of Támasika temperament have been described, A physician should take in hand a patient with an eye towards these mental traits etc. A physician should coolly deliberate upon the different types of temperament described herein and their characteristic features. 75-76.

Thus ends the fourth Chapter of the S'árira Sthánam in the S'us'ruta Samhitá which treats of fœtal development etc.

# CHAPTER V.

Now we shall discourse on the Sáriram which treats of the anatomy of the human body (**Śárira-Śankhyá-Vyákaranam**). 1.

**Definition of Garbha and Śárira :—** The combined semen and ovum (Śukra and Śonita) in the womb, mixed with (the eight categories known as) the Prakriti and (her sixteen modifications known as) Vikára, and ridden in by the **Átmá** (self-consicous self), is called the **fœtus**. There is consciousness in the embryo. The **Váyu** (or the vital force) divides it into Dosha, Dhátu, Mala, etc., limbs, and organs, etc. The **Teja** (or the heat latent in the fecundated matter) gives rise to the metabolism of the tissues ; the **Ápa** (water) keeps it in a liquid state ; the **Kshiti** (earth) is embodied in the shape of its species ; and the **Ákáśa** (ether) contributes to its growth and development. A fully developed fœtus with all its parts, such as the hands, feet, tongue, nose, ears, buttocks etc. and the sense-organs, is called **Śáriram** or body. The body is composed of six main parts, namely, the four extremities (upper and lower), the trunk or middle body, and the head. 2.

**Different members of the body :—**Now we shall describe the Pratyangas or members of the body. The head, the belly (Epigastrium), the back, the navel (umbilical region), the forehead, the nose, the chin, the bladder, and the throat (neck), occur singly ; the ears, the eyes, the nostrils, the eye-brows, the temples, the shoulders, the cheek, the armpits, the breasts, the testes, the sides, the buttocks, the arms, the thighs, and the knee-joints, etc., occur in pairs. The fingers and toes which number twenty in all, and the interior channels (Srotas) of the body, to be presently described, are likewise included within the Pratyangas. These are the different **Pratyangas** or members. 3.

**Enumeration of the different limbs and members of the body :**—The different layers of the skin, the Kalás, the Dhátus (root principles, such as blood, chyle, etc ), the Mala (excrements), the Doshas (morbific principles, such as the Váyu, Pittam, or Kapham), the spleen, the liver, the lungs, the colon and cæcum (Unduka), the heart, the cavities or viscera (Ásáyas), the intestines (Antras), the Vrikkou (Kidneys) the Srotas (internal passages or ducts), the Kandará (nerve trunks), the Jálas (membranes), the Kurchas,* the Rajjus (tendons) the Sevanis (sutures), the Sanghátas (facets), the Simanta, the bones, the joints, the Snáyu (ligament), the Peśi (muscles), the Marmas (vital parts, such as anastomosis of veins and arteries, etc.), the Sira (veins), the Dhamani (arteries), and the Yogaváhini Srotas†, constitute what is collectively called the organism. 4.

**Their number :**—The layers of skin (Tvaka) number seven in all. There are seven connective tissues or fascia (Kalás). The cavities or viscera (Ásayas) are seven in all. The root principles (Dhátu) of the body are seven in number. There are seven hundred Sirá (veins), five hundred Peśi (muscles), nine hundred Snáyu (ligaments), three hundred bones, two hundred and ten Sandhi (joints), one hundred and seven Marmas (vital parts), twenty-four Dhamanis (arteries etc.), three Doshas (morbific principle—such as the Váyu, Pittam,

---

\* Meetings of muscles, ligaments, veins, nerves and bones as at the annular ligament.

† Those, that are in connection with the Dhamani.

and Kapham), three kinds of Mala (excrements) and nine Srota (canals) in all in the human organism, which will be described in detail later on. 5.

The skin, Kalá, the root principles of the body, (Dhàtus) the morbific principles (Doshas) such as the Váyu etc, of the body, liver, spleen, lungs, Unduka (colons), heart and the Vrikkas (kidneys) have been already described (in the preceding chapter). 6.

**The Áŝayas** (cavities or viscera) :—They are named as the **Vátaŝaya** (the receptacle of the bodily Váyu), **Pittaŝaya** (the receptacle of the Pittam), **Śleshmaŝaya** (the receptacle of Śleshmá or Kapham), **Raktaŝaya** (the receptacle of the blood), **Ámaŝaya** (stomach), **Pákvaŝaya** (intestines), and the **Mutráŝaya** (bladder). Females have another Áŝaya (receptacle) in addition to these which is called the **Garbháŝaya** (uterus). The intestines (of an adult) male, measure fourteen cubits (three and a half Vyámas) in length, while those of an adult female measure only twelve cubits. 7—8.

**The Srotas or Channels :**—The nine canals (Śrotas) of the body, such as the ears, the eyes, the mouth, the nostrils, the anus and the urethra, open on the outside. Females have three more such ducts or canals as the two breasts (milk channels) and the one which carries off the menstrual blood. 9.

**The Kandarás :**—The Kandarás number sixteen in all, of which four are in the legs, four in the hands, four in the neck, and four in the back. The Kandarás of the four extremeties extend to the roots of the nails of the fingers and toes. The four Kandarás of the neck, connecting it with the heart, extend down to the penis. The four Kandarás at the back and in the region of the Śróni extend down to the buttocks

(Vimba). These Kandarás terminate above in the head, the thighs, the breast and in the balls of the shoulders respectively (i.e. the Kandarás of the neck terminate above in the head, those of the legs in the thighs, those of the dorsum in the chest, and those of the arms in the shoulders). 10.

**The Jála or Plexuses :**—The Jála or plexuses are of four kinds, such as the **muscular** plexuses, the **Vascular** plexuses, **ligamentous** plexuses, and **bony** plexuses. One of each of the four kinds of plexuses, is found about each of the Manibandda (wrists) and Gulfa (ankles). These four kinds of plexuses intermingle and cross one another in the form of a net-work. The whole body is a chain-work of plexuses. 11.

**The kurchas :**—There are six Kurchas* in all ; of which two are in the hands, two in the feet, one in the neck, and one in the penis. There are four great muscular **cords** or **kajjus** which originate from either side of the spinal column, one pair going inwards and another outwards for the purpose of binding the muscles together.† 12—13.

**The Sevanis or Sutures :**—‡They are seven in number, e. g. five in the head, one in the tongue and one in the genital. An incision should not be made into any of these sevanis. 14.

**The Asthi-Sanghátas :**—The Asthi-sanghátas (collection of a number of bones) are fourteen in

---

\* The Kurchas (clusters or groups) may be made up of muscles, bones, vessels and ligamentous structure—Dallana.

† According to Gayádása four such cords are found on each side of the spinal column and thus totalling eight in all.

‡ **Sevani** evidently means the central tendinous band which looks like a suture from which the muscles on either side arise.

number. Of these one is found in each of the following positions, viz. the two ankles, the two knees and the two groins ; of the remaining eight, six are to be found in similar positions of the upper extremities, namely one in each of the wrists, elbows and axillas ; one is in the cranium and another in the regions of the Trika* (thus making up fourteen in all). 15.

**The Simantas :**—The Simantas number fourteen in all, and are respectively situated about the place of each of the aforesaid Asthi-sanghata. Several authorities assert that there are eighteen Sanghátas.† 16.

**The Bones :**—According to the followers of the **Áyurveda** (general medicine), the entire number of bones in the human body is three hundred and sixty ; whereas **Śalya-Tantram** (the present work) counts only three hundred. Of these, one hundred and twenty are to be found in the (four) extremities, one hundred and seventeen in the pelvis (Śroni), sides (Párśva), back, chest (Urah) and the region of the abdomen (Udara), and sixty-three in the neck and the regions above ; thus numbering three hundred in the aggregate.‡ 17.

---

* "**Trika**" generally means the sacral region, but Dallanan says that here it refers to the meeting of the two clavicles with the breastbone.

† According to them four more Asthi-sangatás are to be found over and above the fourteen already mentioned ; these are—one above the sacrum, one above the chest, one at the junction of the thorax and abdomen, and one at the acromial end (of the Scapula).

‡ Pundita Gangádhara Kaviratna of Murshidabad in his famous commentary, known as the *Tiká-jalpa-kalpa-taru*, in the 7th. chapter of Sárira Sthánam in the Charaka Sambitá states :—

"In the surgical text-book of Suśruta the number of bones in the human body is given to be three hundred in all. Of these, one hundred and eight bones are in the four extremeties ; one hundred and twenty-six in the pelvic cavity (S'roni), sides (Párs'va), back (Prishtha), (**Aksha**) **collar-bones** and breast (Urah) ; and sixty-six in the region

**Bones of the four Extremities:**—There are three bones in each toe of the foot, thus making fifteen bones altogether (in the toes of each leg). Ten bones constitute the Tala (sole), Kurcha (cluster), and Gulpha (ankle) of each leg, and one forms the Páshni (heel); two bones are found in the Janghá (leg); one in the Jánu (knee), and one in the Uru (thigh); thus making thirty bones in one lower extremity. The same number holds good in the case of the other leg as well as in that of the two upper limbs. (Thus the bones in the four extremities are one hundred and twenty in all). 18.

**Bones of the Trunk:**—Five bones form the S'roni (pelvic cavity); of these four are found about the Guda (anus), Bhaga (pubis), and the Nitamva

upward the neck. Thus the total number of three hundred is made up. Now there are three bones in each toe of the feet; this makes fifteen altogether. Seven bones constitute the sole (Tala), cluster (Kurcha), and the ankle (Gulfa). There is one bone in the heel (Páshni), two in the leg (Janghá), one in the knee (Jánu), and one in the thigh (Uru). Thus there are twenty-seven bones in one lower limb. The same number applies to the other lower limb as well as to the two upper limbs. Thus a total number of one hundred and eight bones is made up. There are five bones in the pelvic cavity (S'roni); of these there are two in the hips (Nitamba), and the pubes (Bhaga), anus (Guda) and sacrum (Trika) is constituted with one bone each. There are thirty-six bones in one side (Párs'va) and the same count applies to the other. There are thirty bones in the back (Prishtha); two in the collar-bone (**Akshasanjna**); seventeen in the breast (Ura); eleven in the neck (Griva); four in the wind-pipe (Kantha-nádi); and two in the jaws (Hanu). There are thirty-two teeth. There are three bones in the nose (Násá); two in the palate (Tálu); one each in either cheek (Ganda), ear (Karna) and temple (S'ankha), making six together; and six in the cranium (Sira). Thus a total number of sixty-six bones is made up. (Hence) the total number of three hundred bones is made (with the grand total of the three foregoing totals). Thus the list of bones of a skeleton is described."

(hips), and the fifth one is the Trika or triangular bone (the sacrum). There are thirty-six bones in one Pársva (side), and the same number in the other; thirty in the Prishtha (back), eight in the Urah (chest); and two more known as Akshaka (collar-bone). (Thus making one hundred and seventeen in all). 19.

**Bones above the Clavicles :**—There are nine bones in the Grivá (neck); four in the Kantha-nádi\* (wind-pipe); two in the Hanu (Jaws). The teeth number thirty-two. There are three bones in the nose; one in the Tálu (palate); also one in each Karna (ear), Sankha (temple), and Ganda (cheek), (thus making six in all); six bones form the Sirá (cranium). [Thus making sixty-three in all]. 20.

**Different kinds of Bones and their situations :**—These bones may be divided into five classes (according to their character), such as the Kapála, Ruchaka, Taruna, Valaya and the Nalaka. The bones, situated in the knee-joints, shoulders (Ansa†), hips (Nitamvas), cheeks (Ganda), palate, temples, and the cranium belong to the **Kapála** kind (flat bones). The teeth belong to the **Ruchaka** class. The bones in the nose, ears, throat (trachea) and the socket of the eyes (Akshi-kosha†) are called **Taruna** (cartilages); while those which are found in the palm (wrist), foot (ankle), sides back, chest and regions of the abdomen, belong to the **Valaya** (irregular or curved) class. The remaining

---

\* Tala, Kurcha, and Kantha-nádi are identical with Charak's Sáláká, Sthána and Jatru respectively.

† Though it is asserted here that there exist Taruna bones in the sockets of the eyes (Akshi-kosha) but there is no mention at all in the text, of the presence of any such therein. There is no mention of the shoulder-blade (Ansa) here though it is a part of the skeleton.

bones belong to **Nalaka** class (long-bones, lit.—reed-like or cylindrical). 21.

**Memorable Verses :**—As trees are supported by the hard core inside their trunks, so the body is supported (and kept erect) by the firm bones (which are found in its inside). And since these bones form the pith (Sára) of the human organism, they are not destroyed even after the destruction and falling off of the attached flesh, skin, etc. of the body. Muscles are attached strongly to the bones by means of the veins (Sirás) and ligaments (Snáyus), and are thus kept in position and do not fall off. 22.

**The Sandhis or Joints—(M. T.) :**—The joints may be divided into two kinds according as they are **immovable** (synarthrosis) and **movable** (diarthrosis). Those which are situated at the four extremities as well as in the Kati (waist) and Hanus (jaws) are movable ; the others are known to be unmovable by the learned. There are two hundred and ten articulations (Sandhis) in the human body. Of these sixty-eight are in the four extremities ; fifty-nine in the trunk (Koshtha); and eighty-three in the neck and in the region above it. 23.

**Sandhis of the four Extremities :**— Three joints are found in each toe, two only in the great toe, thus making fourteen in each leg ; one is placed in each ankle, knee-joint and groin, thus making seventeen Sandhis in each leg or thirty-four in the two lower extremities. A similar number is to be found in each of the two upper extremities. 24-25.

**Sandhis of the koshtha and Clavicles :**—There are three Sandhis about the Kapála or flat bone in the Kati (waist, hence pelvis) ; twenty-four in the vertibral column ; twenty-four in the sides ; eight in the chest ; eight in the Grivá (neck) ; three in the Kanthas (windpipe); eighteen in the cords or bands (Nádi) binding the Kloma and the heart ; thirty-two about the roots of the teeth, one in the region of the thyroid (Kákalaka); one in the nose ; two in the eyes ; one in each of the two ears, temples and cheeks (thus making six in all) ; two about the joints of the jaw-bones ; two over the eye-brows ; two above the temples ; five in the Kapála bone of the fore-head and one in the head. 26-27.

**Their forms, distinctions, and locations :**—These joints may be divided into eight different classes (named after the objects which they respectively resemble in shape), namely Kora (hinged or lap-shaped), Udukhala (ball and socket), Sámudga (back of the palm), Pratara (raft), Tunna-sevani (seam-like or dove-tailed), Váyasa-tunda (crow-beak), Mandala (circular), and Sankhá-vartah (involutions of conch-shell). The joints in the fingers, wrists, ankles knee-joints and elbows (Karpura) belong to the **Kora** group. Those in the axilla or shoulder-joint (Kakshá). teeth, and hip (Vankshana) are of the **Udukhala** type. The joints in the region of the anus, vagina, shoulders (Ansa-pitha —i.e glenoid cavity) and hips, belong to the **Sámudga** form The joints in the neck and the spinal columns, belong to the **Pratara** (irregular) type ; while those found in the Kapála bones of the pelvis (Kati) and the forehead, are of **Tunna-sevani** (suture) form. The joints on either side of the cheek-bones (temporomandibular) belong to the **Váyasa-tunda** type. The **Mandala** joints occur in the encircling Nádi of the heart, throat, eyes and Kloma. **Sankhá-varta** joints occur in the bones of the ears and the nostrils. The peculiar features of these different kinds of joints (Sandhis) are evident from their names. 28.

**Metrical Text :**—Only the bone-joints have been enumerated and described ; the joints of muscles ligaments and veins are innumerable. 29.

**The Ligaments (Snáyu) :**—There are nine hundred ligaments (Snáyus) in the human body, of which six hundred occur in the four extremities ; two hundred and thirty in the trunk (Koshtha) and seventy in the neck and upwards. (Of the six hundred ligaments in the four extremities), six ligaments are situated in each toe making thirty (in the toes of each foot) ; thirty in the Tala (soles), Gulpha (ankles), and the Kurcha (ankle-joint) ; thirty in the leg (Janghá) ; ten in the knee-joints (Jánu) ; forty in the Udara (abdomen) ; ten in the groin (Vankshana) ; thus making one hundred and fifty in each leg. The same number is found in the other lower limb and in each of the two upper extremities. (Of the two hundred and thirty ligaments in the trunk), there are sixty in the lumbar region (Kati) ; eighty in the back ; sixty in the sides ; and thirty in the chest. (Of the seventy ligaments to be found in the region above the clavicles) there are thirty six in the neck (Grivá) and thirty-four in the head. Thus the total number of ligaments in a human body is nine hundred. 30—33.

**Memorable Verses :**—Now hear me describe the ligaments (Snáyus). They may be grouped under four distinct heads, viz., Pratánavati (ramifying or branching), Vritta (ring-shaped or circular), Prithu (thick or broad), and Śushira (perforated). The ligaments (Snáyus) which present in the four extremities and the joints belong to the **Pratánavati** type. The Kandarás or large ligaments are of the **Vritta** type ; while those which are found in the stomach (Ámáśaya) or in the intestines (Pakváśaya), and in the bladder belong to the Sushira type. The ligaments of the chest, back, sides and head are of the **Prithu** type. 34—35.

As a boat made of planks and timber fastened together by means of a large number of bindings is enabled to float on the water and to carry cargo; so the human frame being bound and fastened at the Sandhis or joints by a large number of ligaments (Snáyu) is enabled to bear pressure. An injury to, or diseases of, the bones, veins, joints or muscles are not so detrimental to the system as is the case if the Snáyus are affected in any way. Only the physician, who is acquainted with the internal and external ligaments (Snáyus) of the body, is qualified to extract a hidden and imbedded Śalyam (extraneous matter etc.) from any part of the body. 36.

**The Muscles (Peśis) :**—The muscles (Peśis) number five hundred in all, of which four hundred are in the four extremities; Sixty-six\* in the trunk (Koshtha) and thirty-four in the region above the clavicles. 37.

**Muscles in the Extremities :**—There are three muscles in each of the toes, thus making fifteen in the toes of one leg; ten in the anterior part of the foot and the same number (ten) attached to the Kurchcha; ten in the sole and the ankle-bone (Gulpha,—malledi); twenty in the region between the Gulpha and the knee-joint; five in the knee-joint (Jánu); twenty in the thigh (Uru); and ten in the groin (Vankshana); thus making one hundred muscles in all in each leg. The same number is found in each of the other three extremities; (thus making four hundred in all). 38.

**Muscles in the Koshtha :**—(Of the sixty-six muscles in the trunk), three are in the region of the

---

\* Gayádása reads sixty in the trunks and forty above the clavicles.

anus (Pâyu); one in the penis; one in the perineum (Sevani); two in the scrotum; five in each of the haunches (Sphik); two in the top or head of the bladder; five in the abdomen (Udara); one about the umbilicus; five along each side (of the spinal column), on the upper part of the back (making ten in all); six in the sides; ten in the chest; seven around the armpits and shoulders (Akshaka-Ansa); two in the region of heart and stomach (Âmásaya); and six in the region of the liver, spleen and colon (Unduka). 39.

**Muscles of the Head and Neck :**—(Of the thirty-four muscles found in this region), four are in the throat (Grivá); eight in the two jaw-bones (Hanu); one each in the regions of the throat (Kákalaka and Gala); two in the palate; one in the tongue; two in the lips : two in the nose; two in the eyes; four in the cheeks; two in the ears; four in the forehead; and one in the head. Thus the positions and distributions of the five hundred muscles (Pesis) have been described. 40.

**Metrical Text :**—The ligaments, veins, bones and joints etc., of a human body, derive their strength from the fact of their being supported by or covered over by the muscles. 41.

**Extra Muscles in Women :**—Females have twenty extra muscles; ten muscles are to be found about the two breasts, five in each, which (muscles) attain their full growth during puberty; four muscles are present about the parturient passage; and of these (four) two are about the external and two in the internal orifices (of the vagina); three about the region of the os, and three along the passages of the ovum and sperm. The Garbhásáya or uterus is situated in the space bounded by the Pittásaya (small intestine) and Pakvásaya (large intestine) and the fœtus lies in this during the period of gestation.* 42-43.

According to their position in the system, these muscles are found to be thick, slender, small, expanded, circular, short, long, hard, soft, smooth or rough. The muscles cover the veins, ligaments, bones and joints; hence their shape and size are determined by the exigencies (organic structures) of their positions. 44.

**Memorable Verses :**—The muscles which are found in the penis and scrotum of a man as described before correspond to the covering of the uterus in the case of a woman owing to the absence of those organs in her body. The positions and classifications of the veins, channels, Marmas and arteries will be dealt with in a separate chapter. 45-46.

The vagina of a woman resembles the navel of a conch-shell in shape and is possessed of three involuted turns (Ávartas) like the interior of mollusc The uterus (Garbhásaya—fœtal bed) is situated at the third posterior involuted turn. The shape of the uterus resembles the mouth of a Rohit-fish (narrow at the mouth and expanded in the upper end). The fœtus lies in a crouched or doubled up posture in the uterus and thus naturally at the time of parturition its head is presented at the entrance to the vagina. 47-48.

**Superiority of Śalya-Tantram :**—The different parts or members of the body as mentioned before including even the skin cannot be correctly described by any one who is not versed in **Anatomy.** Hence, any one desirous of acquiring a thorough knowledge of anatomy should prepare a dead body and carefully observe (by dissecting it) and examine

---

\* If we read Mutrás'aya (bladder) in place of Pittás'aya it explains the anatomy better —Ed.

its different parts. For a thorough knowledge can only be acquired by comparing the accounts given in the Sástras (books on the subject) by direct personal observation. 49.

**Mode of dissection :**—A dead body selected for this purpose should not be wanting in any of its parts, should not be a person who had lived up to a hundred years (i. e. too old age) or of one who died from any protracted disease or of poison. The excrementa should be first removed from the entrails and the body should be left to decompose in the water of a solitary and still pool, and securely placed in a cage (so that it may not be eaten away by fish nor drift away), after having covered it entirely with the outer sheaths of *Munja* grass, *Kus'a* grass, hemp or with rope etc. After seven days the body would be thoroughly decomposed, when the observer should slowly scrape off the decomposed skin etc. with a whisk made of grass-roots, hair, Kus'a blade or with a strip of split bamboo and carefully observe with his own eyes all the various different organs, external and internal, beginning with the skin as described before. 50—56.

**Memorable Verses :**—The Self, the occult or invisible Lord of the body cannot be detected except with the psychic eye or with that of the mind. He, who has observed the internal mechanism of the human body and is well read in the works bearing on these subjects and has thus all his doubts expelled from his mind is alone qualified in the science of Áyurveda and has a rightful claim to practise the art of healing. 57.

Thus ends the fifth Chapter of the S'árira-sthánam in the Sus'ruta Samhitá which treats of the anatomy of the human body.

# CHAPTER VI.

Now we shall discourse on the Sáriram which specifically treats of the Marmas* or vital parts of the body **(Pratyeka-marma-nirdeśa Śáriram.)** 1.

**Classification of Marmas:**—There are one hundred and seven Marmas (in the human organism), which may be divided into five classes, such as the Mánsa-Marmas, Sirá-Marmas, Snáyu-Marmas, Asthi-Marmas and the Sandhi-Marmas. Indeed there are no other Marmas (vulnerable or vital parts) to be found in the body than the preceding ones. 2.

**Their different numbers:**—There are eleven Mánsa-Marmas (vulnerable muscle-joints); forty-one Sirá-Marmas (similar veins, anastomosis); twenty-seven Snáyu-Marmas (vital ligament-unions); eight Asthi-Marmas (bone-unions) and twenty Sandhi-Marmas (vulnerable joints). 3.

**Their Locations:**—Of these, eleven are in one leg, thus making twenty-two in the two lower extremities. The same number counts in the two hands. There are twelve Marmas in the regions of the chest and the abdomen (Udara); fourteen in the back; and thirty-seven in the region of the neck (Grivá) and above it. 4.

**Names and distributions of Marmas:** —The Marmas which are situated in each leg are known as Kshipra, Tala-Hridaya, Kurchcha, Kurchcha-Sirah, Gulpha, Indravasti, Jánu, Ani, Urvi, Lohitáksha and Vitapa. The twelve Marmas which are situated in the

---

* Places where Veins, arteries, ligaments, joints and muscles unite and an injury to which proves generally fatal.

thorax and the abdomen (Udara) are Guda (anus), Vasti (bladder), Nábhi (umbilicus), Hridaya (heart), Stana-mula (the roots of two breasts), the Stana-Rohita, (muscles of the breasts), the two Apaláps and the two Apastambhas. The fourteen Marmas to be found in the back are the Katika-tarunas (Taruna-bones of the waist), the two Kukundaras, the two Nitamvas (hips), Pársva-Sandhis (the two side-joints), the two Vrihatis, the two Ansa-phalakas (shoulder-blades) and the two Ansas (shoulders). The eleven Marmas to be found in an arm are known as the Kshipra, Tala-Hridaya, Kurchcha, Kurchcha-Sirah, Manivandha, Indravasti, Kurpara, Ani, Urvi, Lohitáksha and Kakshadhara. What is said of the one arm holds good of the other. The Marmas situated above the clavicle regions are known as the four Dhamanis, the eight Mátrikás, the two Krikátikás, the two Vidhuras, the two Phanas, the two Apángas, the two Avartas, the two Utkshepas, the two Sankhas, one Sthapani five Simantas, four Sringátakas and one Adhipati. 5—9.

**The different heads of Marmas:**—Of the aforesaid Marmas, those known as the Tala-Hridaya, Indravasti, Guda and Stana-rohita, are **Mánsa-Marmas.** Those known as Nila-dhamani, Mátriká, Sringátaka, Apánga, Sthapani, Phana, Stana-mula, Apalápa, Apastambha, Hridaya, Nábhi, Pársva-Sandhi, Vrihati, Lohitáksha and Urvi, are **Sirá-Marmas.** Those known as the Ani, Vitapa, Kakshadhara, Kurchcha, Kurchcha-Sirah, Vasti, Kshipra, Ansas, (shoulders), Vidhura and Utkshepa, are **Snáyu-Marmas.** Those known as the Katika-taruna, Nitamva, Ansa-phalaka, Sankha, are **Asthi-Marmas.** The Jánu, the Kurpara, the Simanta, the Adhipati, the Gulpha, the Manivandha, the Kukundara, the Avarta and the Krikátiká are **Sandhi-Marmas.** 10—14.

**Qualitative classes :**—Again these Marmas (vital unions of the body) are under five distinct heads, namely, Sadya-Pránahara, (fatal within twenty-four hours), Kálántara-Pránahara, (fatal within a fortnight or a month), Visalyaghna (fatal as soon as a dart or any other imbedded foreign matter is extracted therefrom), Vaikalyakara, (maiming or deforming) and Rujákar (painful) [according as an injury respectively produces the aforesaid effects]. Of these, nineteen Marmas belong to the Sadya-Pránahara group; thirty-three to the Kálántara-Pránahara group; three to the Visalyaghna group; forty-four to the Vaikalyakara group; and eight to the Rujákara group. 15.

**Memorable Verses :**—To the **Sadya-Pránahara** group (fatal in the course of a day if anyway hurt) belong the four Sringátakas, one Adhipati, the two Sankhas, the eight Kantha-Sirás, the Guda, the Hridaya, the Vasti and the Nábhi. To the **Kálántara-Pránahara** group (fatal later on, if any way hurt) belong the eight Vaksha-Marmas, the five Simantas, the four Tala-Marmas, the four Kshipra-Marmas, the four Indra-vastis, the two Katika-tarunas, the two Pársva-Sandhis, the two Vrihatis, and the two Nitamvas. To the **Visalyaghna** class belong the two Utkshepas and the one Sthapani. To the **Vaikalyakara** (deforming) group belong the Marmas, known as the four Lohitákshas, the four Anis, the two Jánus, the four Urvis, the four Kurchchas, the two Vitapas, the two Kurparas, the two Kukundaras, the two Kakshadharas, the two Vidhuras, the two Krikátikás, the two Ansas (shoulder), the two Ansa-phalakas, (shoulderblades), the two Apángas (tips of eyes), the two Niáls, the two Manyás, the two Phanas and the two Ávartas. A learned physician should know that the two Gulphas, the two Mani-vandhas and the four Kurchcha-Śirah (of the hands and legs), belong to the **Rujákara** group (painful if hurt). A piercing of the Kshipra-Marma ends in an instantaneous death; or death may follow at a later time. 16-21.

Firm unions of Mánsa (muscles), Śirà (veins), Snàyu (ligaments), bones or bone-joints are called Marmas (or vital parts of the body) which naturally and specifically form the seats of life (**Prána**), and hence a hurt to any one of the Marmas invariably produces such symptoms as arise from the hurt of a certain Marma.* 22.

The Marmas belonging to the Sadya-Prànahara group are possessed of fiery virtues (thermogenetic); as fiery virtues are easily enfeebled, so they prove fatal to life (in the event of being any way hurt); while those belonging to the Kálántara-Pránahara group are fiery and lunar (cool) in their properties. And as the fiery virtues are enfeebled easily and the cooling virtues take a considerable time in being so, the Marmas of this group prove fatal in the long run (in the event of being any way hurt, if not instantaneously like the preceding ones). The Viśalyaghna Marmas are possessed of Vàtaja properties (that is, they arrest the escape of the vital Váyu); so long as the dart does not allow the Váyu to escape from their injured interior, the life prolongs; but as soon as the dart is extricated, the Váyu escapes from the inside of the hurt and necessarily proves fatal. The Vaikalyakaras are possessed of Saumya (lunar properties) and they retain the vital fluid owing to their steady and cooling virtues, and hence tend only to deform the organism

---

* Some are of opinion that hallucination, delirium, death, stupor and coma as described in the Sutrast ánam are the results of injuries to thes Mar as.

in the event of their being hurt, instead of bringing on death. The Rujàkara Marmas of fiery and Vátaja properties become extremely painful inasmuch as both of them are pain-generating in their properties. Others, on the contrary, hold the pain to be the result of the properties of the five material components of the body (Páncha-bhautika) 23.

### Different Opinions on the Marmas:—

Some assert that Marmas, which are the firm union of the five bodily factors (of veins, ligaments, muscles, bones and joints), belong to the first group (Sadya-Pránahara); that those, which form the junction of four such, or in which there is one in smaller quantity, will prove fatal in the long run, in the event of their being hurt or injured (Kálántara-Pránahara).* Those, which are the junction of three such factors, belong to the Vis'alya-Pránahara† group; those of the two belong to the Vaikalyakara ‡

---

\* The Marmas, such as Stana-mula, Apalápa, Apastambha, Simanta, Katika-Taruna, PársVa-Sandhi, Vrihati, and Nitamva belonging to the Kálántara-máraka group, are devoid of Mánsa (muscles); and the 'Marmas' known as Stanarohita, Talahridaya, Kshipra, and Indravasti, belonging to the same class, are devoid of Asthi (bones).

† The Utkshepa marma, belonging to the Vis'alya-pránahara group, is devoid of Mánsa (muscles) and Sandhi (joint).

‡ The Sthapani-Marma, belonging to the Vaikalyakara class, is devoid of Mánsa (muscle), S'irá and Snáyu; the Lohitáksha-marma (of the same group) is devoid of Snáyu, Sandhi and Asthi (bones) ; the Jánu-marma (of the same group) is devoid of Mánsa, S'irá and Snáyu; the Urvi-marma (of the said group) is devoid of Asthi, Mánsa and Snáyu ; the Vitapa-marma (of the same class) is devoid of Mánsa, Sirá and Asthi ; the Kurpara-marma (of the same class) is devoid of Mánsa, S'ira, and Snáyu ; the Kukundara-marma (of the same class) is devoid of Mánsa, S'irá and Sandhi ; the Kakshadhara-marma (of the same class) is devoid of S'irá, Asthi, and Sandhi ; the Vidhura-marma (of the said group) is devoid of Mánsa, Sirá and Sandhi ; the Krikatika-marma is devoid of Mánsa, S'irá, and Sandhi ; the Ansa-marma (of the same group) is devoid of Mánsa, Snáyu and Sandhi ; the Ansa-phalaka-marma

group; and those in which only one of them exists belongs to the last or pain-generating type (Rujákara)*.

But the fore going theory is not a sound one, inasmuch as blood is found to exude from an injured joint which would be an impossibility in the absence of any vein, ligament (Snáyu) and muscle being intimately connected with it. Hence every Marma should be understood as a junction or meeting place of the five organic principles of ligaments, veins, muscles, bones and joints. 24-25.

**Metrical text :**—This is further corroborated by the fact that the four classes of Sirá or vessels (which respectively carry the Váyu, Pitta, Kapha and the blood) are found to enter into the Marmas for the purpose of keeping or maintaining the moisture of the local ligaments (Snáyu), bones, muscles and joints and thus sustain the organism.† The Váyu, aggravated by an injury to a Marma, blocks up (those four classes of vessels) in their entire course throughout the organism and gives rise to great pain which extends all over the body. All the internal mechanism of a man (of which a Marma has been pierced into with a shaft or with any other piercing matter) becomes extremely painful, and seems as if it were being constantly shaken or jerked, and symptoms of syncope are found to set in. Hence a careful examination of the affected Marma should

(of the said group) is devoid of Mânsa, Snâyu and Sandhi ; the Nilá, Manyá and Phana Marmas (of the same group) are devoid of Mánsa, Sandhi and Asthi ; the Ávarta-marma is devoid of S'irá, Snâyu and Mânsa ; the Apánga-marma (of the said class) is devoid of Mánsa, Snáyu and Sandhi.

* The Gulpha, Manibandha, and Kurchcha-s'ira Marmas, belonging to the Rujákara group, are devoid of Mânsa, S'irá, Snâyu and Asthi, *i.e.* Sandhi alone is present in these.

† Hence the piercing of a bone is attended with bleeding.

precede all the foregoing acts of extricating a Śalya from its inside. From that similar aggravated conditions and actions of the Pitta and the Kapha should be presumed in the event of a Marma being any way injured or pierced into. 26—29.

A Marma of the Sadyah-Pránahara type being perforated at its edge brings on death at a later time (within seven days), whereas a deformity of the organ follows from the piercing of a Kálántara-Máraka* Marma at the side (instead of in the centre). Similarly, an excruciating pain and distressful after-effects mark a similar perforation of a Marma of the Viśalyaghna† group And a Marma of the Rujákara‡ class produces an excruciating pain (instead of a sharp one) in the event of its being pierced at the fringe. 30.

An injured Marma of the Sadyah-Pránahara type terminates in death within seven days of the injury, while one of the Kálántara type, within a fortnight or a month from the date of hurt (according to circumstances). A case of injured Kshipra-Marma seldom proves fatal before that time (seven days). An injured Marma of the Viśalyaghna or Vaikalyakara group may prove fatal in the event of its being severely injured. 31.

**Marmas of the Extremities :**—Now we shall describe the situation of every Marma. The

---

\* If any of the Marmas of the Kálántara-Pránahara group be deeply perforated, then this perforation is sure to bring on death within a day (*i.e.* it will act like a slightly injured Marma of the Sadyah-Pránahara group).

† Any Marma of the Vis'alyaghna-group, being deeply perforated, brings on death within seven days (*i. e.* it will behave like a slightly injured Marma of the Kálántara-Pránahara class).

‡ Any Marma of the Rujákara class, being deeply perforated (injured), is sure to bring excruciating pain etc , (*i.e* , it will act like a slightly injured Marma of the Vis'alyaghna group).

Marma, known as the **Kshipra***, is situated in the region between the first and the second toes (Tarsal articulation), which, being injured or pierced, brings on death from convulsions. The Marma, known as the **Tala-Hridaya**†, is situated in the middle of the sole of the foot in a straight line drawn from the root of the middle toe. An injury to this Marma gives rise to extreme pain which ends in death. The Marma, known as the **Kurchcha**‡, is situated two fingers' width above from the Kshipra one on each side of the foot. An injury to this Marma results in shivering and bending in of the foot. The Marma called **Kurchcha-Śirah** § is situated under the ankle-joints, one on each side of the foot (Gulpha-Sandhi) ; an injury to it gives rise to pain and swelling of the affected part. A perforation of the **Gulpha-Marma** ||, which is situated at the junction of the foot and the calf, results in pain, paralysis and maimedness of the affected leg. 32-37

An injury to the Marma which is situated in the middle muscle of the calf to the distance of between twelve and thirteen fingers' width from the ankle, and known as the **Indravasti-Marma**,¶ results in excessive hæmorrhage which ends in death. 38.

---

\* It is a Snáyu-Marma (ligament) to the width of half a finger, and belongs to the Kálántara group.

† It is a Mánsa-Marma to the width of half a finger and belongs to the Kálántara group.

‡ It is a Snáyu-Marma to the length of four fingers' width, and belongs to the Vaikalyakara group.

§ It is a Snáyu-Marma, one finger in length and belongs to the Vaikalyakara group.

|| It is a Sandhi-Marma, to the length of two fingers', and belongs to the Vaikalyakara group.

¶ Indravasti measures two fingers in length according to Bhoja and

An injury to or piercing of the **Jánu-Marma**,* situated at the union of the thigh and the knee, results in lameness of the patient. 39.

A piercing of the **Áni-Marma**,† situated on both the sides above three fingers' width from the Jánu (knee-joint), brings on swelling and paralysis (numbness) of the leg. 40.

A perforation of the **Urvi-Marma**,‡ situated in the middle of the Uru (thigh), results in the atrophy of the leg, owing to the incidental hæmorrhage. An injury to the **Lohitáksha-Marma**,‖ situated respectively a little above and below the Urvi-Marma and the Vankshana (groin-joint), and placed near the thigh, is attended with excessive hæmorrhage and causes paralysis (of the leg). 41-42

An injury to the **Vitapa-Marma**,¶ situated between the Scrotum and the Vankshana (inguinal region), brings on loss of manhood or scantiness of semen. Thus the eleven **Sakthi-Marmas** of one leg have been described; those in the other being of an identical nature with the preceding ones. The Marmas in the hands are almost identical with those of the legs, with the exception that **Manivandha, Kurpara** and **Kakshadhara** Marmas

---

Gayádasa, though half a finger in width according to others. It is a Mánsa-Marma and belongs to the Kálántara group.

\* It is a joint-Marma, three fingers in length and belongs to the Vaikalyakara group.

† It is a ligament-Marma, half a finger in length, (three fingers according to Gayàdasa) and is of the Vaikalyakara class.

‡ It is a S'irá-Marma, half a finger in length and of the Vaikalyakara group.

‖ It is a S'irá-Marma, half a finger in length and of the Vaikalyakara group.

¶ It is a Snàyu-Marma to the length of one finger and of the Vaikalyakara group.

occur in the place of the Gulpha, Jánu and Vitapa Marmas respectively. As the Vitapa-Marma is situated between the scrotum and the Vankshana (inguinal region), so the Kakshadhara-Marma is situated between the Vaksha (chest) and the Kaksha (armpit). An injury to these causes supervening symptoms. An injury to the Manivandha-Marma (wrist-marma) results specially in inoperativeness (Kuntha) of the affected hand ; an injury to the Kurpara-Marma ends in dangling (Kuni) of the hand ; and an injury to the Kakshadhara results in hemiplegia. Thus the forty-four Marmas of the upper and the lower extremities have been described. 43-46.

**Marmas on the Thorax etc. :**—Now we shall describe the Marmas, situated in the region of the thorax and the abdomen (trunk). A hurt to the **Guda-Marma**\*, which is attached to the large intestine and serves as the passage of stool and flatus, ends fatally (within twenty-four hours of the hurt). An injury to the **Vasti-Marma**,† situated inside the cavity of the pelvic region and the bladder and composed of small muscles and blood (and which serves as the receptacle of urine), proves fatal within the day, except in the cases of extracting the gravel, only when the injury to the organ is short of complete perforation of both of its walls. The urine oozes out through the aperture in the case where only one of its walls has been perforated, and which may be closed and healed up with proper and judicious medical treatment. An injury to the

---

\* It is a Mânsa-Marma to the length of four fingers' width and belongs to the Sadyo-mâraka class.

† It is a ligament combination (Snáyu-marma) to the length of four fingers, belonging to the Sadyah-Pránhara class.

Nabhi-Marma,* the root of all the Sirâs and situated between the Ámâsaya (stomach) and the Pakvâsaya (intestines) ends in death within the day. 47-50.

A hurt to the **Hridaya-Marma**,† which is situated in the thorax between the two breasts and above the pit of the Ámâsaya and forms the seat of the qualities of Sattva, Rajas and Tamas, proves fatal within the day. An injury to the **Stana-mula-Marmas**,‡ situated immediately below each of the breasts and about two fingers in width fills the Koshtha (thorax) with deranged Kapha, brings on cough, difficult breathing (asthma) and proves fatal. An injury to any of the **Stana-Rohita-Marmas**,§ situated above the nipples of the breasts about two fingers in width, fills the cavity of the Koshtha (thorax) with blood, producing symptoms of cough and asthma, and ends fatally. An injury to the **Apalápa-Marmas**,∥ situated below the Ansa-kuta (balls of the shoulders) and above the sides (meeting of the different branches of the sub-clavicle veins *i.e.* axilla), transforms the blood of the organism into pus and proves fatal thereby. 51-54.

An injury to any of the Vàyu-carrying vessels, known as the **Apastambha-Marma**¶ (meeting of the bifurcated branches of the bronchi lying on both the sides

---

\* It is a S'irá-Marma to the length of four fingers, belonging to the Sadyah-Pránahara class.

† It is a S'irá-Marma to the length of four fingers and of the Sadyah-Pránahara class.

‡ It is a S'irá-Marma, two fingers in length and of the Kálántara class.

§ It is a Mánsa-Marma about half a finger in length and of the Kálántara class. (according to Vgabhata, of the Sadyo-Máraka class).

∥ It is a S'irá-Marma, half a finger in length, and of the Kálántara class.

¶ It is a S'irá-Marma, half a finger in length and belongs to the Kálántara class.

of the breast), fills the Koshtha with the deranged Vâyu (tympanites) accomapanied by cough and dyspepsia, and terminates in death. Thus the twelve Marmas situated in the **thorax** and **abdomen** are described. 55-56.

**Prishtha Marmas :**—Now we shall discourse on the Marmas in the back (of a man). An injury to any of the **Katika-tarunas*** (sacro-iliac articulation), situated in the region of the S'roni (sacrum) on both sides of the spinal column, gives rise to an excessive hæmorrhage and consequent pallor and ends in death. A hurt to any of the **Kukundara Marmas** † (lit :—a hollow—the great sacro-sciatic notch), situated on both sides of the spinal column and in the region slightly below the waist (in the loins), results in complete anæsthesia and inoperativeness of the lower extremities A hurt to the **Nitamva-Marmas**,‡ attached to the side above the Sroni (pelvis) and attached inside to the muscles of the waists, gives rise to Sosha (atrophia) in the lower extremities, weakness and ultimately brings on death. An injury to the **Pârśva-Sandhi-Marmas** § (cælic axes) which are situated just at the middle below the extremities of the sides (Pârśva) and which lies attached at the middle between the loins at their lower regions, feels the Koshtha (abdomen) with the blood and results into death A hurt to the **Vrihati-Marmas** ‖

---

\* It is an Asthi-Marma, half a finger in length and of the Kálántara-máraka class.

† They are Joint-marmas (Sandhi), half a finger in length and of the Vaikalyakara group.

‡ It is a bone Marma, half a finger in length, and of the Kálántara class.

§ It is a S'irá-Marma to the length of half a finger and belongs to the Kálántara class.

‖ They are S'irá-Marmas (arterial anestomsis) to the lengt of half a finger and belong to the Kálántara class.

which commencing from the roots of the breast course round both the sides of the spinal column (Pristha-vamśa), cause excessive bleeding, and the patient dies, as supervening symptoms arise from an excessive loss of blood. An injury to any of the two **Amsa-phalaka-Marmas**\* situated on either side of the vertebral column and connected with the scapula brings on anesthesia or atrophy (Sosha) of the arms. There are two Marmas known as **Amsa-Marmas**† which are situated on either side midway between the neck and the head of the arms and connect the Amsa-Pitha (glenoid cavity) and the Skandha (shoulder). An injury to any of these Marmas is attended with an incapacity of moving the hands. Thus the fourteen Marmas in the back have been described. 57-65.

**The Jatrugata-Marmas :**—Now we shall describe the Marmas which are situated in the regions above the clavicles (Urddhva-Jatru). There are four Dhamani (arteries) about the two sides of the Kantha-Nádi (wind-pipe). Two of them are known as **Nilá**, and the other two as **Manyá**. One Nilá and one Manyá are situated on either side of the larynx, (i.e, anterior and posterior side of the larynx). An injury to any of them produces dumbness, and change of voice (hoarseness), and also the loss of the faculty of taste. ‡ An injury to any of the eight Sirás (arteries), four being on each side of the neck (Grivá), and known as **Sirá-Mátrika-Marmas** §) ends fatally within the day. 65-69.

\* It is an Asthi-Marma, half a finger in length and is Vaikalyakara.

† They are Snáyu-Marmas, half a finger in length and of the Vaikalyakara class.

‡ They are S'irá-Marmas, to the lengrh of four fingers and of the Vaikalyakara class.

§ They are S'irá-Marmas, four fingers in length and of the Sadyo-Máran class.

An injury to any of the two Marmas lying at the junction of the head and neck (Grivá) and known as **Krikátiká*** (transverse process of the arch of the atlas) results in a free movement of the head. A hurt to any of the Marmas attached to the lower end of an ear (posterior extrensic ligament) and known as the **Vidhura†** Marma results in the loss of hearing. An injury to the **Phana-Marmas‡** attached to the interior channels of both the nostrils, results in the loss of the faculty of smell. An injury to the **Apánga-Marmas §** (Anastomosis of the infra-orbital artery) situated below the tips of the eye-brows and about the external corners of the eyes, brings on blindness or defective vision. An injury to the **Ávarta-Marmas ‖** situated above and below the eye-brows, brings on blindness and impaired vision. An injury to the **Śankha-Marmas ¶** (meeting or suture of the temporal, frontal and sphenoid bones—*Pterion*), situated over the tips of the eye-brows and between the ears and the forehead, results in death within the day. The Marmas situated over the two temples (Śankha) and at the border of the hair (sculp) are called **Utkshepa-Marma** (meeting of the posterior and anterior temporal arteries)$. An extraction of a shaft (Śalya) or of any

---

\* They are Sandhi-Marmas, half a finger in length, and of the Vaikalyakara group.

† It is a S'náyu-Marma, and is of the Vaikalyakara class.

‡ They are S'irá-Marmas to the length of half a finger and of the Vaikalyakara class.

§ They are S'irá-Marmas to the length of half a finger and of the Vaikalyakara class.

‖ They are Sandhi-Marmas, to the length of half a finger and of the Vaikalyakara class.

¶ They are Asthi-Marmas to the length of half a finger.

$ They are S'náyu-Marmas, half a finger in length and of the Vis'alyaghna class.

extraneous pointed thing lodged into these Marmas, results in the death of the patient, who, on the contrary, lives as long as the shaft is allowed to remain inside or if the shaft comes out itself (after putrefaction). 70-75.

An injury to the **Sthapani-Marma**\* (nasal arch of the frontal veins), situated in the middle of the eyebrows, ends in the manner of the preceding one. An injury to any of the five joints of the head which are known as the **Simanta-Marmas**†, results in fear, insensibility and madness of the patient and terminates in death. An injury to any of the four **Sringátaka-Marmas**‡ which forms the junction of the four S'irás (nerves), (branches of the facial artery) and soothes the nose, the eyes, the ears and the tongue, proves fatal within the day. An injury to the **Adhipati-Marmas** § (the vertical groove on the frontal bone) which is marked in the inner side of the roof of the cranium by the S'irá-Sannipáta (superior longitudinal sinus), and on the exterior side by the ringlet of the hair (Romávarta) proves fatal within the day. Thus we have described the thirty-seven Marmas, situated in the region above the **clavicles** (Urddhva-Jatru). 76-80.

**Memorable Verses :**—An incision should be made at the spot a finger's width remote from the Urvi, Kurchcha-S'irá, Vitapa, Kaksha and a Párs'va-Marma ; whereas, a clear space of two fingers should

---

\* They are S'irá-Marmas to the length of half a finger and of the Visályaghna class.

† They are Sandhi-Marmas to the length of four fingers and of the Kálántara-Pránahara class.

‡ They are S'irá-Marmas to the length of four fingers and of the Sadyah-Pránahara class.

§ It is a Sandhi-Marma, half a finger in length and of the Sadyah-Pránahara class.

be avoided from its situation in making any incision about the Stanamula, Manivandha or Gulpha-Marma. Similarly a space of three fingers should be avoided from the Hridaya, Vasti, Kurchcha, Guda or Nábhi Marma ; and a space of four fingers should be avoided in respect of the four Śringátakas, five Simantas and ten Marmas in the neck (Nilá etc.) ; a space of half a finger being the rule in respect of the remaining (fifty-six).* Men, versed in the science of surgery, have laid down the rule that, in a case of surgical operation, the situation and dimension of each local Marma should be first taken into account and the incision should be made in a way so as not to affect that particular Marma, inasmuch as an incision, even extending or affecting, in the least, the edge or the side of the Marma, may prove fatal. Hence all the Marma-Sthánas should be carefully avoided in a surgical operation. 81.

The amputation of a hand or a leg may not prove fatal whereas a wound in any of the Marmas situated therein is sure to bring on death. The vessels become contracted in the case of a cut in the leg or in the hand of a man, and hence the incidental bleeding is comparatively scantier. Therefore it is that a cut in any of these parts of the body, however painful, does not necessarily prove fatal, like the lopping off of the branches of a tree. On the contrary, a man pierced into in any such Marmas, as the Kshipra or the Tala, suffers from excessive

---

* Some are of opinion that a surgical operation (in the case of the remaining fifty-six) should be made, leaving a space equal in measurement to the dimensions of a palm (from the affected part). Gayádása, having learnt from Bhoja, explains that a space of two fingers should be left (from the affected part) in making surgical operations of the ten marmas, namely, the two Gulphas, the roots of the two breasts, the four Indravastis, and the two Manivandhas.

hæmorrhage (from the affected part) and attended with an excruciating pain, owing to the derangement of the Váyu, and meets his doom like a tree whose roots have been severed. Hence, in a case of piercing or of injury to any of these Marmas, the hand or the leg should be immediately amputated at the wrist or at the ankle (respectively). 82.

The medical authorities have described the Marmas to have covered half in the scope of Śalya Tantra (Surgery), inasmuch as a person hurt in any of the Marmas dies presently (i. e., within seven days of the hurt). A deformity of the organ is sure to result from an injury to one of these Marmas, even if death be averted by a course of judicious and skillful medical treatment. 83.

The life of the patient is not to be despaired of even in the case of fracture or crushing of a bone of the Koshtha, Śirah and Kapála or perforation of the intestines etc, if the local Marmas are found not to be in any way hurt or affected. Recovery is common in cases of cuts (pierce) in the Sakthi, Bhuja, Páda and Kara or in any other part of the body and even where a whole leg or hand is found to be severed and carried away if the Marmas are not in any way hurt or affected. 84.

These Marmas form the primary seats of the Váyu, the Soma (lunar) and Tejas (fiery principles of the organism), as well as of the three fundamental qualities of Satva, Rajas and Tamas, and that is the reason why a man, hurt in any of the Marmas, does not live. 85.

An injury to a Marma of the Sadyah-Pránahara class (in which death occurs within a day) is attended with the imperfection of the sense organs, loss of consciousness, bewilderment of Manah (mind) and Buddhi (intellect) and various kinds of pain. An injury to a Marma of the Kálántara group (of a person) is sure to be attended with the loss of Dhátus (blood etc.) and various kinds of supervening symptoms (Upadrava) which end in death. The body of a person, hurt in any of the Vaikalyakara Marmas, may remain operative only under a skillful medical treatment; but a deformity of the affected organ is inevitable. An injury to any of the Vis'alyaghna Marmas ends in death for the reasons mentioned above. An injury to any of the Rujákara Marmas gives rise to various kinds of pain in the affected organ, which may ultimately bring about a deformity of the same, if placed under the treatment of an ignorant and unskillful Vaidya (Surgeon). 86.

An injury to the adjacent part of a Marma, whether incidental to a cut, incision, blow (Abhigháta), burn, puncture, or to any other cause exhibits the same series of symptoms as an actually affected one. An injury to a Marma, whether it be severe or slight, is sure to bring deformity or death.* 87.

The diseases which are seated in the Marmas, are generally serious, but they may be made to prove amenable with the greatest care and difficulty. 88-89.

* Gayádása does not read this verse.

Thus ends the sixth Chapter of the S'árira Sthánam in the Sus'ruta Samhitá, which treats of Marmas.

# CHAPTER VII.

Now we shall discourse on the Sáriram which treats of the description and classification of Sirá or vascular system * ( **Sirá-Varnana-Vibhaktináma Sáriram).**

There are seven hundred Sirás (vessels) in the human organism (except those which cannot be counted for their extremely attenuated size). The vessels (Sirás) by their contractibility and expansibility &c, sustain and nourish the organism in the same manner as streamlets and canals serve to keep a field or a garden moist and fruitful. From the principal or central trunk hundreds of small and minute vessels branch off and spread all over the body, just as small or minute fibres are found to emanate from the large central vein of the leaf of a plant. They originate from the umbilical region and thence they spread all over the body upwards and downwards and obliquely.  2.

**Memorable Verses :**—All the Sirás (vessels) that are found in the organisms of created beings, originate from the umbilical region (Nábhi)† and thence they spread all over their bodies. The life of an organic animal is seated in the vessels surrounding its navel which forms their starting point. The navel in its turn rests on or is attached to the Pránas (the life-carrying vessels—nerves attached to it) in the same

---

* The Sanskrita term S'irá denotes Veins, nerves, arteries and lymphatic Vessels as well. Some read *S'irá-Varna* (different colours of the Sirás) in lieu of S'irá-Varnana (description of S'irás).

† Most probably the idea is derived from the appearance of the S'irás in their foetal state.

manner as the nave of a wheel supports the spokes, and the spokes in their turn support the nave. 3-4.

**Principal Śirás:**—Of these Śirás (vessels), forty are principal ones, of which ten are Váyu-carrying Sirás (**nerves**), ten are Pitta-carrying Śirás (**veins**), ten convey Kapha (**lymphatic vessels?**) and ten are blood-carrying Śirás (**arteries**). Of these the Váyu-carrying Śirás, situated in the specific receptacle of that bodily principle (Váta), are again found to branch out in one hundred and seventy five smaller branches (ramifications). Similarly, each of the remaining Pitta-carrying, Kapha-carrying and blood-carrying vessels (Śirás) situated in their specific receptacles, (*i e*, in the receptacles of Pitta, Kapha and spleen and liver respectively) are found to branch out in as many numbers (one hundred and seventy-five),—thus making a total of seven hundred in all. 5.

**Their Specific Locations:**— There are twenty-five Váyu-carrying Śirás (nerves) in one leg and the same count applies to the other. Similarly there are twenty five Váyu-carrying Śirás (vessels) in each of the hands. There are thirty-four Váyu-carrying vessels in the Koshtha (trunk); of these eight occur in the pelvic regions attached with the anus and the penis; two in each of the sides, six in the back, six in the Udara (cavity of the abdomen), and ten in the region of the chest. There are forty-one Váyu-carrying Śirá's (vessels) situated in the region above the clavicles. Of these fourteen occur in the neck; four in the two ears; nine in the tongue; six in the nose and eight in the two eyes. Thus we have finished the description of the one hundred and seventy-five Śirás that carry Váyu. 6.

What has been said of these Váyu-carrying vessels (Śirás) will also hold good to the rest (in blood-carrying,

Pitta-carrying and Kapha-carrying channels in the respective regions of the body), with the exception that in these three cases, ( Pitta, Kapha and blood ) ten occur in the eyes and two in the ears in lieu of eight and four respectively, as in the case of Váyu-carrying Sirás (vessels). Thus we have described the seven hundred Sirás with their branches. 7.

**Memorable Verses**—The Váyu-carrying Sirás :—The Váyu in its normal state and coursing through its specific Sirás (vessels) helps the unobstructed performance of its specific functions *viz*., expansion, contraction, speech, &c., and produces the clearness and non-illusiveness of Buddhi ( intellect ) and the sense-organs, whereas a coursing of the said Váyu in a deranged condition through the aforesaid Sirás (vessels), gives rise to a host of such diseases as are due to the derangement of Váyu. 8.

**The Pitta-carrying Sirás :**—The Pitta in its normal state and coursing through its specific Sirás (vessels) produces the healthy glow of complexion, relish for food, kindling of the appetite, healthfulness and other good effects, characteristic of the Pitta, which however being aggravated and coursing through them gives rise to a host of Pittaja diseases. 9.

**The Kapha-conveying Sirás :**—The Kapha in its normal state and coursing through its specific Sirás (vessels) smoothes and contributes to the firmness of the limbs and joints, improves the strength and produces all other good effects specially belonging to it, whereas the same Kapha, flowing through them in an aggravated condition, ushers in a large number of the Kaphaja distempers of the body. 10.

**The Rakta-carrying Sirás :**—The blood in its normal state and flowing through its specific Sirás (vessels) strengthens the other fundamental principles (Dhátus) of the body, improves the complexion, aids the organ of touch in the proper performance of its functions and produces other functions characteristic of it in the body. Flowing through them in a vitiated condition, it begets diseases which are due to the derangement of the blood. 11.

There is not a single Sirá (vessel) in the body which carries either the Váyu, or the Pitta or the Kapha alone. Hence each of the vessels should be regarded as affording an opportunity for conveying all kinds of the Doshas of the body, for as soon as they are deranged and aggravated they seem to flow through all the Sirás promiscuously Hence they are called **Sarvavahah.** 12.

**Specific colours of the Sirás:**—The vessels which carry the bodily Váyu (nerves) have a vermilion (yellowish red) hue and seem to be stuffed with Váyu. The Pitta-carrying vessels (veins) are coloured blue and felt warm to the touch. The Kapha-carrying vessels are hard, cold to the touch and white-coloured. The blood-carrying vessels (arteries) are red and neither too hot, nor too cold. 13.

Now we shall describe the Sirás (veins) which a surgeon should not pierce or open, inasmuch as it may result in death, or bodily deformity. An intelligent surgeon shall always bear in mind that sixteen out of the four hundred vessels in the extremeties, thirty-two out of the hundred and thirty-six vessels in the trunk and fifty out of the sixty-four vessels in the region above the clavicles, should not be opened or bled on any account. 14-15.

Of the one hundred vessels in a single leg, the one Jáladhará (which is attached to the connective tissue of the Kurchcha-Śirah) as well as the three internal ones, of which two are known as the Urvi-veins and the other as the Lohitáksha, together with the corresponding ones in the other leg and in the two hands, thus making sixteen in all, which are situated in the upper and lower extremeties, should be held unfit for opening. Of the thirty-two veins in the pelvic region (Śroni), eight such, known as the four) Vitapas (two on each side of the testicles) and the four known as the Katika-tarun as (two on each side) should be considered unfit for bleeding or opening. Of the sixteen veins (eight on each side) at the sides, the one which courses upward from each of the two sides and is attached to the Marma known as the **Párśva-Sandh**i, should be considered unfit for similar purposes. Of the twenty-four Śirás which are found in either side of the spinal column, an incision should not be made into any of the two Śirás (on each side) known as the Vrihati and which run upward along either side of it (spinal column). Similarly of the twenty-four Śirás in the abdomen, the two along each of the two sides of symphis pubis should be held unfit for opening or bleeding Of the forty veins in the chest, the two in the heart, two in the root of each breast and two in each of the Stana-rohita (muscle of the breast) and one in each of the Apastambhas and Apalápas, making fourteen in all, should not be opened. Thus thirty-two Śirás in the regions of the back (i e, the sides and the pelvic regions), the abdomen and the chest should be regarded as unfit for opening or other surgical purposes. 16—21.

There are one hundred and sixty-four Śirás in the region above the clavicles. Of these the eight and four (making twelve and respectively known as the eight Mátrikás, the two Nilás and the two Manyás) out of the fifty-six in the neck and the throat, should be regarded as unfit for opening. Similarly the two veins in the two Krikátikás and two in the two Vidhuras, should be held unfit for similar purposes; thus making sixteen in all in the neck. Of the sixteen vessels (eight on each side) of the Hanus (Jaws), the two Sirás about each of the joint of the jaw-bones should never be opened. 22.

Of the thirty-six* vessels in the tongue, sixteen are situated in the under-surface of that organ and twenty in the upper surface; of these the two speech-carrying and the two taste-carrying ones should be held unfit for venesection. Of the twenty-four vessels in the nose, the four adjacent to the nose proper and the one running into the soft palate should be held unfit for similar purposes. Of the thirty-eight vessels in the two eyes, the one situated at each Apánga should not be opened. Of the ten vessels in the two ears, the sound-carrying one in either ear should not be opened. Of the sixty vessels of the nose and eyes coursing through the region of the forehead, the four vessels adjacent to the sculp proper and the Ávarta-Marma should be held unfit for opening or bleeding. One vessel (Sirá) in each of the two Ávartas and the one in the Sthapani-marma should not be opened (on any account). Of the ten vessels in the temple, the one about each temple-joint should be held unfit for opening or bleeding. Of the twelve vessels in the head, the one

---

*Gayí asserts that there are eight each of the Váyu-carrying, Pitta-carrying, Kapha-carrying and blood-carrying S'irás in the region of the neck, thus making a total of 32 in place of 36 of the text.

He also holds that there are 28 in place of 36 S'irás in the tongue, 16 in place of 24 in the nose, 24 in place of 38 in the eyes, 16 in place of 10 in the ears and 8 in place of 10 in the temple. In the counting of the S'irás situate in the other parts of the body, he, however, does not differ from the text.

in each of the two Utkshepa-Marmas, one in each of the (five) Simanta-Marmas and one in the Adhipati-Marma, should be held unfit for the purpose. No incision or opening should be made into any of these fifty vessels situated in the region above the clavicles. 23–31.

**Memorable verses :**—As the stem and leaves etc, of a lotus plant, originated from its bulb, spread over the whole surface of a pool or tank (lit: water), so the vessels emanating from the umbilicus of a man spread over his whole organism. 32.

Thus ends the seventh Chapter of the S'árira Sthánam in the Sus ruta Samhitá which treats of the description and classification of S'irás (Vessels).

# CHAPTER VIII.

Now we shall discourse on the Sáriram which treats of the method of Venesection etc. **(Sirá-Vyadha-Vidhi-Sáriram).** 1.

**Persons unfit for Venesection:**—The vessel or vessels (Sirá) of an infant, an old man, a perched man, one fatigued and emaciated with endocarditis (Kshata-kshina), a person of timid or coward disposition, a person used up with excessive drinking or sexual enjoyments or tired with the troubles of long journey, an intoxicated person, a patient who has been treated with purgatives, emetics or with Anubásana and Ásthápana measures (enemas), a man who has passed a sleepless night, an impotent (Kliva) or emaciated person, an enceinte, or one afflicted with cough, asthma, high fever, phthisis convulsions, paralysis, thirst, epilepsy, or effects of fasting, should not be pierced or opened. Incisions should not be made into those veins (Sirás) which are not fit for opening, or into the fit ones, if invisible; it should be the same with those which cannot be properly ligatured or even if ligatured cannot be raised up. 2.

Diseases which are amenable to acts of venesection have been described before (Sonita-Varnaniya-Adhyáya). Venesection may be performed in the said diseases as well as in those which have not been enumerated in connection with them and also in other cases whether suppurated or unsuppurated, if such a proceeding is deemed necessary and after the application of Sneha and Sveda. Venesection should be made even in the cases declared unfit for it (such as in an infant etc.) in cases of blood-poisoning (such as snake-bite etc.) and in fatal diseases (Vidradhi etc.). 3-4.

**Preliminary rules :**—The patient should be duly fomented (Sveda) and anointed (Sneha) with oily preparations. A liquid* food or diet consisting of articles which are antidotal to the bodily principles (Doshas) which engendered the disease or Yavágu (gruel) should be given to him at first. Then at the proper season (i.e., not in the rainy or winter season etc.) the patient should be brought near the surgeon and made to sit or lie down and the part to be incised upon should be bound, neither too loosely (*e g*, in the extremities etc.) nor too tightly (*e.g.*, in the head etc.), with any of the accessories, such as cloth, linen, skin, the inner fibres of a bark, creepers etc., so as not to create any pain or agitation in his mind. Then the vein should be duly opened with proper instrument (and with a careful regard to the situation of any local Marma). 5

**Metrical text :**—Venesection should not be performed in an extremely cold or hot, cloudy or windy day. It is forbidden to open a vein without necessity or in a healthy person, or in a disease in which such as a proceeding is absolutely prohibited. 6.

**The Yantra-Vidhi :**—The patient whose vein is to be operated upon should be seated on a stool to the height of an Aratni (distance of the elbow from the tip of the small finger) with his face turned towards the sun. He should keep his legs in a drawn up or contracted posture resting his elbows (Kurpara) on his knee-joints and the hands with his two thumbs closed in his fists placed on (the upper ends of) his Manyás (sterno mastoid muscles), Then having cast the binding

---

* A liquid food is recommended for the purpose of liquefying the blood so as to bleed easily.

linen on the two closed fists thus placed on the neck, the surgeon should ask another man from the back side of the patient to take hold of the two ends of the cloth with his left hand having the palm turned upward, and then ask him to tie up with his right hand the bandage round the part, neither too diffusely nor too tightly nor too loosely, so as to raise the vein and to press the bandage round the back for a good out-flow of blood. Then he (surgeon) should perform the operation in the desired spot, the patient having been previously asked to sit with his mouth full of air (*i.e.*, he should confine his breathing till the surgical operation is completed). This proceeding should be adopted in opening any vein of the head, save those which are situated in the cavity of the mouth. 7.

In the case of opening a vein (Sirá) in the **leg**, the affected leg should be placed on a level ground, while the other leg should be held in a somewhat contracted posture, at a little higher place. The affected leg should be bound with a piece of linen below its knee-joint and pressed with the hands down to the ankle. A ligature of the above kind should then be tied four fingers above the region to be incised upon, after which the vein should be opened. 8.

In the case of opening a vein (Sirá) in the arms, the patient should be caused to sit easily and fixedly with his two thumbs closed in his fists (as above). A ligature of the above-mentioned kind (rope etc.,) should be tied (four fingers above the part to be incised upon and the vein opened in the aforesaid manner. The knee-joint and the elbow should be held in a contracted or drawn up posture at the time of opening a vein in a case of Gridhrasi (Sciatica) and Visvachi, respectively. The patient should hold his back raised up and expanded and his head (and shoulders) bent down at the time of opening a vein in the back, shoulders and the Sroni (hips). He should hold his head thrust back and his chest and body expanded at the time of opening a vein in the chest or in the abdomen. 9-12.

He shall embrace his own body with his arms at the time of opening a vein in his sides. The penis should be drawn downward (*i.e.*, in an flaccid state) on a similar occasion in that region. The tongue should be raised up to the roof of the mouth and its fore-part supported by the teeth at the time of opening a vein in its under-surface. The patient should be told to keep his mouth fully open at the time of opening a vein in the gums or in the palate. Similarly a Surgeon should devise proper and adequate means for the purpose of raising up (distinct appearance of) a S'irá (vein) and determine the nature of the bandage to be used therein according to the exigencies (*i.e.*, the health and the kind of diseases of the patient), of each case. 13-17.

An incision to the depth of a barley-corn should be made with a Vrihimukha instrument (into a vein situated) in the muscular parts of the body, whereas the instrument should be thrust only half that depth or to the depth of a *Vrihi* seed in other places (Vrihi here signifies S'ukadhánya as well as Rakta-s'áli). An incision over a bone should be made with the Kuthárika (small surgical axe) to the half depth of a barley-corn. 18-19.

**Memorable Verses :**—An opening should be effected in such a day in the rainy season as would be devoid of the rumblings of a thunder-cloud, during the cold (*i.e.*, in the fourth) part of the day in summer, and at noon in the winter season (Hemanta). These are the only three times of opening a vein. A well and successfully pierced vein bleeds in streams (almost simultaneously with the thrusting of the knife) and spontaneously stops after a Muhurta (a little while). The vitiated blood is seen first to flow out of an opened vein, like the drop of yellow pigment first coming out of a *Kusumbha* flower. Blood does not flow out from an incision made into a vein of an unconscious (Murchchhita), much frightened, or a thirsty patient. An incision of a vein without proper bandaging and raising up is attended with a similar result. 20-23.

A weak person, or one affected with the unusual derangement of the bodily Doshas etc., or one fainted (under operation), should not be subjected to a measure of continuous blood-letting at a time; instead of that, the vein should be opened afresh in the same afternoon or on the following day, or on the third day (as the exigency requires). An intelligent surgeon should not allow the flow of blood to an excess but should stop the flow even with a remnant of the diseased blood in the system and administer soothing internal remedies (Samsamana) for the purification of the diseased remnant. Bleeding to the quantity of a Prastha* measure should be deemed sufficient for a strong and adult patient, stuffed with a large quantity of the deranged Doshas (in the body). 24-26.

The vein should be incised with a Vrihimukha instrument at a distance of two fingers above the seat of the Kshipra-marma in such diseases as Pádadáha, Páda-harsha, Ava-váhuka, Chippa, Visarpa, Váta-rakta, Váta-kantaka, Vicharchiká, Pádadári etc. The mode of opening a vein in the case of Slipada (Elephantiasis)

---

* In medicinal preparations, a Prastha measure is understood to be four seers in the case of liquids, but in cases of excreta due to emetic and purgative measures and of **blood-letting**, a Prastha is meant to be thirteen Palas and a half only.

would be described under the treatment of that disease. In Váta-rogas, such as Kroshtuka-s'irah (Synovites), maimedness (Pangu) and lameness (Khanja), the Sirá (vein) of the Janghá (lower leg-calf), four fingers above the Gulpha, should be opened In cases of Apachi (scrofula), the vein should be opened simultaneously with the appearance of the disease two fingers below the Indravasti-marma. In a case of Gridhrasi (sciatica), the vein should be opened four fingers above or below the Jánu (knee-joint). In a case of goitre, the veins attached to the roots of the Uru (thighs) should be opened. The instructions regarding the opening of a vein in one leg shall hold good in the case of that in the other, as well as in cases of those situated in the two upper extremities (hands), but the speciality is that in a case of enlarged spleen, the vein near the Kurpara-sandhi (elbow-joint) of the left hand or that inside the fourth and the fifth fingers should be opened. Similarly in a case of Yakriddályodara or Kaphodara, the corresponding vein in the right hand should be opened. Several authorities advise the opening of the same vein in cases of cough and asthma* due to the action of the deranged Kapha. 27-35.

In a case of Vis'vachi, the same argument holds good (four fingers above or below the Kurpara-sandhi) as in a case of Gridhrasi. In a case of Pravahiká (diarrhœa) attended with S'ula (colic), the vein within two fingers width around of the Pelvis (S'roni) should be opened. The vein of the penis should be opened in a case of Parikartiká (D R.-Parivartiká), Upadans'a, S'uka-dosha and seminal disorders  The vein on either side of

---

\* Gayi holds that in cases of asthma and cough venesection should be had recourse to only when they are in a mild form.

the scrotum should be opened in a case of hydrocele (Mutra-Vriddhi). 36-39.

The vein four fingers below the navel and on the left side of the Sevani (suture) should be opened in a case of Dakodara (ascites). In a case of internal abscess and colic in the sides (Pleurodynia), the vein in the region between the breast and the left armpit should be opened. Several authorities assert that in a case of Avaváhuka and Váhus'osha (atrophy of the hand), the vein between the Amsas (shoulders) should be opened. In a case of *Tritiyaka* (Tertian) fever, the vein inside the Trika-Sandhi should be opened In a case of *Chaturthaka* fever, a vein joined with either side of and below the shoulder-joint should be opened. In a case of Apasmára, the middle vein adjacent to the joint of the jaw-bones (Hanu-Sandhi) should be opened. In a case of insanity and hysteria\* (Apasmàra), the vein between the temple and the edge of the sculp or those in the Apánga (tips of the eyes), the forehead or the chest should be opened. In cases of the diseases of the tongue and the teeth, the veins on the under-surface (Adho-Jihvá) of the tongue should be opened. In the case of a disease of the palate, the local vein should be opened. In diseases of the ears and specially in a case of inflammatory ear-ache (Karna-S'ula), the vein along the region above the ears should be opened. In diseases of the nose and specially in a case of the loss of the smelling faculty, the vein at the tip of the nose should be opened. In cases of eye-diseases, such as

---

\* Dallana, however, differs here from the text. He says, on the authority of Vágbhata, that the opening of a vein between the temple and the edge of the sculp or those in the Apánga, the forehead and the chest should be recommended in cases of insanity only, and not in the case of of Apasmára as well (as in the text).

Timira (blindness), Akshipáka (ophthalmia) etc., as well as in diseases of the head and in Adhimantha, the veins about the nose, the forehead and the Apánga (the outer canthus of the eyes), should be opened. 40-51.

**Defective Venesection :**—Now we shall describe the twenty kinds of defects relating to an opened vein (Dushta-vyadhana). They are as follows :—Durviddhá, Atividdhá, Kunchitá, Pichchitá, Kuttitá, Aprasrutá, Atyudirná, Ante-abhihatá, Parisushká, Kunitá, Vepitá, Anutthita-viddhá, Sastrahatá, Tiryag-viddhá, Apaviddhá, Avyádhyá, Vidrutá, Dhenuká, Punhpunarviddhá and Marmaviddhá, i.e., incised about the Sirá-marma, the Snáyu-marma, the Asthi-marma and the Sandhi-marma  52-53.

**Their definitions :**—The vein in which an act of venesection is unattended with a satisfactory outflow of blood owing to its being incised with an extremely slender instrument and is marked by an extremely painful swelling in consequence thereof, is called **Durviddhá** (badly incised). The vein in which the incision becomes excessive and no blood comes out properly or enters an internal channel owing to the largeness of the incision, is called **Atividdhá** (over-incised). An opened vein in which the incision has been made in a curving manner and is attended with the foregoing results, is called **Kunchitá** (crooked or contracted). An incised vein presenting a flattened or thrashed appearance on account of its being opened with a blunt knife (Kantha-Sastra) is called **Pichchitá** (thrashed). The vein at the sides of which incisions have been successively made, instead of in its body, is called **Kuttitá** (lacerated) An incised vein, unattended with any bleeding owing to the patient's fright, coldness or loss of consciousness, is called **Aprasrutá** (unbleeding).

A vein with a large incision in its body made with a sharp and flat-edged instrument, is called **Atyudirna** (improperly wide-incised). An opened vein in which blood oozes out in small quantity is called **Ante-abhihata** (struck in the interior). An opened vein in an anæmic patient (marked by a total absence of bleeding and) stuffed with Váyu (lit., as if the flow has been dried up by the Váyu), is called **Parisushka** (dried up). A vein opened but to a quarter part of the proper length and attended with a scanty outflow of blood, is called **Kunita** (partially incised). A vein which trembles owing to its being bandaged at a wrong place and from which blood does not flow out in consequence, is called **Vepita** (quivering). A vein incised without being previously properly raised up and attended with a similar result (i e., absence of blood), is called **Anutthita-viddha**. A vein cut into two and attended with excessive bleeding and inoperativeness of the organ is called **Sastrahata** (knife-cut). A vein incised with an instrument applied slantingly and (consequently) not fully opened, is called **Tiryag-viddha** (obliquely incised). A vein incised several times and (every time) with an improper instrument, is called **Apaviddha** (wrongly incised) A vein unfit for opening (*i.e.*, whose opening has been forbidden in the Sástras), is called **Avyadhya** (unfit for opening). A vein opened carelessly and hastily is called **Vidruta** (erratic). A vein bleeding continuously owing to its being repeatedly pressed and successively opened, is called **Dhenuka**. A vein variously cut owing to its being pierced into the same part with an extremely slender-pointed instrument, is called **Punah-punarvidaha** (repeatedly incised). If a vein in the Snáyu-marmas, the Asthi-marmas, the Sirá-marmas or the Sandhi-marmas be opened, it is called **Marma-viddhá** and in such cases severe pain, emaciation (Sosha) deformity or (even) death may be the result. 54.

**Memorable Verses :**—Practice (even) does not give the necessary skill in surgical operation of the veins etc., as they are naturally unsteady and changing like fishes. Hence a vein should be opened with the greatest care. An opening into the body, made by an ignorant and unskilful surgeon, is attended with the aforesaid dangers and many other distressing symptoms. An act of venesection, properly performed, gives more speedy relief than that derived from the application of medicated oil &c , or of plaster as well. Venesection (bleeding) properly performed is half of the treatment described in surgery like the application of Vasti-karmas (enematic measures) in therapeutics. 55.

A man medically anointed (Sneha-karma), diaphorised (Sveda), vomited (Vamana), purged (Virechana), or treated with both the Vasti-karmas (Anuvásana and Ásthápana) or bled shall forego anger, physical labour, sexual intercourse, sleep in the day time, excessive talking, physical exercises, riding or driving etc., sitting on his haunches, frequent ramblings, exposure to cold, winds and the sun, hardly digestible, uncongenial and incompatible food until the strength is perfectly restored or, according to some authorities, for a month. These subjects will be fully dealt with later on Áturopa-drava-chikitsá, ch.—39). 56.

**Memorable Verses :**—The vitiated blood incarcerated in any part of the body should be abstracted therefrom by scarifying it, by cupping it with a Sirá (pipe), a horn, a gourd, or leeches, or by the opening of a vein respectively, according to the density of the blood. (Others assert that) leeches should be applied in the case of the (vitiated) blood being confined deep into the body, scarification with a surgical instrument should be made in the case of clotted blood, with a pipe in the case of extensive vitiation of the blood throughout the body and with a horn or a gourd in the case of the deranged blood having been seated in the skin. 57-58.

Thus ends the eighth Chapter of the S'árira Sthánam in the Sus'ruta Samhitá which treats of Venesection.

# CHAPTER IX.

Now we shall discourse on the Sáriram which treats of the description of the arteries, nerves and ducts, etc.*
**(Dhamani-Vyákarana-Sáriram).** 1.

There are twenty-four Dhamanies (ducts) in all, and all of them have their origins in the naval region (which includes the whole abdominal region†). Several authorities assert that no arbitrary distinctions should be made among the Síras (veins), Dhamanis (arteries), and the Srotas, (channels), since Dhamanis and Srotas are but different modifications of one original kind of Sírá (vessels). But this opinion is not a sound one inasmuch as they have got different natures, origins and functions and as being described so in the Áyurveda. But owing to their adjacent positions, the existence of several authoritative dicta (Ápta-vák) regarding the oneness of their character, similarity of their functions, and the minute nature of their shape, they appear to be homologous in their action, even amidst the real diversities in their work and office. 2.

Of the twenty-four Dhamanis, which (originally) have their roots in the naval region (Náhhi), ten have upward course, ten have downward course, and four flow laterally or transversely. 3.

**Functions of the up-coursing Dhamanis:**—The ten up-coursing Dhamanis (nerves)

---

\* Sans. Dhama—to be filled with air, so called from the fact of their being distended with air after death.

† So far, as in fœtal life, allantoic arteries and the unbilical veins subserve the purposes of nutrition, excretion, etc , and reflects the rudi. mentary vascular system.

perform such specific functions of the body, as sound, touch, taste, sight, smell, inspiration, sighing, yawning, sneezing, laughter, speech, and weeping, etc., and tend to maintain the integrity of the body. These Dhamanis, reaching the heart, respectively ramify themselves into three branches, thus making thirty (ramifications in all). Ten of these serve the following purposes, *viz*, two serve as the channels of the bodily Váyu, two of the Pitta, two of the Kapha, two of the blood, and two of the Rasa (lymph chyle). Eight of the remaining ones (twenty), serve the following functions, *viz.*, two of them carry sound, two sight or colour, two smell, and two taste. Moreover a man speaks with the help of another two, makes sound with the help of another couple, sleeps through the instrumentality of another pair (couple), and wakes up with the help of another couple. Two of the Dhamanis (ducts) carry the fluid of lachrymation, two of them (ducts), attached to the breasts of a woman, carry milk of her breasts, which, coursing through the breast of a man, convey his seminal fluid. Thus we have described the thirty Dhamanis with their ramifications. These sustain and maintain the integrity (of the limbs and members of the body) above the (line of) umbilicus, such as the Udara, the sides, the back, the chest, the neck, the shoulders and the arms. 4.

**Memorable Verse :**—The up-coursing Dhamanis duly perform the offices stated above. Now I shall describe the specific functions, etc., (*i.e.*, nature, office, and situations, etc.,) of the down-coursing ones. 5.

**Functions of the down-coursing Dhamanis :**—The down-coursing Dhamanis respectively form the channels for the downward conveyance of Váyu (flatus), urine, stool, semen, and catamenial fluid, etc. These Dhamanis reaching down into the Pittásaya (receptacle of the Pitta) separate the serum prepared out of the food and drink through the agency of the local heat (and pitta), and carry it to the remotest parts of the organism maintaining their healthy moisture, supplying them with the necessary principles of nutrition and (ultimately) conveying them to the up-coursing and lateral Dhamanis, in order to be conveyed to the parts traversed by them respectively. Thus they indirectly serve to supply the heart with its quota of healthy Rasa (serus fluid), if not in a direct way. Moreover they tend to separate the effetematter (urine, stool and sweat) from the fully transformed lymph-chyle in the abdomen, the stomach and the small intestines (Ámásaya and Pakvásaya). Each of the down-coursing Dhamanis is found to ramify into three branches at a place midway between the Ámásaya (stomach) and the Pakvásaya (intestines). Thus they number thirty in all. The functions of the ten out of these (thirty vessels) are as follows, *viz.*, two serve to carry Váyu, two Pitta, two Kapha, two blood, and two Rasa (lymph-chyle). Two of these Dhamanis, running into the intestines, carry the food, another two carry the Toya* (watery) part, another two, running into the bladder, serve to carry out the urine (from the bladder), another two carry the semen, and another two serve as the channels of transmission and emission of the same fluid and serve to carry the ovarian discharge in women. The two Dhamanis, attached to the large intestine (Sthulántra), serve as the channels of fæcal matter, while the remaining eight convey perspiration to the lateral-coursing Dhamanis. Thus we have finished describing these thirty Dhamanis with their ramifications. These sustain and maintain the

* This watery part reaching the bladder is transformed into urine.

integrity of the parts of the body below the naval region, such as the Pakvás'aya (Intestine), the waist, the organic principles of stool and urine, the organs of generation, the anus, the bladder, and the lower limbs of the body (Sakthi) (according to their utility in the physical economy of the organism). 6.

**Memorable Verse :**—These down-coursing Dhamanis perform the afore-said functions. Now I shall describe the specific functions (*i.e*, nature, office, and situations, etc.,) of the lateral-coursing Dhamanis. 7.

**Functions of the lateral-coursing Dhamanis :**—The four lateral-coursing Dhamanis, gradually ramifying themselves into hundreds and thousands of branches, simply baffle counting. The net-work of these Dhamanis spreads over the whole orgnism and maintain its integrity. Their exterior orifices are attached to the roots of hairs (pores of the skin) through which they convey the perspiration and the Rasa (serum), thus supplying the body, both internally and externally, with the soothing nutritions (moisture of healthy lymph-chyle). The effects and potencies of the articles of anointment, sprinkling, immersion, and plasters, enter through these orifices into the internal organism through the agency of the heat in the skin, and sensations of a pleasant or painful contact are experienced through their instrumentality. Thus we have finished describing the four lateral-coursing Dhamanis with their ramifications throughout the whole organism. 8.

**Memorable Verses :**—The Dhamanis have got pores in their sides through which they carry the Rasa (lymph-chyle) throughout the organism, like the filaments and fibres of water-lily and lotus. These Dhamanis furnish the self-conscious Ego, confined in the material body, which is the resultant of the combination of the five material elements, with a distinct sensation* peculiar to each of the five sense-organs† and break up the combination (of the five material elements) at the time of death. 9—10.

Now we shall describe the symptoms produced by a **Srota** (duct or channel) pierced at its root or starting point. The ducts or channels respectively conveying the life, the food, the water, (the organic principle of) the Rasa (serum), the blood, the muscles, the fat, the urine, the stool, the semen, and the catamenial blood, naturally fall within the scope of Surgery (Śalya-tantra). Several authorities assert that the Srotas (vessels) are innumerable‡, and perform different functions in their different aspects.

The two Srotas (channels) of **Prána** (bronchi) have their roots in the heart and the Rasa-carrying Dhamanis (pulmonary arteries). An injury to any of these Srotas (vessels) produces groaning, bending down of the body, loss of consciousness (Moha), illusion, and shivering, or may ultimately prove fatal. The **food-carrying** Srotas (Æsophagus) have their roots in the Ámásaya (stomach) and in the food-carrying Dhamanis (intestines). An injury to or piercing of such a duct (Srota), gives rise to tympanites, colic pain, aversion to food, vomiting, thirst, blindness or darkness of vision, or may even end in death. There are two **water-carrying** (Udaka-vaha) ducts or channels which have their roots in the palate and the Kloma, and a piercing of any

---

\* Hearing, touch, smell, taste, and sight.

† Eyes, ears, nose, tongue and skin.

‡ But this science does not take any cognisance of them, since the pain incidental to a piercing of, or an injury to, any of these extremely attenuated channels, must be slight in its character.

of these makes the patient thirsty and ends in his instantaneous death (*i. e*, within seven days) The **serum-carrying** (Rasa-vaha) ducts are two in number and have their roots in (the viscus of) the heart and the serum-carrying Dhamanis (vessels). An injury to or piercing of any of these ducts gives rise to Śosha (consumption) and symptoms identical with those developed by a hurt to the Prána-vaha channels of the body, ending in death. The **blood-carrying** Srotas (channels) are two in number and have their roots in the spleen and the liver, and the blood-carrying Dhamanis (capillaries in general). An injury to any of these channels is attended with pallor, bluishness of complexion, fever, burning sensations, excessive hæmorrhage, and redness of the eyes. The two **muscle-carrying** Srotas (ducts or channels) have their roots in the (Snáyu), nerves Tvak (serum), and the blood-carrying Dhamanis (capillaries). An injury to any of these channels is characterised by swelling, loss or atrophy of the muscles, appearance of varicose veins or may (ultimately) result in death. The **fat-carrying** Srotas (ducts) are two in number and have their roots in the region of the Kati (waist) and the Vrikkas (kidneys). An injury to any of these bring in (a copious flow of) perspiration, oily gloss of the skin, parched condition of the palate, extensive swelling (of the affected locality) and thirst. The two **urine carrying** Srotas (channels) have their roots in the bladder and the penis (urethra). An injury to any of these is marked by constipation or epistaxis in the bladder, retention of urine, and numbness of the genitals. The two **stool-carrying** Srotas (ducts) have their roots in the Guda (anus) and the Pakváśaya (intestines); an injury to any of these is characterised by complete retention of stool (in the bowels), accompanied by a distention of the abdomen, foul smell and intussusception of the intestine (as in a case of enterites). The two **semen-carrying** Srotas (ducts) have their roots in the breasts and the testes. An injury to any of them leads to loss of manhood, delayed emission of semen, or blood-streaked character of that fluid. The two **Ártava-carrying** Srotas (ducts) have their roots in the uterus as well as in the Dhamanis which carry the Ártava (ovarian product). An injury to any of these brings on sterility, suppression of the menses and incapacity for copulation. A cutting to the Sevani (median raphe of the perineum) exhibits symptoms identical with those of a case of injured bladder or anus, described before. A physician may take in hand the medical treatment of a case of a Srota which has been pierced, but he shall not necessarily entertain any hope of ultimate success. (But time works wonders, and such a case may sometimes end in recovery). A case of pierced duct, from which the dart (Śalya, or the like piercing matter) has been extricated, may be medically treated (without holding out any prospect of recovery to the friends of the patient), according to the direction laid down under the head of ulcer (Vrana)   11-12.

**Metrical Text :**—The ducts emanating from the cavity of the heart, other than the Śirás (veins), Dhamanis (arteries), and found to course through the whole body, are called Srotas (lit. channels or currents).   13.

Thus ends the ninth Chapter of the S'árira Sthánam in the Sus'ruta Samhitá which treats of the descriptions of the arteries, ducts and nerves.

# CHAPTER X.

Now we shall discourse on the Sáriram which treats of the nursing and management, etc., of pregnant women from the day of conception till parturition **(Garbhini-Vyákarana-Sáriram).** 1.

**General Rules :**—An enciente, from the first day of conception, should always cherish a clear joyful spirit in a clean body. She should wear clean and white garments, ornaments, &c., engage herself in the doing of peace-giving and benedictory rites and live in devotion to the gods, the Brahmins and her elders and superiors. She should not touch nor come into contact with unclean, deformed or maimed persons, and should forego the use of fetid smelling things, avoid dreadful sights and painful or agitating sounds and the use of dry, stale and dirty food as well as that prepared overnight. Long and distant walks from home, resorts to cremation-grounds or to a solitary retreat, or to a Chaitya\*, and sitting under the shadow of a tree should be absolutely forbidden (to her during the period of gestation) Indulgence in anger, fright or other agitating emotions of the mind should be deemed injurious. To carry a heavy load, to talk in a loud voice and all other things which might occasion injury to the fœtus, (sexual intercourse, &c.) should be refrained from. The practice of constant anointment and the cleansing of the body, &c., (with Ámalaki, Haridrá, etc.—lit. cosmetics) should be given up. All fatiguing exercises should be discontinued and the rules laid down for the

---

\* Chaitya—is a haunted or diefied tree, or according to others a Budhistic monastery.

guidance of a woman in her menses should be strictly adhered to. The couch and the bed of a pregnant woman should be low, soft and guarded on all sides by a number of soft pillows or cushions. The food should be amply sweet, palatable (Hridya),* well-cooked, prepared with appetising drugs and abounding in fluid substances. These rules should be followed up till delivery. 2.

**Special regimen during the period of Gestation :**—During the first three months of pregnancy an enciente should partake of food abounding in sweet, cool and fluid articles. Several medical authorities recommend a food made of Shashtika rice with milk, to be given to her specially in the *third* month of gestation, with curd in the fourth, with milk in the fifth and with clarified butter in the sixth month of pregnancy. Food largely composed of milk and butter, as well as relishing (Hridya) food with the soup of the flesh of *jángala* (wild) animals should be given to her in the fourth, food with milk and clarified butter in the fifth, adequate quantity of clarified butter prepared with (the decoction of) S´vadamshtrá, or gruel (Yavágu) in the sixth ; and clarified butter prepared with (the decoction of) the Prithakparnyádi group in adequate quantities in the seventh month of gestation. These help the foetal development. For the purpose of restoring the Váyu of her body (nervous system) to the normal course and condition and for the cleansing of the bowels, the enciente should be given an Ásthápana (enema), composed of a decoction of Vadara mixed with Valá, Ativalá, S´atapushpá, Palala (flesh), milk, cream of curd, oil, Saindhava salt,

---

* "Hridya" here means the **diet** in which there is an abundance of Ojo-producing (albuminous) properties.

Madana fruit, honey and clarified butter. After that she should have an Anuvásana (enema) made up of oil prepared with milk and decoction of the drugs known as the Madhurádi-gana. This restores the Váyu to its normal course and condition, which brings on an easy and natural parturition unattended with any puerperal disorders. Henceforth up to the time of delivery the enciente should have liquid food (Yavágu) made up of emollient substances (fats) and soup of the flesh of Jángala animals (deer, etc.). If treated on these lines the enciente remains healthy and strong, and parturition becomes easy and unattended with evils. An enciente should be made to enter the lying-in chamber in the **ninth** month of her pregnancy and under the auspices of happy stars and propitious lunar conditions. The chamber of confinement (Sutiká-griha) in respect of a Bráhmin, Kshatriya, Vaiśya and Sudra mother should be raised on grounds respectively possessed of white, red, yellow and black soils, and made of Vilva, Vata, Tinduka and Bhallátaka wood. Couches should be made of these woods respectively in cases of the different social orders. The walls of the room should be well-plastered and the furniture (necessary accessories) should be placed tidy in their proper places. The door of a lying-in chamber should be made to face the south or the east, and the inner dimensions of the room should be eight cubits in length and four in breadth. Religious rites for warding off the visitation of evil spirits and malignant stars should be undertaken at (the door of) the room. 3.

**Signs of imminent parturition**—(M.—T.) :—A looseness of the sides of the abdomen and untying of the umbilical cord of the child (from the cardiac cord of its mother) and a perception of the characteristic pain at the waist would indicate the approach of the time of delivery. A constant and severe pain at the waist and the back, constant (involuntary) motions of the bowels and micturition and mucous discharge from the vulva are the symptoms which are manifest at the time (*i.e.*, a little before) of parturition. 4-5.

**Preliminary Measures :**—Rites of benediction should be performed for the safety of the enciente in her travail and she should be made to pronounce benedictory Mantras surrounded by male babies on all sides. A fruit with a masculine name should be given in her hand. Her body should be anointed with oil and washed with warm water and she should be made to drink largely a gruel (Yavágu) made of articles (which exert a beneficial virtue at the time). Then she should be laid on her back on a soft and sufficiently spacious bed, her head being placed on a pillow and her legs slightly flexed and drawn up. Four elderly ladies with paired finger-nails and skilled in the art of accouchement and with whom she feels no delicacy, should attend and nurse her at the time. 6.

Then after having gently lubricated the mouth of the parturient canal along the natural direction of the pubic hairs (Anuloma) (so as not to create any discomfort in the part) one of them (elderly ladies) should address the enciente as follows :—"O fortunate damsel, try to bear down the child, but do not make such an attempt in the absence of real pain." On experiencing an untying of the umbilical cord of the child, the enciente should gently make such urgings, whenever she will experience pain in the pelvic, pudendal and pubic regions and in the region between the neck of the bladder and the pelvis. Deep urgings should be made on the exit of the fœtus out of the uterus, and after that deeper urgings should be made during the passage of the child through the canal until delivery. 7.

An urging (made by the enciente) in the absence of any real **pain** may lead to deafness, dumbness and deformity of the jaw-bones of the child or subject it to attacks of cough, asthma, consumption, etc., or lead to the diseases of its head, or to the birth of a haunch-backed or deformed child. A case of abnormal presentation (Pratiloma) should be converted into the normal or cephalic one (Anuloma) by version*. 8-9.

In the case of protracted delivery, *e.g.,* an obstruction of the child at the vagina,—the vagina should be fumigated with the fumes of the slough (cast-off skin) of a cobra (snake) or with the fumes of *Pinditaka* (Madana) or the roots of *Hiranyapushpi* (Kantakári) should be tied (round the neck or the waist) or Suvarchala (*Atasi*) or *Vis'alyá* (Pátalá) should be tied round the hand (wrist) and leg (ankle) of the parturient woman. 10.

**Post-parturient Measures :**—The shreds or membranes lying on the body of the child should be removed immediately after its birth and its mouth should be cleansed with clarified butter and rock-salt. Then a linen pad soaked in clarified butter† should be applied on the head of the new-born baby. Then the umbilical cord, after having been slightly drawn out, should be ligatured with one end of a string at a point eight fingers apart from its navel, the other end

---

* The various forms of (Pratiloma) abnormal presentations have been described under Mudha-Garbha Nidánam (Nidán-Sthána—Chap. IX.) and their treatment is to be found in Chikitsá-Sthána—Chap. XV.

† Brahmadeva recommends Valá-Taila instead of clarified butter.

of the string being tied round its neck ; then the umbilical cord should be severed immediately above the ligature. 11.

**Natal Rites :**—Then having sprayed (the face of) the baby with cold water, the post-natal rites should be performed unto it. After that the baby should be made to lick an electuary composed of honey, clarified butter and the expressed juice of *Bráhmi* leaves and *Anantá*, mixed with (half a Rati weight of) gold dust and given with the ring-finger of the feeder. Then the body of the child should be anointed with Valá-taila and it should be bathed in an infusion of the barks of *Kshiri* trees, or in the washings (decoctions) of drugs known as the *Sarvagandha* (Eládi group), or in water in which red-hot gold or silver bar has been immersed, or in a tepid decoction of *Kapittha* leaves, according to the nature of the season, the preponderance of the deranged Doshas in its body and according to its physical conditions. 12.

**Diet for the Child**—(M.—T.) :—The milk in the breasts of a newly parturient woman sets in three or four days after parturition owing to the dilation of the orifices of the milk ducts (galactoferous ducts). Hence the baby should be fed thrice daily (morning, noon and evening) on a handful (child's own hand) of clarified butter and honey mixed with (a Rati weight of) pulverized *Anantá* roots sanctified with Mantras on the first day ; and on the second and third days the child should be fed on clarified butter prepared with the *Lakshaná* (root). On the following (fourth) day the child should be fed on its handful of honey and clarified butter only twice (*i. e.*, in the morning and at noon). (From the evening of fourth day) the mother should first squeeze off a quantity of her milk and then give the child her breast. (This rule should be observed at the time of tending the child every day). 13-14.

**Treatment of the mother :**—The body of the mother should be anointed (after parturition) with the Valá-Taila and treated (both internally and externally) with a decoction of Vàyu-subduing drugs (such as the *Bhadra-Dárvádi* group, etc.). If still there be any abnormality in the condition of the Doshas (the discharge of vitiated blood *i e.*, lochia), the mother should be given to drink a luke-warm solution of treacle mixed with powders of *Pippali, Pippali* roots, *Hasti-pippali, Chitraka* and *S'ringavera,* and the medicine should be continued for two or three days or longer, (if necessary), till the disappearance of the vitiated blood (lochia). When the discharge gets normal (*i e.*, on the appearance of healthy lochia), the mother should be made to take for three days a gruel (Yavágu) prepared with the decoction of the drugs constituting the *Vidári-Gandhádi Gana* and mixed with (a good quantity of) clarified butter or a Yavágu prepared in milk. After that a meal of boiled Sáli-rice and a broth made from the meats of Jángala animals boiled with barley, *Kola* and *Kulattha* pulse, should be prescribed for her, taking into consideration the strength and the condition of her appetite (Agni or digesting power). The mother should observe this regimen of diet and conduct for one month and a half (after delivery). After this period she may be at liberty to choose any food to her liking and revert to her natural mode of living. According to several authorities, however, a woman does not regain her natural temperament of body till the reappearance of the healthy menstruation (after parturition). 15.

A strong but newly delivered woman, born and

bred up in a Jángala country should be given to drink, for three or five nights, either oil or clarified butter in an adequate quantity with an after-potion consisting of the decoction of drugs constituting the group known as the *Pippalyádi Gana.* She should be daily anointed with oil, etc. If, however, of delicate health, she should be made to take, for three or five nights in succession, a medicated Yavágu (gruel) as described in the last para. Thenceforth a diet of demulcent properties should be prescribed for her and her body should be regularly washed with a copious quantity of tepid water. A mother, after parturition, should forego (for a considerable time) sexual intercourse, physical labour and indulgence in irascible emotions,* etc. 16

**Memorable Verses :**—Any disease acquired by a newly delivered mother (Sutiká) by her injudicious conduct of life soon lapses into one of a difficult type (hard to cure); and it becomes incurable if it be due to too much fasting. Hence a wise physician should treat her with such measures as are natural and congenial to her temperament, the time, the place and the nature of the disease, so that she may not be afflicted with any evil effect. 17.

A placenta retained in the uterus causes constipation (Ánáha) of the bowels and distention of the abdomen (tympanites). Hence in such a case her throat should be tickled with a finger covered with hair ; or the exterior orifice of the vagina should be fumigated with the fumes of the cast-off skin of a snake, *Katuka, Alávu, Kritavedhana* and mustard seeds mixed with mustard oil. In the alternative, a plaster of *Lángali*

* Fifteen kinds of emotions as described in the thirty-ninth chapter of the Chikitsá-sthánam.

roots should be applied to the palms and soles of her hands and feet ; or the milky juice of *Snuhi* tree should be applied over her scalp ; or a compound made of pasted *Lángali* roots and *Kushtha* mixed with either wine or the cow's urine should be given her for drink. A Kalka either of *S'áli* roots or of the drugs constituting the *Pippalyádi Gana* mixed with wine (Surá) should be given her for the purpose In the alternative, an Ásthápana (enema) of white mustard seeds *Kushtha* (Kuda), *Lángali*, and the milky juice of *Mahávriksha*, mixed with Surá-manda should be prescribed. (If the above measures fail) an Uttara-Vasti (uterine douche) prepared with the aforesaid drugs and boiled in mustard oil should be applied ; or else the placenta should be removed by the hand lubricated with an oleaginous substance and with the nails clipped off. 18.

**Makkalla and its Treatment :**—The lochia of a newly delivered woman whose organism has become excessively dry on account of profuse use of absorbants or deranged by any other causes,—the lochia being obstructed in its exit by the local Váyu,— gives rise to Granthis (nodules) which may appear below the navel, on the sides of the pelvis about the region of the bladder or of the pubis. Severe piercing pain (Śula) is felt about the region of the navel, the stomach and the bladder and a sensation of pricking with needle and cutting pain in the intestines. At the same time the abdomen becomes distended with the retention of urine. These are the symptoms of **Makkalla**. In such a case, a decoction of the drugs of the *Viratarvádi Gana* mixed with a powdered compound of the *Ushakádi* Gana should be given her. In the alternative, a potion of carbonate of potash (*Yavakshára*) dissolved in tepid water or in clarified butter ; of rock-salt dissolved in the decoction of the *Pippalyâdi* Gana ; of a compound made of the powdered drugs of the latter Gana with Surâ-manda ; of the powders of cardamom and *Pancha-kolas* dissolved in the decoction of the drugs of the *Varunâdi Gana* ; of the powders of pepper and *Bhadradâru* dissolved in the decoction of the *Prithakparnyâdi Gana* ; or of pulverized *Trikatu, Chaturjâtaka* and *Kustumburu* mixed with old treacle ; or of simple Arishta, should be prescribed. 19.

**Management of the Child :**—The baby being wrapped up in silk should be laid on a bed covered with a silken sheet; it should be fanned with the branches of a *Pilu, Nimba, Vadari,* or *Parushaka* tree. A (thin) pad (Pichu) soaked in oil should be constantly kept on the head of the child, and its body should be fumigated with the fumes of drugs (*e.g.,* Vacha, mustard, etc.) potent enough to keep off the (evil) influences of demons and evil spirits. The same drugs should be tied round the neck, hands, legs and head of the infant and the floor of the lying-in room should be kept strewn over with pounded sesamum, mustard, linseed (*Atasi*). A fire should also be kept kindled in the chamber. Measures laid down in the chapter on the nursing of an Ulcer-patient (chapter IX. Sutra.) should be observed in the present case as well. 20.

Then on the tenth day of its birth the parents having performed the necessary rites of benediction and celebrated the occasion with suitable festivities, shall give the child a name of their own choice or one determined by its natal a-trism, etc. 21.

**Lactation and selection of a wet-nurse :**—For the healthy growth of the child a wet-nurse should be selected from among the matrons of its own caste (Varna), and possessed of the following necessary qualifications. She should be of middle stature, neither too old nor too young (middle-aged), of sound health, of good character (not irascible or easily excitable), not fickle, ungreedy, neither too thin nor too corpulent, with lips unprotruded, and with healthy and pure milk in her breasts which should neither be too much pendulent nor drawn up. It should be carefully observed that her skin is healthy and unmarked by any moles or stains, she being free from any sort of crime (such as gambling, day-sleep, debauchery, etc.). She should be of an affectionate heart, and with all her children living.

She should be of respectable parentage and consequently possessed of many good qualities, with an exuberance of milk in her breasts, and not in the habit of doing anything that degrades woman in life. A "Syámá" girl possessed of the aforesaid qualities makes a good wet-nurse. A child nursed at the breast of a woman with upturned or unprominent nipples is apt to be deformed (Karála) in features, while extremely pendulous (large and flabby) breasts may suffocate the child by covering its mouth and nostrils. Having chosen a wet-nurse of the commendable type, the child with its head well-washed should, on an auspicious day, be laid on her lap wrapped in a clean and untorn linen. The face of the child should be turned towards the north, while the nurse should look to the east at the time. Then, after first having a small quantity of the milk pressed out and the breast washed and consecrated with the following Mantras (incantations) the child should be made to suck her right breast. 22.

**Metrical Texts :**—"O, thou beautiful damsel, may the four oceans of the earth contribute to the secretion of milk in thy breasts for the purpose of improving the bodily strength of the child. O, thou with a beautiful face, may the child, reared on your milk, attain a long life, like the gods made immortal with drinks of ambrosia". 22.

A child nursed at the breast of any and every woman for want of a nurse of the commendable type, may fall an easy prey to disease, owing to the fact of the promiscuous nature of the milk proving incongenial to its physical temperament. The milk of a nurse not being pressed out and spelled off at the outset may produce cough, difficulty of breathing, or vomiting of the child, owing to the sudden rush of the accumulated milk into its throat choking up the channels. Hence a child should not be allowed to suck in such milk. 23.

The loss or suppression of the milk in the breasts of a woman is usually due to anger, grief, and the absence of natural affection for her child, etc. For the purpose of establishing a flow in her breast, her equanimity should be first restored, and diets consisting of Sáli-rice, barley, wheat, Shashtika, meat-soup, wine (Surá), Souviraka, sesamum-paste, garlic, fish, *Kas'eruka*, *S'ringátaka*, lotus-stalk, *Vidári-kandá*, *Madhúka* flower, *S'atávari*, *Nalikà*, *Alávu*, and *Kála-S'áka*, etc., should be prescribed. 24.

**Examination, etc., of milk :**—The breast-milk of a nurse or a mother should be tested by casting it in water. The milk which is thin, cold, clear, and tinged like the hue of a conch-shell, is found to be easily miscible with water, does not give rise to froths and shreds, and neither floats nor sinks in water, should be regarded as **pure** and **healthy**. A child fed on such milk is sure to thrive and gain in strentgh and health. A child should not be allowed to take the breast of a hungry, aggrieved, fatigued, too thin, too corpulent, fevered, or a pregnant woman, nor of one in whom the assimilated food is followed by an acid reaction, or of one who is fond of incongenial and unhealthy dietary, or whose fundamental principles are vitiated. A child should not be given the breast until an administered medicine is assimilated in its organism, lest this should give rise to a violent aggravation of the pharmacological action of the medicine, as well as of the deranged Doshas (Váyu, Pitta, etc ), and the refuse matters (Malas) of its body. 25.

**Memorable Verses :**—The Doshas (Váyu, Pitta and Kapha) of a wet-nurse are aggravated by ingestion of indigestible or incompatible food, or of those articles which tend to derange the Doshas of the body, and hence her milk may be vitiated. A child, fed on the vitiated milk of a woman, vitiated by the deranged Doshas owing to injudicious and intemperate eating and living, falls an easy prey to physical disease. An intelligent physician in such a case should devise means for the purification of the milk as well as of the deranged Doshas which account for such vitiation (inasmuch as the medication of the child alone will not produce any satisfactory effect). 26-27.

**Infantile diseases and their Diagnosis :**—A child constantly touches its diseased part or organ and cries for the least touch (by another of that part of its body). If the seat of disease be its head, the child cannot raise nor move that organ and remains with its eyes closely shut. A disease seated in its bladder gives rise to retention of urine, thirst, pain and occasional fainting fits. A retention of urine and stool, discolouring of complexion, vomiting, distention of the abdomen, and gurgling in the intestines indicate the seat of the disease to be its Koshtha (colon). A constant crying (and the child's refusal to be consoled) would signify that the diseased principle (morbiferous diathesis) extends all through its organism. 28.

**Treatment of Infants :**—Medicines laid down under the head of a particular disease should likewise be prescribed in the case of its appearance in a child or an infant ; but then only the remedies of mild potency and those which do not tend to disintegrate the bodily fat and Kapha should be given in adequate doses (according to age, etc) as mentioned hereafter and administered through the vehicle of milk and clarified butter, to a child living on milk alone, while the nurse also is to take the same medicines as well.* In the case of a child fed both on milk and (boiled) rice (*Kshiránnáda*,i.e., living on both solid and liquid food) the medicine should be administered both to the child and its wet-nurse. In the case of a child living on solid food only, decoctions (Kasháya) etc. should be given to the child and not to the nurse. Medicines to the quantity of a small pinchful may be prescribed for a suckling who has completed its first month of life. Kalkas (medicated pastes) should be given to a child fed on both milk and rice to the size of a stone of a plum-fruit (Kola), and the dose for a child fed on rice (solid food) only being to the size of a plum (Kola) † 29.

* Milk and clarified butter being congenial to the constitution of infants should be used as vehicles for drugs in their cases but, these are not necessary in the case of the nurse.

† According to several other authorities, the dosage in the case of children is to be regulated as follows :—

In the case of a child, one month old, drugs should be given in the form of an electuary through the vehicle of milk, honey, syrup, clarified butter, etc.,—the dose being one Rati (about two grains) at first, and gradually increased by a Rati a month, till it completes one year. After this time the dose is to be one Máshá (about twenty grains) for each year of age till he is fifteen.

This dosage, however, does not apply in the present age.—Ed.

**Metrical Texts :**—In the case of any disease of a child nursed at the breast, the breasts of the nurse should be plastered with the pastes of drugs recommended by physicians for the particular malady (instead of giving the drugs to the child), and the child made to suck the same. The use of clarified butter is not beneficial to a child on the first day of an attack of Váta-jvara (fever due to the derangement of the bodily Váyu), within the first two days of an attack of Pittaja fever, and within the first three days of that of Kaphaja fever. But the use of clarified butter may be prescribed for an infant fed on milk and boiled rice, or on boiled rice alone, according to requirements. 30-31.

In case of fever a child should be given no suck at all, lest the symptoms of thirst might develop. Purgatives, Vastis, or emetics are forbidden in the disease of children, unless the disease threatens to take a fatal course. 32.

If the local Váyu aggravated by the waste of brain-materials (Mastulunga), bends down the palate bone of a child attended with an excessive thirst and agony, clarified butter boiled with (the decoction and Kalka of) the drugs of the Madhura Gana, should be used both internally and externally, and the patient should as well be treated with spray of cold water (to stimulate him). The disease in which the navel of a child becomes swollen and painful, is called **Tundi**. It should be remedied by applying fomentations, medicated oils, Upanáhas, etc., possessed of the virtue of subduing the Váyu. A suppuration of the anal region (**Guda-páka**) of a child should be treated with Pittaghna (Pitta-destroying) measures and medicines. Rasánjana used internally and externally (as an unguent) proves very efficacious in these cases. 33-35.

**Infantile Elixirs :**—Clarified butter cooked with (the decoction and Kalka of) white mustard seeds, *Vachá, Mánsi, Payasyá, Apámárga, S'atávari, Sárivá, Bráhmi, Pippali, Haridrá, Kushtha* and *Saindhava* salt should be given to an infant fed exclusively on milk. Clarified butter prepared with (the docoction and Kalka of) *Madhuka* (Yashtimadhu), *Vacha, Chitraka, Pippali* and *Triphalá* should be given to an infant fed both on milk and (boiled) rice (solid and liquid food). Clarified butter boiled with (the decoction and Kalka of) Dasamula, milk, *Tagara, Bhadradáru, Maricha,* honey, *Vidanga, Drákshá* and the two sorts of *Bráhmis* should be given to an infant fed on (boiled) rice (solid food) By these the health, strength, intellect and longivity of the child is improved. 36-37.

A child should be so handled or lifted as not to cause any discomfort. A baby should not be scolded, nor suddenly roused up (from sleep), lest it might get awfully frightened. It should not be suddenly drawn up nor suddenly laid down, lest this should result in the derangement of its bodily Váyu. An attempt to seat it (before it has learnt to sit steadily), may lead to haunch-back (Kyphosis). Lovingly should a child be fondled and amused with toys and play-things. A child unruffled by any of the above ways becomes healthy, cheerful and intelligent as it grows older. An infant should be guarded against any exposure to the rains, the sun, or the glare of lightning. He should not be placed uuder a tree or a creeper, in low lands, and in lonely houses or in their shades (caves) ; and it should be protected from the malignant influences of evil stars and occult powers. 38.

**Metrical Texts :**—A child should not be left (alone) in an unclean and unholy place, nor under the sky (uncovered place), nor over an undulating ground, nor should it be exposed to heat, storm, rain, dust, smoke and water Milk is congenial to the organism of a child, *i e.,* it is its proper food Hence in the absence of sufficient breast-milk, the child should be given the milk of a cow or of a she-goat in adequate quantities. 39.

In the sixth month of its birth the child should be fed on light and wholesome boiled rice. A child should always be kept in an inner apartment of the house, and religious rites should be performed on its behalf for the propitiation of evil deities, and it should be carefully guarded against the influences of evil stars. 40.

**Symptoms when a malignant star, etc., strikes :**—The child looks frightened and agitated, cries, becomes unconscious at times, wounds himself or its nurse with its teeth and finger-nails, gnashes its teeth, crooks, yawns, or moves its eye-brows with upturned eyes, vomits frothy matter, bites its lips, becomes cross, passes loose stool mixed with shreds of mucus, cries in an agonised voice, becomes dull in complexion, becomes weak, does not sleep in the night, does not suck the breast as before, or emits a fishy, bug-like or mole-like smell from its body—these are the general symptoms exhibited by a child under the influence of a malignant star or planet which will be specifically described later on in the Uttara-Tantra 41.

**Education and Marriage :**—The education of a child should be commenced at a suitable age and with subjects proper to the particular social Varna or order it belongs to. On attaining the twenty-fifth year he should marry a girl of twelve. A conformity to these rules, is sure to crown him with health, satisfaction, progeny and a capacity for fully discharging the religious rites and paying off his parental debts. 42.

**Metrical Texts :**—An offspring of a girl below the age of **sixteen** by a man below **twenty-five** is usually found to die in the womb. Such a child, in the event of its being born alive, dies a premature death or else becomes weak in organs (Indriyas). Hence a girl of extremely tender age should not be fecundated at all. An extremely old woman, or one suffering from a chronic affection (of the generative organ), or afflicted with any other disease, should not be likewise impregnated. A man with similar disabilities should be held likewise unfit. 40-44.

A fœtus, on the point of being miscarried on account of the above-mentioned causes, produces pain in the uterus, bladder, waist (Kati), and the inguinal regions (Vamkshana) and bleeding. In such a case, the patient should be treated with cold baths, sprays of cold water and medicated plaster (Pradeha) &c., at the time, and milk * boiled with drugs constituting the *Jivaniya* group, should be given to her for drink. In case of unusual movements of the fœtus in the womb, the enciente should be given a drink of milk boiled with the drugs of *Utpaládi Gana*, for soothing and making it steady in its place. 45.

A fœtus being displaced from its normal position produces the following symptoms, viz , pain or spasms in the back and the sides (Párs'va), burning sensation, excessive discharge of blood and retention of urine and fœces A fœtus changing place or shifting from one place to another, swells up the abdomen (Koshtha). Cooling and soothing measures should be adopted in such cases. 46.

---

* Jivaniya drugs two Tolás, milk sixteen Tolás and water sixty-four Tolás, to be boiled and reduced to sixteen Tolás, *i e.*, to weight of the milk.

**Medical Treatment :**—In a case of pain under the circumstances, the enciente should be made to drink a potion consisting of milk boiled with *Mahá-saha, Kshudrasahá, Madhuka* flower, *S'vadanstrá* and *Kantakári*, mixed with sugar and honey. In the case of retention of urine, the patient should be made to drink a potion of milk boiled with drugs known as the *Dárvádi Gana* (mixed with sugar and honey). In the case of A'náha (retention of stool attended with distention of the abdomen), a potion consisting of milk boiled with asafetida, *Sauvarchala* salt, garlic and *Vacha* (mixed with honey and sugar) should be given. In cases of excessive bleeding, linctus made of the powdered chamber of a Koshthágáriká insect*, *Samangá, Dhátaki* flowers, *Navamáliká, Gairika*, resin and *Rasánjana*, or of as many of them as would be available, mixed with honey, should be licked. In the alternative, the bark and sprouts of the drugs known as the *Nyagrodhádi Gana* mixed with boiled milk should be administered, or a Kalka of the drugs of the Utpaládi group mixed with boiled milk should be used, or a Kalka of S'áluka, S'ringátaka and Kas'eru mixed with boiled milk should be given. As a further alternative, the enciente may be made to eat cakes made of powdered Sáli rice with the decoction of Udumbara fruit and Audaka-kanda, mixed with honey and sugar. A piece of linen or a plug soaked in the expressed juice of the drugs of the Nyagrodhádi group should be inserted into the passage of the vagina. 47.

In a case of pain unattended with bleeding, the enciente should be made to drink a potion composed of milk-boiled with *Madhuka* (Yashtimadhu), *Devadáru* and

---

\* There is a kind of insect which makes its chamber with earth generally under the ceiling or on the walls. This earth should be used.

*Payasyá* ; or with *As'mantaka, Satávari* and *Payasyá* ; or with the drugs of the group of *Vidárigandhádi* Gana ; or with *Vriháti, Kantakári, Utpala, S'atávari, Sárivá, Payasyá* and *Madhuka* (Yashtimadhu). These remedies speedily applied tend to alleviate the pain and make the fœtus steady in the womb. 48.

After the fœtus has been steadied by the aforesaid mesaures, a diet consisting of (boiled rice and) cow's milk, boiled with the dried tender fruits of *Udumvara*, should be prescribed for the patient. In the event of **miscarriage,** the patient should be made to drink a Yavágu (gruel) of the *Uddálaka* rice, &c., cooked with the decoction of the Páchaniya group (Pippalyádi) and devoid of all saline and fatty matter, for a number of days corresponding to that of the month of gestation. Old treacle mixed with the powdered drugs of the Dipaniya group (Pancha-kola), or simply some Arishta (Abhayárishta, etc.), should be given, in the event of there being pain in the pelvis, bladder and abdomen. 49.

The internal ducts and channels (Srotas) stuffed with aggravated Váyu lead to the weakening (Laya) of the fœtus and, if the state continues, it leads even to its death. Hence the case should be treated with mild anointing measures, etc., (Sneha-karma, etc.,) and gruels made of the flesh of the birds of the Utkros'a species and mixed with a sufficient quantity of clarified butter, should be given to her. As an alternative, Kulmásha * boiled with Másha, sesamum and pieces of dried (tender) Vilva fruit should be given her, after which she should be made to drink, for a week, honey and Máddhvika (a kind of weak wine). At the non-delivery of the child

---

* "Kulmásha" may mean either Kulattha pulse or half boiled wheat, barley, etc.

even after the lapse of the full term of gestation, the enciente should be made to thrash corn with a pestle in an Udukhala or mortar (husking apparatus) or should be made to|sit or move (on legs or by conveyance), on an uneven ground. 50.

Atrophy of a fœtus in the womb should be ascribed to the action of the deranged Váyu. This is detected by the comparatively lesser fulness of the abdomen of the enciente and slow movement of the fœtus in the womb. In such a case, the enciente should be treated with milk, with the Vrimhaniya (of restorative and constructive properties) drugs, and with meat-soup.* 51.

A combination of ovum and semen affected by the deranged Váyu in the womb, may not give rise to a successful fecundation (living impregnated matter), but leads to a distention of the abdomen (as in pregnancy), which again, at any time, may disappear of itself. And this is ascribed by the ignorant to the malignant influence of Naigamesha (spirits). Such an impregnated matter, sometimes lying concealed in the uterus, is called Nágodara, which should be treated with the remedies laid down under the head of Lina-Garbha (weak fœtus). 52.

Now we shall discourse on the management of pregnancy according to the months (period) of gestation.

**Metrical Texts:**—The following receipes, such as, (1) Madhuka (Yashtimadhu), S'ákavija, Payasyá, and Devadáru ; (2) As'mantaka, black sesamum, pippali, Manjishthá, Támra-valli and Śatávari ; (3) Vrikshádani, Payasyá, Latá (Durvá), Utpala and Sáriva ; (4) Anantá, Sáriva, Rásná, Padma, and Madhuka (Yashtimadhu) ;

* The particle "cha" in the text signifies the use of any other constructive tonic.

(5) Vrihati, Kantakári, Kás'mari, sprouts (S'unga) and barks of milk-exuding trees (as, Vata, etc.), and clarified butter† ; (6) Pris'ni-parni, Valá, S'igru, S'vadanshtrá and Madhuparniká ; and (7) S'ring'taka, Visa (stalks of lotus), Drákshá, Kas'aru, Madhuka (Yashtimadhu), and sugar ; should successively be given with milk* to an enciente, from the first to the seventh month of her gestation, in the case of a threatened miscarraige or abortion. 53.

An enciente should be made to drink milk boiled with the roots of Kapittha, Vrihati, Vilva, Patola, Ikshu and Kantakári, (in case of impending or threatened miscarraige) in the eighth month of her pregnancy. In the ninth month (and under similar conditions), the potion should be made up of Madhuka (Yashtimadhu), Ananta-mula, Payashá and Sáriva. In the tenth month (and under similar conditions), a potion consisting of milk boiled with Sunthi and Payasyá is beneficial, or, in the alternative, may be given a potion made up of milk with Sunthi, Madhuka (Liquorice) and Devadáru. The severe pain would vanish and the fœtus would continue to develop safely in the womb, under the aforesaid mode of treatment. 54–57.

A child born of a woman, who had remained sterile (not-conceived) for a period of six years (Nivritta-prasavá)* after a previous child-birth, becomes a short-lived one. 58.

* Chakradatta reads "Visam" (stalks of lotus) instead of "Ghritam" (clarified butter).

† If a conception does not occur in a woman for a period of more than five years after a child-birth, she is called **Nivritta-prasavá**.

* Sivadása also says that powders of these drugs should be given with boiled milk, but he adds that some authorities recommend these drugs to be boiled in milk according to Kshira-páka-vidhi.

Application of mild emetic medicines, (though forbidden in the case of a pregnant woman), may be resorted to, in the case of a fatal disease, (even in that stage). A diet consisting of sweet and acid things should be prescribed for her, so as to bring the deranged Doshas to the normal state ; mild Samsamaniya (soothing and pacifying) medicines should be applied and food and drink consisting of articles mild in their potency, predominently sweet-tasting and not injurious to the fœtus, should be advised and mild (external) measures not baneful to the fœtus should be resorted to, according to the requirements of the case. 59.

**Memorable Verses :**—The growth, memory, strength and intellect of a child are improved by the use of the four following medicinal compounds, used as linctus (Prás'a), viz., (1) well-powdered gold, Kushtha, honey, clarified butter and Vacha ; (2) Matsyákshaka* (Bráhmi), Sankha-puspi, powdered gold, clarified butter and honey ; (3) Arkapuspi, honey, clarified butter powdered gold and Vacha ; and (4) powdered gold, Kaitaryyah (Mahá-Nimba), white Durbá,† clarified butter and honey. 60.

Thus ends the tenth Chapter of the S'árira Sthánam in the Sus'ruta Samhitá, which treats of the nursing and management etc. of pregnant women.

\* Some, however, explain Matsyákshaka to be *Dhustura;* others again say it is a kind of red-flowered shrub grown in the Ánupa country.

† The word "S'veta," in the Text, may either be adjective to "Durvá" and mean "white" or it may mean white Vacha or white Aparajitá or white Durvá.

---

# Here ends the Śárira Sthánam.

# THE SUŚRUTA SAMHITÁ

## CHIKITSÁ-STHÁNAM.

(Section of Therapeutics).

## CHAPTER I.

Now we shall discourse on the medical treatment of the two kinds of inflamed ulcers (**Dvivraniya Chikitsitam**). 1.

Ulcers may be grouped under two heads according as they are **Idiopathic** or **Traumatic** in their origin. The first group includes within its boundary all ulcers that are caused through the vitiated condition of the blood or the several deranged conditions of the Váyu, Pitta and Kapha, or are due to their concerted action (Sannipáta), while the second group embraces those which are caused by the bites of men, beasts, birds, ferocious animals, reptiles or lizards, or by a fall, pressure and blow, or by fire, alkali, poison, or irritant drugs, or through injuries inflicted by pointed wood, skeletal bones\*, horns, discus, arrows, axes, tridents, or *Kuntas* (a kind of shovel), or such other weapons. Although both these classes of ulcers possess many features in common, they have been grouped under two distinct heads on account of the diversity of their origin, the difference in remedial measures to be adopted in their treatment, and the variation in their

\* Fragments of broken pottery.—Dallana.

strength and tenacity. Hence the chapter is called **Dvivraniya.** 2.

In all cases of **traumatic ulcers,** cooling measures should be at once resorted to, just after (the fall or blow or stroke), for the cooling of the expanding (radiating) heat of the incidenta' ulcer, in the manner laid down in respect of (the pacification of enraged) Pitta, and a compound of honey and clarified butter should be applied on the wounded locality for the adhesion (Sandhána) of the lacerated parts, [and for the pacification, i e, restoration to normal state, of the local blood and Váyu aggravated through an obstruction of their passage]. Hence arises the necessity of making the two-fold classification of ulcers. After that (a week) a traumatic ulcer should be treated as an idiopathic one (to all intents and purposes', inasmuch as it is found to be associated with deranged Váyu, Pitta or Kapha Hence at that stage the medical treatment of both the forms of ulcer is (practically) the same. 3.

In short, ulcers are further subdivided (particularly) into fifteen groups, according to the presence of the morbific diathesis (deranged Váyu, Pitta Kapha and blood therein), either severally or in combinations as described (before) in the Chapter on Vrana-Prasna (Sutra Sthánam. Ch. XXI). Several authorities, by adding the simple uncomplicated ulcers (unassociated with any of the morbific principles of the deranged Váyu, Pitta, &c.) to the list, hold the number of types to be sixteen. (Practically they are innumerable, according to the combinations made of the deranged Váyu, etc. and the different **Dhátus** of the system). 4.

Symptoms of ulcer may be divided into two kinds *viz.*, **General** and **Specific.** Pain is the general characteristic (of all forms of ulcer), while the symptoms, which are exhibited in each case according to the virtue of the deranged Váyu, Pitta, etc, involved therein, are called the Specific ones. A **Vrana** is so named from its etymology (the term being derived from the root Vrana—to break) and signifies a cracked or broken condition (of the skin and flesh of the afflicted part) of the body. 5.

**The Vátaja-Ulcer :**—The ulcer assumes a brown or vermilion colour and exudes a thin, slimy and cold secretion, largely attended with tension, throbbing and a sort of pricking and piercing pain (in its inside), which seems as if being expanded and extended. This type of ulcer does not extend much and is characterised by a complete destruction of the tissue (flesh). **The Pittaja ulcer** is rapid in its growth. It assumes a bluish yellow colour, exudes a hot secretion resembling the washings of Kimśuka flowers, and is attended with burning, suppuration and redness, being surrounded with eruptions of small yellow-coloured pustules. The **Kaphaja ulcer** is found to be extended and raised around its margin and is accompanied by an irresistible itching sensation. It is thick and compact (in its depth), covered with a large number of vessels and membranous tissues (Śirá-snáyu-jála), grey in colour, slightly painful, hard and heavy, and exudes a thick, cold, white and slimy secretion. **The Raktaja ulcer** (resulting from a vitiated condition of the blood) looks like a lump of red coral. It is often found to be surrounded by black vesicles and pustules and to smell like a strong alkali. It becomes painful and produces a sensation, as if fumes were escaping out (of it). Bleeding (is present) and the specific symptoms of the Pittaja type are likewise found to supervene. 6—9.

**The Váta-Pittaja Type :**—An ulcer due to the concerted action of the deranged Váyu and Pitta is marked by a pricking and burning pain and a red or vermilion colour. A sensation of fumes arising out of it (is also felt) and the ulcer exudes a secretion which partakes of the characteristic colours of both the deranged Váyu and Pitta. An itching and piercing pain is felt in the ulcer due to the combined action of the deranged Váyu and Kapha (**Kapha-Vátaja type**), which becomes heavy and indurated, constantly discharging a cold, slimy secretion. An ulcer resulting from the deranged condition of the Pitta and Kapha (**Kapha-Pittaja type**) becomes heavy, hot and yellow. It is marked by a burning sensatian and exudes a pale, yellow-coloured secretion. An ulcer marked by the aggravated condition of the deranged Váyu and blood (**Váta-Raktaja type**) is dry and thin and is largely attended with a piercing pain and anæsthesia. It exudes blood or a vermil-coloured secretion and is marked by the combined hues respectively peculiar to the deranged Váyu and blood. An ulcer due to the combined action of the deranged Pitta and blood (**Rakta-Pittaja type**) is marked by a colour which resembles the surface cream of clarified butter. It smells like the washing of fish, is soft, spreading (erysipelatous), and secretes a hot blackish matter. An ulcer due to the combined action of the deranged Kapha and blood (**Kapha-Raktaja type**) is red-coloured, heavy, slimy, glossy and indurated. It is usually marked by itching and exudes a yellowish bloody secretion. An ulcer due to the concerted action of the deranged Váyu, Pitta and blood (**Váta-Pitta-Raktaja type**) is marked by a sort of throbbing, pricking and burning pain. It discharges a flow of thin yellowish blood and produces a sensation, as if fumes were escaping (out of its cavity). An ulcer due to the concerted action of the deranged Váyu, Kapha and blood (**Váta-Sleshma-Raktaja type**) is usually attended with itching, throbbing and tingling sensations and thick, grey, blood-streaked discharge. An ulcer associated with the deranged Kapha, Pitta, and blood (**Kapha-Pitta-Raktaja type**) is largely attended with redness, itching, suppuration and burning sensation. It emits a thick, greyish, bloody secretion. An ulcer marked by the concerted action of the deranged Váyu, Pitta and Kapha (**Sánnipátika**) is attended with diverse kinds of pain, secretion, colour, &c., peculiar to each of these types. An ulcer associated with the combined action of the deranged Váyu, Pitta, Kapha and blood (**Váta-Pitta-Kapha-Raktaja type**) is attended with a sensation, as if it were being burnt and lacerated. It is largely accompanied by throbbing, itching sensation, a sort of pricking and burning pain, with complete anæsthesia in the locality; redness, suppuration, various other kinds of colour, pain and secretion are its further characteristics. 10—20.

An ulcer (Vrana) which is of the same colour with the back of the tongue, soft, glossy, smooth, painless, well-shaped and marked by the absence of any kind of secretion whatsoever, is called a clean ulcer (**Suddha-Vrana**). 21.

**Therapeutics :**—The medical (and surgical) treatment of a **Vrana** (ulcer) admits of being divided into sixty * different factors, such as,—Apatarpana (fasting or low diet), Álepa (plastering), Parisheka (irrigating or spraying), Abhyanga (anointing), Sveda

* **N.B.** Authorities, however, differ in enumerating these factors, although every one of them sticks to the total number of sixty.

(fomentations, etc.), Vimlápana (resolution by massage or rubbing), Upanáha (poultice), Páchana (inducing suppuration), Visrávana (evacuating or draining), Sneha (internal use of medicated oils, ghrita, etc.), Vamana (emetics), Virechana (purgatives), Chhedana (excision), Bhedana (opening—e.g., of an abscess), Dárana (bursting by medicinal applications), Lekhana (scraping), Áharana (extraction), Eshana (probing), Vyadhana (puncturing—opening a vein), Vidrávana (inducing discharge), Sivana (suturing), Sandhána (helping re-union or adhesion), Pidana (pressing), Sonitásthápana (arrest of bleeding), Nirvápana (cooling application), Utkáriká (massive poultices), Kasháya (washing with decoctions), Varti (lint or plug), Kalka (paste), Ghrita (application of medicated clarified butter), Taila (application of medicated oil), Rasa-kriyá (application of drug-extracts), Avachurnana (dusting with medicinal powders), Vrana-Dhupana (fumigation of an ulcer), Utsádana (raising of the margins or bed of an ulcer), Avasádana (destruction of exuberant granulation), Mridu-Karma (softening), Dáruna-Karma (hardening of soft parts), Kshára-Karma (application of caustics), Agni-Karma (cauterization), Krishna-Karma (blackening), Pándu-Karma (making yellow-coloured cicatrices), Pratisárana (rubbing with medicinal powders), Roma-sanjanana (growing of hairs), Lomápaharana (epilation), Vasti-karma (application of enemas), Uttara-Vasti-karma (urethral and vaginal injections), Vandha (bandaging), Patradána (application of certain leaves—vide Infra), Krimighna (Vermifugal measures), Vrimhana (application of restorative tonics), Vishaghna (disinfectant or anti-poisonous applications), Siro-virechana (errhines), Nasya (snuff), Kavala-dhárana (holding in the mouth of certain drug-masses for diseases of the oral cavity or gargling), Dhuma (smoking or vapouring), Madhu-sarpih (honey and clarified butter), Yantra (mechanical contrivances, e g , pulleys, &c.), Áhára (diet) and Rakshá-Vidhána (protection from the influence of malicious spirits). 22.

Of these, Kasháya, Varti, Kalka, Ghrita, Taila, Rasa-kriyá and Avachurnana are the measures for the cleansing (Sodhana) of an ulcer and for helping its granulation (Ropana). The eight acts (from Chhedana to Sivana) are surgical operations. We have already spoken of such acts as Sonitásthápana, Kshára-karma, Agni-karma, Yantra, Áhára, Rakshá-vidhána and Vandha-Vidhána (in the Sutra-sthána). Later on, we shall discourse on Sneha, Sveda, Vamana, Virechana, Vasti, Uttara-vasti, Siro-virechana, Nasya, Dhuma, and Kavala-dhárana. Of the remaining measures we shall speak in the present chapter. 23.

There are six kinds of swellings (Sophas), as described before, and the following eleven measures, commencing with Apatarpana and ending in Virechana, should be regarded as their cure. These are the proper remedies for a swelling and do not (cease to be efficacious in, nor) prove hostile to cases of swelling which are transformed into ulcers. The other measures should be deemed as remedial to ulcers but Apatarpana is the first, general and principal remedy in all types of swellings (Sophas). 24.

**Memorable Verses :**—Apatarpana (fasting) should be prescribed in the case of a patient, full of enraged Doshas, as well as, in one having his organic principles (Dhátus) and refuse matters (Malas) of the system, deranged by them, for the purpose of bringing them to their normal condition, with a regard both to their nature and to the strength, age, &c., of the patient. Persons afflicted with diseases which result from the up-coursing of the deranged Váyu (Urdhva-váta) such as cough, asthma, &c., or with thirst, hunger, dryness of the mouth and fatigue, as well as old men, infants, weak persons, men of timid dispositions and pregnant women should never fast. A swelling and an extremely painful ulcer should be respectively treated with a proper medicated plaster at the very outset. The pain in such a case will yield to the medicinal plaster as a blazing room or house is readily extinguished by means of steady watering. Such plasters not only give comfort to the patient (by removing the pain and leading to the absorption of the swelling), but heaves up the bed of the sore or the ulcer and contributes to its speedy purification and healing up (granulation). 25—28.

In the case of a swelling brought on by the deranged Váyu, the affected part should be washed or sprinkled (Parisheka) with a warm lotion of clarified butter, oil, Dhányámla and essence of meat or with a decoction of the drugs that tend to pacify the enraged Váyu and to relieve the pain. A swelling due to the action of the deranged **Pitta** or **blood** or to the effect of a blow or poison should be washed or sprinkled with a lotion of milk, clarified butter, honey and sugar dissolved in water, the expressed juice of sugar-cane and a cold decoction of the drugs of the Madhura group (Kákolyádi-gana) and the Kshira-Vrikshas. A **Kaphaja** swelling on the body should be washed or sprinkled with a luke-warm lotion of oil, cow's urine, alkaline solution, wine (Surá), Sukta and with a decoction of drugs that destroy the deranged Kapha. 29—31.

**Metrical Text :**—As a fire is put out by jets of water, so the fire of the deranged morbific principles (Doshágni) of the body are speedily subdued and put down by the application of (medicinal lotions) washes. 32.

An anointing (Abhyanga), duly prescribed and used with a full regard to the nature of the aggravated Doshas, leads to their pacification (restoration to the normal condition) and to softness (subsidence) of the swelling. 33.

**Metrical Texts:**—An application of an anointment (Abhyanga) should precede the measures of fomentation, resolution, &c , while it should follow all evacuating measures, &c. A painful, extended and indurated swelling, as well as an ulcer of a similar nature, should be fomented, while an act of Vimlápana (resolution by gentle massage) should be done in respect of a fixed or unfluctuating swelling attended with little or no pain whatsoever. A wise physician should first annoint and foment the part and then gently and slowly press it with a bamboo-reed or with the back of his thumb or palm. A non-suppurated swelling or one that is partially suppurated should be treated with poultice (Upanáha), which would lead to its resolution or suppuration, as the case might be. A swelling, not resolved or not subsiding even after the adoption of the measures beginning with Apatarpana and ending in Virechana (in the given list), should be caused to suppurate with the drugs enumerated in the chapter of Misraka, such as curd, whey, wine (Surá), Sukta and Dhányámla (a kind of fermented paddy gruel). They should be formed into a paste and the paste should be cooked into an efficacious poultice-like composition (Utkáriká), and mixed with salt and oil or clarified butter, it should be applied over the affected part (swelling) and bandaged with the leaves of an Eranda plant. The patient should be allowed to take a wholesome (*i e.*, which does not produce Kapha) diet as soon as suppuration would set in (in the swelling). 34-39.

**Blood-letting :**—Blood-letting should be resorted to in a case of newly formed swelling for its resolution and for alleviating the pain. Bleeding (**Visrávana**) is recommended in the case of an ulcer which is indurated, marked by a considerable swelling and inflammation and is reddish black or red-coloured, extremely painful, gagged in its shape and considerably extended at its base (congested), specially in the case of a poisonous ulcer, for the subsidence of the pain and for warding off a process of suppuratiou therein, either by applying leeches or by opening (a vein in the locality) by means of an instrument. An ulcer-patient of a dry or parched temperament affected with distressing supervenients or ulcer-cachixia or who is weak should be made to drink an emulsive potion cooked with (a decoction of) appropriate drugs. A patient afflicted with an ulcer with an elevated margin and attended with swelling and specially marked by the presence of the deranged Kapha and by a flow of blackish red blood should be treated with emetics. Ulcer-experts recommend purgatives to a patient afflicted with an old or long-standing ulcer, attended with a deranged condition of the Váyu and Pitta. An **excision** should be made into an ulcer which refuses to suppurate and which is of a hard and indurated character attended with sloughing of the local nerves and ligaments (Snáyu). An **opening** or excision (Bhedana) should be made into an ulcer (Vrana) in the inside of which pus has accumalated and makes it heave up and which not finding any outlet consequently eats into the underlying tissues and makes fissures and cavities. 40-46.

Measures which contribute to a spontaneous bursting by medicinal applications (**Dárana**) of a swelling should be adopted in the case of an infant or an old or enfeebled patient, or of one incapable of bearing the pain (of a surgical operation), or of a person of a timid disposition, as well as in the case of a woman, and in the case of swellings which appear on the vulnerable parts (Marmas) of the body. Remedies which lead to the spontaneous bursting of a swelling should be applied by a wise physician to a well-suppurated swelling drawn up and with all its pus gathered to a head ; or an alkaline substance should be applied on its surface and a bursting should be effected when the Doshas are found to be just aggravated by the incarcerated pus. 47.

An ulcer which is indurated, whose edges are thick and rounded, which has been repeatedly burst open, and the flesh of whose cavity is hard and elevated, should be scarified by a surgeon ; or, in other words, an indurated ulcer should be deeply scarified, one with thick and rounded edges should be excessively scarified, while the one which has been repeatedly burst open should be entirely scraped off. An ulcer with a hard and elevated bed should be scraped evenly and longitudinally along the length of its cavity. In the absence of a scarifying instrument, the act should be performed with a piece of Kshauma (cloth made of the fibres of an Atasi plant), a linen (Plota) or a cotton pad (Pichu), or with such alkaline substances as nitrate of potash, Samudra-phena, rock-salt, or rough leaves of trees (e. g., those of Udumbara, &c.). 48.

The cavities or courses of a sinus, or of an ulcer which had any foreign matter lying imbedded in its inside, or which takes a crooked or round about direction, as well as of the one formed into cavities within its interior, should

---

\* This scraping off of the ulcer should be done by an instrument of Surgery and not by any rough leaf or the like, mentioned hereafter.

be probed by gently introducing the tender fibres of bamboo sprouts (Karira), a (lock of) hair, a finger, or an indicator into its inside. The course of a sinus occurring about the anus or in the region of the eyes (Netra-Vartma) should be probed with the slender fibres of Chuchchu, Upodiká, or Karira, in the event of their mouths being narrow and attended with bleeding. The Sálya (incarcerated pus, etc.) should be extricated, whether the mouth of the sinus is constricted or otherwise, in conformityw ith the directions laid down before on that behalf. In diseases amenable to acts of puncturing (Vyadhana), the knife should be inserted into the seat of the disease to a proper depth and extent, to be determined by its situation in the body, and the Doshas (pus, etc.) should be let out, as stated before. Ulcers with a wide mouth, unattended with any symptoms of suppuration, and occurring in a fleshy part of the body, should be sutured up, and the adhesion (Sandhána) of the edges should likewise be effected, as directed before. A plaster composed of drugs (capable of drawing out and secreting the pus), as described before, should be applied around the mouth of an ulcer seated in any of the Marmas (vulnerable parts), or full of pus in its inside, with a narrow-mouthed aperture. The plaster should be removed when dry, and should not be applied on the orifice of the ulcer, as it would, in that case, interfere with the spontaneous secretion of pus (Dosha). 49-54.

An excessive hæmorrhage incidental to such acts, as excessive hurting of the vein, etc., should be arrested with suitable styptic* measures and remedies (Sonitàsthápana).

---

* Styptic measures are of four kinds—Sandhàna, Skandana, Páchana, and Dahana. See Sutra-Sthánam, Chap. XIV.

An ulcer attended with fever, suppuration and burning sensation due to the excited state of the deranged Pitta and congestion of blood should be allayed (Nirvápana—literally putting out) with suitable and proper medicinal remedies. It should be allayed with compounds made up of the proper cooling drugs (of the Miśraka chapter), pasted with milk and lubricated with clarified butter. Cooling plasters (Lepa) should then be applied as well. 55-56.

An ulcer whose flesh is eaten away, which discharges a thin secretion, or is non-suppurating in its character, and is marked by roughness, hardness, shivering and the presence of an aching and piercing pain, should be fomented with a poultice-like efficacious preparation (**Utkáriká** )cooked with the drugs of Váyu-subduing properties, those included within the Amla-varga, and those which belong to the Kákolyádi group, and with the oily seeds (such as linseed, sesamum, mustard, castor, etc.). An indurated, painful, fætid, moist and slimy ulcer should be washed with a disinfectant or purifying lotion consisting of a decoction of the drugs mentioned before for the purpose. 57-58.

Plugs or lints plastered with a paste of the purifying drugs (enumerated before) should be inserted into an ulcer with any foreign matter (e.g., pus) lying embedded in it, or into one with a deep but narrow opening, or into one situated in a fleshy part of the body. An ulcer full of putrid flesh and marked by the action of the highly deranged Doshas (Váyu and Kapha) should be purified with a paste of the aforesaid available drugs making up the plug. An ulcer of a Pittaja origin, which is deep-seated and attended with a burning sensation and with suppuration, should be purified with the application of a medicated clarified butter, prepared with the purifying drugs with an admixture of Kárpása-phala*. An intelligent Surgeon should purify an ulcer with raised flesh, and which is dry and is attended with scanty secretion with an application of medicated mustard oil. An indurated ulcer, refusing to be purified with the foregoing medicated oils, should be purified with a duly prepared decoction of the drugs enumerated before (Sutra. chap. 38,—the Sálasárádi group) and prepared in the following manner of **Rasa-kriyá**. A decoction of the said drugs duly prepared should be saturated with an after-throw of *Haritála, Manahs'ilá, Kásisa* and *Saurâshtra* earth, and well compounded together ; the preparation should also be mixed with the expressed juice of *Mátulunga* and with honey. The medicine thus prepared should be applied to the ulcer on every third or fourth day. 59.

Deep† and foul-smelling ulcers covered with layers of deranged fat (phlegmonous ulcer) should be purified by the learned physician with the powders of the drugs with which the purifying plug or the lint has been enjoined to be plastered (Ajagandhá, &c.). Decoctions of the drugs which are possessed of the virtue of setting in a process of granulation (**Ropana**) in an ulcer, such as *Vata*, &c., as stated before, should be used by a surgeon (Vaidya) after it had been found to have been thoroughly purified. Medicated plugs, composed of drugs possessing healing properties (such as, *Soma, Amritá, As'vagandhá, etc.*) should be inserted in deep-seated ulcers, when cleansed and unattended with pain. 60-62.

---

\* The total weight of the purifying drugs should be equal to that of the Kárpása-phala alone and they should be boiled together with four times their qnantity of clarified butter and with sixteen times of water.

† There is a different reading of "Agambhira" in place of "Gabhira," but Gayi thinks the emendation undesirable.

A Kalka or a levigated paste of sesamum and honey (mentioned in the Misraka Chapter) should be applied for the purpose of healing up an ulcer situated in a muscular part from which all putrid flesh has been removed or sloughed off and which exhibited a clear cavity. This paste (of sesamum) tends to allay the deranged Váyu through its sweet taste, oleaginousness and heat-making potency; subdues the deranged Pitta through its astringent, sweet and bitter taste and proves beneficial even in the case of the deranged Kapha through its heat-producing potency and bitter and astringent taste. An application of the levigated paste of sesamum mixed with the drugs of purifying and healing properties tends to purify and heal up an ulcer. An application of the levigated paste of sesamum mixed with honey and *Nimba*-leaves leads to the purification of sores; whereas an application of the same paste (*i e*, sesamum, honey and leaves of *Nimba*), mixed with clarified butter tends to heal up the ulcer. Several authorities atribute the same virtue to a barley-paste.[*] Levigated pastes of barley and of sesamum (or a paste of barley mixed with sesamum) contribute to the resolution or subsidence of a non-suppurated swelling, fully suppurate one which is partially suppurated, lead to the spontaneous bursting of a fully suppurated one, and purify as well as heal up one that has already burst out. 63-65.

An ulcer, which is due to the effects of poison, vitiated blood, or aggravated Pitta, and which is deep-seated or is of traumatic origin, should be healed up with a medicated clarified butter prepared with the drugs of healing virtues (Ropaniya—enumerated before) and milk. An ulcer marked by an aggravated condition of the deranged

---

[*] Jejjada and Gayadása interpret the term to mean "barley-paste mixed with sesamum."

Váyu and Kapha should be healed up with the application of an oil, boiled and prepared with the proper purifying drugs mentioned before. 66 67.

Rasa-kriyá* with the two kinds of *Haridrá* should be resorted to for the purpose of healing up an ulcer, in which bandaging is forbidden (such as those due to the deranged Pitta or blood, or to blow, &c., or to the effects of poison), and an ulcer appearing on the moveable joints, which, though exhibiting all the features of a well-cleansed sore, has not been marked by any process of healthy granulation†. Healing medicinal powders should be used in the case of an ulcer which is confined to the skin, and is firm-fleshed and marked by the absence of any irregularity in its shape (*i.e.*, not uneven in its margin). The mode of applying medicinal powders, as stated in the Sutra-sthána, should be adopted in the present instance. 68-69.

The healing and purifying measures described above should be deemed equally applicable to, and efficacious in cases of ulcers in general with regard to their Doshas (both idiopathic and traumatic). The success of these measures has been witnessed in thousands of cases and has been recorded in the Sástras (authorised works on medicine). Hence they should be used as incantations without any doubt as to their tested and infallible efficacy. An intelligent physician should employ the drugs, mentioned before, in any of the seven forms (either in the shape of a decoction, or a

---

* The decoction of *Triphalá* and the drugs of the Nyagrodhádi group should be duly prepared, filtered and then condensed to the consistency of treacle. Powders of *Haridrá* and Dáru-haridrá should be then thrown into it. In the end, the whole preparation should be well-stirred, mixed with honey and applied. This is what is called **Rasa-kriyá**.

† Several editions read "though cleansed yet ungranulating ulcers."

plug, or a paste, or through the medium of medicated oils and clarified butter, or in the shape of Rasa-kriyá, or as powders), according to the requirements of each case. 70.

The drugs which constitute the two groups of Panchamulas (major and minor), as well as those of the Váyu-subduing group, should be employed in the case of an ulcer due to the aggravated **Váyu** in any of the seven forms —decoction, etc. Similarly the drugs which are included within the groups of Nyagrodhádi or Kákolyádi should be used in any of those seven forms, in the case of an ulcer due to the aggravated **Pitta** (for the purification and healing thereof). Drugs which form the group of Áragvadhádi, as well as those which have been described as heat-making in their potency, should be used in any of those seven aforesaid forms, in the case of an ulcer due to the deranged **Kapha**. The drugs of two or three of those groups, should be combinedly used in any of those seven forms, in connection with an ulcer marked by the aggravated condition of any **two** or **three** of the deranged Doshas respectively. 71-74.

**Fumigation :**—Vátaja ulcers with severe pain and secretion should be fumigated with the fumes of *Kshauma*, barley, clarified butter and other proper fumigating substances [such as turpentine and resin (gum of Sála tree)]. 75.

**Utsádana-Kriyá** ( Elevation ) **:**—Medicated plasters (consisting of *Apámárga, As'vagandhá*, etc.) and medicated clarified butter (prepared with the same drugs should be used in ulcers (due to the aggravated Váyu and marked by the absence of any secretion, and affecting a considerably smaller area or depth of flesh, as well as in those (due to the deranged and aggravated Pitta and) seated deep into the flesh, for the purpose of raising up (filling up) the beds or cavities thereof. Meat of carnivorous animals should be taken in the proper manner by the patient, inasmuch as meat properly partaken of in a calm and joyful frame of mind adds to the bodily flesh of its partaker. 76.

**Avasádana** (destruction of super-growths):—Proper drugs or articles (such as sulphate of copper, etc.) powdered and pasted with honey should be applied for destroying the soft marginal growths of an ulcer found to be more elevated than the surrounding surface of the affected locality. 77.

**Mridu-Karma** (softening):—In respect of indurated and fleshless (not seated in a part of the body where flesh abounds) ulcers marked by a deranged condition of Váyu, softening measures (with the help of repeated applications of lotions and plasters composed of sweet and demulcent substances mixed with salt in a tepid or luke-warm state) and blood-letting* should be resorted to. Sprinkling (Seka) and application of clarified butter or oil prepared with the Váyu-subduing drugs should also be resorted to. 78.

**Dáruna-karma:**—The employment of hardening measures (Dáruna-karma) is efficacious in connection with soft ulcers and in the following manner. Barks of *Dhava, Priyangu, As'oka, Rohini,* Triphalá, *Dhátaki* flowers, *Lodhra* and *Sarjarasa*, taken in equal parts and pounded into fine powders, should be strewn over the ulcer, i.e., the ulcer should be dusted with the same. 79.

**Kshára-Karma** (Potential cauterization):—The measure of applying alkali should be adopted for the

---

\* Blood-letting should be resorted to in the event of any vitiated blood being found to have been involved in the case ; but in the event of a similar participation of any deranged Kapha, oils and lotions composed of the Váyu-destroying drugs should be made use of.

purification of the sore of a long-standing ulcer which is of an indurated character with its margin raised higher (than the surrounding skin), and is marked by itching and a stubborn resistance to all purifying medicines. 80.

**Agni-Karma** (actual cauterization) :—An ulcer incidental to an act of lithotomic operation allowing the urine to dribble out through its fissure, or one marked by excessive bleeding, or in which the connecting ends have been completely severed, should be actually cauterised with fire. 81.

**Krishna-Karma :**—The blackening of a white cicatrix, which is the result of a bad or defective granulation, should be made (after the complete healing up of the ulcer) in the following manner. Several *Bhallátaka* seeds should be first soaked in the urine of a cow (and then dried in the sun, this process should be repeated for seven days consecutively), after which they should be kept (a week) immersed in a pitcher full of milk. After that the seeds should be cut into two and placed in an iron pitcher. Another pitcher should be buried in the ground with a thin and perforated lid placed over its mouth, and the pitcher containing the seeds should be placed upon it with its mouth downward (so that the mouths of the two pitchers might meet), and then the meeting place should be firmly joined (with clay). This being done a cow-dung fire should be lit around the upper pitcher. The oily matter (melted by the heat) and dribbling down from the Bhallátaka seeds into the underground pitcher should be slowly and carefully collected. The hoofs of village animals (such as horses, etc.) and those which live in swamps (Ánupas— such as buffaloes, etc.) should be burnt and pounded together into extremely fine powder. The oil (of the Bhallátaka seeds collected as above) should then be mixed with this powder, and applied to the white cicatrix. Similarly, the oily essence of the piths of some kinds of wood, as well as of some kinds of fruit (*Phala-sneha*) prepared in the manner of the Bhallátaka oil (and mixed with the powdered ashes of hoofs) should be used for the blackening of a cicatrix. 82-83.

**Pándu-karana :**—The natural and healthy colour (Pándu) of the surrounding skin should be imparted to a cicatrix which has assumed a black colour owing to the defective or faulty healing up of the sore in the following manner. The fruit of the *Rohini*\* should be immersed in goat's milk for seven nights and, afterwards finely pasted with the same milk, should be applied to the skin. This measure is called **Pándu-karana** (imparting a yellow or natural skin-colour to the cicatrix). To attain the same result, the powder of a new earthen pot, *Vetasa* roots, *S'ála* roots, Sulphate of iron, and *Madhuka* (Yashti-madhu) pasted together with honey may be used. As an alternative, the hollow rind of the *Kapittha* fruit, from which the pulp has been removed, should be filled with the urine of a goat together with Kásisa (Sulphate of iron), *Rochaná*, Tuttham (Sulphate of copper). *Haritála, Manahs'ilá,* scrapings of raw bamboo skin, Prapunnáda (seeds of Chákunde), and Rasánjana and buried a month beneath the roots of an *Arjuna* tree after which it should be taken out and applied to the black cicatrix. The shell of a hen's egg, *Kataka, Madhuka,* (Yashti-madhu), sea-oysters and crystals† (pearls according to Jejjata and Brahmadeva) taken in equal parts should be pounded and pasted with

---

\* Rohini, according to some commentators, means a kind of Haritaki ; according to others, it means Katu-tumbi.

† Burnt ashes of sea-oysters and pearls etc., should be used.

the urine of a cow and made into boluses which should be rubbed over the cicatrix.* 84-87.

**Roma-sanjanana**—hair-producers :— The burnt ashes of ivory and pure *Rasánjana* (black antimony) pounded (and pasted with goat's milk) should be applied to the spot where the appearance of hair (*Lomotpatti*) is desired. An application of this plaster would lead to the appearance of hair even on the palms of the hands. Another alternative is a pulverised compound consisting of the burnt ashes of the bones, nails, hair, skin, hoofs and horns of any quadruped, over a part of the body, previously anointed (rubbed) with oil, which would lead to the appearance of hair in that region. And lastly, a plaster composed of Sulphate of iron, and tender *Karanja* leaves pasted with the expressed juice of *Kapittha*, would be attended with the same result. 88—90.

**Hair-depilators :**—The hair of an ulcerated part of the body found to interfere with the satisfactory healing up of the ulcer, should be shaved with a razor or clipped with scissors, or rooted out with the help of forceps. As an alternative, an application of a plaster consisting of two parts of pulverised (burnt ashes of) conch-shell and one part of *Haritála* (yellow orpiment or yellow oxide of arsenic) pasted with Śukta (an acid gruel) over the desired spot, would be attended with the same result A compound made of the oil of **Bhallátaka** mixed with the milky exudation of Snuhi, should be used by an intelligent physician as a depilatory measure. As an alternative, the burnt ashes of the stems of plantain leaves and *Dirghavrinta* (Śyonáka) mixed with rock-salt, *Haritála* and the seeds of Śami,

---

* This also is a remedy for giving a natural colour to the skin.

pasted with cold water, should be deemed a good hair-depilatory.* A plaster composed of the ashes of the tail of a domestic lizard, plantain, Haritála (oxide of arsenic), and the seeds of *Ingudi* burnt together and pasted with oil and water, and baked in the sun may also be used for the eradicating of hair in the affected locality. 94-95.

**Vasti-Karma :**—A medicated Vasti (**enema**) should be applied to the rectum in the case of an ulcer marked by an aggravated condition of the deranged Váyu which is extremely dry and is attended with an excruciating pain occurring specially in the lower region of the body. A measure of **Uttara-vasti** (Vaginal or Urethral syringe) should be adopted in the cases of strictures and other disorders connected with urine, semen and menstruation, as well as in cases of gravel † in case these are due to an ulcer. An ulcer is purified, softened and healed up by **bandaging** leaving no room for the apprehension of a relapse. Hence bandaging is recommended. 96-98.

**Patradána** (application of leaves on an ulcer) :— Leaves possessed of proper medicinal virtues taking into consideration the particular Dosha and season of the year should be tied (over the medicinal plaster applied) over an ulcer of non-shifting or non-changing character and not affecting a large depth of flesh and which refuses to be healed up owing to its extreme dryness. An ulcer of the deranged Váyu should be tied over with the leaves of the *Eranda, Bhurja, Putika,* or *Haridrá* plants as well as with those of the *Upodiká* and *Gámbhári.* An ulcer marked by an aggravated condition

---

\* According to some this may be used internally for the purpose.

† D. R. Some read "Tathánile" in place of "Aśmari-vrane." "Tathánile" means and in cases of (aggravated) Váyu.

of the deranged Pitta, or incidental to a vitiated condition of the blood, should be tied in the aforesaid manner with the leaves of the *Kás'mari*, the *Kshira* trees (milk-exuding trees), and aquatic plants. An ulcer due to the deranged and aggravated Kapha, should be tied over with the leaves of the *Páthá, Murvá, Guduchi, Káka-máchi, Haridrá* or of the *S'ukanásá*. Only those leaves which are not rough, nor putrid, nor old and decomposed, nor worm-eaten and which are soft and tender should be used for purposes of **Patradána**.* The rationale of such a procedure (Patra-vandha) is that the leaves tied by an intelligent physician in the manner above indicated serve to generate heat or cold and retain the liniment or medicated oil in their seat of application. 99-102.

**Vermifugal :**—The germination of **worms** due to flies in an ulcer is attended with various kinds of extreme pain, swelling and bleeding in case the worms eat up the flesh. A decoction of the drugs of the *Surasádi* gana proves efficacious as a wash and healing medicine in such a case. The ulcer should be plastered with such drugs as the bark of *Saptaparna, Karanja, Arka, Nimba,* and *Rájádana* pasted with the urine of a cow, or washed with an alkaline wash (for expelling the vermin from it). As an alternative, the worms should be brought out of the ulcer by placing a small piece of raw flesh on the ulcer. These vermin may be divided into twenty groups or classes, which will be fully dealt with later on. (Uttara-Tantram—ch. 54). 103.

**Vrinhanam** (use of restorative and constructive tonics) :—All kinds of tone-giving and constructive measures should be adopted in the case of a patient

---

* The leaf which does not poison the Sneha and the essence of the medicinal drugs placed in a folded piece of linen (and applied over an ulcer is the proper leaf and) should be used for tying over the paste.

weak and emaciated with the troubles of a long-standing sore, taking full precaution not to tax his digestive powers. **Anti-toxic** (Vishaghna) medicines and measures and symptoms of poisonings will be described under their respective heads in the Kalpa-Sthánam. 104-105.

**Śiro-virechana and Nasya :**—Śiro-virechana measures (errhines) shou'd be resorted to by skilful physicians in respect of ulcers situated in the clavicle regions and marked by itching and swelling. The use of medicated (fatty) **snuff** (Nasya) is recommended in cases where the ulcers would be found to be seated in the regions above the clavicles and marked by an aggravated condition of the deranged Váyu, pain, and absence of the oily matter. 106-107.

**Kavala-dhárana :**—Medicated gargles (consisting of decoctions of drugs) of purifying or healing virtues either hot or cold\* (according to requirements) should be used in the case of an ulcer in the mouth, for the purpose of alleviating the Doshas therein, for allaying the local pain and burning, and for removing the impurities of the teeth and the tongue. 108.

**Dhuma-pána :**—Inhaling of smoke or vapours (of medicated drugs) should be prescribed in cases of ulcers of the deranged Váyu and Kapha attended with swelling, secretion and pain and situated in the region above the clavicles. Application of **honey** and **clarified butter**, separately or mixed together should be prescribed in cases of extended or elongated ulcers which are traumatic or incidental in their character (Sadyo-Vrana) for allaying the heat of the ulcer and for bringing about its adhesion. **Surgical instruments** should be used in connec-

---

\* Hot gargles are recommended in cases of ulcers of the deranged Váyu and Kapha while cold ones in cases of ulcers of the aggravated Pitta and blood.

tion with an ulcer which is deep-seated but provided with a narrow orifice and which is due to the penetration of a S'alya (shaft) and which could not be removed with the hand alone. 109-111.

The **diet** of an ulcer-patient should in all cases be made to consist of food which is light in quantity as well as in quality, demulcent, heat-making (in potency) and possessed of appetising properties.* **Protective rites** should be performed for the safety of an ulcer-patient from the influences of malignant stars and spirits with the major and the minor duties (Yama and Niyama) enjoined to be practised on his behalf. 112-113.

The causes of ulcers are six† ; their seats in the body number eight‡ in all ; the features which characterise them are five §. The medicinal measures and remedies in respect of ulcers are sixty ‖ in number. And these ulcers are curable with the help or co-operation of the four necessary factors (the physician, the medicines, the nurse and the patient). 114.

The comparatively smaller number of drugs which I have mentioned (under the heads of Ropana, S'odhana, etc., in the present chapter) from fear of prolixity, may be increased in combination with other drugs or substances of similar virtue, (digestionary transformation and potency, etc.) without any apprehension

---

* See Chap. XIX.—Sutra-Sthánam.

† The six causes of an ulcer are Váyu, Pitta, Kapha, Sannipáta, S'onita aud Ágantu.

‡ The eight seats of an ulcer are Tvak, Mánsa, S'irá, Snáyu, Sandhi, Asthi, Koshtha and Marma.

§ The five symptoms of an ulcer are due to Váta, Pitta, Kapha, Sannipáta and Ágantu. The symptoms due to S'onita being identical with those due to Pitta, are not separately counted.

‖ The sixty medicinal measures and remedies are those described before in the present chapter.

of doing any mischief thereby. Recipes consisting of rare or a large number of drugs or ingredients, should be made up with as many of them as would be available in the absence of all of them, as mentioned in the present work. A drug belonging to any particular Gana or group if separately described as non-efficacious to any specific disease, should be omitted whereas a drug not belonging to a group may be added to it if it is elsewhere laid down as positively beneficial thereto. 115-117.

**Upadrava :**—The distressing supervening symptoms which are found to attend a case of **ulcer,** are quite different from those of an **ulcer-patient.** Those which confine themselves solely to the ulcer are five in all— smell, colour, etc., and those which are exclusively manifest in the patient are fever, diarrhœa, hiccup, vomiting, fainting fits, aversion to food, cough, difficult breathing, indigestion and thirst. The medical treatment of ulcers though described in detail in the present chapter, will be further dealt with in the next chapter on **Sadyo-Vrana.** 118-120.

Thus ends the first Chapter of the Chikitsita-Sthánam in the Sus'ruta Samhitá which deals with the treatment of the two kinds of ulcer.

# CHAPTER II.

Now we shall discourse on the medical treatment of recent or traumatic wounds or sores **(Sadyovrana-Chikitsá).** 1,

**Metrical Texts:** —The holy Dhanvantari, the foremost of the pious and the greatest of all discoursers, thus discoursed to his disciple Sus'ruta, the son of Vis'vámitra. 2.

**Different shapes of Sores :**—I shall describe the shapes of the various kinds of Vrana (sores or wounds) caused by weapons of variously shaped edges in the different parts of the human body. Traumatic ulcers have a variety of shapes. Some of these are elongated, others are rectangular, or triangular, or circular, while some are crescent shaped, or extended, or have a zigzag shape, and some are hollow in the middle like a saucer, and lastly some have she shapes of a barley corn (bulged out at the middle). An abscess or a swelling, due to the several Doshas and which spontaneouly bursts out, may assume any of the aforesaid forms, while the one effected by a surgeon's knife should never have a distorted or an improper shape. A surgeon thoroughly familiar with the shapes of ulcers is never puzzled at the sight of one of a terrible and distorted shape. 3—5.

Physicians of yore have grouped these variously shaped traumatic ulcers under six broad sub-heads, such as the Chhinna (cut), Bhinna (punctured or perforated), Viddha (pierced), Kshata (contused), Pichchita (crushed), and the Ghrishta (mangled or lacerated) according to their common features and I shall describe their symptoms. 6.

**Their definitions:**—A traumatic ulcer which is oblique or straight and elongated is called a **Chhinna** (cut) ulcer, while a complete severance of a part or member of the body is also designated by that name. A perforation of any of the cavities or receptacles of the body by the tip of a Kunta, spear, Rishti, or a sword or by a horn, attended with a little discharge, constitutes what is called a **Bhinna** (punctured) wound or ulcer. The Ámáśaya (stomach), the Pakváśaya (intestines), the Agnyáśaya (gall-bladder?), the Mutráśaya (urinary bladder), the Raktáśaya (receptacle of blood), the heart, the Unduka and the lungs constitute what is called the **Koshtha** (viscus). A perforation (of the wall of any) of the Áśayas causes it to become filled with blood which is discharged through the urethra, the anus, the mouth or the nostrils and is attended with fever, thirst, fainting fits, dyspnœa, burning sensations, tympanites, suppression of stool, urine and flatus (Váta) with an aversion for food, perspiration, redness of the eyes, a bloody smell in the mouth, and feted one in the body and an aching pain in the heart and in the sides. 7—10.

Now hear me discourse on (their) detailed symptoms. A perforation of the wall of the **Ámáśaya** (stomach) is marked by constant vomiting of blood, excessive tympanites and an excruciating pain. A perforation of the **Pakváśaya** fills it with blood and is attended with extreme pain, a heaviness in the limbs, coldness of the sub-umbilical region, and bleeding through the (lower) ducts and orifices of the body. Even in the absence of any perforation, the Antras (intestines) are filled with blood through the small pores or apertures in their walls in the same manner as a pitcher with its mouth firmly covered may be filled through the pores (in its sides), and a sense of heaviness is also perceived in their inside. 11-13.

A wound or an ulcer caused by any sharp pointed Salya (shaft) in any part of the body other than the aforesaid Ásayas with or without that Salya being extricated is called a **Viddha** (pierced one). An ulcer which is neither a cut nor a perforation or puncture but partakes of the nature of both and is uneven is called a **Kshata** (wound). A part of the body with the local bone crushed between the folds of a door or by a blow becomes extended and covered with blood and marrow and is called a **Pichchita** (thrashed) wound or ulcer. The skin of any part of the body suffering abrasion through friction or from any other such like causes and attended with heat and a secretion is called a **Ghrishta** (mangled or lacerated) wound or ulcer. 14-17.

**Their Treatment :**—A part or member of the body any wise cut, perforated, pierced or wounded which is attended with excessive bleeding and with the local Váyu enraged or aggravated by the incidental bleeding, or hæmorrhage will occasion excruciating pain. Potions of Sneha (oily or fatty liquids) and using the same as a washing (in a lukewarm state) should be advised in such cases. Preparation of Vesaváras and other Krisarás largely mixed with oil or clarified butter should be used as poultices and fomentations with the Másha pulse, etc., and the use of oily ungents and emulsive Vastis (enematas)* prepared with decoctions of Váyu-subduing drugs should be applied. A crushed or thrashed wound or abrasion is not attended with any excessive bleeding an absolute absence whereof, (on the contrary) gives rise to an excessive burning sensation and suppuration in the affected part. Cold washes and cooling plasters should be used in these cases for the alleviation of the

* Snehapána is recommended when the ulcer is in a region above the umbilicus and Vasti-karma when the ulcer is in a subumbilical region.

burning and suppuration as well as for the cooling of the (incarcerated) heat. What has been specifically said of these six forms of ulcers, or wounds should be understood to include the treatment of all kinds of traumatic wounds or ulcers as well. 18—20.

**Treatment of cuts or incised wounds &c :**—Now we shall discourse on the medical treatment of **Chhinna** cuts. An open mouthed ulcer on the side of the head* should be duly sutured as described before and firmly bandaged. An ear severed or lopped off should be sutured in the proper way and position and oil should be poured into its cavity. A Chhinna cut on the Krikatiká (lying on the posterior side of the junction of the neck and the head) and even if it allow the Váyu † (air) to escape through its cavity should be brought together and duly sutured and bandaged in a manner (so as not to leave any intervening space between'. The part thus adhesioned should be sprinkled with clarified butter prepared from goat's milk. The patient should be made to take his food lying on his back, properly secured or fastened with straps (so that he might not move his head and advised to perform all other physical acts such as, urination, defecation etc, in that position). 21-24

In the case of a lateral and wide-mouthed wound (sword-cut, etc.) on the extremeties, the bone-joints should be duly set and joined together as instructed before and the wound should be sutured and speedily bandaged in the manner of a Vellitaka bandage, or

---

* Several commentators explain those that are situated either on the head or on the sides.

† The dictum that a hurt on any of the wind-carrying sounding channels is pronounced to be incurable, should not be supposed to hold good in the present case.

with a piece of skin or hide in the Gophaná or such other form as would seem proper and beneficial and oil should be poured over it. In the case of a wound on the back the patient should be laid on his back, while in the case of its occurring on the chest the patient should be laid on his face.* 25-27.

In the case of a hand or a leg being carried away or completely severed the wound should be cauterised with the application of hot oil and bandaged in the manner of a **Kosha** bandage and proper healing medicines should be applied. An oil cooked with the eight drugs *Chandana, Padmaka, Rodhra, Utpala, Priyangu, Haridrá, Madhuka,* (Yasthimadhu) and milk, forms one of the most efficacious healing (**Ropana**) agents A Kalka of the thirteen drugs—*Chandana, Karkatákhya,* the two kinds of *Sahá* (Mugáni and Masháni), *Mánsi,* (D.R.— Máshahva, Somáhva), *Amritá, Harenu, Mrinála Triphalá, Padmaka* and *Utpala* should be cooked in oil mixed with milk (four times that of oil) and the three other kinds of oily matter (lard, marrow and clarified butter) and this medicated oil should be used for sprinkling over a wound of this type for the purpose of healing (Ropana). 28.

**Medical Treatment of Bhinna :—** Henceforth we shall deal with the medical treatment of **Bhinna** (excised) wounds. A case of an excised eye (Bhinna) should be given up as incurable. But in the case where an eye (ball) instead of being completely separated would be found to be dangling out (of its

---

* For the complete elimination of the deranged Dosha *i.e.*, pus, etc , of the wound invloved in the case—Jejjata.

He who has got a wound on his back should be laid on his face and he who has got an ulcer on his breast should be laid on his back— Differeut Reading Gayi.

socket) the affected organ should be re-instated in its natural cavity in a manner so as not to disturb the connected Śirás (nerve arrangements) and gently pressed with the palms of the hand by first putting a lotus leaf on its (eye) surface. After that the eye should be filled (Tarpana) with the following (D.R,— Ájena in place of "Anena"—i.e., prepared from goat's milk) medicated clarified butter, which should be as well used in the form of an errhine. The recipe is as follows :—Clarified butter prepared from goat's milk, *Madhuka*, *Utpala*, *Jivaka* and *Rishavaka* taken in equal parts should be pasted together, and cooked with sixteen seers of cow's milk and four seers of clarified butter.* The use of the medicated Ghrita thus prepared should be regarded as commendable in all types of occular hurt or injury. 29.

In the case of a perforation of the abdomen marked by the discharge of lumps or rope-like Varti (fat) through the wound, the emitted or ejected fat-lump should be dusted with the burnt ashes (D. R. – powders) of astringent woods (such as *Manu*, *Arjuna*, etc.) and black clay (pounded together). A ligature of thread should then be bound round the fat-lump and the fat-lump cut off with a heated instrument. Honey should then be applied and the wound (Vrana) should then be duly bandaged. The patient should be caused to drink clarified butter after the full digestion of his injested food. Instead of this Ghrita, milk prepared

---

* Several authorities, however, say that equal parts of clarified butter prepared from goat's milk and from cow's milk should be taken and cooked with 16 seers of cow's milk and with the four drugs as a Kalka.

But Gayi recommends only four seers of clarified butter prepared from goat's milk cooked with 16 seers of cow's milk and the four drugs as a Kalka.

medicinally with *Yashti-maddu*, *Lákshá* and *Gokshura*, mixed with (a proper quantity of) sugar and castor oil (as Prakshepa)*, is equally commendable for the alleviation of the pain and the burning sensation, (in the wound or ulcer). The fat-lump (pariental fat) aforesaid causes a rumbling sound with pain in the abdomen and may prove even fatal in the event of its being left uncut. The medicated oil to be mentioned hereafter in connection with Medaja-Granthi should be applied in such cases. 30-32

Foreign bodies (Śalya) piercing into any of the Koshthas after having run through the (seven layers of) skin, whether passing through the veins, etc , (muscles, nerves, bones or joints, or not, produces the distressing symptoms described before (Ch. III.—Sutra). The blood (of the affected chamber or receptacle) in such case lies incarcerated therein in the event of its failing to find an outlet and causes a pallor of the face and a coldness of the extremities and of the face in the patient. Respiration becomes cold, the eyes red-coloured, the bowels constipated and the abdomen distended. The manifestation of these symptoms indicates the incurable character of the disease. 33-34.

* This explanation is given on the authority of old Vágabhata. Dallana, however, explains the verse in a different way. He explains it to mean two different preparations of milk—one with Vashti-madhu and mixed with sugar and castor oil as a Prakshepa and the other with Gokshura and mixed with Lákshá and castor oil as a Prakshepa.

A third interpretation would make three preparations of milk prepared separately with Yashti-madhu, Lákshá and Gokshura—sugar and castor oil being mixed in the first (as Prakshepa) and castor oil alone in the second and third.

A fourth preparation would be to prepare the milk separately with Yashtimadhu, Lákshá and Gokshura as in the preceding case—without the addition of castor oil (as Prakshepa).

Emesis is beneficial in the case where the blood would be found to be confined in the Ámásaya (stomach). Purgatives should unhesitatingly be prescribed where the blood would be found to have been lodged in the Pakvásaya (intestines) and Ásthápana measures without oil should be employed with hot, purifying (Sodhana) substances (such as the cow-urine, etc.) The patient should be made to drink a Yavágu (gruel) with Saindhava salt and his diet should consist of boiled rice mixed with the soup of barley, *Kola* and *Kulalttha* pulse divested of oil. 35-36.

In a case of a perforation or piercing of any of the bodily Koshthas attended with excessive hæmorrhage or bleeding, the patient should be caused to drink (a potion of animal) blood and such a case marked by the passage of stool, urine, etc., through their proper channels of outlet and by the absence of fever and tympanites and other dangerous symptoms, (Upadrava), may end in the ultimate recovery of the patient. 37-38.

In a case of a perforation of the Koshtha (abdomen) where the intestines have protruded or bulged out in an untorn condition, they should be gently re-introduced into the cavity and placed in their original position, and not otherwise. According to others, however, large black ants should be applied even to the perforated intestines in such a case and their bodies should be separated from their heads after they had firmly bitten the perforated parts with their claws. After that the intestines with the heads of the ants attached to them should be gently pushed back into the cavity and reinstated in their original situation therein. The bulged out intestines should be rinsed with grass, blood and dust, washed with milk and lubricated with clarified butter and gently re-introduced into the cavity of the abdomen with the hand with its finger nails cleanly paired. The dried intestines should be washed with milk and lubricated with clarified butter before introducing it into their former and natural place in the abdomen. 39-41.

In a case where the intestines could be but partially introduced, the three following measures should be adopted. The interior of the throat of the patient should be gently rubbed with a finger [and the urging for vomiting thus engendered, would help the full introduction of the intestines into the abdominal cavity]. As an alternative, he should be enlivened with sprays of cold water; or he should be caught hold of by his hands and lifted up into the air with the help of strong attendants and shaken in a manner that would bring about a complete introduction of the intestines into the natural position in the abdominal cavity. They should be so introduced as to press upon their specific (Maladhará) Kalá (facia). 42-43.

In a case where the re-introduction of the intestines into the abdominal cavity would be found to be difficult owing to the narrowness or largeness of the orifice of the wound, it should be extended or widened with a small or slight incisiona ccording to requirements, and the intestines re-introduced into their proper place. The orifice or mouth of the wound should be forthwith carefully sutured as soon as the intestines would be found to have been introduced into their right place. Intestines dislodged from their proper seat, or not introduced into their correct position, or coiled up into a lump bring on death. 44-46.

**Subsequent Treatment :**—[After the full and correct introduction of the intestines] the wound should be bandaged with a piece of silk-cloth saturated with clarified butter, and the patient should be given a draught of tepid clarified butter (D. R. tepid milk) with castor oil for an easy passage of the stool and downward coursing of the Váyu (spontaneous emission of the flatus). Then, for its healing up (Ropana), a medicated oil, prepared with the bark of the *Asvakarna, Dhava, S'álmali, Mesha-s'ringi, S'allaki, Arjuna, Viddri,* and *Kshiri* trees and *Vald* roots should be applied to the wound. For a year the patient should live a life of strictest conticence and forego all kinds of physical exercise. 47—48.

The legs and the eyes of the patient should be washed and sprinkled with water in the event of the **bursting** out of the **testicles** which should be introduced into their proper place within the scrotum, and sewn up in the manner of a Tunna-sevani (raised seam). The scrotum should be bandaged in the shape of a **Gophaná-Vandha** and a restraining apparatus (Ghatta-Yantra) placed round the waist of the patient (to guard it against its oscillations or hanging down). The wound should not be lubricated with any kind of oil or Ghrita inasmuch as it would make the wound moist and slimy. The wound should be healed with a medicated oil prepared with *Káldnusári, Aguru, Elá, Játi* flower, *Chandana, Padmaka, Manahs'ilá, Devadáru, Amrita* and sulphate of copper (pounded together). 49-50.

A plug of hair should be inserted into a wound on the head, after having extracted the foreign matter therefrom, with a view to arrest the exuding of the brain matter (Mastulunga) which invariably proves fatal to the patient through the aggravation of the deranged Váyu in consequence thereof. The hairs of the plug should be taken out one by one as the healing process progresses (granulation). An oleaginous medicated plug or lint should be inserted into a wound on any other part of the body, which should be treated with the measures and remedial agents laid down in connection with a traumatic ulcer after having first allowed the vitiated blood to escape. 51-52.

The medicated oil known as the **Chakra-taila**\* should be poured (frequently applied) by means of a slender pipe into an ulcer (wound) which is deep-seated but narrow-mouthed, after first letting out the vitiated blood†. An oil duly prepared and boiled with *Samangá, Haridrá, Padmá, Trivarga‡ Tuttha, Vidanga, Katuka, Pathyá, Guduchi* and *Karanja* acts as a good healing (Ropana) agent (in these cases). The use of an oil prepared with *Tális'a, Padmaka, Mánsi, Harenu, Aguru, Chandana,* and the two kinds of *Haridrá, Padma-vija, Us'ira* and *Yashti-madhu* acts as a good healing remedy in cases of traumatic ulcers. 53-55.

A cut wound (**Kshata**) should be treated with its own specific measures and remedies, while a bruised one (**Pichchita**) should be treated (to all intents and purposes) as a case of Bhagna (bone-fracture). The first treatment of a mangled or contused wound (**Ghrishta**) is to extinguish pain, after which it should be dusted with the powder of proper medicinal drugs (such as *S'ála, Sarja, Arjuna,* etc.). 56-57.

In the case of a dislocation of any part of the body, caused by a fall (from a tree), or in the event of having been run over or trampled down (Mathita—by a carriage or by a beast), or of being wounded (by a blow, etc.),

---

\* The oil just pressed out of an old oil-mill or squeezed out of the chips of wood belonging to an old one, in the manner of the **Anu-taila** to be described hereafter, is called the **Chakra-taila**.

† The vitiated blood should first be let out for fear of putrefaction of the ulcer.

‡ Triphalá, Trikatu and Trimada are called **Trivarga**.

the patient should be kept immersed in a large tank (Droni) of oil and the diet should consist of the soup or essence (Rasa) of meat. A man fatigued (from the labours of a journey), or hurt at any of the **Marmas**, should be likewise treated with the preceding measures. 58.

Oil or clarified butter should be always administered as drinks, washes or external healing applications for an ulcer-patient with a due regard to his temperament and the nature of the season. Medicated Ghritas, yet to be mentioned in connection with the medical treatment of a Pittaja abscess, should be used as well in the case of a traumatic ulcer (according to its respective indications). A physician should wash a traumatic ulcer, attended with an aching pain either with a Valá-oil or tepid clarified butter (according to the nature of the season and the temperament of the patient).* 59—61.

An oil cooked with *Samangá, Rajani, Padmá* (Bhárgi), *Pathyá*, sulphate of copper, *Suvarchalá, Padmaka, Lodhra, Yashti-madhuka, Vidanga, Harenuka, Tális'apatra, Nalada (Jatámánsi)*, (red) *Chandana, Padmakes'ara, Manjishthá, Us'ira, Lákshá*, and the tender leaves of *Kshiri* trees, *Piyála* seeds, raw and tender *Tinduka* fruit, or with as many of them as would be available, should be regarded as a good healing remedy in respect of all non-malignant traumatic sores or ulcers. Applications of astringent, sweet, cooling and oily medicines should be used for a week in a case of a traumatic ulcer (Sadyo-vrana), after which those mentioned before, in the Chapter of Divraniya, should be adopted 62—63.

* With oil in autumn and in the case of a patient of Rakta-pitta temperament, and with Valá-oil in winter and in the case of one of a Váta-kapha temperament.

**Treatment of Dushta-Vrana:**—In the case of a malignant ulcer (Dushta-Vrana) emetics, errhines, purgatives, Ásthápana, fasting, specific sorts of diet (composed of bitter, pungent and astringent things) and blood-letting, should be prescribed (according to the requirements of each case). The ulcer or sore should be washed with the decoctions of the drugs of both the Áragvadhádi and the Surasádi ganas, and an oil cooked with a decoction of the said drugs should be applied to the wound for the purification (Śodhana) thereof. As an alternative, an oil boiled and prepared in an alkaline water or solution (four times that of oil) with a Kalka of alkaline substances (such as Ghantápáruli, Paláśa, etc.) should be used for that end Oil cooked with *Dravanti* (Śatamuli, according to certain authorities, Mushika-parni according to others), *Chiravilva, Danti, Chitraka, Prithvikā Nimba-leaves, Kásisa, Tuttha, Trivrit, Tejovati, Nili* (indigo), the two kinds of *Haridrá*, Saindhava salt, *Tila, Bhumi-Kadamba, Suvahá, Śukákhyá, Lángaláhvá, Naipáli, Jálini, Madayanti, Mrigádani, Sudhá, Murvá, Arka, Kitári, Haritála*, and *Karanja*, or with as many of them as would be available, should be used for the purification (of a malignant sore or ulcer). If found applicable, a medicated Ghrita prepared and cooked with the foregoing drugs and substances as Kalka should be used for the same purpose. In the case of a malignant ulcer, due to the aggravated Váyu, the purifying remedy should consist of a Kalka of Saindhava salt, *Trivrit* and castor leaves. In the case of a (malignant) Pittaja sore, the remedy should consist of a Kalka of *Trivrit, Haridrá, Yashtimadhu* and *Tila*. In the case of a malignant ulcer, caused by the aggravated **Kapha**, the purifying remedial agent should consist of *Tila, Tejohvá, Danti, Svarjiká* and *Chitraka* roots. An ulcer brought on owing to the presence of the virus of **Meha** or **Kushtha** in the system, measures and remedies mentioned under the treatment of Dushta-vrana should be adopted and used. 64—68.

The recognised school of physicians, which recognises these six types of traumatic sores, does not add to the list, herein mentioned, other types of ulcers, whereas vain pedagogues try to swell it with a larger number of types by adding connotative prefixes and suffixes to the names of the aforesaid six. It is mere vain-gloriousness on their part to say so, since all the other types that they can devise are but single instances and can be made to fall under one of these six general heads. Hence there should be only six kinds (of traumatic sores) and not more. 69.

Thus ends the second Chapter of the Chikitsita Sthánam of the Sus'ruta Samhitá which deals with the treatment of Sadyo-Vrana (traumatic sores).

# CHAPTER III.

Now we shall discourse on the medical treatments of fractures and dislocations (**Bhagnas**). 1.

**Metrical Texts :**—A fracture or dislocation (Bhagna) occurring in a person of a Vátika temperament, or of intemperate habits, or in one who is sparing in his diet, or is affected with such supervening disorders (as fever, tympanites, suppression of the stool and urine, &c.) is hard to cure.* A fracture-patient must forego the use of salt, acid, pungent and alkaline substances and must live a life of strictest continence, avoid exposure to the sun and forego physical exercises and parchifying (devoid of oleaginous) articles of food. A diet consisting of boiled rice, meat-soup, milk, † clarified butter, soup of *Satina* pulse and all other nutritive and constructive food and drink, should be discriminately given to a fracture-patient. The barks of *Udumbara, Madhuka, As'vattha, Palás'a, Kakubha, Bamboo, Vata* or *Sála* trees should be used as splints (**Kuśa**). *Manjishthá, Madhuka,* red sandal wood and *Sáli*-rice mixed with S'ata-Dhauta clarified butter (*i.e.,* clarified butter

---

\* Jejjata does not read the first verse, but Gayi does.

† As a general rule, milk should not be prescribed to a patient suffering from an ulcer (Vrana) in general ; but a case of fracture forms an exception thereto. Some authorities hold that tepid milk may be given to a fracture-patient, if there be no ulcer (Vrana). Others, on the contrary, are of opinion that milk should not, in any case, be given to a fracture-patient for fear of suppuration and the setting in of pus.

Others, however, take "Kshira-sarpih" to be a compound word and explain the term to mean the clarified butter prepared from milk (as distinguished from that prepared from curd).

But experience tells us that in cases of excessive weakness or emaciation, milk may be given without any hesitation—Ed.

washed one hundred times in succession) should be used for **plastering** the fracture. 2-6.

**Bandage :**—Fractures should be (dressed and) bandaged once a week in cold weather, on every fifth day in temperate weather (*i.e.*, in spring and autumn), and on every fourth day in hot weather (*i.e.*, in summer), or the interval of the period for bandaging should be determined by the intensity of the Doshas involved in each individual case. An extremely loose bandage prevents the firm adhesion of a fractured bone, a light bandage gives rise to pain, swelling and suppuration of the local skin, &c. Hence in cases of fractures, experts prefer a bandage which is neither too tight nor too loose. 7-8.

**Washings :**—A cold decoction of the drugs of the *Nyagrodhádi* group should be used in washing (the affected part), whereas in the presence of (excessive) pain, (the part) should be washed with milk boiled with the drugs of the (minor) *Pancha-mula,* or simply with the oil known as the Chakra-taila made lukewarm*. Cold (or warm) lotions and medicinal plasters (Pradehas) of Dosha-subduing drugs should be prescribed with due regard to the nature of the season and the Doshas involved in each case 9-10.

A preparation of milk † from a cow, delivered for the first time, boiled with the drugs of the *Madhurádi* group and mixed with powdered shellac and clarified butter (as an afterthrow) should be given (when cold) to a fracture-patient as a beverage every morning. In a case of

---

\* In winter and where the aching pain is present due to Váyu and Kapha.

† Consisting of the drugs of the Kákolyádi group weighing two Tolás, milk sixteen Tolás, water sixty-four Tolás, boiled together with the water entirely evaporated.

fracture attended with ulcer on the part, an astringent plaster plentifully mixed with honey and clarified butter should be applied ; and the rest (diet and regimen of conduct) should be as laid down in the case of a (simple) fracture. 11-12.

**Prognosis :** —A case of fracture occurring in a youth or a person with slightly deranged Doshas or in winter, is held to be easily curable (with the help of the aforesaid medicines and diet). A fractured bone in a youth is joined by the aforesaid treatment in the course of a month, in two months in the case of a middle-aged man and in three months in one of old age. 13-14.

An elevated and fractured joint should be reduced by pressing it down, while one hanging down should be set by raising it up, by pulling it in the case of its being pushed aside, and by reinstating it in its upward (proper) position in the event of its being lowered down. An intelligent physician should set all dislocated (Bhagna) joints, whether fixed or movable, by the mode of reduction, known as Ánchhana, Pidana, (pressure), Sankshepa and Vandhana (bandaging). 15-16.

**Treatment :**—A crushed or dislocated joint should not be shaken (*i.e.*, should be kept at rest) and cold lotions or washes and medicated plasters (Pradeha) should be applied to the part. A joint is spontaneously reset to its natural or normal state or position after the correction of its deformity incidental to a blow or hurt having been effected. The fractured or dislocated part should be first covered with a piece of linen soaked in clarified butter. Splint should then be placed over it and the part properly bandaged. 17-19.

**Treatment of fractures in particular limbs :**—Now we shall discourse on the measures to be adopted in fractures occurring in each particular limb. In the case of a **nail-joint**, being in any way crushed or swollen by the accumulation of the deranged blood (in the locality), the incarcerated blood should be first let out with the help of an awl (Árá) and the part should be plastered with a paste of Sáli-rice. A finger or **phalanx** bone put out of joint or fractured should be first set in its natural position and bandaged with a piece of thin linen and should be then sprinkled over with clarified butter. In the case of a fracture in the **foot** the fractured part should be first lubricated with clarified butter, then duly splinted up, and bandaged with linen. Such a patient should forego all kinds of locomotion. In the case of a fracture of the **knee-joint** or **thigh-bone** the affected part should be lubricated with clarified butter and carefully pulled straight, after which it should be splinted with barks (of Nyagrodha, etc.) and bandaged with clean linen. In case of the fracture projecting out a **thigh-bone** should be reset with the help of a circular splint and bandaged. In the case of Sphutita (cracked) or Pichchita (bruised) thigh-bone, the part should be also bandaged in the aforesaid manner. 20-24.

In a case of a fracture in the Kati (Ilium-bone), it should be reduced by the fractured bone being raised up or pressed down (as the case may be) and the patient should then be treated with Vasti (enematas of medicated oils or Ghritas*). In the case of a fracture of one of the **rib-bones** (Pársaka), the patient should be lubricated with clarified butter. He should then be lifted up (in a standing posture) and the fractured rib (bone), whether left or right, should be relaxed by being rubbed with clarified butter. Strips of bamboo or pad

---

\* In the Nidána-Sthána—Chap. XV., 9—it is stated that a case of fracture in the Kati should be given up (Varjjayet). Jejjata, however, explains "Varjjayet" as "hard to cure."

(Kaválika) should be placed over it and the patient should be carefully laid in a tank or cauldron full of oil with the bamboo splint duly tied up with straps of hide. In the case of a dislocation of the **Amsa-Sandhi** (shoulder-joint), the region of the Kaksha (arm-pit) should be raised up with an iron-rod (Mushala) and the wise physician should bandage the part, thus reduced, in the shape of a Svastika (8-shaped) bandage. A dislocated **elbow-joint** should be first rubbed with the thumb, after which it should be pressed with a view to set it in its right place by fixing and expanding the same. After that the affected part should be sprinkled over with any oleaginous substance. The same measures should be adopted in the case of a dislocation of the **knee**-joint (Jánu-sandhi), the **wrist-joint** (Gulpha-sandhi) and the **ankle-joint** (Mani-vandha). 25-29.

In the case of fractured bones in the palms of the hands, the two palms* should be made even and opposed, and then bandaged together and the affected parts should be sprinkled with raw and unmedicated oil (Áma-taila). The patient should be made later first to hold a ball of cow-dung, then a ball of clay and then a piece of stone in his palms and so on, with the progressive return of strength (to the affected parts). In a case of a fracture of the Akshaka, the affected part should be first fomented and then reduced by raising it up with a Mushala (iron-rod) in the arm-pit or by pressing it down (as the case may be) and should be firmly bandaged. A case of fractured **arm-bone** should be treated according to the directions given in the case of a fractured thigh-bone. 30-32.

---

* The text has "*Ubhe tale same kritvá.*" Jejjata explains "Ubhe tale" to mean "palms of the hands and soles of the feet ;" Gayá Dása explains it to mean "the palms of both the hands."

In the case of a bending (twisting) or intussusception of the **neck** downward, the head should be lifted up by putting the fingers into the hollow (Avatu) above the nape of the neck and at the roots of the jaw-bones (Hanu).* Then the part should be bandaged with a piece of linen after having evenly put the splint (Kuśa round the neck). The patient should be caused to lie constantly on his back for a week. In a case of a dislocation of the joints of the **jaw-bones** (Hanu), the jaw-bones should be fomented and duly set in their right position, bandaged in the manner of a Panchángi-vandha, and a Ghrita boiled and prepared with (the Kalka and a decoction of) the Madhura (Kákolyádi) and Váyu-subduing (Chavyádi) groups should be used as errhines by the patient. 33-34.

A tooth of a young person, not broken but loose, should be plastered with a cooling paste on its outside after having pressed out the accumulated blood at the root. The tooth should be sprinkled or washed with cold water and treated with drugs having Sandhániya (adhesive) properties † The patient should be caused to drink milk with the help of a lotus stem. The loose tooth of an old man should be drawn. A nose sunk down or depressed (by a blow) should be raised up with the help of a rod or director, while it should be straightened in a case of simple bending. Then two tubes, open at both ends, should be inserted into the nostrils (to facilitate the process of breathing) and the organ should be bandaged and sprinkled with clarified butter. In the case of (the cartilage of) the ear being broken, the organ should be rubbed with

---

\* According to Gayi, the lifting up of the head by putting fingers in the *Avatu* and in the *Hanus* should be made in cases of bending and intussusception of the neck respectively.

† Honey, clarified butter, and drugs of the Nyagrodhádi group.

clarified butter straightened, and evenly set in its right position and bandaged. Measures and remedial agents mentioned in connection with Sadyo-vrana, should be likewise adopted and employed in the present instance. 37.

In a case of a fracture of the bone of the forehead unattended by any oozing out of brain matter, the affected part should be simply rubbed with honey and clarified butter and then duly bandaged. The patient should take clarified butter for a week * 38.

Cooling plasters and washes should be applied to a part of the body, swollen but not in any way ulcerated on account of a fall or a blow. In the case of a fracture of the bone in the leg and in the thigh, the patient should be laid down on a plank or board and bound to five stakes or pegs in five different places for the purpose of preventing any movements of his limbs. The distribution of the (bindings) pegs in each case should be as follows. In the first case (fractured leg-bone), two on each side of the two thighs making four and one on the exterior side of the enguinal region of the affected side. In the second case (fracture of knee-joint) two on each side of the ankle-joints making four and one on the side of the sole of the affected leg. The same sort of bed and fastenings should be used in cases of fractures and dislocations of the **pelvic-joint**, the **spinal column**, the **chest** and the **shoulders**†. In cases of long-standing dislocations, the joint should be lubricated with oily or lardaceous applications, fomented and softened (with

* In the case of such an emission or oozing out a plug of bristles or hair as described in the preceding chapter and remedial agents laid down in connection therewith, should be used.

† The principle of splintering and bandaging may be profitably compared with those followed in Agnur's splint.

proper medicinal drugs) in the manner mentioned above in order to reduce it to its natural state. 39-40.

. In the case of a faulty union of a (fractured) bone lying between two joints (**Kánda-bhagna**), the union should be again disjointed, and the fractured bone should again be set right and treated as a case of ordinary fracture. In the case where a fractured bone would be found to have protruded out of the ulcerated part and dried, it should be carefully cut off near the margin of the (incidental) ulcer,(so as not to create a fresh ulcer on any other spot of the affected part) and subsequently treated as a case of fractural ulcer. A fracture occurring in the upper part of the body should be treated with applications of Mastikya-Śirovasti [oil-soaked pads on the head] and pourings of oil into the cavity of the ears. Potions of clarified butter,* errhines and Anuvásana (enematas) should be prescribed in cases of fractures in the extremeties. 41-43.

**Gandha-Taila :**—Now we shall discourse on the recipe of a medicated oil, capable of bringing about the union of fractured bones. A quantity of black sesamum-seeds (tied up into a knot with a piece of linen) should be kept immersed at night in a stream of running water and taken out and dried in the sun (for seven consecutive days). It should then be saturated with cow's milk (at night and dried in the sun, during the second week). During the third week the sesamum-seeds should be saturated with a decoction of Yashti-madhu (at night) and dried in the sun the next day. Then (during the fourth week) it should be again saturated with cows milk and dried and powdered. The said sesamum-

---

\* According to Jejjata, not only Anuvásana-enematas but potions of clarified butter and errhines also should be prescribed in cases of fractures in the extremetics.

powder and powder of the drugs, constituting the Kákolyádi Gana as well as *Yasthi-madhu, Manjishthá, Sárivá, Kushtha, Sarja-rasa, Mánsi, Deva-dáru,* (red) *Chandana,* and *S'atapushpá* should be mixed together. Then a quantity of cow's milk boiled with the aromatic drugs (of the Eládi group) should be used with the preceding pulverised compound for the purpose of pressing out the oil therefrom. The oil thus pressed out should be boiled in four times the quantity of cow's milk with the drugs such as *Elá, S'álparni, Tejapatra, Jivaka, Tagara, Rodhra, Prapaundarika, Kálánusári,* (Tagara), *Saireyaka, Kshira-Vidári, Anantá, Madhuliká, S'ringátaka,* and those of the aforesaid list (Kákolyádi group and *Yasthi-madhu,* etc., up to *S'atapushpá*) pasted together. The oil should be duly cooked over a gentle fire and is called the **Gandha-Taila**. This oil should be administered with good results in possible ways (e.g., as potions, liniments, unguents and errhines) to a fracture-patient. Its efficacy is witnessed in cases of convulsions, hemiplegia, parchedness or atrophy of the palate, in Ardita (facial paralysis) as well as in Manyá-stambha (Paralysis or stiffness of the neck), in diseases of the head (cephalagia), in ear-ache in Hanu-graha, in deafness and in blindness and in emaciation due to sexual excesses. Administered in food or drink, or employed as a liniment, in Vasti-karma (enemata measures) or as an errhine, it acts as a sovereign restorative. Rubbed over the neck, chest and shoulders, it adds to the strength and expansion of those parts of the body, makes the face fair and lovely like a full-blown lotus and imparts a sweet

\* There should be three parts of sesamum powder and one part of the powders of Kákolyádi, Vashti-madhu, Manjishthá, etc. (combined). But śiva Dàsa says that four parts of sesamum-powders should be taken.

fragrance to the breath. It is one of the most powerful remedial agents in disorders of the aggravated Váyu (diseases of the nervous system). It may be used even by kings and for them it should be specially prepared. 44-45.

The expressed oil of the seeds of the Trapusha, Aksha and Piyála should be cooked with a decoction of drugs of the Madhura group (Kákolyádi gana) and with ten times the quantity of milk. A quantity of lard if available, should be poured into it (during the process of cooking). It is an excellent medicated oil and used as a potion for anointing, and as an errhine, Vasti-karma and washes, it speedily brings about the union of fractured bones. 46.

A physician should exert his utmost to guard against the advent of any suppurative setting in in a fractured bone, since a suppuration of the local veins, nerves and muscles is difficult to cure  A complete union of a fractured joint should be inferred from its painless or unhurt character, from its full and perfect development (leaving no detectable signs of its once fractured condition), from the absence of all elevation (unevenness) and from its perfect freedom in flexion and expansion, etc. 47-48.

Thus ends the third Chapter of the Chikitsita Sthánam in the Sus'ruta Samhitá which deals with the medical treatment of fractures and dislocations.

# CHAPTER IV.

Now we shall diseourse on the medical treatment of nervous disorders (**Váta-vyádhi**). 1.

**Metrical Texts :**—The patient having been made to vomit in the event of the deranged Váyu being incarcerated (lodged) in the **Ámaśaya** (stomach), a pulverised compound known as the Shad-Dharana-yoga (a compound of six Dharanas or twenty-four Máshá weight) with tepid water should be administered to him for seven days. A compound made up of *Chitraka, Indra-yava, Páthá, Katuka, Ativishá, Abhayá* (taken in equal parts) together is known as the **Shad-Dharana-yoga**\* and contains the properties of subduing an attack of Váta-vyádhi. 2-3.

In the event of the aggravated Váyu being incarcerated in the **Pakvaśaya** (intestines), purgatives of fatty matters (Sneha-Virechana, i.e ,Tilvaka-Sarpih,etc ), and Śodhana- Vasti of purifying drugs (with decoctions and Kalka of fatty matters) and diet (Práśa) abounding in salt† or saline articles should be prescribed. In the case of the aggravated Váyu being incarcerated in the **Vasti** (urinary bladder), diuretic (lit. bladder-cleansing) measures and remedial agents should be resorted to. Anointing with medicated oils, Ghritas, etc., application of poultices (Upanáha) compounded of Váyu-subduing drugs, massage, and plasters (Álepa) of similar properties are the remedies in cases where the aggravated Váyu is lodged in the **internal ducts** or channels such

---

\* One Dharana is equal to four Máshás.

† Sneha-Lavana and Kánda-Lavana, etc.

as the ears, etc., of the body. Blood-letting (venesection) is the remedy where the aggravated Váyu would be found to be confined in the **skin, flesh, blood** or **veins** (Sirás). Similarly, application of fatty matters (Sneha), actual cauterization, massage, application of poultices and binding of ligatures should be the remedies where the aggravated Váyu would be found to have become involved in the **Snáyu** (ligaments), **joints and bones** Where the aggravated Váyu would be found to have become situated in the bone, the skin and flesh of that part of the body should be perforated with a proper surgical instrument (Árá-Sastra) and the underlying bone should be similarly treated with an awl. A tube open at both ends should be inserted into the aperture, thus made, and a strong physician should suck the aggravated Váyu from out of the affected bone by applying his mouth to the exterior open end of the tube. 4-9.

In the case of the aggravatd Váyu having contaminated the **semen**, measures and remedies for seminal disorders (Sukra-dosha)* should be employed. The intelligent (physician) would take recourse to measures, such as blood-letting, immersion or bath in a vessel (full of Váyu-subduing decoctions), fomentation with heated stones, as well as in the manner of Karshu-Sveda, vapour-bath in a closed chamber (Kuti sveda), anointment, Vasti-Karmas, etc., in the event of the aggravated Váyu having extended throughout the whole organism; whereas bleeding by means of a horn (cuffing) should be regarded as the remedy when the aggravated Dosha

---

* Treatments, such as, the purification of the semen, etc., and the use of medicines for making Aphrodisia (Váji-karana) and for the remedy of the disordered urinary organ (Mutra-dosha) should be adopted and employed.

would be found to have been confined in any parti u'ar part of the body.* 10-12.

In the event of the aggravated Váyu being connected either with the **Pitta** or the **Kapha**, such a course of treatment should be adopted as would not be hostile to the two other Doshas. Blood-letting (in small quantities) should be resorted to several times in a case of complete ænesthesia (Supta-Váta) and the body should be anointed with oil mixed with salt and chamber-dust (Agára-dhuma) Milk boiled with a decoction of the drugs of the Pancha-mula group, acid-fruits (Phalámla), meat-soup or soup of (well-cooked) corn (Dhánya) with clarified butter are beneficial in cases of Váta-roga. 13-15.

**Sálvana-Upanáha :**—A poultice composed of the drugs of the Kákolyádi group, the Váyu-subduing drugs (those of Bhadra-dárvádi and Vidárigandhádi groups), and all kinds of acid articles† (such as, Kánjika, Sauvira, fermented rice-gruel, etc.), the flesh of animals which live in swamps (Ánupa) or in water (Audaka)‡, oil, clarified butter and all kinds of lardaceous substances, mixed together and saturated with a profuse quantity of salt and then slightly heated is known by the name of **Sálvana**. A person suffering from any form of Váta roga should be always treated with such Sálvana poultices (Upanáha). The poultice should be applied to such part of the body as is

---

\* It is to be understood that measures and remedies laid down under the head of Sarvánga-gata should be used when the Váyu would be found to be diffused throughout the whole organism instead of being confined to any specific part.

† According to others it means all kinds of acid-fruits, etc.

‡ Chakradatta reads "सानुसमांसः सुखिन्नः" (well-cooked with the flesh of "Ánupa" animals) in place of सानूपौदकमांसस्तु ।

numbed, painful or contracted and the affected part should be firmly bandaged thereafter with a piece of Kshauma* linen or woollen cloth. As an alternative, the affected part should be plastered (and well rubbed) with the ingredients of the Sálvana-Upanáha and inserted into a bag made of cat or mungoose skin or that of a camel or deer hide. 16.

The aggravated Váyu, if located in the shoulders, the chest, the sacrum (Trika) or the Manyá, should be subdued by emetics and errhines judiciously employed. Siro-Vasti should be applied to the head of the patient as long as it would take one to utter a thousand Mátrás (a short vowel sound), more or less, as the case may require, where the aggravated Váyu would be found to have located itself in the head, (if necessary) blood-letting should be resorted to. As a mountain is capable of obstructing the passage of the wind, so the Sneha-Vasti (oily enema) is alone capable of resisting the action of the aggravated Váyu whether it extends throughout the whole system or is confined to a single part. 17-19

**Measures beneficial to Váta-Vyádhi:**
—An application of Sneha, fomentations, anointment of the body, Vasti, oily purgatives, Siro-vasti, the rubbing of oils on the head, oily fumigation, gargling with tepid oil, oily errhines, the use of meat-soup, milk, meat, clarified butter, oil and other lardaceous articles (of food), all kinds of acid fruits, salt, lukewarm washes, gentle massage, the use of saffron, *Agura, Patra, Kushtha, Elá, Tagara,* the wearing of woollen, silken, cotton or any other thick kind of garments, living in a warm room or in one not exposed to the wind or in an inner chamber, the use of a soft bed, basking in the glare of fire, entire sexual abstinence, these and such like other things

* Some read it as Válka, *i.e.*, made up bark.

should be generally adopted by a patient suffering from Váta-roga 20.

**The Tilvaka-Ghrita :**—A paste (Kalka) of the following drugs, viz, *Trivrit, Danti, Suvarna-kshiri, Saptalá, Samkhini, Triphalá* and *Vidanga*, each weighing an Aksha (two tolás), and **Tilvaka**-roots and *Kampillaka*, each weighing a Vilva (eight tolás), a decoction of Triphalá and curd, each weighing two Pátras * (thirty-two seers) and clarified butter, weighing sixteen seers, should be duly cooked together. Medical authorities recommend this Tilvaka Ghrita as an oily purgative in cases of Váta-roga. Asoka-Ghrita and Ramyaka-Ghrita are prepared in the same manner, (viz., by substituting Asoka and Ramyaka respectively for Tilvaka). 21.

**The Anu-Taila :**—The log of a long-standing wooden oil-mill should be cut into small chips and then thrashed and boiled in water in a large cauldron. The globules of oil that will be found floating on the surface of the boiling water should be skimmed off either with the hand or with a saucer The oil thus collected should then be cooked with the Kalka of Váyu-subduing drugs as in the preparation of a medicated oil. This oil is known as the **Anu-Taila** The use of this oil has been advised by medical authorities in cases of Váta-roga. This oil is so named from the fact of its being pressed out of small chips of oily wood (as described above). 22.

**The Sahasra-páka-Taila :**—The wood of drugs belonging to the group of Mahá-pancha-mula should be collected in large quantities and burnt on a

---

* Pátra means 64 Palas, i e., 8 seers, but in cases of liquids the weight should be doubled,

plot of land, so as to make the soil black. The fire should be kept burning one whole night ; on the following morning on the extinction of the fire the ashes should be removed and the ground, when cool, should be soaked with one hundred Ghatas (six thousand and four hundred seers) of oil cooked with the drugs of the *Vidári-gandhádi group* and with the same quantity of milk and kept in that condition for one night more. On the next morning the earth should be dug up, down to the stratum found to have been soaked with the oil and the soil should then be dissolved in warm water in large cauldrons for the purpose. The oil that will be found floating on the surface of the water should be skimmed off with both hands and kept in a safe basin. Then the decoction of the Váyu-subduing drugs (the Bhadra-dárvádi group), meat-juice, milk, fermented rice-gruel (each taken in a quantity measuring a quarter part of that oil) should be taken one thousand times and each time should be boiled with the oil. Váyu-subduing and aromatic drugs and spices, in the northern (trans-Himálaya) and southern (Deccan) countries, should be thrown into it and boiled with the oil. The boiling should be completed within the period during which it could be properly done. Then after the completion of the cooking, conch-shells should be blown, Dundubhis should be sounded, umbrellas should be held open, chowries should be blown into it and a thousand Bráhmins should be treated with repasts. The oil so sacredly prepared should be stored carefully in golden, silver or earthen pitchers. This oil is called the **Sahasrapáka-Taila** and is of irresistible potency and fit even for the use of kings. **Śatapáka-Taila** is also prepared in the above manner (with the aforesaid ingredients) by cooking it one hundred times only. 23.

**The Patra-Lavana :**—The green leaves of the *Eranda* plants and those of the trees known as *Mushkaka, Naktamála, Atarushaka, Putika, Áragvadha* and *Chitraka* should be thrashed with (salt of equal quantity) in an Udukhala (a hand thrashing mill) and placed in an earthen pitcher, saturated with oil or clarified butter. Having covered the mouth of the pitcher with a lid, it should be plastered and burnt in fire of cow-dung. The medicine thus prepared (with the help of internal heat) is called the **Patra-Lavana**. Medical experts advise the application of this medicine in cases of Váta-roga. 24.

**The Kánda-Lavana :**—Similarly, *Snuhi*-twigs, *Brinjal* (Vártáku), and *S'igru*-bark (taken in equal parts) and rock-salt (of equal weight as the entire drugs) should be thrashed and kept in a pitcher. Oil, clarified butter, lard and marrow should be added to it equal in weight with salt and then having covered the mouth of the pitcher with a lid, it should be plastered and burnt in a fire of cow-dung (as before) The use of this medicated salt which is called the **Kánda-Lavana** or **Sneha-Lavana** is recommended by experts in Váta-roga. 25.

**The Kalyánaka-Lavana :**—The following drugs with their roots, leaves and twigs, *viz., Gandira, Palása, Kutaja, Vilva, Arka, Snuhi, Apámárga, Pátalá, Páribhadra, Nádeyi, Krishnagandhá Nipa, Nimba, Nirdahani, Atarushaka, Nakta-málaka, Putika, Vrihati, Kantikari, Bhallátaka, Ingudi, Baijayanti, Kadali, Varshábhu, Hrivera, Kshuraka, Indraváruni, Svetamokshaka* and *Asoka* should be gathered in a green condition and mixed with (as large a quantity of) rock-salt and having thrashed them in an Udukhala should be burnt in a hermetically sealed pitcher as above, after which it should be filtered (twenty times) and boiled in the manner of alkaline preparations At the close of the boiling, powders\* of the drugs of the *Hingvádi* or Pippalyádi group should be mixed with it. This medicine is called the **Kaláynaka-Lavana** and is specially efficacious in all cases of Váta-roga and is applicable both in food and drink in cases of Gulma, enlarged spleen, impaired digestion, indigestion, hæmorrhoids, intestinal worms, aversion to food and cough. 26

**Memorable Verse :**—The remedy proves efficacious in Váta-roga through its heat-making potency, power of liquifying and secreting the deranged Doshas and of restoring and correcting them as well. 27.

Thus ends the fourth Chapter of the Chikitsita Sthánam in the Sus'ruta Samhitá which deals with the treatment of Váta-Vyádhi.

---

\* The total weight of these powders should be one-fourth of the weight of the rock-salt taken in the course of the preparation.—Dallana.

# CHAPTER V.

Now we shall discourse on the chapter which deals with the medical treatment of **Mahá-Váta-Vyádhi.** 1.

Several authorities group the disease Váta-Rakta under two different sub-heads, such as superficial and deep-seated. But such a classification is arbitrary and unscientific, inasmuch as this disease first manifests itself on the surface (layer of the skin) like Kushtha and gradually invades the deeper tissues of the body. Hence there are no (two) forms of this disease. 1–2.

**Causes of Váta-Rakta :**—The Váyu of the body is enraged or agitated by such causes as wrestling with a man of superior and uncommon physical strength, etc., while the blood is vitiated by such causes as constant over-eating of edibles which are of difficult digestion and heat-making in their potency or ingestion of food before the digestion of the previous meal. The Váyu thus enraged and agitated enters into the blood-carrying channels of the body and being obstructed in its passage, becomes mixed with the vitiated blood. The deranged Váyu and the blood thus combine to give rise to a disease characterised by the specific symptoms of each, which is known as **Váta-Rakta.** The characteristic pain, which at first confines itself to the extremities, gradually extends over the whole body.

**Premonitory symptoms of Váta-Rakta :**—The disease is ushered in with a pricking pain, a burning and an itching sensation (in the affected part), a swelling, roughness and numbness (anæsthesia) of the diseased locality, throbbing of the veins, ligaments, nerves and arteries, a weakness in the thighs and sudden appearance of red or brownish circular patches on the palms of the hands and soles of the feet, fingers and heels, etc., (A. R.—wrists). If neglected and immoderately treated in its premonitory stages, the disease soon develops its characteristic symptoms in succession, which have been described before ; whereas (a lifelong) deformity (of the affected part) is the penalty for neglecting it (in its fully patent or devoloped stage). 3.

**Memorable Verse :**—Men of a mild and delicate constitution, as well as those who are (inordinately) stout or sedentary in their habits or are addicted to unwholesome and incompatible food, etc., are generally found to be susceptible to an attack of **Váta-Rakta.** 4.

**Prognosis :**—A physician is advised to take in hand the medical treatment of a Váta-Rakta-patient who has as yet not lost much strength and muscle, nor is afflicted with thirst, fever, epileptic fits, dyspnœa, cough, numbness (of the affected part), aversion to food, indigestion, extension and contraction of the limb, as well as of a person who is strong and temperate in his living and can afford to pay for the diet and other necessary accessories of the treatement. 5.

**Preliminary remedial measures :**—In the first stage of the disease the blood, having become vitiated owing to its being obstructed in its course (by the unusually agitated Váyu in the system), should be gradually and not profusely bled, except when the body would be found to have become extremely dry or to have lost its natural healthful glow or complexion through the action of the aggravated morbific principle (Váyu), for fear of further aggravating the Váyu. Emetics, purgatives, and Vasti (enemas), etc., should be administered and the patient should be made to take a diet consisting of old and matured clarified butter (and boiled rice), in the case where the aggravated condition of the deranged Váyu would be found to predominate. As an alternative, he should be made to drink a potion consisting of goat's milk mixed with half its quantity of oil, with two Tolá weight of *Yashti-madhu* or goat's milk cooked with *Pris'niparni* (two Tolá weight) with honey and sugar (added after cooking), or cooked with *S'unthi, S'ringátaka,* and *Kas'eruka,* or cooked with *S'yámá, Rásná, Sushavi, Pris'niparni, Pilu, S'atávari, S'vadamshtrá* and *Das'a-mula.* 6

Oil, cooked with the addition of milk previously boiled with the decoction of *Das'a-mula* of eight times its own weight and a Kalka of *Madhuka, Mesha-s'ringi* (A. R. Śárngashtá), *S'vadamshtrá, Sarala, Bhadra-dáru, Vachá* and *Surabhi* pasted together, should be administered in drinks, etc., (viz, anointment, sprinkling, etc.). As an alternative, the oil cooked with the decoction of *S'atávari, Mayuraka, Madhuka, Kshira-Vidári, Valá, Ati-valá* and *Trina-pancha-mula,* with the paste of the drugs belonging to the *Kákolyádi* group, or the oil* cooked with the decoction and a Kalka of Valá for a hundred times should be prescribed for the patient. The affected part should be washed with the milk, boiled with the roots of the Váta-hara (Váyu-subduing) drugs (*i.e.,* Dasa-mula), or simply with Amla (gruel, etc.), or a plaster composed of barley, *Madhuka, Eranda* (castor) and *Varshábhu* (pasted together and heated), should be applied to the part. 7.

**Plasters, etc. :**—Barley, wheat, sesamum, Mudga pulse aud Másha pulse should be taken in equal

---

* According to Jejjata Ácháryya, the "Valá-Taila", which is administered in the medical treatment of Mudha-garbha, should be prescribed in this case.

parts and pounded separately; and the paste of the following drugs, viz., *Kákoli, Kshira-kákoli, Jivaka, Rishabhaka, Valá, Ati-valá, Visa-mrindla* (lotus stem), *Pris'niparni, Mesha-s'ringi, Piyála, S'arkará* (sugar), *Kas'eruka, Surabhi,* and *Vachá* should be mixed with each of the preceding powders and each of these compounds (so formed) should be boiled with milk, oil, lard, marrow and clarified butter. The five compounds, thus prepared, are called **Páyasas**, which should be applied as a hot poultice (Upanáha) to the affected part; or an **Utkárika**, made of the pulp of oily fruit (seeds) * (prepared by cooking them with milk) should be applied; or powders of wheat, barley, sesamum, Mudga pulse, or Másha pulse, and Ves'avára, made of various kinds of fish and flesh, should be used as a plaster. *Vilvapes'iká, Tagara, Deva-dáru, Saralá, Rásná, Harenu, Kushtha, S'ata-pushpá, Elá, Surá* and cream of milk-curd pasted together, should be applied to the affected part as a plaster (**Upanáha**). As an alternative, the expressed juice of Mátulunga, mixed with Kánjika, Saindhava salt and clarified butter, pasted together with the root of the *Madhu-s'igru* and with sesamum,† should be used in a similar way. The preceding remedies should be administered in a case of **Váta-Rakta** marked by a preponderance of the aggravated Váyu. 8.

**Váta-Rakta with a preponderance of Pitta :**—In cases of Váta-Rakta where the Pitta preponderates, the patient should be made to drink a potion consisting of a decoction of *Dráksha, Áragvadha, Katphala, Kshira-vidári, Yashti-madhu, Chandana* and *Kás marya* sweetened with a quantity of sugar and honey.

---

\* Such as sesamum, castor-seed, linseed, Vibhitaka-seeds, etc.

† Some say that a paste of sesamum only should be used as a separate plaster.

As an alternative, a decoction of *S'atávari, Yashti-madhu, Patola, Triphalá,* and *Katu-rohini,* or a decoction of *Guduchi,* or a decoction of the drugs belonging to the Chandanádi group, which are possessed of virtues for allaying pittaja fever, should be administered to the patient, sweetened with sugar and honey. Clarified butter, cooked and prepared with a decoction of bitter and astringent drugs* also proves beneficial in such cases. 9.

The affected part should be washed (Parisheka) with a decoction of *Visa-mrinála, Chandana* and *Padmaka* (taken in equal parts and) mixed with half its quantity of milk. As an alternative, the affected part should be sprinkled with a compound composed of milk, the expressed juice of *Ikshu* (sugar-cane), honey, sugar, and washings of rice (taken in equal parts) ; or with curd-cream, honey, and Dhányámla (fermented paddy-gruel), mixed with a decoction of grapes and *Ikshu* ; or the affected part should be anointed with clarified butter cooked with the drugs of the Jivaniya group, or with the clarified butter washed a hundred times in water, or with clarified butter cooked with the Kalka of the Kákolyádi group. 10.

Pradeha (plaster) composed of *S'áli, Shashtika, Nala, Vanjula, Tális'a, S'rigátaka, Galodya, Haridrá, Gairika, S'aivala, Padma-káshtha,* leaves of *padma* (lotus), pasted with *Dhányámla* and mixed with clarified butter, should be applied to the affected part. This plaster (Pradeha) may be applied lukewarm even in cases of Váta-Rakta, marked by a preponderance of the aggravated Váyu. All the remedial measures (laid down above) may also

---

* D. R.—Sweet, bitter, and astringent drugs.

Bitter drugs—Patoládi group ; Kasháya drugs—Triphaládi group ; sweet drugs—Kákolyádi group.

be advantageously applied in cases marked by a preponderance of the vitiated blood, with this exception that cold plasters and repeated blood-lettings should be resorted to in the latter (Raktaja-Váta-Rakta). 11.

**Váta-Rakta with a preponderance of Kapha:**—In cases where the Kapha preponderates, the patient should be made to drink a potion consisting of a decoction of *Haridrá* and *Ámalaka*, sweetened with honey; or a decoction of *Triphalá*, or a Kalka of *Madhuka, S'ringavera, Haritaki* and *Tikta-rohini* mixed with honey. As an alternative, *Haritaki* and treacle with either cow's urine or water, should be given to him.

The affected part or limb should be sprinkled or washed with cow's urine, oil, alkaline water, Surá, Sukta, or with a decoction of Kapha-destroying drugs. A hot decoction of the drugs constituting the Áragvadhádi group may be used with benefit in sprinkling the affected part. The body of the patient should be lubricated or anointed with clarified butter, boiled with the cream of milk-curd, cow's urine, wine, *S'ukta* and with the Kalka of *Yashti-madhu, Sárivá* and *Padma-káshtha*. A plaster (Pradeha), composed of pounded sesamum, mustard seed, linseed and barley (taken in equal parts) and mixed and pasted with *S'leshmátaka, Kapittha, Madhu-s'igru* and cow's urine, and *Yava-kshára* should be applied (hot to the seat of the disease) 12-13.

**The Five Pradehas :**—(1) A paste of white mustard seed, (2) that of sesamum and As'vagandhá, (3) a similar paste of *Piyála, S'elu* and *Kapittha* bark, (4) that of *Madhu-s'igru, Punarnavá* and (5) a paste of *Vyosha, Tiktá, Prithakparni* and *Vrihati*, these five kinds of Pradehas should be separately pasted with alkaline water and (any of them) applied lukewarm to the affected locality. 14.

As an alternative, a plaster composed *S'álaparni, Pris'niparni, Vrihati* and *Kantakári*, pasted together with milk and mixed with Tarpana,* should be applied (to the seat of the disease). In cases of Váta-Rakta involving the concerted action of two or three of the Doshas, the remedy consists in applying such drugs in combination as are possessed of the efficacy of subduing the action of each of them. 15.

**Guda-Haritaki and Pippali-Vardhamána Yogas :**—*Haritaki* with treacle may be used in all types of Váta-Rakta. As an alternative, the patient should be enjoined to use *Pippali*, pasted with milk or water, every day (in the following way).† The number of *Pippali* should be increased by five or ten respectively on each successive day till the tenth day of its use ; after which period the number of *Pippali* should be decreased (by a similar number) on each suceessive day till it is reduced to the original five or ten. The patient should live on a diet of milk and rice only (during the entire course of this treatment). This medicine which is known as the **Pippali-Vardhamána**,‡ proves efficacious in cases of Váta-Rakta, chronic fever (Vishama-Jvara), aversion to food, jaundice, enlarged spleen, piles, cough, asthma, œdema, phthysis, loss of appetite, heart-disease and ascitis. 16.

Clarified butter, cooked in milk with the paste of the drugs of the Jivaniya group, should be used in

* Flour of barley or fried grain, dissolved in water, is known as **Tarpana.**

† The dosage should begin originally with five or ten Pippalis according to the strength of the patient.

‡ Maharshi Charaka mentions this **Yoga** in the chapter on Rasáyana and prescribes it also in the treatement of Udara. Chakradatta mentions the use of this medicine in the treatment of liver and spleen and of fever.

anointing (the body of the patient). A plaster, composed of *Sahá, Sahadevá, Chandana, Murvá, Mustá, Piyála, S'atávari, Kas'eru, Padma-kástha Yashti-madhu, S'ata-pushpá* (A. D. Vidári) and *Kushtha*, pasted together with milk and mixed with the cream of clarified butter, should be applied (hot) to the affected locality. A plaster composed of *Saireyaka, Atarushaka, Valá, Ati-valá, Jivanti* and *Sushavi*, pasted together with the milk of a she-goat, should be likewise applied (to the seat of the disease). As an alternative, the diseased locality should be plastered with the pastes of *Kás'marya, Yashti-madhu* and *Tarpana* mixed together; or it should be treated with Pinda-Taila, prepared by cooking *Madhu-chchhishta* (bee's wax), *Manjishthá*, resin, and *Ananta-mula* in milk\* (and oil taken together). 17-20.

In all cases of Váta-Rakta, old and matured clarified butter boiled with the expressed juice of Ámalaka should be prescribed as drinks. The affected part should be washed or sprinkled with old and matured clarified butter, boiled with a decoction and paste (Kalka) of the drugs belonging to the *Kákolyádi* group, or with those of the *Jivaniya* group, or with the decoction of *Sushavi*, or of Káravellaka. The Valá-Taila† should be used for sprinkling and immersing purposes, and as drink and Vasti-karma (enemas).

**Diet :**—The diet should consist of articles made of old and matured S'áli or Shashtika rice, wheat or barley, taken with milk ‡ or with the soup of Mudga

---

\* Milk four times of oil should be taken.

† The "Valá-Taila" described in the medical treatment of Mudha-garbha, ch. XV.

‡ In the case of Váta-roga with preponderant Pitta, the patient should take the food with milk; in the preponderance of Váyu, with the soup of Jángala meat; and in the preponderance of Kapha, with Mudga-soup, devoid of any acid combination.

pulse or flesh of Jángala animals and devoid of any acid combination.* 21.

Frequent blood-letting should be resorted to and measures, such as, emetics, purgatives, Ásthápana and Anuvásana should be adopted in cases of the aggravated Doshas† (involved in the case). 22.

**Memorable Verses :**—A case of Váta-Rakta of recent growth, proves readily amenable to the remedial measures described before. Long-standing, *i.e*, chronic cases (of Váta-Rakta) are never perfectly cured, but can only be palliated. The application of poultices (Upanáha), of medicinal washes or sprinkles (Parisheka), hot-plasters, anointings (Abhyanga), spacious and comfortable bed-chambers which do not admit of too large an influx of air, shampooing, and the use of soft and pleasant beds and soft pillows, are chiefly recommended in a case of Váta-Rakta ; whereas physical exercise, sexual intercourse, display of anger, the use of heat-making, saline, acid and difficultly digestible food and eatables producing effuse serus or slimy matter in the bodily channels, and sleep in the day-time (should be deemed extremely injurious and hence) should be studiously refrained from. 23.

**The Medical Treatment of Apatánaka :**—The medical treatment of a patient suffering from **Apatánaka** (hysterical convulsions), not exhibiting fixedness of gaze and arched eye-brows, with an absence

---

\* In the case of Váta-roga, with a preponderance of Pitta, the patient should take his food with milk ; in the preponderance of Váyu, with the soup of Jángala meat ; and in the preponderance of Kapha, with Mudga-soup, devoid of any acid combination.

† In the preponderance of Kapha, emetics should be employed ; in the preponderance of Pitta, purgatives should be given ; and in the preponderance of Váyu, Anuvásana and Ásthápana measures should be resorted to.

of perspiration, quivering, delirium and the numbness of genitals, found not to fall on the ground but capable of being supported on his arms (Akhattá-páti) and whose trunk is not bent or arched on its posterior (dorsal) side (Vahiráyáma), may be attempted (with success). The body of the patient should be first anointed with emulsions (Sneha) and then fomented; strong medicated snuff should then be administred for purifying (the accumulated mucus in) the head. After that the patient should be made to drink a clear potion prepared of clarified butter, cooked in combination with a decoction of the drugs constituting the Vidári-gandhádi group, extract of meat, milk and milk-curd, so as to arrest the further expansion of the deranged Váyu into the system.

**Traivrita Ghrita :**—A decoction of the Váyu-subduing drugs, such as, *Bhadra-dárvádi*, etc., barley, *Kulattha* pulse, *Kola*, and the flesh of the Ánupa and Audaka animals with the Pancha-Vargas* should be

---

\* According to Jejjata, "Pancha-Vargam" means the flesh of the five kinds of Ánupa animals, *viz.*, Kulachara, Plava, Kos'astha, Pádin and Matsya (fishes).

The reading here is doubtful. The term "Audaka" in the compound word " Sánupaudaka-mámsam " seems to be redundant, inasmuch as "Audaka" animals are included in the " Ánupa " class. (Sutra, chap. XLVI. Page 487, Vol I). In this case the word " Pancha-vargam " also seems to be only an explanation of the term "Ánupa" meaning the fiive kinds of Ánupa flesh, and it seems to have surreptitiously crept into the body of the text from the marginal notes of some authoritative manuscript copy of the book. If, however, we are to abide by the current reading of the book, "Pancha-Varga" cannot mean the five kinds of flesh in the presence of the word "Audaka" mentioned separately, as Jejjata would have it. In that case it can only mean either the five groups of Pancha-mulas, viz., the major Pancha-mulas, the minor Pancha-mulas, the Valli-Pancha-mulas, the Kantaka-Pancha-mulas and the Trina-Pancha-mulas. (Sutra, chap. XXXVIII, Pages 355-6, Vol. I), as some would explain it to mean. Others, however, prefer the reading as it is and explain the term "Pancha-Varga" to be the five kinds of medicinal drugs mentioned before in the sentence,

made. The decoction, thus prepared, should be mixed with milk and fermented rice-gruel, etc., and then cooked with an adequate quantity of clarified butter, oil, lard and marrow by casting Kalka (paste) of the Madhura (Kákolyádi group) into it This Traivrita-Ghrita* (lit. consisting of clarified butter with three other lardaceous articles), thus prepared, should be administered to Apatánaka-patients in potions and diet, in effusions and immersions, in anointings and errhines, as well as in Anuvásana measures. Diaphoretic measures should be applied according to the prescribed rules. In a case marked by an unusually aggravated condition of the Váyu, the patient should be made to stand neck-deep in a pit tolerably warmed or heated with burning husks, and cow-dung. As an alternative, Palás'a leaves should be strewn over a hot stone-slab or over a hot oven, after having sprinkled wine over them, and the patient should be laid full length upon these leaves, or fomentations should be made with *Ves'avára*, *Kris'ara* and *Páyasa*. 24—25.

An oil, cooked in combination with the expressed

viz., the Váthaghna drugs, Yava, Kola, Kulattha and flesh. Others, again, mean by the term "Pancha-varga" the five parts, viz., leaf, fruit, flower, bark and root, of the Váthaghna drugs mentioned in the sentence.

We have, however, the authority of Vágbhata and Chakradatta in our side to accept the first view that the term "Audaka" is redundant, inasmuch as they have not read the word "Audaka" in their compilations. —Ed.

* According to Dallana, four seers of clarified butter, oil, lard and marrow (each weighing one seer), sixteen seers of Kánji, etc., sixteen seers of milk, sixteen seers of the decoction and one seer of the Kalka (paste) should be taken in its preparation. But Gayádása is of opinion that four seers of milk should be taken instead of sixteen seers.

Four seers of Ghrita, etc., four seers of milk, six seers of Kánji, six seers of the decoction and one seer of the Kalka (paste) are generally taken by experienced physicians in its preparation.—Ed.

juice of *Mulaka, Eranda, Sphurja, Arjaka, Arka, Saptalá* and *S'amkhini* should be used in washing (Parisheka), etc., the body of an Apatánaka-patient. Potions consisting of sour **Dadhi** (milk-curd) mixed with powdered pepper and *Vachá*, or of oil, clarified butter, lard, or honey, mixed with the same things and taken in an empty stomach, prove curative in cases of Apatânaka. 26.

These remedial measures are applicable in cases of Apatánaka when the action of the aggravated Váyu alone preponderates. In a case involving the concerted action of two or more of the Doshas, drugs, remedial to each of them, should be combinedly employed. Medicinal liquid errhines (*Avapida*) should be employed after the subsidence of a severe attack The fat or lard of a cock, crab, Krishna-fish, porpoise or of a boar should be taken* by the patient. As an alternative, he should be made to drink (a potion consisting of) milk boiled with Váyu-subduing drugs (Das'a-mula, etc.), or a gruel (Yavágu) composed of barley, *Kola, Kulattha*-pulse and *Mulaka*, cooked with curd, oil and clarified butter. Oily purgatives, Ásthápana and Anuvásana measures, should be employed if the paroxysm does not subside even in ten days. Medicines and remedial measures laid down under the head of Váta-vyádhi and the process of Rakshá-karma, should be likewise adopted (in cases of Apatánaka). 27.

**Treatment of Pakshághata :**—A physician is enjoined to take in hand the medical treatment of a patient laid up with Pakshághátá, unattended by a discolouring of the skin, but having pain in the affected part, and who habitually observes the rules of

---

* Vriddha Vágbhata recommends external application with these lards,

diet and regimen and who can afford to pay for the necessary accessories. The affected part should be first anointed and then fomented. Mild emetics and purgatives should be subsequently employed for the purpose of cleansing the system. Medicated Anuvásana and Ásthápana measures should then be employed, after which the general directions and remedial measures, laid down under the treatment of Ákshepaka, should be followed and employed at the proper time Applications of the Mastikya-Śiro-vasti with the Anu-taila for anointing the body, of the articles of Sálvana-Sveda for the purpose of poulticing, and of the Valá-taila as an Anuvásana measure, are the marked features of the medical treatment of this disease, and should be followed carefully for a continuous period of three or four months. 28.

These preceding remedies as well as dry fomentations (Ruksha-sveda) and errhines, which possess the virtue of subduing the deranged Váyu and Kapha should be likewise employed in cases of **Manyá-stambha.** 29

**Treatment of Apatantraka :**—Fasting is prohibited in cases of patients suffering from Apatantraka (Apoplectic convulsions). Emetic, Ásthápana and Anuvásana measures are likewise forbidden. The passage of respiration should be blown open by violent breathings in the event of its being choked up with an accumulation of the deranged Váyu and Kapha The patient should be made to drink a potion consisting of *Tumburu, Pushkara, Hingu, Amla-vetasa, Haritaki* and the three (officinal) kinds of salts, with a decoction of barley.* As an alternative, four seers of clarified

* Chakradatta quotes this in the chapter on the treatment of colic (s'ula), but does not read 'Amla-vetasa' there.

butter, cooked in combination with sixteen seers of milk, two Pala weight of Sauvarchala salt and fifty of Haritakis should be prescribed for the use of the patient. All other remedial agents, possessing the virtue of subduing the deranged Váyu and Kapha should be likewise employed. 30.

**Treatment of Ardita :**—A patient suffering from Ardita (facial Paralysis) should be treated with the measures and remedies laid down under the head of Váta-vyádhi in the event of his being found to be sufficiently strong and capable of affording the necessary expenses for his treatment. Errhines, Mastikya-Śiro-vasti, inhalation of the smoke (Dhuma-pána) from medicated drugs, poulticing (Upanáha), unguents and Nádi-sveda, etc., are the special features of the medical treatment of this disease. After that, a decoction should be made of the drugs constituting the groups of · *Trina-Pancha-mula, Mahá-Pancha-mula, Kákolyádi* and *Vidári-gandhádi* groups, aquatic bulbs, and the flesh of animals which are aquatic in their habits (Audaka) and those which frequent swampy places (Ánupa), by boiling them together with a Drona measure of milk and double the quantity of water. The decoction should be considered boiled when three quarter parts of its original weight of the liquid has been evaporated and should then be strained. The decoction thus prepared should be boiled with a Prastha measure of oil (four seers) and be removed from the fire when the oil is well mixed with the milk. The compound (oil and milk) thus prepared should be allowed to cool down and then churned. The churned off cream (Sneha) should be again boiled with the drugs of the Madhura (Kákolyádi) group, Másha-parni and milk (four times that of the original oil). This medicated oil is known as the **Kshira-Taila** and should be administered as potions and unguents, etc, to an Ardita-patient The above preparation with clarified butter in the place of oil is known as the **Kshira-sarpih** and it should be used as an Akshi-tarpana (eye-lotion). 31—32.

Venesection should be duly resorted to in the affected parts, according to the directions given before, in cases of Sciatica, Gridhrasi, Visvachi (Synovitis of the knee-joints), Kroshtuka-sirah, Khanja (lameness), Pangula, Váta-kantaka, Páda-dáha, Páda-harsha, Ava-váhuka and Vádhiryya and in cases where the deranged Váyu would be found to be seated in a Dhamani. Measures and remedies laid down under the head of Váta-vyádhi should be adopted, except in a case of Ava-váhuka. 33.

The expressed juice of green ginger, made lukewarm after mixing it with (equal quantities of) oil, honey and Saindhava salt, should be poured into the cavity of the ear in a case of (acute) ear-ache. As an alternative, the urine of a she-goat, or oil and honey, or oil with the urine (of a cow) mixed with the expressed juice of *Mátulunga*, pomegranate and tamarind, or the oil boiled and prepared with Surá, Takra, Sukta, salt and the urine (of a cow), should be poured into the cavity of the ear; fomentation should be given (to the interior of the affected organ) after the manner of Nádi-sveda. The remedial measures for Váta-vyádhi should be resorted to. We shall, however, revert to the subject in the Uttara-Tantra. 34.

The patient should be made to drink a potion of Sneha-Lavana* dissolved in an adequate quantity of water, or the powders of the Pippalyádi group (with an

---

* Sneha-Lavana has been described in Chap. 4. (treatment of Váta-vyádhi) para. 24.

adequate quantity of water), or clarified butter, thickened or saturated with pulverised asafœtida and Yava-kshára (Carbonate of Potass), in cases of **Tuni** and **Prati-tuni**. Applications of Vastis should also be resorted to. 35.

In a case of **Ádhmána** (Tympanites), the remedy should consist in the applications of powders of the Dipaniya (appetising) group, of suppositories (Phala-varti), Vastis and digestive drugs (Páchaniya group). The patient should also be advised to observe a rigid fast and his abdomen should be fomented with hot palms. After that he should break his fast with boiled rice prepared with appetising (Dipana) drugs such as, Dhányaka, Jiraka, etc. Similarly, a case of **Pratyádhmána** should be treated with fasting, emetics and appetising drugs. Cases of **Ashthilá** or **Pratyashthilá** should be treated as a case of Gulma and internal abscess, to all intents and purposes. 36-38.

**Hingvádi-Vati :**—A compound consisting of asafœtida, *Trikatu*, *Vachá*, *Ajamodá*, *Dhanyá*, *Ajagandhá*, *Dádimba*, *Tintidi*, Páthá, Chitraka, Yava-kshára, *Saindhava* salt, *Vid* salt, *Sauvarchala* salt, *Svarjikákshára*, *Pippali-mula*, *Amla-vetasa*, *S'athi*, *Pushkara-mula*, *Hapushá*, *Chavyá*, *Ajáji* and *Pathyá*, powdered together and treated many times with the expressed juice of *Mátulunga* in the manner of Bhávaná* saturation, should be made into boluses, each weighing an Aksha (two Tolás) in weight. One (such) pill should be taken (in an empty stomach) every morning in all diseases of the deranged Váyu. This compound proves curative in cough, asthma, internal tumour (Gulma), ascites, heart-disease,

---

\* "Bhávaná" consists in soaking a powder or a pulverised compound with the expressed juice or decoction of any drugs or with any liquid and in getting it dry (generally). This process should be cotinued many times (generally seven times) in succesion.

tympanites, aching pain at the sides, in the abdomen and in the bladder, in cases of an aversion to food, retention of stool, strangunary, enlarged spleen, piles, Tuni and Prati-tuni. 39.

**Memorable Verses :**—From the symptoms or leading indications, exhibited in each case and from a close examination thereof, it should be inferred whether the Váyu alone has been deranged or whether it has combined with any other Dosha, or has affected any other fundamental principle (Dhátu) of the organism as well ; and the medical treatment should follow a course, so as not to prove hostile to the **Doshas** or the **Dhátus** (organic principles) implicated in the case, in its attempt to subdue the aggravated Váyu. In a case of cold, compact and painful swelling (appearing in any part of the body) owing to the combination of the deranged Váyu with fat, the treatment should be identical with that of a swelling in general. 40-41.

**Uru-stambha :**—The deranged Váyu, surcharged with the local fat and Kapha gives rise to a swelling in the region of the thigh which is known as **Uru-stambha ;** others designate it as **Ádhya-Váta**. This disease is marked by lassitude and an aching pain in the limbs, by the presence of fever, horripilation and somnolence and by a sensation of coldness, numbness, heaviness, and unsteadiness in the thighs, which seem foreign to the body. 42.

**Its Treatment :**—The patient should be made to drink a potion consisting of the pulverised compound known as the Shad-dharana-yoga ; or of the drugs constituting the Pippallyádi group, dissolved in (an adequate quantity of) hot water without using any oleaginous substance ; or a lambative, composed of pulverised *Triphalá* and *Katuka* mixed with honey, should be used; or a potion, consisting of Guggulu or S'ilájatu dissolved in cow's urine, should be administered. These compounds subdue the aggravated Váyu surcharged with deranged fat and Kapha and prove curative in heart-disease, an aversion to food, Gulma and internal abscesses. A medicinal plaster composed of *Karanja* fruits and mustard seeds, pasted with a copious quantity of cow's urine should be applied hot to the affected part, which may be as well fomented with cow's urine mixed with alkali (Kshára); or the locality should be shampooed with articles devoid of any oily substance. The **diet** of the patient should consist of old and matured Syámáka, Kodrava, Uddála and Sáli rice with the soup of dry Mulaka or Patola, or of the flesh of animals of the Jángala group cooked without clarified butter or vegetables (*S'áka*) cooked without salt. The use of oil and of lardaceous substances in general (Sneha-karma) should, however, be prescribed after the deranged fat and Kapha have (totally) subsided. 43.

**Therapeutic properties of Guggulu:** —Guggulu is aromatic, light, penetrating into the minutest parts of the body, sharp, heat-making in potency, pungent in taste and digestion, laxative, emulsive, slimy, and wholesome to the heart (Hridya). **New Guggulu** is an aphrodisiac and a constructive tonic. **Old Guggulu** is anti-fat and hence reduces corpulency. It is owing to its sharpness and heat-making potency that Guggulu tends to reduce the Váyu and the Kapha; it is its laxativeness that destroys the Malas (refuge deposits in the Srotas) and the deranged Pitta; its aroma removes the bad odours of the **Koshtha**; and it is its subtle essence that improves the appetising faculty. Guggulu should be taken every morning with a decoction of *Triphalá*, *Dárvi* and

*Patola* or with that of *Kus'a* roots\*; it may also be taken with an adequate quantity of cow's urine, or with alkaline† or tepid water. The patient should take boiled rice with soup, milk, or extract of meat after the Guggulu has been digested. Diseases such as internal tumour (Gulma), urinary complaints (Meha), Udávarta, ascites, fistula-in-ano, worms in the intestines, itches, an aversion to food, leucoderma (Śvitra), tumour and glands (Arvuda), sinus, Ádhya-Váta, swelling (œdema), cutaneous affections (Kushtha) and malignant sores and ulcers readily yield to it, if used for a month (with the observance of the regimen of diet and conduct laid down previously). It also destroys the deranged Váyu incarcerated in the Koshtha, bones and joints, just as a thunderbolt will destroy trees. 44.

Thus ends the fifth Chapter of the Chikitsita Sthánam in the Sus'ruta-Samhitá which deals with the medical treatment of Mahá-Váta-Vyádhi.

\* Some explain that a third decoction should be that of Triphalá, Dárvi, Patola and Kus'a grass taken together.—Dallana.

The decoctions may be prepared separately with Triphalá, Dárvi, Patola and Kus'a.—*Ed*.

† Some read "Kshira" (milk) in the place of "Kshára" (alkali).

# CHAPTER VI.

Now we shall discourse on the medical treatment of Hæmorrhoids (**Arśas**). 1.

The remedial measures in hæmorrhoids may be grouped under four subheads; namely, the employment of (active) medicinal remedies, the application of an alkali (into the seat of the disease), actual cauterization (of the polypii) and surgical operation. A case of recent origin involving the action of the Doshas to a slight degree and uncomplicated with any grave or dangerous symptom and complication may prove amenable to medicine alone. Deep-seated polypii, which are soft to the touch and markedly elevated and extended (external—D R), should be treated with alkaline applications, while those which are rough, firm, thick and hard should be cauterized with fire. Polypii which are raised, exuding and slender at the roots should be surgically treated. Hœmorrhoids which are held amenable to medicine and are not visible (to the naked eye) should be treated with the help of medicines alone. Now, listen to the procedure to be adopted- in- the treatment of Arśas which would require alkaline applications, a cauterization, or a surgical operation. 2.

**Application of Kshára:**—The body of the patient suffering from hæmorrhoids, in the event of possessing sufficient strength, should be anointed and duly fomented. He should be made to eat warm but demulcent food (Anna) in a fluid state (of a gruel-like consistency) to alleviate the excessive pain incidental to the action of the deranged Váyu. In a season neither too hot nor too cold, and when the sky is cloudless, he should be placed in a raised up position in a clean and well-equipped place on a plain slab or on a clean bed with his head resting on the lap of an attendant and the anal region exposed to the sun. In this position the waist should be made to elevate a little and to rest on a cushion of cloths or blankets. The neck and the thighs of the patient should be drawn out, and then secured with trappings and held fast by the attendants so as not to allow him to move. Then a straight and slender-mouthed instrument (somewhat like the modern rectal speculum), lubricated with clarified butter, should be gently inserted into the rectum and the patient should be asked to strain down gently at the time. After seeing the polypus (through the speculum), it should be scraped with an indicator and cleansed with a piece of cotton or linen after which an alkali should be applied to it. The exterior orifice of the instrument should be closed with the palm of the hand after this application and kept in that manner for a period that would be required to utter a hundred words.

Then after having cleansed the polypus, a fresh application should be made according to the strength of the alkali and the intensity of the aggravated Doshas involved in the case. Further application of the alkali should be stopped and the polypus washed with fermented rice-gruel (Dhányámla), curd-cream, Sukta, or the juice of acid fruits, in the event of its having been found to have become a little flabby, bent down, and to have assumed the colour of a ripe Jambu fruit. After that it should be cooled with clarified butter mixed with *Yashti-Madhu*, the trappings should be removed and the patient should be raised up and placed in a sitting posture in warm water and refreshed with sprays of cold water, or, according to some authorities, with warm water. Then the patient should be made to lie in a spacious chamber, not exposed to the blasts of cold winds (specially), and advised as regards his diet and regimen. Each of the remaining polypii, if any, should be cauterized with the alkaline application at an interval of seven days. In case of a number of polypii, those on the right side should be first cauterized and then those on the left, and after that those on the posterior side ; and lastly those that would be found to be in front. 3.

Polypii, having their origin in the deranged **Váyu** and **Kapha**, should be cauterized with fire or alkali ; while those, which are the outcome of the deranged **Pitta** and vitiated **blood** should be treated with a mild alkali alone. A perfect and satisfactory cauterization (**Samyag-dagdha**) of a polypus should be understood from such symptoms as, restoration of the bodily Váyu to its normal condition, relish for food, keenness of the appetite, lightness of the body and improvement in strength, complexion and pleasure. An over-cauterized (**Ati-dagdha**) polypus gives rise to such symptoms as, cracking of the region of the anus, a burning sensation (in the affected locality), fainting, fever, thirst, and profuse hæmorrhage (from the rectum), and consequent complications ; while an insufficiently cauterized (**Hina-dagdha**) polypus is known by its tawny brown colour, smallness of the incidental ulcer, itching, derangement of the bodily Váyu, discomforts of the cognitive organs and a non-cure of the disease. 4.

A large polypus, appearing in a strong person, should be clipped off (with a knife) and cauterized with fire. As regards an external polypus full of extremely aggravated Doshas (Váyu, Pitta, Kapha and blood) no

Yantra should be used, but the treatment should consist of fomentation, anointing, poulticing, immersion, plastering, evacuating measures (Visráva), cauterization with fire and alkali and a surgical operation. Measures laid down under the head of Rakta-pitta should be resorted to in cases of hæmorrhage (from the seat of affection). Remedies mentioned in connection with dysentery (Atisára) should be employed in cases of a looseness of the bowels; whereas in cases of constipation of the bowels oily purgatives should be administered, or the remedies for Udávartta should be adopted. These rules shall hold good in the cases of treating (cauterization, etc.) a polypus occurring in any part of the body whatsoever. 5.

A polypus should be caught hold of and an alkali should be applied thereto with a Darvi, or a brush (Kurcha), or an indicator (Saláká). In a case of a prolapsus of the anus, cauterization should be made without the help of any Yantra (speculum).

**Diet :**—In all types of hæmorrhoids, the diet should consist of wheat barley, Shashtika rice or Sáli rice, (boiled) and mixed with clarified butter, to be taken with milk, Nimba-soup, or Patola-soup. The patient should be advised to take (his meal) with *Vástuka, Tanduliyaka, Jivanti, Upodiká, As'va-valá,* tender *Mulaka, Pálanka, Asana, Chilli, Chuchchu, Kaláya, Valli,* or any other *S'ákas* (pot-herbs), according to the nature of rhe Doshas involved in the case Any other oleaginous, diuretic, laxative and appetising (Dipana) diet possessing the virtue of curing piles should also be prescribed. 6.

After the cauterization of the polypus, as well as in a case where no cauterization would be necessary, the body of the patient should be anointed with clarified butter and oil, etc., and measures both **general** and **specific** (mentioned below and in accordance with the Dosha or Doshas involved) should be employed for the purpose of improving the digestive powers and to alleviate any aggravation of the **Váyu**. He should be made to drink a potion consisting of clarified butter cooked with the Váyu-subduing and appetising (Dipana) drugs* (Kalka and Kvátha) mixed with the powders of Hingu, etc , (described in the treatment of Mahá-Váta-vyádhi, chapter. V). In a case of **Pittaja-Arśas**, clarified butter prepared by cooking it with the drugs of the *Pippallyádi* and *Bhadra-dárvádi*† groups, should again be cooked with the decoction of Prithakparnyádi group and the Kalka of the Dipaniya (Pippallyádi) group, and given as a potion to the patient. In a case of hæmorrhoid due to the action of the deranged blood ‡ (**Raktárśas**), the clarified butter should be cooked with a decoction of *Manjishthá, Murungi*, (D. R. Surangi), &c., while in a case of one due to the action of the deranged **Kapha**, the clarified butter should be cooked with a decoction of the drugs constituting the *Surasádi* group. The supervening distresses should be alleviated by the remedial measures peculiar to each of them 7.

Cauterization with fire or with an alkali or any surgical

---

\* Such as the decoction of the drugs of the Bhadra-darvádi (Váyu-subduing) and Pippalyádi (Dipaniya) groups. This Ghrita should be prescribed in a **Vátaja Arśas**.

† The epithet "Bhadra-dárvádi-pippallyádi" in the phrase "Bhadra-dárvádi-pippallyádi-sarpih" seems to be included into the body of the text through an accident. In our opinion, it is only an annotation of the phrase "Dipaniya-Váta-hara-siddha" occurring in the last sentence.—*Ed.*

‡ The Kalkas of the Pippallyádi group should also be taken in the preparation of the two kinds of medicated clarified butter to be used in Raktárs'as, and Pittárs'as.—*Dallana.*

operation in the present disease should be effected by introducing the Yantra (speculum) into the rectum (with the utmost care, inasmuch as an error happening in any of these cases may bring on impotency, swelling (Sopha), a burning sensation, epilepsy, rumbling in the intestines, retention of stool and urine, dysentery, diarrhœa, or may ultimately end in death. 8.

**Rectal Speculum :**—Now we shall describe the dimensions of the Yantras (and the materials of which they are made of). The instrument may be made of iron, ivory, horn or wood. It should be made to resemble the teat of a cow. In the case of a male patient, it should be four fingers in length and five fingers in circumference ; whereas in the case of a female patient, the length should be commensurate with that of the palm of the hand (of the same length as before—D. R.) and six fingers in circumference. The instrument should be provided with two separate apertures in its inside, one for seeing the interior of the rectum and the other for applying an alkali, or actual cautery (Agni) to the polypus, since it is impossible to apply fire and alkali through the same aperture. The circumference of the aperture in the upper three fingers of the instrument should be like that of a thumb. There should be a bulb-like protrusion of the same width, at the bottom, and above it a space of half a finger's width. Thus we have briefly described the shape of the instrument. 9-10.

**Álepa** (plasters) **:**—Now we shall describe the plasters to be applied to the hæmorrhoids (to cause their spontaneous dropping off). The first consists of pulverised turmeric mixed with the milky exudation of the *Snuhi tree*. The second contains of the cock-evacuations and pulverised *Gunjá*, turmeric and *Pippali* pasted with the urine and bile of a cow. The third is compounded of *Danti, Chitraka, Suvarchiká* and *Lángali* pounded together and made into a paste with cow's bile. The fourth consists of *Pippali*, rock-salt, *S'irisha*-seeds and *Kushtha* pasted with the milky juice of an *Arka*, or *Snuhi* plant. An oil cooked in combination with *Kásisa* (sulphate of iron), *Haritála* (yellow orpiment), rock-salt, *As'vamáraka, Vidanga, Putika, Kritavedhana, Jambu, Arka, Uttamárani, Danti, Chitraka, Alarka* and *Snuhi*-milk, and used as an unguent, leads to the falling off of the polypus. 11

**Internal piles :**—Now we shall describe the remedial measures which bring about the falling off of the invisible (internal) hæmorrhoids. The patient should take *Haritaki* with treacle every morning ; or a hundred *Haritakis* should be boiled in a Drona measure of cow's urine and the patient, observing a strict continence, should take with honey every morning as many of them as suit his constitution ; or he should be made to take every day a paste made of the roots of *Apámárga* with the washings of rice and with honey. *S'atávari* pasted with an adequate quantity of milk or (a Karsha measure of) the powders of *Chitraka* mixed with a copious quantity of good *Sidhu* wine, or a gruel (Mantha) (neither extremely thick nor thin), or powdered barley or wheat mixed with Takra and *Bhallátaka* powder, should be administered without any salt. A quantity of Takra should be kept in an earthen pitcher, plastered inside with a paste of *Chitraka* roots, and given to the patient in food and drinks whether fermented or not. A Takra should also be separately prepared as in the preceding manner with *Bhárgi, Ásphotá*, barley, *Ámalaka* and *Guduchi* and administered similarly ; this is called the **Takra-kalpa** (butter-milk compound). 12.

A medicated Takra should also be prepared with *Pippali*, *Pippali-mula*, *Chavya*, *Chitraka*, *Vidanga*, *S'unthi* and *Haritaki*, in the manner described above, (and given to the patient), who should abstain from taking any solid food, but live only on (this) Takra for a period of one full month ; or he should be given milk boiled with a decoction of *S'ringavera*, *Punarnavá* and *Chitraka*, or a condensed decoction (Phánita) of the bark of *Kutaja* roots mixed with an after-throw of the powdered drugs of the *Pippalyádi* group and honey. The patient should be made to partake of the medicinal compound known as the **Hingvádi-churna**,* described in the chapter on Mahá-Váta-vyádhi, and be made to live either on milk, or on Takra. As an alternative, he should take *Kulmásha* boiled in Kshárodaka (alkaline water) prepared from *Chitraka*-roots and made saline with a liberal after-throw of Yava-kshára ; or he should take milk boiled with the Kshárodaka (alkaline water) prepared from *Chitraka*-roots, or Kulmásha boiled with the alkaline water prepared from the ashes of burnt *Palása* ; or he should drink frequent potions of clarified butter mixed with the alkali made of the ashes of either *Patola*, *Apámárga*, *Vrihati*, or *Palásá* wood ; or drink Takra mixed with the Kalka of the roots of *Kutaja* and of *Vandáka* ; or take the alkaline water of *Putika* mixed with a Kalka of *Chitraka*, *Putika* and *Nágara* ; or use the clarified butter boiled in an alkaline solution† with the powdered drugs of the *Pippalyádi* group,

---

\* In a preponderance of Váyu and Kapha, Takra should be taken as diet ; whereas milk should be taken in a case of the preponderance of vitiated blood.

† During the period when the above mentioned alkaline preparations are used, the diet of the patient should consist of clarified butter, milk and meat-soup for fear of the loss of the Ojo-Dhátu,

added to it by way of an after-throw; or he should take every morning one or two Palas of black sesamum (according as required), with cold water. These measures prove remedial in cases of hæmorrhoids and tend to improve the digestion. 13.

**Dantyarishta:**—A Tulá weight\* (twelve seers and a half) of the following drugs, *viz.*, *Das'a-mula*, *Danti*, *Chitraka* and *Haritaki* should be boiled with four Drona measures of water till reduced to one quarter part (one Drona). The decoction, thus prepared, should be cooled down, filtered, mixed with a Tulá measure of treacle and preserved into a receptacle which formerly contained clarified butter, which should then be kept buried for a month in a heap of unthrashed barley At the close of this period an adequate dose of this preparation should be given to the patient every morning. This medicine proves beneficial in cases of hæmorrhoids, chronic diarrhœa (Grahani), jaundice, obstinate constipation of the bowels (Udávartta) and in an aversion to food. It is also a good stomachic agent.

**Abhayárishta**† :—Two Pala weight of each of the following drugs, *viz.*, *Pippali*, *Maricha*, *Vidanga*, *Elaváluká* and *Lodhra*, five ‡ Pala weight of *Indra-váruni*, ten Pala weight of the inner pulps of the *Kapittha* fruit, half a Prastha measure (one Prastha is equal to two seers) of *Haritaki* and one Prastha weight of *Ámalaki*, boiled together with four Drona measures of

---

\* Some are of opinion that one Tulá weight of each of the drugs should be taken; but Gayadása does not say so.

† Charaka also reads this under the name of Abhayárishta.

‡ Experienced physicians recommend two and a half Pala weight of Indra-Váruni in lieu of five Palas for its astringent taste. Charaka, however, recommends only "half a Pala."

water until reduced to one quarter of its quantity. This decoction should be filtered (through a piece of linen) and cooled down, after which two Tulá weight of treacle should be added to it. The whole preparation should be then kept in a receptacle which formerly contained clarified butter, and be kept buried half a month in a heap of unthrashed barley. After the lapse of the said period, the patient should be made to drink (an adequate quantity of) this preparation every morning according to his strength. This Arishta proves curative in cases of an enlarged spleen, impaired digestion, chronic diarrhœa (Grahani), Arśas, heart-disease, jaundice, cutaneous affection, ascites, Gulma, œdema (Śopha), and worms in the intestines, and improves the strength and complexion of the body. 14

Anointing (Sneha-karma), fomentation, use of emetics and purgatives and the application of Anuvásana and Ásthápana measures should be employed in cases of hæmorrhoids due to the action of the deranged **Váyu**.* The use of purgatives is recommended in the **Pittaja** type; soothing or pacifying (Samsamana) measures in the **Raktaja** type ; and *S'ringavera* and *Kulattha* in the type caused by the action of the deranged **Kapha**. All the preceding remedies should be combinedly employed when the concerted action of all the Doshas would be detected. As an alternative, milk boiled with the proper drugs may be administered in every case. 15.

**Bhallátaka-yoga**† :—Now we shall describe the mode of using **Bhallátaka** in cases of hæmorrhoids.

---

\* Some are of opinion that the Rishis do not read this line But as Gayadása explains it, so Dallana, he tells us, also does the same.

† A physician should apply this medicine after a due consideration and according to the physical condition of the patient.

A ripe and fresh Bhallátaka should be cut into two, three or four pieces and a decoction should be made of them in the usual way The patient should be made to drink four Tolá weight of this cold every morning after lubricating or anointing his tongue, palate and lips with clarified butter, and should take his chief meal with milk and clarified butter in the afternoon. The number of Bhallátakas in preparing the decoction should be increased by one every day till the fifth day, (and the quantity of the decoction to be drunk by the patient should be similarly increased). After that, the number of Bhallátakas (and consequently the quantity of the decoction to be taken) should be increased by five every day. This method should be followed till the number of the Bhallátakas reaches **seventy**, after which it should be decreased every day by five until it is reduced to **five** Bhallátakas only (and five Śukti measures of the decoction). Subsequently the number of Bhallátaka (and the dose) should be diminished by **one** (and one Śukti measure respectively) every day, until it is reduced to the original **one** (and one Śukti measure). By taking a thousand Bhallátakas in this manner, one may get rid of an attack of any kind of Kushtha and Arśas, and, having become strong and healthy, may live for one hundred years. 16.

**Other forms of Bhallátaka-yoga :—** The oil extracted from or pressed out of Bhallátakas, in the manner laid down in the chapter on Dvi-vrana, should be taken in a dose of one Śukti (four Tolás) every morning. The patient, as in the preceding case, should take his meal ( of boiled rice, milk and clarified butter) after the digestion of the oil with a similar good effect. As an alternative, oil should be extracted from the marrow of Bhallátakas and the patient, after cleansing his system with emetics and purgatives, etc., and regulating his diet in the order of Peyá, etc. should enter into a spacious chamber, protected from the blasts of the winds and take two Palas, or one Pala weight of the oil according to his strength  A meal of boiled rice, milk and clarified butter, etc., should be taken after the oil had been fully digested. The oil should be continued, in this way, for a month, the regimen of diet should be strictly observed for a period of three months and the patient should abstain from anger, etc, during this period. The use of this oil, in the above mentioned way, not only ensures a radical cure of the disease with all its complications, but would increase the duration of life to a hundred years with the glow of youth and health and with an increment in the powers of memory, retention and wisdom. The application of this oil for every one month will extend one's life for a period of one hundred years  In the same way a continuous use for ten months would enable him to live for a thousand years. 17

**Memorabie Verses :**—Vrikshaka (Kutaja) and **Bhallátaka*** prove as much curative in cases of all kinds of hæmorrhoids, as **Kshadira** and **Vijaka** are effective in cases of cutaneous affections (Kushtha). **Cauterization** with fire, or with an alkali, proves as much palliative in cases of external hæmorrhoids as **turmeric** proves soothing in those of Prameha. 18-19.

Medicated Ghritas, appetising drugs, electuaries, medicinal wines, Ayaskriti and Ásava should be prescribed in cases of hæmorrhoids, according to the nature and intensity of the Doshas involved

---

\* Boiled with sixteen times of water in the event of the Bhallátaka being dry, otherwise with eight times of water only.

therein. Voluntary suppression of any natural urgings of the body, sexual intercourse, riding on horse-back, etc., sitting on the legs and such diets as would aggravate the Doshas, should be avoided in cases of hæmorrhoids. 20-21.

Thus ends the sixth Chapter in the Chikitsita Sthánam of the Sus'ruta Samhitá which deals with the medical treatment of Ars'as.

# CHAPTER VII.

Now we shall discourse on the medical treatment of urinary calculus, etc. (**Aśmari**). 1.

**Metrical Texts :**—Aśmari (urinary calculus, etc) is a dangerous disease and is as fatal as death itself. A case of recent origin (acute) proves amenable to **medicines,** while an enlarged or chronic one requires **surgical operations.** The remedial measures, in the order of anointing, etc., should be employed in the first or incipient stage of the disease, whereby the entire defects with their causes (*i.e.*, roots of the disease) would be radically cured. 2.

**Treatment of Vátaja Aśmari :**—Clarified butter cooked with a decoction of *Páshánabheda, Vasuka, Vas'ira, As'mantaka, S'atávari, S'vadamstrá, Vrihati, Kantakárika, Kapotavamka, A'rtagala, Kakubha\*, Us'ira, Kubjaka, Vrikshádani, Bhalluka, Varuna, S'áka-phala,* barley, *Kulattha, Kola* and *Kataka* fruits and with the Kalka of the drugs constituting the group of *Ushakádi,* speedily brings about the disintergration of As'mari (urinary calculi, etc.) due to the action of the deranged **Váyu.** Milk, Yavágu (gruel), a decoction, soup, or an alkali, properly prepared with the above Váyu-subduing drugs should also be administered as food and drink in the above cases. 3.

**Treatment of Pittaja Aśmari :**—Similarly a medicated clarified butter cooked with the

---

\* Chakradatta reads "Kopotavaktrá" in place of "Kapotavamka" "Kánchana" in place of "Kakubha"; and "Gulmaka" in place of "Kubjaka " From an examination of Dallana it appears that "Kachchhaka" is also a reading of "Kakubha."

decoction of *Kus'a, Kás'a, S'ara, Gundrá, Itkata, Morata, As'mabhid, S'atávari, Vidári, Váráhi, S'áli-mula, Trikantaka, Bhalluka, Pátalá, Páthá, Pattura, Kuruntiká, Punarnavá\*, S'irisha*, with the paste (Kalka) consisting of *S'ilájatu, Madhuka* (flower) and the seeds of *Indivara*†, *Trapusha* and *Ervdruka*, would speedily bring about the disintegration of **Pittaja** As'mari (calculi, etc.). An alkali, Yavágu (gruel), soup, a decoction, or milk, properly prepared with the above Pitta-subduing drugs, should also be prescribed as food and drink in these cases. 4.

**Treatment of Kaphaja As'mari :—** The use of medicated clarified butter prepared from the milk of a she-goat†† and cooked with the paste (Kalka) of the drugs constituting the *Varunádi* group‡, *Guggulu, Elá, Harenu, Kushtha*, the *Bhadrádi* group, *Maricha, Chitraka, Suráhvá* and the *Ushakádi* group, leads to the speedy disintegration and expulsion of the As'mari (stone, etc.) due to the action of the deranged **Kapha**. So also the use of an alkali, Yavágu (gruel), soup, milk, or a decoction, properly prepared with the above Kapha-subduing drugs, is recommended as food and drink in such cases. 5.

A potion consisting of the powdered fruit of the *Pichuka, Amkola, Kataka, S'áka* and *Indivara* mixed with treacle§

---

\* Chakradatta reads "Punarnave" *i.e.*, both the kinds of Punarnavá.

† Jejjata explains "Indivara" as 'Nilotpala.' But Gayádása does not support this.

‡ Some say that "Aja-sarpih" is superfluous. Chakradatta reads "गणे वरुणकादौ च गुग्गुल्वेलाहरेणुभिः" in place of "गणो वरुणकादिस्तु गुग्गुल्वेला-हरेणव" meaning thereby that the decoction of the Varunádi-gana is to be used. Chakradatta's reading seems to be the correct one and is observed in practice with good results.—Ed.

§ The quantity of treacle, to be taken, should be equal to the entire quantity of the powders : and hot water should be used —Dallana.

and water proves beneficial in cases of **Gravel** (S'arkará). The bones of the Krauncha, camel and ass, as well as the drugs known as *S'vadamshtrá*,* *Tálamuli, Ajamodá, Kadamba*-roots and *Nágara* pounded together and administered through the vehicle of wine (Surá) or hot water, leads to the disintegration of S'arkará (gravel). The milk of an ewe mixed with powdered *Trikantaka*-seeds and honey should be used for seven days for the disintegration and separation of an As'mari. 6-7.

**Alkaline Treatments :**—An alkali should be prepared from the ashes of the drugs used in the preparation of the aforesaid medicated clarified butters, by dissolving and filtering them in ewe's urine The alkali should then be slowly boiled with an alkali similarly prepared from the dung of domestic animals, with the powders of *Trikatu* and the drugs of the *Ushakádi* group thrown into them as an after-throw. It proves curative in cases of stone, Gulma, and gravel. Alkalies† from burnt bark of sesamum, *Apámárga*, plantain, *Palás'a* and barley taken with the urine of an ewe destroy the gravel (S'arkará). As an alternative, the alkalies of *Pátalá* and *Karavira* should be used in the preceding manner. 8-9.

Two Tolá (Aksha) weights of the pastes of *S'vadamstrá, Yashti-madhu* and *Bráhmi* (mixed with ewe's urine) should be given to the patient ; or the expressed juice of the *Edaká, S'obhánjana* and *Márkava* (with the said urine) should be given, or a potion consisting of the pasted roots of the *Kapotavamka* with Kánjika, or Surá, etc., should be administered. Milk boiled with the aforesaid drug (Kapotavamka) should be taken by a patient

---

\* Some explain it as "Gokshura-seeds" and others as "Markataka-seeds."

† Four or six Tolá weight of an alkali should be dissolved and filtered for a number of times before use.

in case there is pain (in urinating). Milk boiled with *Triphalá* or *Varshábhu* should be administered as a drink and a decoction of the drugs of the *Vira-tarádi* group should be employed in all these cases.* 10.

A physician should have recourse to the following measures (surgical operations) in cases where the above-mentioned decoctions, medicated milk, alkalies, clarified butter and Uttara-vasti (urethral syringe) of the aforesaid drugs, etc., would prove ineffective. Surgical operations in these cases do not prove successful even in the hands of a skilful and experienced surgeon; so a surgical (Lithotomic) operation should be considered a remedy that has little to recommend itself. The death of the patient is almost certain without a surgical operation and the result to be derived from it is also uncertain. Hence a skilled surgeon should perform such operations only with the permission of the king. 11-12.

**Modes of Surgical Operations :**—The patient should be soothed (Snigdha) by the application of oleaginous substances, his system should be cleansed with emetics and purgatives and be slightly reduced thereby; he should then be fomented after being anointed with oily unguents; and be made to pertake of a meal. Prayers, offerings and prophylactic charms should be offered and the instruments and surgical accessories required in the case should be arranged in the order laid down in the Agropaharaniya chapter of the present work (Sutra-sthánam, ch. V.). The

---

\* Dallana recommends the use of Triphalá boiled with milk in cases of pain accompanying Pittaja As'mari, while that boiled with Varshábhu is advised to be given for the alleviation of pain in a case of Vátaja or Kaphaja As'mari. The drugs of Vira-tarádi group should be used with milk, clarified butter, a decoction, Yavágu (gruel), food, etc., and also for bath, immersion, etc.

surgeon should use his best endeavours to encourage the patient and infuse hope and confidence in the patient's mind. A person of strong physique and un-agitated mind should be first made to sit on a level board or table as high as the knee-joint. The patient should then be made to lie on his back on the table placing the upper part of his body in the attendant's lap, with his waist resting on an elevated cloth cushion. Then the elbows and knee-joints (of the patient) should be contracted and bound up with fastenings (S'átaka) or with linen. After that the umbelical region (abdomen) of the patient should be well rubbed with oil or with clarified butter and the left side of the umbelical region should be pressed down with a closed fist so that the **stone** comes within the reach of the operator. The surgeon should then introduce into the rectum, the second and third fingers of his left hand, duly anointed and with the nails well pared. Then the fingers should be carried upward towards the rope of the perineum *i.e*, in the middle line so as to bring the stone between the rectum and the penis, when it should be so firmly and strongly pressed as to look like an elevated Granthi (tumour), taking care that the bladder remains contracted but at the same time even.

**Prognosis-M. Text :**—An operation should not be proceeded with nor an attempt made to extract the stone (Śalya) in a case where, the stone on being handled, the patient would be found to drop down motionless (*i e.*, faint) with his head bent down, and eyes fixed in a vacant stare like that of a dead man, as an extraction in such a case is sure to be followed by death. The operation should only be continued in the absence of such an occurrence.

An incision should then be made on the left side

of the raphe of the perineum at the distance of a barley-corn and of a sufficient width to allow the free egress of the stone. Several authorities recommend the opening to be on the right side of the raphe of the perineum for the convenience of the operation. Special care should be taken in extracting the stone from its cavity so that it may not break into pieces nor leave any broken particles behind (i.e., inside the bladder), however small, as they would, in such a case, be sure to grow larger again. Hence the entire stone should be extracted with the help of an Agravaktra Yantra (a kind of forceps the points of which are not too sharp). 13.

**Lithotomic Operation in a female :—** In a woman, the uterus (Garbhás'aya) is adjacent to the urinary bladder, hence the stone should be removed by making an oblique and upward incision, otherwise a urine-exuding ulcer might result from the deep incision in that locality. Any hurt to the urethra during the operation would be attended with the same result even in a male patient. An incision made only on one side of the organ in a disease other than that of stone, baffles all attempts at healing ; while an ulcer incidental to an incision made on both its sides, should be deemed incurable An ulcer incidental to an incision made on either side of the bladder in extracting a stone might be healed up, inasmuch as medicinal potions and fomentations, etc., employed for the healing of a surgical wound, lead to the healing of the wound in the bladder ; secondly because the surgical opening is only made large enough for the extraction of the stone as recommended in the authoritative books ; and thirdly because an increase in the quantity of urine contributes to an increase in the size of the stone and hence a slight secretion of that fluid or employment of diuretic Peyás, etc., are not attended with any injurious effects.

**Post-Surgical Measures :**—After the extraction of a stone, the patient should be made to sit in a Droni (cauldron) full of warm water and be fomented thereby. In doing so the possibility of an accumulation of blood in the bladder will be prevented ; however if blood be accumulated therein, a decoction of the Kshira-trees should be injected into the bladder with the help of a Pushpa-netra (urethral Syringe). 14-15.

**Memorable Verse :**—Stones and the accumulated blood in the bladder would be speedily expelled by means of injecting a decoction of the Kshira-trees into it with the help of a Pushpa-netra (urethral Syringe). 16.

For the clearance of the urinary passage, a treacle solution should be given to the patient ; and after taking him out of the Droni, the incidental ulcer should be lubricated with honey and clarified butter. A Yavágu, boiled with the drugs* possessed of the virtue of cleansing or purifying the urine, and mixed with clarified butter, should be given to the patient in a warm state every morning and evening for three consecutive days.

After that period a diet (meal) of rice well boiled and mixed with milk and a large quantity of treacle, should be given (to the patient) in small quantities for ten days for the purification of the blood and the secretion of urine as well as for the purpose of establishing secretion in the ulcer. The patient should be made to partake of a diet (of rice) with the soup of the flesh of Jángala animals and the expressed juice of acid fruits after the lapse of these ten days. 17.

* The urine-purifying drugs are the Trina-Panchamulas, Gokshura, Kásamarda, Páshánabheda, etc.

After that period, the body of the patient should be carefully fomented for ten successive days by applying any warm oleaginous substance or with any warm medicinal fluid (Drava-Sveda) As an alternative, the ulcer should be washed with the decoction of (the bark of) the *Kshira-Vrikshas*. A paste of Rodhra, Madhuka, Manjishthá and Prapaundarika (pounded together), should be applied then to the ulcer. A medicated oil or Ghrita cooked with turmeric and the preceding drugs should be applied to the ulcer. The accumulated blood in the affected part should be removed with the help of a Uttara-vasti (urethral Syringe). The ulcer should be cauterized with fire in the manner described before in the event of the urine not flowing through its natural passage after the lapse of seven days. After the urine takes its natural course, Uttara-vasti, Ásthápana and Anuvásana measures should be employed with the decoction of the drugs belonging to the *Madhura-Varga*.

A seminial stone or gravel (S'arkará) spontaneously brought down into the urinary passage should be removed through the same passage. The urethra should be cut open and the stone should be extracted with a hook (Vadiśa) or any other instrument in the case of its not being expelled out by the passage. The patient should refrain from sexual intercourse, riding on horse back or on the back of an elephant, swimming, climbing on trees and up mountains and partaking of indigestible substances for a year even after the healing of the ulcer. 18.

**Parts to be guarded in Lithotomic Operations:**—The Mutra-vaha (urine-carrying) and the S'úkra-vaha (semen-carrying) ducts or channels, the Mushka-srotas (cords of the testes), the Mutra-praseka (urinary) channels, the Sevani (the raphe of the perineum), the Yoni (uterus, vagina, etc.), the Guda (rectum) and the Vasti (bladder) should be carefully guarded at the time of performing a lithotomic operation. Death results in the event of the urine-carrying channels being in any way hurt during the operation owing to an accumulation of urine in the bladder. Similarly, any hurt or injury to the semen-carrying ducts at the time, results in death or in impotency of the patient; a hurt to the cords of the testes begets an incapacity of fecundation; a hurt to the urinary ducts leads to a frequent dribbling of urine; while a hurt to the Yoni (uterus, vagina, etc.), or to the raphe of the perineum gives rise to extreme pain The symptoms which characterise a hurt to the rectum or to the bladder have been described before. 19.

**Memorable Verses:**—The surgeon who is not well cognisant of the nature and positions of the Marmas or vulnerable parts seated in the eight Srotas (ducts) of the body such as, the raphe of the perineum, the spermatic cords, the cords of the testes and the corresponding ones in females (Yoni), the anal region, the urinary ducts, the urine-carrying ducts, and the urinary bladder and is not practiced in the art of surgery brings about the death of many an innocent victim. 20.

Thus ends the seventh Chapter of the Chikitsita Sthánam in the Sus'ruta Samhitá which deals with the treatment of Urinary calculus.

# CHAPTER VIII.

Now we shall discourse on the medical treatment of Fistula-in-ano, etc., **(Bhagandara)**. 1.

The disease admits of being divided into five different groups, of which the two, known as S'ambukávarta and S'alyaja (traumatic), should be regarded as incurable, and the rest as extremely difficult to cure. 2.

**The General Treatment :**—The eleven* kinds of remedial measures commencing with Apatarpana up to purgatives (as described under the treatment of Dvi-vrana) should be employed as long as any fistular ulcer would remain in an insuppurated stage The patient should be soothed by the application of medicated oil, etc., and his body should be fomented by immersing him in a receptacle of warm water, etc as soon as suppuration would set in (and even after the ulcer had burst). Then having laid him on a bed and bound his hands and thighs with straps as described under the treatment of Hæmorrhoid, the surgeon should examine closely as to where the mouth of the fistula is directed, outward or inward, and whether the ulcer itself is situated, upward or downward. Then the whole cavity or receptacle of pus (sinus) should be raised up and scraped out with an Eshani (indicator or probe). In a case of inter-mouthed fistula, the patient should be secured with straps (as before described) and asked to strain down. An incision should then be made by first directing the indicator when its mouth would become visible from the outside. Cauterization

---

* Apatarpana, Álepa, Parisheka, Abhyanga, Sveda, Vimlápana, Upanáha, Páchana, Visrávana, Sneha, and Vamana.

with fire or an alkali is a general remedial measure which may be resorted to in all the types of this disease. 3-4.

**Specific Measures—M. Texts :**—In cases of the Śataponaka type all the small Vranas about the anus should be first incisioned and the principal sinus in the locality should not be looked after until these small ones had been healed up. The connected abscesses should be respectively incisioned on the external side, while the unconnected ones should not be opened at the same time in order that they may not run into one another and be thus converted into a wide-mouthed ulcer. The urine and the fæcal matter are found in each case to flow out of the cavity of such a wide-mouthed ulcer ; and aching pains in the rectum and a rumbling sound in the abdomen, due to the action of the aggravated Váyu, are experienced. Such a case is enough to confound even a well-read and experienced physician. Hence the mouth of a fistula of the Śataponaka type should not be opened with a broad incision.

**Forms of incision :**—An experienced surgeon should know that the Lángalaka, Ardha-Lángalaka, Sarvatobhadraka and the Gotirthaka forms of incision should be the different shapes of incision, in a case of a many-mouthed S'ataponaka. An incision equal in its two sides is called the **Lángalaka** (curvilineal), while the one with one arm longer than the other is named the **Ardha-Lángalaka.** An incision made in the region of the anus in the shape of a cross (crucial) and a little removed from the raphe of the perineum, is called the **Sarvatobhadraka** by men conversant with the shapes of surgical incisions. An incision made by inserting the knife in one side is called the **Gotirthaka** (longitudinal). All exuding (bleeding) channels in the affected region should be cauterized with fire by the surgeon.

A case of the Śataponaka type occurring in a person of timid disposition or of delicate constitution, is extremely difficult to cure. Medicinal fomentations endowed with the virtue of arresting secretion and alleviating pain, should be quickly applied (to the seat of the disease). Fomentations with Kriśará, or Páyasa (porridge), made with the aforesaid Svedaniya (diaphoretic) drugs with a decoction of the drugs constituting the *Vilvádi* group, *Vrikshádani* and roots of the castor-plant mixed and boiled together with the flesh of the Láva, Vishkira (a kind of bird) and that of animals living in swampy or marshy land or aquatic in their habits or Grámya animals, and then kept in an oily pitcher and applied in the way of a Nádi-Sveda (fomentation through Nádi or pipe), should be at once applied to the seat of the ulcer. Sesamum, castor-seeds, linseed, *Másha*-pulse, barley, wheat, mustard-seeds, salts and the Amla-Varga (see Rasa-Vijnániya chapter) should be boiled in a saucer and the affected part or ulcer should be fomented therewith. After being fomented, the patient should drink (a potion consisting of) *Kushtha*, salts (the five officinal kinds of salts) *Vachá*, *Hingu* and *Ajamoda* taken in equal parts and mixed with (an adequate quantity of) clarified butter, grape-wine (Márdvika), Kánjika (Amla), Surá or Sauviraka.\* Subsequent to that, the ulcer should be wetted with the *Madhuka*-oil and the rectum should be washed with medicated oils which would alleviate pain due to the action of the deranged and aggravated Váyu. The preceding medicinal remedies tend to bring about the outflow or evacuations of stool and urine through their natural channels or courses, and undoubtedly alleviate all acute and supervening distresses which specifically mark

---

\* By the use of this potion the digestive power is increased.

the progress of the disease. We have described the treatment of a case of fistula-in-ano of the Sataponaka (sieve) type ; now listen to me about the treatment of the Ushtragriva (camel's neck) type of the disease. 5.

**Treatment of Ushtra-griva :**—The ulcer should first be searched with a probe or director and, after an operation, an alkali should be applied to it. To remove all sloughed off or sloughing flesh and membranes cauterization with fire is forbidden. [The fissures of pus (sinuses) and sloughed off flesh should be first drawn out]. A plaster of clarified butter and pasted sesamum should then be applied to it, and the ulcer duly bandaged. Clarified butter should be constantly applied over the bandage which should be removed on the third day. Cleansing or disinfecting (S'odhana) measures should then be used by the surgeon, according to the Doshas involved in the ulcer, and the successive healing (Ropana) measures resorted after its being properly purified (S'odhana). 6

**Treatment of Parisrávi :**—In a case of the Parisrávi (exuding) type, where there is bleeding and secretion from the ulcer, the sinus and the cavities of pus should be first removed and then cauterized with an alkali or with fire by an intelligent surgeon. The region of the anus should then be kept wet by the sprinkling of lukewarm **Anu-toila** (described in the chapter on Váta-vyádhi) Warm plasters, or poultices, mixed with *Yavakshára* and the urine (of a cow) should then be applied. Decoction of the emetic drugs as the seeds of *Madana*, etc.), should also be sprinkled slightly on the affected part. The ulcer when found to be softened and nearly free from pain and secretion (owing to the preceding measures) should be searched with a probe and the principal sinus should be cut open and again completely cauterized with fire or with an alkali. The incisions should be made in the shape or form of a Kharjura-patra (leaf of the date-palm), Ardha-chandra (half-moon), Chandra-chakra (moon's disc), Suchi-mukha (needle's mouth), or Avámmukha (with downward mouth). After that the ulcer should be purified with mild cleansing or disinfecting remedies (as described above)  7.

In the case of an infant cauterization with fire or with an alkali, the use of strong purgatives and surgical operations are forbidden in the case of the disease (Bhagandara), whether outer mouthed or inter-mouthed. Medicinal remedies calculated to be mild, though keen in their efficacy, should be used in such cases. A plug or a Varti in the shape of a wick and made of powdered *Áragvadha, Haridrá* and Kálá, mixed with honey and clarified butter, should be inserted into the ulcer for purifying purposes. This medicinal compound speedily brings about the healing of a sinus, just as the wind will drive away a cloud.  8—9

**Treatment of Ágantuka Bhagandara :**—The sinus in a fistula of traumatic origin should be carefully cut open by a surgeon (with a knife) and cauterized, according to the rules laid down, with a red-hot Jambvoshtha (instrument) or with a red-hot director (Saláká). Vermifugal remedies should be applied to it, and measures laid down in connection with the extraction of a Salya from the body should be carefully resorted to.  10.

**Treatment of Tridoshaja Bhagandara :**—A case of Bhagandara, due to the concerted action of the **three Doshas**, should be treated without holding out any hope of recovery tot he patient's people, or should be given up as hopeless. The measures and remedies mentioned above should be adopted in succession in all types of Bhagandara. In the event of there being any pain in it, owing to the insertion of a knife or to any other surgical operation, luke-warm Anu-taila should be applied. As an alternative, the drugs possessed of the virtue of subduing the deranged Váyu (Bhadra-dárvádi and Erandádi groups) should be boiled in a pot covered by a lid having a hole or aperture on its top ; then the patient with his rectum anointed with oil, etc., should be made to sit in such a way over the said covered pot that the seat of the disease may be fomented with the warm fumes escaping through that aperture ; or Nádi-sveda should be applied to the affected region through a pipe in a recumbent posture to alleviate the pain. As an alternative, a hot bath should be prescribed for the alleviation of the pain. **Sálvana Upanáha** (described in connection with the treatment of Váta-vyádhi and that with the skins of the Kadali Mriga, Lopáka and Priyaka, should be applied to the affected locality to subdue the pain. A potion of the drugs or substances such as, *Trikatu, Vachá, Hingu,* salt (five kinds of salt) and *Dipyaka*, should be administered with wine, Kánjika, Sauviraka and Kulattha-Soup, etc   11-12.

*Jyotishmati, Lángalaki, S'yámá, Danti, Trivrit, Tila, Kushtha, S'atáhvá, Golomi, Tilvaka, Giri-karniká, Kásisa* and the two kinds of *Kánchana-kshiri*, compose the group which is possessed of the virtue of purifying (a fistular sore). (The decoction of these substances should be applied for the purification of the ulcer). The sore of a fistula may be filled (healed) up by the application of (a compound of) *Trivrit, Tila, Nágadanti, Manjishthá* and rock-salt pasted together with milk and honey. A plaster (Kalka) consisting of *Rasánjana*, turmeric, *Dáru-haridrá, Manjishthá, Nimba* leaves, *Trivrit, Tejovati* and *Danti* proves curative in a case of sinus. The drugs known as *Kushtha*, *Trivrit*, *Tila*, *Danti*, *Pippali*, *Saindhava*, honey, turmeric, Triphalá and sulphate of copper (Tuttha) are efficacious in purifying an ulcer. 13-16.

Oil* cooked (slowly) with *Pippali*, *Yashti-madhu*, *Lodhra*, *Kushtha*, *Elá*, *Harenu*, *Samangá* (Baráha-kránta), *Dhátaki* flower, *Sárivá*, the two kinds of *Haridrá*, *Priyangu*, *Sarja-rasa*, *Padmaka*, *Padmá-kes'ara*, *Sudhá*, *Vachá*, *Lángaliká*, wax, and *Saindhava* should be regarded as a potent remedy in healing up the ulcer and curing fistula-in-ano. This remedy proves beneficial in cases of scrofula (Ganda-málá), Meha, ulcers and in the Mandala type of cutaneous affections as well. The drugs which constitute the *Nyagrodhádi* group are efficacious in disinfecting (Śodhana) and healing up an ulcer. A medicated oil or Ghrita prepared with the preceding drugs proves curative in a case of fistula-in-ano. Similarly a medicated oil duly cooked and prepared with the roots of *Trivrit*, *Danti*, *Haridrá*, and *Arka*, as well as with Vidanga, *Triphalá*, milk of both *Snuhi* and *Arka*, honey and wax should be applied, as it is specifically efficacious in a case of Bhagandara. 17-19.

**Syandana Taila :**—Oil slowly cooked and prepared (in the manner aforesaid) with *Chitraka*, *Arka*, *Trivrit*, *Páthá*, *Malapu* (Kákodumbara), *Karavira*, *Sudhá* (Snuhi), *Vachá*, *Lángalaki*, *Saptaparna*, *Suvarchiká* and *Jyotishmati*, is called the **Syandana-Taila** and should be constantly applied in a case of Bhagandara. It is efficacious in purifying, healing and imparting a natural skin-colour to the cicatrix. A learned and experienced physician should adopt the remedial measures for this disease according to the procedure laid

---

* Four seers of oil, one seer of the drugs and sixteen seers of water should be taken at the time of preparation.

down under the treatment of Dvi-Vrana, when there is any ulcer (vrana) in existence. 20.

The bulb-like protrusion above the hole of the instrument (speculum), mentioned in connection with the treatment of Arśas, should be removed and the instrument, now in the shape of a half-moon, should be used by an experienced surgeon in the treatment of a case of fistula-in-ano. The patient should refrain from sexual intercourse, physical exercise, riding, anger, and the use of heavy and indigestible articles of food for a full period of one year even after the healing up of the ulcer in a Bhagandara. 21—22.

Thus ends the eighth Chapter of the Chikitsita Sthánam of the Sus'ruta-Samhitá which deals with the treatment of Bhagandara.

# CHAPTER IX.

Now we shall discourse on the medical treatment of cutaneous affections in general (**Kushtha**). 1.

A cutaneous disease (Twag-dosha) originates through injudicious conduct of life such as, partaking of large quantities of unwholesome food, or taking it before the previously eaten one is digested (*i.e*, eating too often), indulgence in incompatible articles of fare, voluntary suppression of the natural urgings of the body, and improper application of medicated oil, clarified butter, or other lardacious articles. It is attributed even to the dynamics of sinful acts done by a man in this or in some prior existence. 2.

**Conduct of diet and regimen :**—A person afflicted with any kind of skin disease should refrain from taking meat, lard, milk, curd, oil, *Kulattha* pulse, *Másha* pulse, *Nishpáva*, preparations and modifications of sugarcane juice, acid substances, incompatible food, meals taken before the complete digestion of the preceding one, unwholesome and indigestible food, or food causing a burning sensation and some kind of internal secretion, day-sleep and sexual intercourse. 3.

**Regulation of diet and conduct :**— The old and matured grain of *S'áli*, *Shashtika*, barley, wheat, *Koradusha*, *S'yámáka*, *Uddálaka*, etc., boiled and taken along with the soup (Supa) or a decoction\* (Yusha)

---

\* An unsalted decoction of any substance not seasoned with any spices whatever is called **Yusha,** while the one salted and seasoned with spices is called **Supa.** In preparing the soup of any pulse, all husks should be carefully thrashed out and the grain should be slightly fried before boiling.

of either *Mudga* pulse or *Ádhaki* pulse mixed with *Nimba* leaves and *Arushkara* are wholesome in a case of Kushtha. Preparations of any of the aforesaid grains may be taken with *Manduka-parni, Avalguja, Atarushaka* and *Rupiká* flowers cooked in mustard oil or clarified butter, or with the soup prepared of the articles of the *Tikta-varga* (bitter group, mentioned in the Sutra-sthánam). The cooked flesh of Jángala animals, devoid of all fatty matter, should be given to a patient, habituated to the use of meat diet. The medicated oil, known as the **Vajraka-Taila** should be used for anointing the body. A decoction of the drugs of the *Áragvadhádi* group should be used for rubbing (Utsádana) purposes. Decoctions of **Khadira** should be employed in drinks, baths, washes, etc. The preceding rules are intended to regulate the diet and regimen of one suffering from Kushtha (cutaneous affections). 4.

**Preliminary Treatment :**—In the premonitary stages of the disease the system should be cleansed by the application of both emetics and pur-. gatives. When the disease is found to invade the **Tvak**\* only, a plaster prepared of the purifying drugs should be applied to the affected parts ; blood-letting and the use of medicinal decoctions and purifying and disinfecting plasters are the remedies to be employed when the desease would appear to infect the **blood**:. The same remedies and Arishta, Mantha, Prása, etc , should be employed when the disease would be found to have invaded the principle of the **Mámsa** (muscles). Palliation and temporary respite are the only cure that can be offered in a case of the sin-begotten type† of the

---

\* Tvak here means Rasa or serum.

† The type of Kushtha affecting the principle of **Medas** (fat) is generally supposed to be sin-begotten.

disease which is the **fourth** (in order of enumeration) and that even is purely contingent on the willingness and capacity of the patient to conform to a strict regimen of diet, conduct and dress. Blood-letting and purifying measures (emetics and purgatives) should be resorted to in such a case and then the special medicinal remedies prepared from **Bhallátaka†, Śilájatu, Guggulu, Aguru, Tuvaraka, Khadira,** and **Asana** and the **Ayaskriti** should be used in accordance with the prescribed rules. The disease in its **fifth** form (is found to invade the **bones** and) should be given up as incurable. 3-6.

**Treatments of Doshaja Types :**—In the first stage of Kushtha, the patient should be treated in accordance with the prescribed maxims (rules) of Sneha-pána. In a case of **Vátaja-Kushtha**, oil or clarified butter, cooked with (a decoction and Kalka of) *Mesha s'ringi, S'wadamshtrá, S'arngashtá, Guduchi* and the drugs included in the group of *Das'amula* should be used as drink and ointment. In cases of the **Pittaja** type, the patient should be made to drink (a potion consisting of) clarified butter prepared with (a decoction and Kalka of) *Dhava, As'vakarna, Kakubha, Palás'a, Pichu-mardha, Parpataka, Madhuka, Rodhra* and *Samangá.* In the **Kaphaja** type, clarified butter cooked with (a decoction and Kalka of) *Piyála, S'ála, Áragvadha, Nimba, Saptaparna, Chitraka, Maricha, Vacha* and *Kushtha* should be prescribed.

---

\* Bhallátaka-preparations have been described in the treatment of Ars'as, preparations of S'ilájatu, Guggulu, Aguru and Tuvaraka in the treatment of Prameha-pidaká, and Khadira, Asana and Ayaskriti preparations in the treatment of Mahá-kushtha.

† Oil should be used in a case of Kapha-predominance, whereas clarified butter in that of Pitta-predominance. Others assert that clarified butter should be used for drinking purposes and oil for anointments.

The clarified butter cooked with (a Kalka and a decoction of) *Bhallátaka, Abhayá* and *Vidanga*, or (the medicinal oils known as) the Tuvaraka Taila and the Bhallátaka Taila should be used in all types of Kushtha. 7-8.

**The Mahá-tikta Ghrita :**—A paste or Kalka should be made by pounding equal parts of *Saptaparna, Áragvadha, Ativishá, Páthá, Katu-rohini, Amritá, Triphalá, Patola, Pichu-marda, Parpataka, Durálabhá, Tráyamáná, Mustá, Chandana, Padmaka, Haridrá, Upakulyá, Vis'álá, Murvá, S'atávari, S'áriva, Indra-yava, Átarushaka, Shadgranthá (vacha), Madhuka, Bhu-nimba* and *Grishtiká\**. This paste (Kalka) should be cooked with four times its own weight of clarified butter, with the juice of *Ámalaka*, weighing twice as much as the clarified butter and with water weighing four times the quantity of the *Ámalaka* juice. It should be constantly stirred (with a ladle), while being cooked. This medicated Ghrita is called the **Mahá-tikta Ghrita**, which proves curative in Kushtha, chronic fevers, hæmorrhage, heart-disease, insanity, Apasmára, Gulma, postular eruptions, menorrhagia, goitre, scrofula, elephantiasis, jaundice, erysipelas, impotency, itches and Pámá, etc. 9

**The Tikta-Sarpih :**—Two Pala weight of each of the following drugs, *viz., Triphalá, Patola, Pichumarda, Atarushaka, Katu-rohini, Durálabhá, Tráyamáná* and *Parpataka†* should be taken and boiled together in a Drona measure of water. The boiling should be continued till it is reduced to one fourth of its original quantity. Then half a Pala weight of each of the following drugs, viz., *Tráyamáná, Musta, Indra-yava,* (red)

---

\* Chakradatta does not read "Grishtiká" but read "Us'ira" instead. He also takes both the kinds of "Haridrá," of "Upakulyá" (Pippali) and of "Sárivá".

† Chakradatta reads "Nis'á" in addition to the above drugs.

*Chandana, Kirátá* and *Pippali* should be pasted together. This pasted Kalka and the decoction should be cooked with a Prastha measure of clarified butter. The medicated Ghrita thus prepared is called the **Tikta-Sarpih.** Diseases such as Kushtha, chronic fever, Gulma, Hæmorrhoids, Grahani, edema, jaundice, erysipelas and impotency readily yield to the curative efficacy of this Ghrita. 10.

**Medicinal Plasters for Kushtha :—** Having first soothed the patient with any of the preceding medicated clarified butters and having his body fomented, the surgeon should have recourse to the venisection. One, two, three, four, or five śirás (veins) of the patient may be opened (according to the circumtances). The raised or elevated patches on the skin should be scraped off, or should be kept constantly covered with a medicinal plaster. As an alternative, the characteristic patches of the disease should be first rubbed with the substance known as the *Samudra-phena* or with the leaves of *S'áka, Goji,* or *Kákodumbara* and a plaster (Lepa) composed of *Lákshá. Sarja-rasa, Rasánjana, Prapunnáda, Avalguja, Tejovati* and the roots of *As'va-máraka, Arka, Kutaja,* and *Árevata,* pasted with the urine or bile of a cow, should be applied to them ; or Svarjiká, sulphate of copper, sulphate of iron, *Vidanga,* Agára-dhuma, *Chitraka, Katuka, Sudhá,* turmeric and Saindhava pounded together with the urine or bile of a cow should be applied to the diseased localities.

As an alternative, the alkali prepared from the ashes of *Palás'a* wood in the prescribed manner, should be boiled with the powders of the preceding drugs ; it should be removed from the oven after reducing it to the thickness or consistency of a Phánita and used in plastering (the diseased patches) ; or a plaster composed of *Jyotishka*-fruits,. *Lákshá, Maricha, .Pippali* and the leaves of the *Játi* flower pasted together ; or a plaster composed of yellow orpiment, *Manah-s'ilá*, the milky juice of *Arka*, sesamum, *S'igru* and *Maricha*, pasted together ; or a plaster composed of *Svarjiká, Kushtha*, sulphate of copper, *Kutaja, chitraka, Vidanga, Maricha* and *Manah-s'ilá* pasted together; or a plaster of *Haritaki, Karanjiká, Vidanga*, white mustard seeds, rock-salt, *Gorochaná, Somarája* and *Haridrá* pasted together should be applied to the diseased localities.

**Metrical Text :**—The preceding seven medicinal plasters are possessed of the virtue of destroying or curing Kushtha in **general.** Now hear me deal with the remedies to be **specifically** employed in cases of ringworm **(Dadru)** and leucoderma **(Svitra)**. 11.

**Treatment of Dadru :**—A plaster composed of *Kushtha*, mustard seeds, *S'ri-niketa, Haridrá, Trikatu* and the seeds of *Chakra-marda* and of *Mulaka* pasted together with Takra (butter milk ?) should be applied to the ringworm. The disease is found to readily yield to the curative efficacy of a medicinal plaster, composed of *Saindhava, Chakra-marda* seeds, treacle, *Kes'ara* (Vakula), and *Tárksha-s'aila* (Rasánjana) pasted together with expressed *Kapittha* juice. Preparations of *Hemakshiri, Vyádhi-gháta* (Áragvadha), *S'irisha, Nimba, Sarja, Vatsaka* and *Aja-karna* (a species of Sarja) should be used in cases of ringworm of a virulent type for baths (D. R. Drinks),* plasters and rubbing. 12.

**Treatment of Svitra :**—In cases of Svitra and Pundarika, the patient should be made to drink a lukewarm decoction prepared with equal parts of the

---

* In drinks or baths, a decoction should be used and in plasters and rubbings the ingredients should be pasted with **Takra** and the expressed juice of Kapittha.

roots of *Bhadrá* (Udumbara) and *Malapu*. The use of this potion would produce blisters on the patches. These blisters should be treated, after their bursting, with a plaster (Pralepa) composed of the ashes of the burnt skin of leopards and elephants and made into a thin paste with (mustard) oil. A plaster composed of the insect known as the Puti and the Kshára (alkali) of *Áragvadha* should be found to be the best remedy for Śvitra. 13

All kinds of Śvitra are found to readily yield to the application of a medicinal plaster made of the black ashes of a well-burnt cobra (Krishna-Sarpa) pasted with the oil of *Vibhitaka*. The white ashes of the said cobra mixed with one and a half time of its own weight of water should be filtered seven times in the manner of preparing an alkali. Mustard oil* should be cooked with this alkaline water weighing four times as much. An application of this oil proves curative in cases of Śvitra. 14.

The *Prapunnáda* seeds, *Kushtha* and *Yashti-madhu* should be pasted together with clarified butter. The plaster thus prepared should be given to a domestic white cock, purposely kept without food for a day and a half when it would evince any sign of hunger after the period. The dung of the said cock should then be collected after a full digestion of the said medicated drugs and applied as plasters on the affected patches for a month. It would bring about the cure (even) of internal† Śvitras. 15.

Well burnt ashes of the dung of an elephant‡, mixed

---

\* This is the best medicine for curing S'vitra.

† The internal S'vitras are those under the blisters produced by the application of the remedy mentioned first in the list.

‡ S'ivádàsa, the commentator of Chakradatta, says that some read जलगन्धजे in place of गजलङ्के in which case it would mean "S'amatha."

with elephant's urine, should be filtered several times (twenty-one times or seven times) after the manner of an alkaline preparation. A Drona measure of this alkaline solution should be boiled with the seeds of the *Somarájí* weighing a tenth part thereof. This compound should be taken down from the oven as soon as it assumes a glossy hue and should then be made into boluses. Having rubbed the diseased patches of Śvitra, a plaster of these boluses should be applied to them which would soon assume a healthy and natural complexion. 16.

The leaves and bark (Dala-tvacham) of the *Ámra* (mango) and the *Haritaki*\* should be well soaked in a decoction of the same drugs (after the manner of a Bhávaná-saturation) and made into Vartis (*i.e*, plugs). These Vartis should again be well soaked in the milky exudation of the *Vata* tree and lighted (with mustard oil) in a copper vessel used as an Indian lamp. The lamp black, thus produced, should be collected and well soaked in a decoction of *Haritaki*. Kilása (a particular kind of Kushtha) is destroyed, if rubbed with this preparation for several times after having been lubricated with mustard oil.† 17.

---

\* According to some, both the leaves and bark of the "Ámra" and of the "Haritaki" should be taken.

† The leaves and bark respectively of the *A'mra* and the *Haritaki* should be taken in the preparation. The whole stanza seems to be of faulty construction. Dallana, in his commentary, says that some read the fourth line as "तं लेन सिक्तं कटुना समस्तमालिपयेदेवमुपैति शान्तिम् ॥" This seems to be a better reading. It removes the difficulty in the construction, but it omits also the word "Kilása" from the text. This, however, is also an improvement, inasmuch as this preparation seems to be a remedy for **Śvitra** (which is only a variety of Kilása) like the preceding and the following ones; and it seems unlikely that Sus'ruta would introduce a remedy for **Kilása** in general in the special treatment of S'vitra.

A case of leucoderma would (undoubtedly) yield to the curative virtue of a medicinal plaster composed of *Somarâji* seeds, *Mâkshika*, *Kâkodumbara*, *Lâkshâ*, powdered iron, *Pippali* and *Rasânjana*, taken in equal parts and black sesamum equal to their combined weight, pasted with the bile of a cow and applied to the diseased patches. Similarly, a case of Śvitra would prove amenable to the application of peacock's bile, or of burnt *Hrivera* mixed with the said bile. 18.

Various types of Śvitra are cured with the application of either of the two following medicinal plasters. The first consists of *Tuttha* (sulphate of copper), *Haritâla* (yellow oxide of arsenic), *Katukâ*, *Trikatu*, *Simha* (Rakta-Sobhânjana), *Arka*, *Karavira*, *Kushtha*, *Avalguja*, *Bhallâtaka*, *Kshirini*, mustard seeds and *Snuhi*; and the second consists of the leaves of the *Tilvaka*, *Arishta* (Nimba), *Pilu* and *Âragvadha* pasted together with the seeds of the *Vidanga* and *Karavira* and *Haridrâ*, *Dâruharidrâ*, *Vrihati* and *Kantakâri*. 19.

**Nila-Ghrita :**—*Vâyasi*, *Phalgu* and *Tiktâ* each weighing one hundred Palas, two Prastha measures of powdered iron, three Âdhaka (eight seers) measures of *Triphalâ* and two Âdhaka measures of *Asana* should be boiled together with three Drona measures of water. This decoction should be taken down when reduced to one quarter of its original measure and cooked again with a quantity of clarified butter (weighing a quarter part of the former (decoction) and with a Kalka consisting of *Indra-yava*, *Trikatu*, *Tvak*, *Deva-dâru*, *Âragvadha*, *Pârâvata-padi*, *Danti*, *Vâkuchi*, *Kes'ardhva* (Vakula) and *Kantakâri*. The patient should be made to drink this medicated clarified butter when the disease would be found to have attacked the **Dhâtus** (fundamental principles of the organism), or to have become involved in the aggravated **Doshas** of the system. The diseased patches should be rubbed with it, in the event of the affection being found to be confined to the Tvak (skin) alone. Even the type of Kushtha, commonly held to be incurable, has been found to prove amenable to the use of this medicated clarified butter, which is known as the Nila-Ghrita. 20.

**Mahá-Nila-Ghrita :**—A Tulá* weight of the drugs known as *Triphalá, Tvak, Trikatu, Surasá, Madayantiká, Váyasi* and *Áragvadha* and ten Pala weights of each of the drugs known as *Kákamáchi, Arka, Varuna, Danti, Kutaja, Chitraka, Dáru-haridrá* and *Kantakári* should be boiled together with three Drona measures of water. This decoction, boiled down or reduced to six Prastha measures, should be again boiled with the watery secretion of cowdung, cow's urine, milk, curd and clarified butter, each weighing an Ádhaka, and with the Kalka (weighing one-fourth as much of clarified butter) of *Bhu-nimba, Trikatu, Chitraka, Karánja*-fruit, *Niliká, S'yámá, Avalguja, Pilu, Nilini* and *Nimba*-flowers. It is a curative for Kushtha. The rubbing of the diseased patches with this Ghrita imparts a healthy and natural colour to the skin in cases of S'vitra or white leprosy. It also cures diseases like fistula-in-ano, worms in the intestines and Ars'as. It is known as the **Mahá-Nila-Ghrita.**† 21.

A compound consisting of cow's urine, *Chitraka, Trikatu* and honey should be kept for a fortnight in a

---

\* A Tulá is equal to a hundred Palas or twelve seers and a half of our modern measure.

† Dallana, in his commentary, says that the two Ghritas (Nila and Mahá-Nila) seem to be spurious (Anársha). But he has included them in his commentary as Jejjata and Gayadása have read and explained them before him.

closed earthen pitcher which formerly contained clarified butter. A Śvitra-patient would do well to take this medicine after this period. He should also observe the rules of diet and regimen of a Kushtha-patient. The application of a Lepa (medicinal plaster), prepared by pasting the tender twigs of the *Putika, Arka, Snuhi, Aragvadha* and of the *Játi* flower with cow's urine, would prove curative in cases of Śvitra, ringworm, ulcer, bad types of hæmorrhoids and sinus. 22-23.

In case the foregoing medicinal remedies prove ineffective, the patient should be duly **bled** for the purpose of letting out the vitiated blood from the system, and after sufficiently recouping his strength (after blood-betting) his body should be anointed with clarified butter. Copious vomitings should be induced with the help of strong **emetics** and the patient should be treated subsequently with a judicious administration of **purgatives** (so as to remove the aggravated **Doshas** from the system). The aggravated Doshas of the body, not being fully expelled from the organism of a Kushtha-patient by means of the preceding emetic and purgative measures, tend to extend all over the organism and the disease in consequence thereof is sure to lapse into one of an incurable type. Hence the aggravated Doshas should be fully eliminated from the organism. 24-25.

Emetics should be administered to a Kushtha-patient once a fortnight and Sramsana (purgatives) once a month. He should be bled twice a year though not profusely and medicated snuffs should be administered to him every fourth day. 26.

Internal application of *Haritaki, Trikatu* and treacle (prepared from the juice of the sugarcane) mixed with oil would lead to the early recovery of a case of Kushtha,

As an alternative, he should use a lambative medicinal compound of *Amalaka, Aksha, Pippali* and *Vidanga* mixed with honey and clarified butter. Or he should take a Pala weight of *Haridrá* with an adequate quantity of cow's urine every day for a month in order to get free from Kushtha; or the same quantity of the fine powder of *Pippali* or of *Chitraka* should be given to him through the same vehicle and for the same period which would cure him of Kushtha. The same quantity of the fine powder of *Rasánjana* should be given through the said vehicle and in the same manner for a period of one month and the same should also be repeatedly applied externally. 27-28.

The bark of *Arishta* (Nimba) and *Sapta-parni, Lákshá, Musta, Das'a-muli, Haridrá, Dáru-haridrá, Manjishthá, Áksha, Vásaka, Deva-dáru, Pathyá, Chitraka Trikatu, Ámalaki* and *Vidanga* taken in equal parts and pounded together should be mixed with powdered *Vidanga* weighing as much as the total weight of the preceding drugs; the patient should be made to take a Pala weight of this pulverised compound every day (for a month), or he should be made to drink (in adequate doses) a Drona measure of medicated clarified butter, cooked with the powders of *Triphalá* and *Trikatu*. As an alternative, *Áksha-pida* should be boiled in a Drona measure of cow's\* urine. Clarified butter, cooked in this preparation may be used, as a remedy for Kushtha. An adequate quantity of old and matured clarified butter should be boiled with *Áragvadha, Sapta-parna, Patola, Vrikshaka, Naktamála, Nimba,* the two kinds of *Haridrá* and *Mushkaka*. This medicated Ghrita,

---

\* Cow's urine and water in equal parts should be taken according to some commentators. Dallana, however, recommends cow's urine only and no water.

thus prepared, would lead to the destruction of Kushtha.* 29-30.

Drugs such as *Rodhra, Nimba, Padma-káshtha, Rakta-chandana, Sapta-parni, Aksha, Vrikshaka* and *Vijaka* should be administered in the bath† of the patient in the event of there being any burning sensation; or a potion consisting of honey and pasted *Tri-bhandi* (Trivrit) should be given to him. Old and matured Mudga, boiled in the decoction‡ of *Nimba* and mixed with oil, should be given to the patient as drink where sloughing would be detected in the diseased localities. A decoction of *Nimba* or that of *Arka, Alarka* and *Sapta-chchhada* should be given him if there be any worms in the diseased locality. The affected part of the body should be plastered over with the roots of the *As'va-mára* and *Vidanga,* pasted with cow's urine, in the event of its being eaten away by the worms. Cow's urine should be sprinkled over the diseased locality and all food (of the patient) should be given with the powders of **Vidanga**. 31-32.

As an alternative, the affected parts should be rubbed with the oil of *Karanja,* mustard, *S'igru,* or *Kos'ámra,* or with an oil (any one of the preceding oils) cooked with (a decoction of) pungent, bitter and heat-producing substances. Measures laid down under the head of **Dushta-Vrana** (malignant ulcer) should be resorted to in a case where the aforesaid remedies would fail to produce any beneficial effect. 33.

* Dallana says that the authorship of this remedy should not be attributed to Sus'ruta, inasmuch as Jejjata does not mention it in his commentary.

† The drugs are to be boiled in water in which the patient should take his bath.

‡ The decoction should be prepared in the manner of "Shadanga-kalpa."

**Vajraka-Taila :**—The roots of *Sapta-parna*, *Karanja*, *Arka*, *Málati*, *Karavira*, *Snuhi*, *S'irisha*, *Chitraka* and *Ásphotá* as well as of *Visha* (aconite root), *Lángala*, *Vajrákhya* (mica), sulphate of iron, *Haritála*, *Manah-s'ilá Karanja*-seeds, *Trikatu*, *Triphalá*, the two kinds of *Haridrá*, white mustard-seeds, *Vidanga* and *Prapunnáda* should be pasted together with the urine of a cow. The paste thus prepared should be cooked in an adequate quantity of oil.* This oil known as the **Vajraka-Taila**, used as uguents, proves remedial to Kushtha etc., sinus and malignant ulcers in general. 34.

**Mahá-Vajraka Taila :**—The drugs and substances known as white mustard-seeds (Siddhárthaka), the two kinds of *Karanja*, the two kinds of *Haridrá*, *Rasánjana*, *Kutaja*, *Prapunnáda*, *Sapta-parna*, *Mrigádani Lákshá*, *Sarja-rasa*, *Arka*, *Ásphotá*, *Áragvadha*, *Snuhi*, *S'irisha*, *Tuvara*, *Kutaja*, *Arushkara*, *Vacha*, *Kushtha*, *Vidanga*, *Manjishthá*, *Lángali*, *Chitraka*, *Málati*, *Katutumbi*, *Gandháhvá*, *Mulaka*, *Saindhava*, *Karavira*, *Grihadhuma*, *Visha* (aconite), *Kampillaka*, *Sindura* (mercuric oxide), *Tejohvá* and sulphate of copper should be taken in equal parts and made into a paste. This paste (Kalka) should be cooked with either *Karanja*-oil or mustard-oil†, both of which have great curative potency, with double the quantity of cow's urine. It may also be prepared with sesamum-oil, but in this case four times as much of cow's urine should be taken. As an anointment it is undoubtedly efficacious in a case of Kushtha of whatsoever type as well as in cases of scrofula, fistula-in-ano, sinus and malignant ulcers. This oil is known by the

---

* S'ivadása, the commentator on chakradatta, asserts, on the authority of Vágbhata, that the oil should be sesamum-oil and it should be boiled with cow's urine.

† According to Gayadása mustard-oil should be used.

name of **Mahá-Vajraka** oil and is possessed of supreme and unquestionable efficacy. 35.

The drugs which constitute the *Lákshádi* group should be pasted with an adequate quantity of cow's urine and cooked* with sesamum-oil and mixed with Pitta (cow's bile). The oil, thus prepared, should be preserved for a week inside the body of a *Katukáládvu*. The oil should be taken out (after this period) and the patient should use it both internally and externally (in an adequate quantity). After doing this, he should expose himself to the heat of the sun whereby all the Doshas would be eliminated from his organism. After the complete elimination of the Doshas from the system, the patient should be removed from the sun and bathed with a decoction† of *Khadira*, and a gruel, prepared with the decoction of *Khadira*, should be given him as diet. Similarly, oil or clarified butter boiled and prepared with the drugs constituting the *Sams'odhana* group (mentioned in chap. xxxix, Sutra.) or with the drugs possessing anti-Kushtha properties should be used as hot plasters and rubbings (in the diseased localities) Purgatives should be administered every morning with good results. The preceding remedies should be taken and continued for five, six, seven, or eight days, or till the Doshas of the system producing the disease are not perfectly eliminated. As an alternative, camel's urine and after its full digestion, camel's milk should be taken. Even parasitic types of Kushtha are sure to disappear within six months (under the course of this treatment). 36.

---

\* In cooking the oil, cow's urine weighing four times of oil should be taken.—Dallana.

† The decoction of Khadira in the bath as well as in the preparation of the gruel should be prepared after the manner of Shadanga-Kalpa.—Dallana.

A Kushtha-patient desirous of being perfectly cured should constantly use preparations of **Khadira** in his drinks, food, bath, etc. Khadira, if properly used, is potent enough to curb the virulence of the disease in the same proportion as the latter is in invading the successive strata of the human organism and ultimately in bringing on the death of the patient. 37.

The paring of the nails and shaving the hair off, light physical exercise, the use of wholesome food, regularity in using medicines, abstinence from wine, women and meat-diet are the rules of conduct which should be strictly observed by a patient affected with Kushtha. With the strict observance of the above rules a Kushtha-patient may be expected to recover. 38.

Thus ends the ninth Chapter of the Chikitsita Sthánam in the Sus'ruta Samhitá which deals with the medical treatment of Kushtha.

## CHAPTER X.

Now we shall discourse on the medical treatment of major cutaneous affections (**Mahá-Kushtha**).* 1.

**Metrical Text :**—An intelligent physician should have recourse to the following medicinal compounds in virulent types of Kushtha, urinary complaints (Meha), diseases due to the action of the deranged and aggravated Kapha and general œdima of the body and also in respect of inordinately corpulent persons wishing to reduce their obesity. 2.

**Mantha-Kalpas :**—Pounded barley-corn should be saturated with the urine of a cow and kept in a large bamboo basket (Kilinja) for the whole night; and should then be dried in the sun on the following day. This process should be continued for seven consecutive days. At the close of this period it should be fried in an earthen vessel (Kapála) and then ground to fine powder (Śaktu). The powder, thus prepared should be given every morning to a person afflicted with Kushtha (leprosy), or any urinary complaint (Prameha) through the medium of a decoction of the drugs included within the *S'álasárádi* group, or of the *Kantaki* (thorny) † trees, and mixed with a pulverised compound of *Bhallátaka, Prapunnáda, Avalguja, Arka, Chitraka, Vidanga* and *Musta* weighing a fourth part of the **S'aktu**. Barley-corn should, in the same manner, be soaked in a

---

\* Kushtha which affects the deeper tissues and fundamental principles of the body is called Mahá-Kushtha.

Gayi interprets the term "Mahá-Kushtha" as signifying those seven types of Kushtha which cannot be attributed to any detectable cause.

† Vadara, Khadira, Arimeda, Snuhi, etc.

decoction of the drugs constituting the *S'ála-sárádi* or the *Áragvadhádi* groups, or barley-corn should be given to a cow to eat and the undigested barley-corn passed with the cow-dung should be collected. This barley-corn should then be fried and powdered in the form of Saktu. This powder should be mixed with a pulverised compound of *Bhallátaka*, etc., mentioned above, and given to the patient through the medium of a decoction of any one of the *Khadira, Asana, Nimba, Rája-Vriksha, Rohitaka* and *Guduchi*, sweetened with honey and sugar, and acidified with grapes, or the expressed juice of pomegranate and *Amla-vetasa* and then mixed with rock-salt. This is the method of preparing all kinds of **Manthas**. 3.

Articles of food made of barley-corn in the form of Dháná, Lunchaka, Kulmásha, Apupa, Purnakosa, Utkáriká,\* Sashkuliká, Kunári† and Konáli, etc., should be given as diet. Preparations of wheat and Venu-yava (seeds of bamboo) after the manner of barley preparations should also be recommended as a proper food. 4 5.

**Medicated Arishtas :**—Now we shall describe the mode of preparing **Arishtas** (applicable in cases of Kushtha). Six Pala weight of each of the following drugs, viz., *Putika, Chavya, Chitraka, Deva-dáru, Sárivá, Danti* and *Trikatu*, and one Kudava weight of *Vadara* and *Triphalá* should be powdered. An earthen jar or pitcher, which formerly contained clarified butter, should be purified‡ and plastered inside with a compound

\* Gayadása reads Chitrá (a kind of soup) before "Utkáriká.'

† Dallana does not read "Konáli" but says that some read "Konáliká' in place of "Kunári" both of which are synonyms. We have, however, both the terms in our text.

‡ The jar should be purified or disinfected by fumigation with the medicinal drugs such as *Nimba-leaves,* Guggulu, etc.

of honey, clarified butter and powdered *Pippali*. Then the pulverised compound, mentioned above, together with seven Kudava measures of water*, half a Kudava measure of iron-powder, and half a Tulá weight of treacle, should be poured into the said jar which should then be tightly covered with a lid and placed under a heap of barley for seven days (for fermentation). After this period, it should be taken out and the patient should be made to take some of it (every day) according to his physical capacity. This Arishta (fermented liquor) cures Kushtha, obesity, urinary complaints (Meha), jaundice and œdima. Arishtas may also be similarly perpared from the drugs included in the *S'ála-sáradi*, the *Nyagrodhádi* or *the Áragvadhádi* group. 6.

**Medicated Ásavas :**—Now we shall describe the mode of preparing Ásavas. The ashes of burnt *Palás'a* should be dissolved in hot water and duly filtered. Three parts of this (alkaline) water, subsequently cooled, and two parts of Phánita (molasses) should be mixed together and fermented in the manner of preparing **Arishta†.** Ásavas may be similarly prepared with the alkali made of the ashes of sesamum plants (described in connection with the treatment of As'mari —Chapter. VII), or with the drugs constituting the *S'álasárádi*, the *Nyagrodhádi*, or the *Áragvadhádi* groups, or with cow's urine as in the preceeding manner. 7.

**Medicated Surás :**—Now we shall describe the process of preparing Surás (wines). A decoction should be duly made of *S'ims'pá* and *Khadira* woods with *Uttamárani*, *Bráhmi* and *Kos'átaki* boiled together

---

\* Jejjata recommends twenty-eight Pala weight of water, but Gayadása does not support this.

† Powders of Putika, Chitraka, etc., mentioned in connection with the preparation of Arishtas should be likewise added to it.—Dallana.

in water*. Then Surá-kinva (the drug which is used to cause the fermentation in the manufacture of spirits) should be mixed with the above decoction and the compound distilled in the usual officinial method. The liquor thus prepared is called **Surá**. Surás may be similarly prepared. from the drugs of the *S'ála-sárádi*, the *Aragvadhadi*, or the *Nyagrodhádi* groups. 8.

**Medicated Avalehas** (lambatives) :—Now we shall describe (the method of preparing) medicated Avalehas (lambatives). A decoction should be prepared with the Sára (essential parts) of *Khadira, Asana, Nimba, Rája-vriksha* and *S'ála*. † Fine powders of the same drugs should be mixed with the above (decoction) and boiled again. The compound should be removed from the fire neither thick nor thin. The patient should be made to lick a handful ‡ of the compound mixed with honey and be made to abstain from taking any meal in the morning. Similar preparations may be made (**Avaleha**) from the drugs of the *S'ála-sárádi*, the *Áragvadhádi*, or the *Nyagrodhádi* groups. 9.

**Medicinal Churnas :**—Now we shall describe the process of preparing pulverised compounds. A Prashtha measure of the powdered Sára of the trees belonging to the *S'ála-sárádi* group should be

---

\* One part of S'iṁs'apa', one of Khadira and a third of Uttamárani, Bráhmi and Kos'átaki should be taken. Tulá weight of the drugs and four Drona measures of water should be boiled and reduced to one Droṅa. —Dallana.

† Gayá lása does not read "S'ála" in the list.

‡ Though the word "Pánitala" means a "Karsha" *i e.*, two Tolás, yet as there is the word "Purnam" inserted after it, so a handful should be understood here by this term.—Dallana. It should be observed, however, that the difference in the two interpretations is ultimately immaterial.—Ed.

many times (i. e., seven days) saturated with the decoction of the drugs of the *Áragvadhádi* group (and dried). Then the prepared compound should be taken with the vehicle of the decoction of the drugs of the said *S'álasárádi* group. A pulverised compound (*Churna*) may be as well prepared in the above manner from the fruits of the *Nyagrodádhi* group or from the flowers of the *Áragvadhádi* group. 10.

**Medicinal Ayaskriti :**—Now we shall describe the process of preparing an Ayaskriti (iron compound). Thin leaves of steel should be plastered with the (five officinal kinds of) salts and heated in fire a of dried cow-dung. When red-hot, they should be immersed in a decoction of *Triphalá* and the drugs of the *S'ála-sárádi* group. The above process should be repeated sixteen times in succession after which they should be heated and burnt in a fire of Khadira wood. When cooled down, the iron foils should be pounded into fine powder and passed through a piece of thick linen. The patient should be made to take this powder with honey and clarified butter in an adequate dose suiting his capacity. After the digestion of the medicine, he should take such a meal as is not hostile to hisparticular disease and is devoid of salt and acid articles. The use of a Tulá measure of this medicinal iron preparation in the above manner leads to the recovery of Kushtha, Meha (urinary complaints), obesity, œdima, jaundice, insanity and epilepsy and makes the patient live for one hundred years. The use of each additional Tulá weight of the preparation adds a century to the duration of the user's life. This is the mode of medically preparing all kinds of **Loha** (zinc, copper, lead and gold). 11-12.

**Aushadha Ayaskriti :**—A ball of iron (weighing fifty Palas) heated and made red-hot in a fire of Khadira wood should be cooled by immersing it in a cauldran (Droni), made of (green) Palása wood and containing (five-hundred Palas of) Svarasa (expressed juice*, of Trivit, S'yámá, Agnimantha, Samkhini, Kevuka, Lodhra, Triphalá, Palás'a and Simsapá. The iron mass should be thus heated and cooled twenty one times in succession; finally the iron ball should be immersed and boiled in the expressed juice of the foregoing drugs over a fire of cow-dungs. It should be removed from the fire when only a quarter part of the liquid would remain. It should now be filtered and the mass of iron should be again heated in the fire mixed with the same liquid and boiled again; when the cooking is nearly complete, (it should be removed from the fire and) a pulverised compound of the drugs included in the *Pippalyádi* group together with honey and clarified butter each weighing double the quantity of the iron mass or ball should be mixed with the same. When cooled down, this preparation should be preserved in a well-sealed iron-pitcher. The medicine, thus prepared, should be given to the patient according to his capacity but not less than a Śukti (half a Pala) or a Prakuncha measure (one Pala). After the digestion of this medicine, a diet should be given to the patient determined by the nature of his disease. This is called the **Aushadha Ayaskriti** and it cures even the incurable types of Kushtha and urinary complaints (Meha), reduces obesity, impairs œdima and improves the impaired digestive functions.

* Old and experienced physicians explain "*Svarasam*" to be the decoction as well. Gayadása says that a decoction of one Drona weight of the drugs, boiled in four Drona weight of water and reduced to its quarter part should be taken. Dallana says that if the expressed juice of the drugs be not available, then a cold infusion of one Ádhaka weight of the powdered drugs should be taken,

It is specially efficacious in cases of phthisis (Rája-Yakshmá). A proper and regular use of this remedy increases the duration of life to a hundred years. 13.

**Mahaushadha-Ayaskriti :**—A decoction of the drugs of the *S'ála sárádi* group should be poured in a Droni (vessel) made of *Palás'a* wood. Sheets of iron should be made red-hot and cooled down (twenty one times) by immersing them into the said decoction of the drugs of the *S'ála-sárádi* group. The interior part of an earthen pitcher should be disinfected (with fumigation). Then the iron foils and the powder of the drugs of the *Pippalyádi* group together with treacle and honey should be added and preserved in the earthen pitcher with its mouth well-covered with a lid for a period of one month (in winter) or a fortnight (in summer). This preparation is called the **Mahaushadha-Ayaskriti** and an adequate quantity of it should be given to the patient after the lapse of the said period. Similar preparations of (iron) may be made with a decoction of the drugs of the *Nyagrodhádi* or *Árevatádi* (Áragvadhádi) group. 14.

**The Khadira Vidhána :**—Now we shall describe the **Khadira** preparations. The earth around the central root of a middle-aged Khadira tree, grown in a commendable soil and not worm-eaten, should be dug out and the central and principal root of the tree should be cut open. An iron pitcher should be placed under the tree so that the secreted juice may collect into it through the main root. The outer surface of the tree should be completely plastered with a paste of clay and cow-dung (mixed together). It should then be treated with a fire fed with faggots mixed with cow-dung so that the glutinous secretions of the Khadira tree would naturally settle down into the pitcher (through the principal root). When the pitcher is filled up, the juice should be collected and filtered and then kept in another vessel with its lid carefully closed and sealed. The extract so preserved should be taken in proper doses with honey, clarified butter and the expressed juice of *Ámalaka*. The patient should be made to take such diet and observe such regimen of conduct, as has been prescribed in connection with the use of **Bhallátaka** compounds, after the digestion of the medicine. A Prastha measure of this remedy gradually taken by a man enables him to live a hundred summers. 15.

**Khadira-Sára-Kalpa :**—A decoction made by boiling a Tulá weight of the essential part (Sára) of the Khadira tree with a Drona measure of water and boiled down to a sixteenth part of its original quantity should be kept in a vessel with its mouth tightly closed. An adequate quantity of this decoction should be taken every day with honey, clarified butter and the expressed juice of *Ámalaka*. The present method should be adopted with the extract from the essential parts (Sára) of all other medicinal trees. 16.

Every morning the patient should be made to take an adequate dose of the powders of **Khadira-sára**, or its decoction, until a Tulá weight is consumed, or he should be made to take a potion of the clarified butter churned from the milk of a ewe and cooked in a decoction of Khadira-sára. As an alternative the expressed juice or a decoction of *Amrita-valli*, or clarified butter cooked with that juice or decoction, should be taken every morning. The patient should every afternoon take a meal of boiled rice with clarified butter and *Ámalaka*-soup. A constant use of this remedy and a conformity to the foregoing diet for a month would lead to a radical cure of any type of Kushtha. 17.

Oils pressed out of black sesamum and *Bhallátaka*, clarified butter, the expressed juice of *Ámalaka* and the decoction of the drugs of the *S'ála-sárádi* group, each weighing a Drona measure, and a Pala weight of each of the following drugs, viz., *Triphalá, Trikatu,* the pith or marrow of *Parusha* fruit, *Vidanga* seed, *Chitraka, Arka, Avalguja, Haridrá, Dáru-haridrá, Trivrit, Danti, Indra-yava, Yashti-madhu, Ativishá, Rasánjana* and *Priyangu*, should be boiled together in the manner of cooking medicated oil, etc. (Snehapáka Vidhána). When well cooked, this medicated compound should be strained (through a piece of clean linen) and carefully preserved (in an earthen pitcher with its mouth well closed with a lid). The system of the patient should be well cleansed (with appropriate emetics and purgatives) and a Pala weight of this preparation, mixed with honey, should be given to him every morning. After the digestion of this medicine, he should be made to take a light meal of rice well cooked with a decoction of the *Khadira-wood* and mixed with clarified butter, and the soup (Yusha) of *Ámalaka* or *Mudga* unseasoned with salt. A Drona measure (of this compound), gradually taken in the aforesaid manner by a patient taking a (light) decoction* of Khadira (instead of water), would ensure a speedy recovery from all types of Kushtha and enable the patient to witness a hundred summers (on earth) in the full enjoyment of sound health and intellect. 18.

---

\* The decoction of Khadira-wood for drink should be prepared after the manner of Shadanga-pániya preparation.—Ed.

**Memorable Verse :**—An intelligent physician may prepare a thousand varieties of medicated remedies, such as Surás, Ásavas, Arishtas, Lehas (lambatives), powders and Ayaskritis (metal-preparations) with the aforesaid drugs and in the manner described above. 19.

Thus ends the tenth Chapter of Chikitsita Stha'nam in the Sus'ruta Samhitá which deals with the medical treatment of Mahá-Kushtha.

# CHAPTER XI.

Now we shall discourse on the medical treatment of the diseases of the urinary tracts **(Prameha).** 1.

This disease may be ascribed to two causes, such as the congenital (Sahaja) and that attributable to the use of injudicious diet. The first type (Sahaja) is due to a defect in the seeds of one's parents and the second is originated from the use of unwholesome food. The symptoms, which mark the first of these two types, are emaciation and a dryness (of the body), diminished capacity of eating, too much thirst and restlessness; while the symptoms, which usually attend the latter type of the disease, are obesity, voracity, gloss of the body, increased soporific tendency and inclination for lounging in bed or on cushions. A case of emaciation, etc., (viz., the first kind of Prameha) should be remedied with nutritious food and drink, etc., whereas Apatarpana, etc., (fasting, physical exercise, depletory measures etc.), should be adopted in cases of obesity viz., the second kind of (Prameha). 2.

**Forbidden Articles of Food & Drink:** —All patients suffering from Prameha should forego the use of (the different species of wine and fermented liquor known as) Sauviraka, Tushodaka, Sukta, Maireya, Surá, and Ásava, water, oil, clarified butter, milk, any modification of the expressed juice of sugarcane, cakes, milk-curd, acid, Pánaka\*, the flesh of domestic and aquatic animals and of those which frequent swamps or marshy places   3.

---

† Made of sugar, lemon-juice, or fermented rice-gruel boiled together.

**Articles of diet:**—The use of sufficiently old and matured, *S'áli* and *Shashtika* rice, barley, wheat, *Kodrava, Uddálaka*, with the different preparations of *Chanaka, Ádhaki, Kulattha* or *Mudga* pulse is recommended ; or the meal should be taken with the *S'ákas* (potherbs) of bitter or astringent taste cooked with the oils of *Nikumbha, Ingudi*, mustard or linseed oil ; or with the soup of the lean flesh of Jángala animals which are possessed of anti-diuretic properties cooked without any clarified butter and unseasoned with any acid juice. 4.

**Preliminary Treatment :**—The patient should be first anointed with any of the oils (of Nikumbha, Ingudi, Sarshapa, Atasi, etc.); or with the medicated clarified butter\* cooked with the drugs of the *Priyangvádi* group and should also be treated with strong emetics and purgatives†. After the application of purgatives, an Ásthápana measure with a decoction of the drugs of the *Surasádi* group, mixed with honey and Saindhava salt and with the powders of *S'unthi, Bhadradáru* and *Musta* by way of an after-throw, should be resorted to. (On the eighth day) in a case attended with a burning sensation, a decoction of the *Nyagrodhádi* group without (*ie*, mixed with a little quantity of) Sneha (oil or clarified butter) should be used (in the manner of an Ásthápana).

**The five Medicinal remedies :**—After cleansing the system, the expressed juice‡ of *Ámalaka* mixed with *Haridrá* (powder) and honey should

---
\* The patient should be anointed with the medicated clarified butter in a case of Pittaja-meha.

† Emetics in cases of **Kaphaja-meha** and purgatives in those of **Pittaja-meha**, should be applied.

‡ This is also found in Charaka and has been quoted by Chakradatta in his compilation.

be administered. As an alternative, a decoction* of *Triphalá, Vis'álá, Deva-dáru* and *Musta* or an Aksha (two Tolá) measure of the Kalka (powders)† of *S'ála, Kampillaka* and *Mushkaka* (both of them) sweetened with honey and the expressed juice of *Ámalaka* should be taken; or powders‡ of the flowers of *Kutaja, Kapittha, Rohita, Vibhitaka* and *Saptaparna* (should be taken with honey, Haridrá and the expressed juice of Ámalaka), or a decoction of the roots, leaves, barks, flowers and fruits of *Nimba, Áragvadha, Saptaparna, Murvá, Kutaja, Soma-vriksha, Palás'a* should be given to the patient. All cases of Meha are often found to yield to the use of any of these five medicinal preparations. 5.

**Specific Treatments:**—Now we shall specifically describe the course of treatment to be adopted in each particular type of the disease (Prameha). A decoction of *Párijáta* should be given in a case of **Udaka-meha;** a decoction of *Vaijayanti* in that of **Ikshu-meha;** a decoction of *Nimba* in a case of **Surámeha;** a decoction of *Chitraka* in a case of **S'ikatámeha;** a decoction of *Khadira* in a case of **S'anairmeha;** a decoction of *Páthá* and *Aguru* in a case of **Lavana-meha;** a decoction of *Haridrá*

---

* This is quoted by Chakradatta but he reads " दारुनिश्रा " in place of " देवदारु " and does not mention the use of the expressed juice of Ámalaka. The practice, however, is to follow the recipe of Chakradatta.

† The third Yoga of the text is also quoted by Chakradatta but no addition of Haridrá powder is prescribed there. Chakradatta is more generally followed in the case.

‡ The fourth Yoga of the text is found also in Charaka although with some variation. Charaka adds the flowers of Kampilla and S'ála in the list, but does not recommend the use of Haridrá powder nor of the expressed juice of Ámalaki as the medium of taking the medicine. Charaka, however, is quoted *verbatim* by Chakradatta and is followed in practical use,

and *Dáru-haridrá* in a case of **Pishta-meha**; a decoction of *S'aptaparna* in a case of **Sándra-meha**; a decoction of *Durvá*, *S'aivála*, *Plava*, *Hatha-karanja* and *Kas'eruka*, or that of *Kakubha* and red-sandal wood in a case of **Śukra-meha**; and a decoction of *Triphalá*, *Áragvadha* and *Drákshá* mixed with honey in a case of a **Phena-meha**. All decoctions, to be employed in the foregoing ten types of **Kaphaja-meha**, should be sweetened with honey (slightly sweetened with honey—D. R).

**Treatment of Pittaja Prameha :**—In the Pittaja types of the disease, a decoction of the drugs of the *S'ála-sárádi* group or that of *As'vattha* should be administered in a case of **Nila-meha**; similarly a decoction of *Rája-vriksha* should be given in a case of **Haridrá-meha**; a decoction of the *Nyagrodhádi* group, mixed with honey, in a case of **Amla-meha**; a decoction of *Triphlá* in a case of **Kshára-meha**; a decoction of *Manjishthá* and (red) Chandana in a case of **Manjishthá-meha**; and a decoction of *Guduchi*, seeds of *Tinduka*, *Kás'marya* and *Kharjura*, mixed with honey, in a case of **Śonita-meha\***. 6.

**Palliative Measures :**—Now we shall describe the palliative measures to be adopted even in cases of incurable types of the disease. A Kalka compound of *Kushtha*, *Kutaja*, *Páthá*, *Hingu* and *Katu-rohini* should be taken with a decoction of *Guduchi* and *Chitraka* in a case of **Sarpir-meha**. A patient afflicted with an attack of **Vasá-meha** should be made to drink a decoction of *Agni-mantha* or of *S'ims'apá*. Similarly a decoc-

---

\* Honey should be added to all oi these decoctions prescribed in cases Pittaja-meha.—Dallana.

† Honey should also be added to these decoctions prescribed in cases of Vátja Meha —Dallana.

tion of *Khadira, Kadara* and *Kramuka* should be given in a case of **Kshaudra-meha** ; a decoction of *Tinduka, Kapittha, S'irisha, Palás'a, Páthá, Murvá,* and *Dusparsá* (Durálabhá) mixed with honey,* or the Kshára, (alkaline water) prepared from the ashes of the bones of an elephant, horse, hog, ass or camel, in a case of **Hasti-meha.** A gruel (Yavágu prepared in the manner of Shadanga-kalpa) with a decoction of aquatic bulbs and sweetened with milk and the juice of sugarcane should be prescribed in a case attended with a burning sensation. 7.

**Medicinal Arishtas, Ásavas, Yavágus, etc. :**—Likewise Arishtas, Ayaskritis, lambatives and Ásavas should be prepared (in the manner hereinbefore described) with *Priyangu, Anantá, Yuthiká, Padmá* (Bhárgi), *Tráyantiká, Lohitiká, Ambashthá,* bark of pomegranate, *S'ála-parni,* (D.R.—Tála-parni), *Padma* (lotus), *Tunga, Kes'ura, Dhátaki, Vakula, S'almali, S'ri-veshtaka* and *Mocharasa,* should be administered to the patient. As an alternative, similar preparations made of *S'ringátaka, Gilodya,, Mrinála, Kas'eruka, Madhuka, A'mra, Jambu, Asana, Tinis'a, Arjuna, Katvanga, Lodhra, Bhallátaka, Charmi-vriksha, Giri-karniká, S'ita-s'iva, Nichula, Dádima, Aja-karna, Hari-vriksha, Rájádana, Gopaghontá* and *Vikamkata* should be prescribed. Different preparations of Yavágu, etc. should be given to the patient as diet. A gruel (Yavágu) cooked with the decoction of the preceding medcinal drugs or (only these) decoctions should be given to the patient as drinks.

Potions of any of the aforesaid Ásavas thickened with an admixture of powdered *Páthá, Chitraka* and *Haritaki* and sweetened with a liberal quantity of honey

---

* Jejjata interprets it as grape-wine, but Gayadasa does not support this view.

should be prescribed for a rich or royal patient of injudicious conduct and refusing to take medicines; or he should be made to drink frequent potions of Mádhvika liquors (prepared from honey) * with meat roasted on gridiron over a charcoal fire. Food and drinks mixed with honey, *Kapittha* and pepper should be prescribed for him. 8.

The powdered dung of a camel, a mule, or an ass should be administered to him in food ; he should take his meal with soups saturated with a compound of asafœtida and Saindhava salt or with mustard preparations (Rága). * His food and drink should be fragrant and well flavoured with ingredient not incompatible with the nature of the disease. 9-10.

The practice of regular physical exercise, wrestling, active sports, riding on a horse or an elephant, long walks, pedestrial journeys, practising archery, casting of javelines, etc., should be resorted to in a case where the disease has made a decided advance. 11.

A poor and friendless patient should live on alms, lead a life of perfect continence like an ascetic, forego the use of shoes and umbrella and walk a hundred Yojanas† or more on foot without staying for more than one night at a single village. A rich man (suffering from Prameha) should live on *S'ydma'ka, Kapittha, Tinduka* and *As'mantaka* and live among the deer. He should constantly follow the tracks of cows and take their dung and urine (for food and drink). A Bráhman patient should live on the grain, spontaneously fallen from plants, constantly study the Vedas and draw

---

\* Some read "आर्कैः" i e. potherb ( of mustard ) in place of "रागैः ।"

† A Yojana is equal to eight miles.

chariots occupied by Bráhmanas.* A patient belonging to the lower orders of society (Sudras, etc.) should be made to sink wells (under such circumstances) and the strength of a weak or emaciated patient should be preserved (with nutritive diets, etc.). 12.

**Memorable Verse :**—A poor patient, carefully following these directions of his medical advisers without the least demur or delay, should be able to get rid of the disease (Prameha) in the course of a year or even in less than that time. 13.

Thus ends the eleventh Chapter of the Chikitsita Sthánam in the Sus'ruta Samhitá which deals with the medical treatment of Prameha.

---

* Some explain the phrase "ब्रह्मरथमुपधारयेत्" to mean that he should retain in his memory (the teachings of) the Vedas..—Dallana.

# CHAPTER XII.

Now we shall discourse on the medical treatment of the abscesses or eruptions which mark the sequel of a case of Prameha (**Prameha-Pidaká**). 1.

The nine kinds of abscesses (Pidakás), such as Saráviká, etc., have been described before. Of such abscesses those, appearing in a strong person but small in size, affecting (only) the Tvak (skin) and the flesh, soft to the touch, slightly painful, easily suppurative and after a time bursting, are curable. 2.

Patients suffering from Prameha and afflicted with the above kinds of abscesses (Pidakás) should be treated (in the following manner). Measures, such as fastings (Apatarpana), etc., decoctions * (of Vata, etc.) and the urine of a she-goat, should be employed in the incubative stage of the disease. The urine, perspiration and the Sleshmá (sputum, etc.), soon acquire a sweetish taste, if the aforesaid preliminary measures are not resorted to and if the patient goes on using sweet articles of food in utter disregard of the instructions, thus developing fully the specific indications of Prameha. In this stage the system of the patient should be cleansed (Sams'odhana) with both emetics and purgatives. If the disease is not checked (even at this stage) with the aforesaid measures (emetics and purgatives), the aggravated Doshas of the body go on increasing in intensity and tend to affect or vitiate the flesh and the blood and produce an inflamatory swelling of the body, or bring on other supervening distresses

---

* Astringent drugs of fig-tree (Vata-tree), etc.—D. R.

in their train, venesection as well as the aforesaid remedies and measures should be resorted to in such cases. 3.

The swelling increases in size attended with excessive pain and burning sensation, if the aforesaid remedies be not employed at this stage of the disease. Surgical operations and other remedial measures, described in connection with abscesses or inflammatory swellings (Vrana) in general, should be resorted to in such cases. If these be not done (at this stage), the pus eats into the deeper tissues of the locality, creates large cavities in its inside, and is accumulated there and the abscess (Vrana) becomes incurable.* Hence a case of Prameha should be remedied at its very outset. 4-6.

**Dhánvantara-Ghrita :**—Ten Pala weight of each of these drugs, *viz., Bhallátaka, Vilva, Ambu,* roots of *Pippali, Udakiryyá, Prakiryyá*†, *Varshábhu, Punarnavá*‡, *Chitraka, S'athi, Snuhi, Varunaka, Pushkara, Danti* and *Haritaki* and one Prastha measure of each of the following, viz., barley, *Kola* and *Kulattha* pulse should be boiled with a Drona measure of water. The decoction should be boiled down to its quarter part, removed from the fire, and strained. It should then be cooked with a Prastha measure (four seers) of clarified butter with half a Pala weight of each of the following drugs, *viz., Vachá, Trivrit, Kampilla, Bhárgi, Nichula, S'unthi, Gaja-Pippali, Vidanga* and *S'irisha* as Kalka.

* On the failure of the above treatment it would spontaneously burst out and secrete pus and force its way inside, which would lead gradually to widen its mouth or fissure, and help its running into an incurable stage.—Dallana.

† "Udakiryá and Prakiryá" are the two kinds of Karanja.

‡ "Varshábhu and Punarnavá" are the two kinds of Punarnavá (*i.e.,* red and white).

It is called the **Dhánvantara-Ghrita*** and covers within the range of its therapeutic application Meha (urinary diseases), swelling, (S'otha), Kushtha, Gulma, Ascites, hæmorrhoids, enlargement of the spleen, carbuncles (Pidaká) and abscesses. 7.

Ordinary purgatives fail to produce any satisfactory effect in cases of Madhu-Meha owing to the excessive accumulation and pervasion of **Medas** (fat) in the organism of the patient. Hence strong Śodhana (purgatives) should be employed in such cases. In all types of Meha, attended with **Pidaká** (eruptions or abscesses) and other complications, the perspiration and expectorations, etc. of a Prameha-patient acquire a sweet taste and smell like that of honey. Hence they are technically known as **Madhu-Meha** (to all intents and purposes . **Fomentation** (of any kind) is forbidden in the case of a patient suffering from Madhu-Meha, since it might lead to the gradual emaciation of his frame by drying up the organic fat (**Medas**), which is usually found to abound in his organism. The aggravated Doshas of the body fail to make an upward passage in the organism of a Prameha-patient, owing to the weakness of the channels of chyle, blood, Kapha and Pitta (as well as for an exhausted condition of the nerves in his body) and the Doshas are thus forced to course in and confine themselves into the lower part of the body where their incarceration helps the easy formation of **Pidakás** (abscesses), etc Such a Pidaká should be remedied with the measures described in connection with Vranas, as soon as the process of suppuration would set in; whereas

* According to Dallana, the introduction of this medicated Ghrita into the text is an interpolation. Since Jejjata has not explained it in his commentary, Dallana does not explain it. Chakradatta, however, mentions this Ghrita in his compilation, though with some additions and alterations under the treatment of Prameha.—Ed.

it should be treated as a swelling in its unsuppurated stage. Medicated oils should be likewise employed for the purposes of healing (Ropana), etc. 8.

A decoction of the drugs of the *Áragvadhádi* group should be used for the purpose of raising up (Utsádana) the cavity of the incidental ulcer; that of the S'ala-sára'di group should be used for sprinkling purposes; that of the drugs of the *Pippalyádi* group should be given as food and drinks. A pulverised compound of *Páthá, Chitraka, S'árṃgashtá, Kshudra, Vrihati, S'árivá Soma-valka, Saptaparna, Áragvadha* and *Kutaja* roots mixed with honey should be internally given to the patient.

**S'ála-sárádi Avaleha :**—A decoction of (one hundred Pala weight of) the drugs of the *S'ála-sárádi* group should be made by boiling it (in sixteen times the weight of water) down to a quarter part (of the water) and then duly filtered (through a piece of linen). It should be cooked again very carefully, so that it may not be burnt; powders of *Ámalaka,\* Rodhra, Priyamgu, Danti,* black-iron and copper should then be added to it just before the completion of the cooking, so that it may be reduced to the consistency of an **Avalcha** (lambative). It should then be removed from the fire and kept in a closed earthen pitcher. The patient should take an adequate dose of this medicine as it is a sovereign remedy for all types of Prameha. 9.

**Naváyasa-Churna :**—Equal parts of the powders of the following nine drugs, viz., *Triphalá, Chitraka, Trikatu, Vidanga* and *Musta,* and nine parts

---

\* Chakradatta reads "S'ivá" in place of "Ámalaka" and does not include "Priyamgu" in the list. According to some commentators the total weight of the after-throw (Prakshepa) would be a quarter part of the total weight of the drugs boiled ; whereas, according to others, the different drugs for Prakshepa would weigh one Pala each.

of powdered black-iron* should be mixed together and taken in adequate doses with honey and clarified butter. This is called the **Navayasa Churna**, which proves curative in abdominal obesity, improves the impaired digestion and acts as a prophylactic against hæmorrhoids, swelling, jaundice, Kushtha, indigestion, cough, asthma and Prameha, etc. 10.

**Lohárishta :**—A decoction of the drugs of the *S'alá-sárádi* group should be made by boiling it down to a quarter part (of the original quantity of water) Then it should be duly filtered ; when cooled, a quantity (*i.e.*, fifty Pala weight) of Mákshika-honey† should be added to it. A quantity of purified treacle‡ reduced to the consistency of Phánita as well as fine powders of the drugs of the *Pippalyádi* group should be mixed with it. A strong and well cleansed (earthen) pitcher satu-

---

\* Charaka and Chakrapáni Datta insert this medicine among the curatives of " Pa'ndu-roga ". S'ivadása (the commentator) advises to take " Mandura-iron" instead of " black-iron ". In the practical field also we derive great and good effects in cases of spleen and liver diseases and specially in cases of infantile liver and heart diseases.—Ed.

† Dallana says that fifty Pala weight of each of the two substances—Madhva'sava and Pha'nita, and twenty-five Pala weight of each of the following substances , viz., the powders of the drugs of the Pippalyádi group and steel-foils, should be taken in preparing it. But Gayadása explains that such a quantity of old and matured honey should be mixed with the decoction as will sweeten it ; the same quantity of old and matured Phánita treacle should be taken ; the powders of Pippalyádi group should be added to it till it gets a slight astringent (Katuka) taste.

Some commentators, however, hold that the honey, the powders of the drugs of the Pippalyádi group and of the steel-foils should be each a quarter part of the decoction in weight.

Dallana explains the term "Madhu" as the A'sava prepared of honey. Gayadása, however, explains it simply as honey.

‡ The Phánita should be refined by dissolving it in the decoction of the drugs of the S'ála-sárádi group and then filtere .—Dallana,

rated with clarified butter should be purified (in the usual way) and its interior plastered with coating of honey and powdered *Pippali* made into a thin paste. The medicinal compound prepared as above should be kept in the pitcher. After that, thin foils of steel made red-hot in a fire of Khadira wood should be immersed into the compound prepared before. Then the pitcher with the steel-foils immersed into its contents should be kept buried in a heap of barley for three or four months or until the steel-foils are entirely eaten away by the medicine and the characteristic flavour is produced. It should be used in proper doses every morning and a suitable diet should be given to the patient after its use. It reduces fat, improves the impaired digestion and proves efficacious in cases of swellings, internal tumours, Kushtha, Meha, jaundice, dropsy of the spleen (Plihodara), chronic fever, and excessive urination (dribbling of urine). This preparation is called **Lohárishta*** and it is a highly efficacious remedy. 11.

---

\* The recipe of Lohárishta, according to Vágbhata, is as follows :— The drugs of the Asanádi group (which corresponds with Sus'ruta's S'ála-sárádi group), each weighing twenty Palas, should be boiled in eight Dronas of water down to a quarter part of its weight. Two hundred Pala weight of treacle and half an Ádhaka (four seers) of honey and the powders of the drugs of the Vatsakádi group (which corresponds with the Pippa-lyádi group of Sus'ruta), each weighing one Pala, should be mixed with the above decoction when cooled. A (new earthen) pitcher should be plastered inside with (an adequate quantity of) Pippali-powder and honey, the outer side being plastered with shellac. The above preparation should now be poured into this pitcher which should be kept in a heap of barley. A fire should be kindled with Khadira charcoal. Thin iron-foils should be alternately heated in this fire and immersed in the above preparation until the iron-foils are powdered. Vágbhata gives the name of Ayaskriti to this preparation.

We, however, follow Vágbhata in the preparation of this Arishta with good results..—Ed.

**Traits of cure :** —The cure of Prameha-patients should be understood from the non-slimy and unturbid condition of the urine and from its clear transparent aspect and bitter or pungent taste. 12.

Thus ends the twelfth Chapter of the Chikitsita Sthánam in the Sus'ruta Samhitá which deals with the medical treatment of Prameha-Pidaká.

# CHAPTER XIII.

Now we shall discourse on the medical treatment of Diabetes **(Madhu-Meha)**. 1.

**Metrical Text :**—The intelligent physician should adopt the following course of treatment in the case of a Madhu-Meha-patient abandoned as incurable by other physicians. 2.

**Śilájatu, its origin and properties :—** A kind of gelatinous substance is secreted from the sides of the mountains when they have become heated by the rays of the sun in the months of Jyaishtha and Áshádha. This substance is what is known as the Śilájatu and it cures all distempers of the body.

The presence of the six kinds of metal, such as tin, lead, copper, silver, gold and black-iron, in their essential form in the substance (Śilájatu), may be detected by their respective smell and hence it is known to the people by the name of **Shad-Yoni** (lit.—having six different origins). The taste of this shellac-coloured substance has the same taste (Rasa) and potency (Virya) as the metal to whose essence it owes its origin. It should be understood that as tin, lead and iron, etc., are progressively more and more efficacious, so the different varieties of Śilájatu, originated from the essence of tin, lead, iron, etc., are progressively more efficacious in their application.

All kinds of Śilájatu have a bitter and pungent taste with an astringent after-taste (Anu-rasa), are laxative, pungent in their digestionary reaction, heat-making in their potency and possessed of absorbing and purifying (Chhedana) properties. Of these what looks black and glossy, is heavy and devoid of sandy particles, as well as what smells like the urine of a cow, should be considered as the best. This best kind of Śilájatu should be infused with the decoction of the drugs of the Śála-sárádi group after the manner of Bhávaná saturation (for ten, twenty or thirty days). Then after cleansing the body (by the application of emetics and purgatives), it should be taken every morning (by the patient in adequate doses), well pasted with Sárodaka.* He should further be made to take a meal of boiled rice mixed with the soup of the flesh of animals of the Jángala group after the medicine had been fully digested. 3-4.

A Tulá measure of this hill-begotten panacea (Śilájatu), when gradually taken, (in adequade doses) tends to improve the strength and complexion of the body, cures an attack of Madhu-Meha and enables the user to witness a hundred summers on earth, free from disease and decay. Each Tulá weight of this medicine, taken successively, adds a century to the duration of human life, while ten Tulá measures extend it to a thousand years. The regimen of diet and conduct during the period of its use should be identical with that described in connection with the use of the **Bhallátaka** compounds. Cases of Meha, Kushtha, epilepsy (Apasmára), insanity, elephantiasis, poison-begotten distempers, phthisis, ædema, hæmorrhoids, Gulma (internal tumours), jaundice and chronic fever, prove readily amenable to the curative efficacy of Śilájatu. Indeed there is no such bodily distemper

---

\* It is evident from the reading of Chakradatta that "Sárodaka" means a decoction of the drugs of the **Śála-sárádi** group. But Dallana explains it as "Pancha-sárodaka" which is quite unintelligible. In practice, also, Chakradatta is followed.—Ed.

which does not yield to its highly curative virtues. It acts as a potent solvent in cases of long-standing Sarkará (gravel) in the bladder as well as of stone. Silájatu should be treated (soaked and dried) with appropriate medicinal drugs by stirring it up with the same. 5.

**The Mákshika Kalpa:**—The metal known as **Mákshika** (iron-pyrites), which grows in the river Tápi and which copes with the divine ambrosia in its highly therapeutic properties, may be also used in the same way and under the same sort of preparation. The metal is divided into two classes according to its colour, as **Svarna**-Mákshika (gold-coloured) and Rajata-Mákshika (silver-coloured). Of these the first has a sweet taste while the second is acid. Both of them prove efficacious in cases of decrepitude, Kushtha, Meha, jaundice and consumption. A person using Silájátu and Mákshika (in the manner prescribed above) should refrain from taking pigeon-flesh and *Kulattha* pulse (during his life-time). 6.

The following measures should be adopted by an experienced physician in the case of a patient suffering from (Meha and) Kushtha and who has a firm faith in medicines and is desirous of existence (life) and in whose case the curative efficacy of Pancha-karma* has been baffled. 7.

**The Tuvaraka Kalpa:**—The Tuvaraka plants which grow on the shores of the Western Sea (Arabian Sea) are constantly tossed about by the winds raised by the waves of the sea. The pith or marrow of the seeds (lit.—fruits) of these plants should be care-

---

\* Some take the term in its ordinary sense to mean the five measures of emetics, purgatives, etc. ; but Dallana would explain it as the measures adopted in the treatment of the Kushtha affecting the bone which is the fifth Dhátu in the system.

fully collected in the rainy season while they ripen and should be subsequenly dried and pounded. The oil should be either pressed out of these seeds in a mill in the manner of preparing sesamum oil, or squeezed out (of a press bag) like that used in the case of *Kusumbha* flowers. The oil should be boiled over a fire so as to have its inherent watery particles completely evaporated. Then it should be taken down from the fire and kept in a pitcher and then buried for a fortnight in a heap of well dried cowdung. The patient (in the meantime) should be duly anointed, fomented and treated with cleansing remedies (i.e., emetics and purgatives).* He should wait a fortnight (after the administration of the aforesaid measures) and wait for a period of four meals† (i.e., two days) more ; and on the next morning he should drink a portion of the oil in adequate doses (two Tolás) under the auspices of favourable astral combinations in the lighted fortnight of the month. He should be made to recite, at the time of his taking the fourth dose, a Mantra which runs as follows :—
"Cleansest and purifiest, O Thou potent essence of seed-marrow, all the essential principles of (my) vital organism. The deity who knows no decay and suffers no change and who weilds a discus, a mace and a conch-shell in his arms, commands thee on that behalf "

The Doshas in both the upper and the lower parts of a patient's body are cleansed with the help of this **oil**

---

\* The **Kapha** should be first reduced with emetics ; and after a fortnight, the **Pitta** with purgatives. A fortnight after the use of purgatives, a potion of the Tuvarka oil should be administered inasmuch as it is a Sams'odhaka (cleansing) remedy.

† On the sixteenth day after the administration of the cleansing measures, as well as on the morning of the seventeenth day, the patient should take his meals as usual. On the evening of the seventeenth day no meal should be taken. On the following morning the oil should be taken.

(which should be given to the patient in the morning); while a cold gruel, unseasoned* with salt and not mixed with any emollient substance (oil or clarified butter) should be given to him in the afternoon. The use of this oil should be repeated in the same manner for five days in succession, and the patient should avoid anger, etc., and live on *Mudga* soup (Yusha) and boiled rice for a fortnight. A five days' use of this oil would ensure the cure of every types of Kushtha (and Madhumeha). 8-9.

The foregoing (Tuvaraka) oil should be boiled and prepared with a decoction of **Khadira** weighing three times the quantity of the oil and taken internally with patience for a month for the same purpose. The patient should anoint his body with the same and then take his meals in the prescribed form. A Kushtha-patient (as well as a Meha-patient) suffering from hoarseness, red-eyes and with worm-eaten and emaciated limbs should be speedily treated with this oil as an anointment and a drink. Regular potions of the above medicinal (Tuvaraka) oil taken with honey, clarified butter and a decoction of Khadira and a diet consisting of the soups of bird's flesh (during its course) would enable the user to live for a period of two hundred years. A use of this oil as errhines (Nasya) for a period of fifty consecutive days would enable the user to witness three hundred years on earth, in the full enjoyment of bodily vigour and a youthful glow of complexion, as well as with a very powerful retentive memory.

A regular use (in an adequate dose) of the pith of **Tuvaraka** cleanses the system of the patient and is a most potent remedy in cases of Kushtha and Meha. 10.

* A little quantity of salt and of oil or clarified butter may be given.

The pith (inner pulp of the seeds) of the Tuvaraka burnt in a closed vessel (Antar-dhuma) should be mixed with Saindhava-salt, *Anjana*\* and *Tuvaraka* oil. This prepared compound, used as a collyrium, is efficacious in cases of eye-diseases, such as night-blindness, Arman, Nili, Kácha-roga (dimness of sight) and Timira. 11.

Thus ends the thirteenth Chapter of the Chikitsita Sthánam in the Sus'ruta Samhitá which deals with the treatment of Madhu-Meha.

\* Dallana recommends the three things, viz., the pith of the Tuvaraka, the Saindhava-salt and the Rasánjana to be mixed and burnt together in a closed Vessel.

# CHAPTER XIV.

Now we shall discourse on the medical treatment of dropsy with an abnormal condition of the abdomen **(Udara).** 1.

Of the eight different types of Udara, described before, those severally known as the Vaddha-guda and the Parisrávi should be understood as incurable, the rest being equally hard to cure. Hence the medical treatment of all cases of Udara (abdominal dropsy) should be resorted to without holding out any positive hope of recovery. The first four types of the disease (as metioned in the list of enumeration), may prove amenable to medicine ; but the rest would require **Surgical** treatment. All the types of the disease, however, would, with the progress of time, require a surgical operation, or (attaining an incurable stage) they may have to be abondned. 2.

**Diet of articles forbidden :**—A patient, afflicted with an attack of Udara, should forego the use of heavy (indigestible), or emollient fare, of all kinds of meats and of those that produce a state of extreme dryness in the system, or produce a slimy secretion from the channels (of the Doshas and the vital principles) of the body, or give rise to a sort of digestionary acid reaction (acid transformation in the stomach) and refrain from bathing and using effusions. Meals consisting of well cooked *S'áli* rice, barley, wheat, or *Niváva* seeds should be the daily diet of such a patient. 3.

**Treatment of the Vátaja type :** – In a case of Vátaja Udara, the body of the patient should be anointed with clarified butter cooked with the drugs of the *Vidári-gandhádi* group, while the one cooked with

*Tilvaka* should be used as purgatives (Anuloma). A compound made of a copious quantity of oil of *Chitrá* seeds, mixed with a decoction of the drugs of the *Vidári-gandhádi* group, should be used as Ásthápana and Anuvásana measures. The **Sálvana Upanáha** (poultice) should be applied to the abdomen. Milk cooked with the drugs of the *Vidári-gandhádi* group, or the soup of the flesh of Jángala animals should be given to the patient with his meal and the affected region should be frequently fomented. 4.

**Treatment of the Pittaja Type :—** In a case of Pittaja Udara, the patient should be anointed with clarified butter cooked with the drugs of the Madhura (Kákolyádi) group. Similarly, clarified butter cooked with *S'yámá, Triphalá* and *Trivrit* should be used as purgatives and the decoction of the drugs of the *Nyagrodhádi* group, mixed with a copious quantity of sugar, honey and clarified butter, should be used as Anuvásana and A'sthápana measures. The abdomen should be poulticed with Páyasa (porridge prepared with rice and milk) and the diet should consist of boiled rice and milk, cooked with the drugs of the *Vidári-gandhádi* group. 5.

**Treatment of the Kaphaja Type :—** In a case of Kaphaja Udara, the patient should be anointed with clarified butter, cooked with the decoction of the drugs of the *Pippalyádi* group. Likewise, clarified butter, cooked with the milky juice of *Snuhi* plants, should be used as purgatives ; and the decoction of the drugs of the *Mushkakádi* group, with a copious quantity of *Trikatu,* cow's urine, Kshára (Yava-kshára) and oil, should be applied as Anuvásana and Ásthápana measures. A poultice (Upanáha) prepared of *S'ana* seeds, *Atasi* seeds, *Dhátaki* (flower), mustard, *Mulaka* seeds and *Kinva* should be applied (hot) to the abdomen. The diet should consist of (boiled rice well-mixed with) *Kulattha* soup (Yusha), profusely seasoned with powdered *Trikatu*, or of Páyasa ; and the abdomen should be frequently fomented. 6.

**Treatment of Dushyodara :**—In a case of Dushyodara, the patient should be treated without giving any hope of a positive cure. Purgatives with clarified butter, cooked with the expressed juice of the *Saptalá* and *S'amkhini*, should be first administered (continuously) for a fortnight or even a month ; or clarified butter, cooked with the milky juice of the *Mahávriksha*, and with wine and cow's urine, should be similarly used as a purgative. A Kalka made up of the roots of the *As'vamáraka, Gunjá* and *Kákádani* mixed with wine (Surá), should be given after the bowels had begun to move freely. As an alternative, a Krishna-Sarpa (black lance-hooded cobra) should be enraged to bite a sugarcane and this piece of sugarcane should be given to the patient to chew (and suck) ; or the fruits of creepers (Valli-phala) should be used (in the preceding manner) ; or poisonous[*] roots and bulbs should be prescribed, whereby the disease may be cured or may take a different turn. 7.

**Memorable Verse :**—A case of abdominal dropsy (Udara) of whatsoever type should be presumed to have its origin in an aggravation of the bodily Váyu and an accumulation of fæcal matter in the bowels ; hence frequent use of **Anulomana** (purgatives, etc.) is recommended in this disease. 8.

---

[*] If this be not done, the patient is sure to die ; but it is not certain whether he would get any relief from this treatment. It being, however, possible in some cases to save the life of a patient by the application of this medicine, it should be used, as the last resort with the permission of the king.—Dallana.

**General Treatment :—** Now we shall describe a few general medicinal compounds (which may be used with advantage in cases of Udara). They are as follows ;—Castor oil with milk or with the urine of a cow should be taken for a month or two. No **water** should be taken during the period, or the patient should forego the use of **water** and all other food, but drink only the urine of a she-buffalo and (cow's) milk ; * or he should live upon the milk of a she-camel alone, foregoing the use of rice and water and submit himself to a course of **Pippali** for one month in the manner described before (under the treatment of Mahá-Vátavyádhi),† or take the oil of the *Nikumbha* with *Saindhava-salt* and powdered *Ajamodá* dissolved in it. The said oil (of Nikumbha), cooked with a hundred Pátra weight of the expressed juice of *A'rdraka* and *S'ringavera* (fresh ginger), should be applied in the event of there being any S'ula (colic pain), due to the action of the deranged and aggravated Váyu. Milk, boiled with the expressed juice of *S'ringavera* (fresh ginger), should be taken. A paste-compound of *Chavya* and *S'ringavera,* or a paste-compound of *Sarala, Deva-dáru* and *Chitraka* (with milk), or a paste-compound of *Murangi, S'álaparni, S'yámá* and *Punarnavá* (with milk), or the oil of *Joytishka* seed, mixed with milk, *Svarjiká* and Asafœtida, should be administered to the patient. 9

He should take *Haritaki* with treacle, or a thousand *Pippali* soaked (twenty one times) with the milky juice of the *Snuhi* plant (in the manner of Bhávaná saturation), should be gradually consumed. Powdered *Pippali* and

---

\* The milk here, says Dallana on the authority of Jejjata, should be buffalo's milk. But, according to Vágbhata and S'ivadása, the commentator of Chakradatta, cow's milk should be used.—Ed.

† The Pippalis shohld be taken with milk only in the present instance,

*Haritaki* should be soaked with the milky juice of the *Snuhi* plant (and dried in the sun). Utkáriká should now be preapared with this compound and given to the patient. 10.

**The Haritaki Ghrita :**—A Prastha measure of powdered *Haritaki* should be mixed with an Ádhaka measure of clarified butter and heated over a charcoal fire by stirring it up quickly with a ladle ; when well mixed, the compound should be poured into an earthen pitcher, which should be kept well corked and buried in a heap of barley for a fortnight. The pitcher should then be taken out and the compound should be strained and cooked again with an adequate * quantity of the decoction of *Haritaki, Kánjika* (fermented rice-gruel) and curd. The patient should use this medicine for a month or a fortnight in proper doses and with adequate vehicles. 11.

**The Mahá-vriksha Ghrita :**—A quantity of the milky juice (one fourth of the cow's milk in quantity) of the *Mahá-vriksha* (Snuhi plant), should be boiled with cow's milk. Then it should be removed from the oven, cooled down and churned (with a churning rod). The butter thus prepared and cooked again with the milky exudations of the *Mahá-vriksha* (and an adequate quantity of water) should be given to the patient for a month or a fortnight in adequate doses and with proper vehicles. 12.

**The Chavyádi Ghrita :**—Half a Karsha (one Tolá) measure of each of the following drugs, *viz., Chavya, Chitraka, Danti, Ativishá, Haridrá, S'amkhini, Trivrit* and *Trikatu*, together with an eight Karsha measure of the inner pulps of the fruit (seeds) of the *Rája-vriksha,*

---

* Each of the three things (liquids) should be four times as much as the clarified butter.

two Pala weight of the milky juice of the *Mahá-vriksha*, eight Pala weight of cow's milk and eight Pala weight of cow's urine, should be cooked* with a Prastha measure (four seers) of clarified butter. The medicated Ghrita, thus prepared, should be given in convenient doses to the patient for the period of a month or a fortnight. 13.

The aforesaid three Ghritas (Haritaki-Ghrita, Mahá-vriksha-Ghrita and Chavyádi-Ghrita) and the Tilvaka-Ghrita (mentioned in the chapter dealing with Váta-vyádi) should be employed, whenever purgatives would be necessary in cases of Udara, internal tumour (Gulma), abscess, Ashthilá, Ánáha, Kushtha, insanity and epilepsy. 14.

Constant use of (cow's) urine or (any kind of) Ásava, Arishta or wine, cooked with the milky exudation of *Mahá-vrikshá*, † is recommended. A decoction of purgative drugs, thickened with an admixture, in copious quantity, of powdered *S'unthi* and *Deva-dáru*, may be used with advantage in this desease.

**Ánáha Varti :**—A Pala weight of the emetic and purgative drugs and the same weight of the fine powders of the drugs of each of the *Vachádi*,. *Pippalyádi* and the *Haridrádi* group, and all the officinal kinds of salt should be mixed (with four or eight times that of) the urine (of a cow, buffalo, etc.). Then this (mixture) compound should be boiled and cooked over a gentle fire with a Prastha measure of the milky juice of *Mahá-vriksha*

---

* In the absence of any mention about the quantity of water to be added, four times as much of water should be added for the completion of the preparation according to the general maxim.—Ed.

† Dallana explains the sentence as follows :—

ÁsaVas, Arishtas and Surás should be prepared with urine (instead of the liquid i.e., water) and the milky exudation of Mahá-vriksha (as an after-throw), and should be constantly used.

by constantly stirring it with a ladle. Precaution should be taken so that the Kalkas may not be scorched or burnt. This medicinal compound, when properly prepared, should be removed from the fire and when cooled should then be made into pills (Gutiká), each being an Aksha (two Tolás) in weight. These pills should be given once, twice or thrice daily according to the exigency of the case and the capacity of the patient for a period of three or four consecutive months. The medicine is known as the **Ánáha-varti,** and is specially beneficial in cases of Mahá-vyádhi, and is equally efficacious in destroying intestinal worms. These pills, if regularly used, prove beneficial in cases of cough, asthma, Kushtha, parasites, catarrh, indigestion, aversion to food and Udávarta. 15.

**Second Ánáha-Varti :**—The inner pulp of the seeds of *Madana* fruits with *Kutaja, Jimutaka, Ikshváku* (bitter gourd), *Dhámárgava, Trivrit, Trikatu,* mustard seed and rock-salt, should be pasted together with either the milky juice of *Mahá-vriksha* or with the urine of a cow; and the paste should be made into thumb-shaped plugs (**Varti**). In a case of Ánáha of the patient already suffering from Udara, the outer end of his rectum should be lubricated with oil and salt and one or two of the plugs should be inserted therein. The application of this **Ánáha-varti** should as well be applied in cases of Udávarta, due to a suppression or retention of stool, urine, and Váta (flatus) and in cases of tympanites (Ádhmána) and distention of the abdomen (Ánáha). 16.

**Treatment of Plihodara :**—In a case of Plihodara,* applications of Sneha (oil, etc.) and Sveda

---

* Dropsical swelling of the abdomen owing to an enlargement of the spleen.

(fomentations) should be made and the patient should be fed on boiled rice mixed with milk-curd. Then the vein (Śirá) inside the elbow of his left hand, should be duly opened. The spleen should be rubbed with the hand for the proper out-flow of its deranged blood (for the relief of that enlarged organ). Then having properly cleansed his system, the physician should advise the patient to take the alkali of marine oyster-shells through the medium of milk. As an alternative, *Yava-kshára* should be given to him with *Sauvarchiká* and *Hingu,* or with filtered alkali (made with the ashes) of *Paláśa* wood. As an alternative, the alkali of *Párijátaka, Ikshváku* and *Apámárga,* mixed with oil, should be prescribed; or the decoction of *S'obhánjana,* mixed with *Chitraka, Saindhava* and *Pippali,* or the alkali of *Puti-karanja,* filtered with *Kánjika* and mixed with a copious quantity of *Vid* salt (black salt) and powdered *Pippali* should be administerd. 17.

**Shat-palaka Ghrita :**—One pala weight of each of the following drugs, viz, *Pippali, Pippali-roots, Chitraka, S'unthi, Yava-kshára* and *Saindhava* should be cooked with one Prastha measure of clarified butter and the same quantity of milk*. The medicated Ghrita thus prepared is called the **Shat-palaka-Ghrita.** It is highly efficacious in cases of an enlargement of the spleen, impaired digestion, Gulma, dropsy, Udávarta, swelling (Śvayathu), jaundice, cough, asthma, catarrh, Urdhva-Váta and Vishama-Jvara. In cases of Udara attended with impaired digestion, the **Hingva'di Churna** should be prescribed. These measures should be as well employed in a case of an enlargement of the liver (Yakrit), but the speciality is that the vein (inside the elbow) of

---

\* The practice, in this case, is to add twelve Seers (three prastha measures) of water to the Prastha measure of milk at the time of cooking.

the right hand (instead of the left hand) should be opened in this case 18.

**Metrical Text :**—After slightly bending down the wrist (of the left hand), the vein in connection with the thumb of the left hand should be cauterized with a (burning) Sara for the purpose of giving relief in a case of enlarged spleen. 19.

**Treatment of Vaddha-gudodara, etc. :**—In cases of the **Vaddha-guda** (Entertis) and the **Parisrávi** types of Udara, the patient should be first treated with emulsive measures and fomentations and then anointed with a sneha. Then an incision should be made on the left side of the abdomen below the umbilicus and four fingers to the left of the line of hair which stretches downward from the navel. The intestine to the length of four fingers should be gently drawn out; any stone, any dry hardened substance (Scybalum ?), or any hair found stiffing to the intestine should be carefully examined and removed. Then the intestine should be moistened with honey and clarified butter. It should then be gently replaced in its original position and the mouth of the incision in the abdomen should be sewn up. 20.

**Treatment of Parisrávi-Udara :**—In cases of the **Parisrávi** type of Udara, the obstructing matter should be similarly removed (from the intestines), as in the preceding case, and the secreting intestine should be purified. The (two ends of the severed intestines should be firmly pressed and adhered together and large black ants should be applied to these spots to grip them fastly with their claws. Then the bodies of the ants having their heads firmly adhering to the spots, as directed, should be severed and the intestines should be gently reintroduced into their original position (with the severed heads of the ants adhering to the ends of the incision) and sutured up, as in the preceding case. A union or adhesion of the incidental wound should then be duly effected. The seam should now be plastered with black earth mixed with Yashtimadhu and duly bandaged. The surgeon should cause the patient to be removed to a chamber protected from the wind and give him the necessary instructions. The patient should be made to sit in a vessel full of oil or clarified butter and his diet should consist only of milk. 21.

**Treatment of Udakodara :**—A patient afflicted with **Jalodara** (ascites) should be first anointed with medicated oils, possessed of Váyu-subduing virtues, and fomented with hot water. Then his friends and relatives should be asked to hold him firmly by his arm-pits, when the surgeon would make a puncture with a surgical instrument, known as the Vrihi-mukhá, on the left side of the abdomen below the umbilicus, to the breadth of the thumb in depth and at a distance of four fingers to the left of the dividing line of hairs in the abdomen. Simultaneously with that, a metal tube or a bird's quill, open at both ends, should be introduced through the passage of the puncture to allow the morbific fluids (Doshodoka), accumulated in the abdomen, to ooze out. And then having removed the tube or the quill, the puncture should be lubricated with oil and Saindhava salt and bandaged in the manner described in connection with the bandaging of ulcers.

The entire quantity of the morbific fluid should not be allowed to ooze out in a single day, inasmuch as thirst, fever, aching of the limbs, dysentery, dyspnœa and a burning of the feet (Páda-dáha) might supervene in consequence, or as it might lead to a fresh accumulation of matter in the abdomen, in the event of the patient being of a weak coustitution. Hence it should be gradually tapped at intervals of three, four, five, six, eight, ten, twelve, or of even sixteen days. After the complete outflow of the fluid, the abdomen should be firmly tied with a piece of flannel, silk-cloth or leather, inasmuch as this would prevent its flatulent distention.

**Diet :**—For six months the patient should take his food only with **milk** or with the soup (Rasa) of Jángala animals.

The diet* for the next three months should consist of (meals taken with) milk diluted (and boiled) with an equal quantity of water or with the soup of flesh of animals of the Jángala group seasoned with the juice of acid fruits. During the next three months it should consist of light and wholesome meals. This rule observed for a year brings about a cure. 22.

**Memorable Verse :**—Skilled physicians should prescribe boiled milk and the soup of the flesh

---

\* The use of water is forbidden during these nine months.

During the first six months, drinking, washing, etc., should be done with milk or the soup of Jángala animals. After this period, the said purposes should be served with half-diluted milk or meat-soup seasoned with the juice of acid fruits. Water may be used during the period of the next three months —Dallana.

Vágbhata following Charaka says :—

The patient should live only on milk for six months. After this period, he should live on porridge (Peyá) boiled with milk ; and for the next three months he should live on boiled S'yámá-rice with milk, or with the soup of meat seasoned with the juice or acid fruits and mixed with clarified butter and a small quantity of salt.

The water of tender and green cocoanuts is used in cases of Udara in place of pure drinking water with benefit.—Ed.

of animals of the Jángala group as food and drink in all cases of Udara and use these as Ásthápana measures and as purgatives as well. 23.

Thus ends the fourteenth Chapter in the Chikitsita Sthánam of the Sus'ruta Samhitá which deals with the treatment of Udara.

# CHAPTER XV.

Now we shall discourse on the (surgical and medical) treatment of the cases of difficult malpresentation of the fœtus and of difficult labour (**Mudha-Garbha**). 1.

The extraction of a fœtus, acting (in the womb) as an obstructing Śalya (foreign matter lodged in the body), is the most difficult of all surgical operations, inasmuch as actual contact or actual manipulation is the only means accessible to a surgeon in the region of the pelvic cavity, the spleen, the liver, the intestines and the uterus. All surgical acts in respect of the fœtus or the enceinte, such as lifting up, drawing down, changing of postures (version), excision, incision, the cutting of limbs and section, pressure, the straightening and the perforating of the abdomen, could not be done otherwise than by actual contact of the hand, which may sometimes prove fatal to the fœtus or to the enceinte. Hence the king should be first informed (as success in these cases is often uncertain) and all acts should be performed with the greatest care and coolness.

We have stated before that the fœtus is generally presented in cases of difficult labour in **eight** different postures or forms. The obstruction of the child in the passage of parturition (Garbha-Sanga) may be effected in three different ways, owing to its head, shoulders or hips being presented in a wrong way and held fast in the passage. Every care should be taken and no pains spared to bring a child alive into the world, which is not already dead in the womb. The sacred verses (Mantras), possessing of the virtue of bringing out the fœtus, should be recited in the hearing of the enceinte in the case of a failure in the first attempts at effecting parturition. The mantras are as follows. 2.

**Metrical Texts :**—"O thou beautiful damsel, may the divine ambrosia' and the Moon god with Chitrabhánu and the celestial horse Uchchaih-Sravas take their residence in thy room ; may this water-begotten nectar, help thee, O lady, in swiftly casting off thy womb. May the Sun, the Vásavas and the Wind-god (Pavana) in the company of the saline Ocean give thee peace. The incarcerated beasts have been freed from their fastenings and binding chords. The Sun god has freed his rays of light. Freed from all danger, come, O, come, O child, and rest in peace in these precincts." 3.

Proper and useful medicinal remedies should also be employed for the delivery of the child.

**Postures of the Fœtus :**—In the case of the fœtus being dead in the womb, the enciente should be made to lie on her back with her thighs flexed down and with a pillow of rags under her waist so as to keep it a little elevated. Then the physician should lubricate his (own) hand with a compound consisting of earth, clarified butter and (the compressed juice of) *S'allaki*, *Dhanvana* and *S'álmali* and inserting it into the passage of parturition (Yoni) should draw out the dead fœtus (downward with the hand). 4.

In the case of a leg-presentation (**Sakthi**), the fœtus should be drawn downward by pulling its legs. In case where a single leg (Sakthi) is presented, the other leg of the fœtus should be expanded and then it should be drawn downward.

In the case of the presentation of the **buttocks** (Sphik) (breech presentation), the buttocks should be first pressed and lifted up and then the fœtus should be drawn downward by the -legs. In the case of a **longitudinal** presentation (the child coming stretched cross-wise) like a belt and arrested in the passage, its lower extremities should be pushed upward with the hand and the child should be drawn out with its upper part (*viz.*, the head, etc.), thus pointed downward, and brought straight into the passage of parturition. In a case of the head being hung back a little on one side, the shoulder should be lifted up by pressing it (with the hand) after chafening it, so as to bring the head at the door of the passage and the child should be drawn straight downward Similarly in the case of the presentation of the two **arms**, the shoulder should be lifted up by pressing it (with the hand) and, the head being brought back to the passage, the child should be drawn downward. The remaining two kinds of false presentation 'Mudhagarbha) previously described (in the eighth Chapter of the Nidána Sthána) should be considered as irremediable. The applications of instruments (Sastra) should be the last resort when such manipulatory measures would fail. 5.

**Metrical Text :**—But even in such irremediable (Asádhya) cases, surgical operations should not be made if the fœtus could be detected alive in the womb, as such a course (as the cutting of the fœtus, etc.) would fatally end both as regards the child and its mother. 6.

**Operations involving destruction of the Fœtus—Craniotomy :**—In cases where there would be any necessity of using an instrument for the purpose of delivery, the enciente should be encouraged (with hopes of life) before making the surgical operation. The head or skull of the child in such cases should be severed with the knife known as the Mandalágra or the Anguli-śastra ; then having carefully taken out the particles of the skull-bone (Kapála), the fœtus should be drawn out by pulling it at its **chest** or at the **shoulder** with a Śanku (forceps). Where the head would not be punctured and smashed, the fœtus should be drawn out by pulling it at the **cheeks** or the **eye-sockets**. The hands of the fœtus should be severed from the body at the shoulders, when they (the shoulders) would be found to have been obstructed in the passage and then the fœtus should be drawn out. The abdomen of a child, dead in the womb, should be pierced and the intestines drawn out, in event of the former being swollen into a flatulent (Váta) distension like a leather bag (for holding water), as such a procedure would remove the stiffness of its limbs, and then it should be drawn out. The bones of the thighs (Jaghana-kapála) should be first cut out and removed, where the fœtus would be found to have adhered fast to the passage with its thighs (Jaghana). 7.

**Metrical Texts :**—In short, that part of the body of the fœtus should be severed and removed which |prevents its (fœtus) withdrawal from the womb and the life of the mother should be saved at all hazards. The different types of false-presentations should be ascribed to the abnormal coursing of the deranged **Váyu** (in the uterus), and hence an intelligent physician should adopt, after careful considerations, proper remedies (for its pacification). An intelligent physician should not waste a single moment in drawing out the fœtus, as soon as it would be found to be dead in the womb, since neglect in such cases leads to the instantaneous death of the mother, like an animal dying of suffocation. An erudite physician, well-versed in anatomy, should use in such cases a Mandalágra instrument for the purpose of cutting out (the fœtus), since a sharpe-edged Vriddhi-patra may sometimes hurt the mother during the operation. 9-19.

A non-falling placenta (**Apará**) should be extracted in the way indicated before or the enciente should be firmly pressed and the placenta extracted with the hand. Her body should be constantly shaken or her shoulders constantly rubbed at the time (of extracting the placenta after lubricating the passsage of parturition with oil. 11.

**After-measures :**—Thus having extracted the S'alya (fœtus), the body of the mother should be washed with warm water and anointed with oil, etc Oil should also be copiously applied to the passage of parturition,* as it would soften the **Yoni** and alleviate the pain therein. After that, powdered *Pippali*, *Pippali-roots*, *S'unthi*, *Elá*, *Hingu*, *Bhárgi*, *Dipyaka*, *Vachá*, *Ativishá*, *Kásná* and *Chavya* should be given in a Sneha (clarified butter, etc.), for the (proper) discharge (*i.e.*, purification) of the Doshas (lotia) and for the alleviation of the pain. A plaster, or a decoction, or a pulverised compound of the said drugs without the addition of any Sneha (clarified butter, etc.) may also be given to her. As an alternative, the physician should ask the parturient woman to take *S'áka*-bark, *Hingu*, *Ativishá*, *Páthá*, *Katu-rohini* and *Tejovati* prepared and administered in the preceding manner. Then for three, five or seven days, Sneha (clarified butter, etc.) should again be given ; or the patient should be asked to take well prepared Ásavas and Arishtas at night time. A decoction of the bark of *S'irisha* and *Kakubha* should be used for washing (Áchamana†) purposes and the other supervening distresses (*i e.* complications) should be remedied with proper medicines. 12-A.

---

* The oil should be introduced into the vaginal canal by means of **Pichu**, *i e.*, cotton plugs soaked in oil, etc.

† This decoction should be specially used for washing the uterus (Yoni).—Ed.

**Diet and regimen of conduct :**—The mother should always be neat and clean and subjected to a course of a small quantity of wholesome and emollient diet and to daily anointments and fomentations ; and she should be advised to renounce all anger. Milk cooked with the Váyu-subduing drugs should be used for the first ten days. Meat-soup should then be prescribed for another such period, after which a diet should be prescribed according to the patient's health and nature. This regimen should be observed for a period of four months, after which, the patient would be found to have regained her health, strength and glow of complexion, without any complications, when the medical treatment, etc , should be discontinued 12-14.

The following Valá-Taila should be used for applying into the Yoni (Vagina, etc.), for anointing the body and for drinking and eating purposes (i.e., along with other food) as well as for Vasti-Karma, as the oil is highly efficacious in curbing the action of the deranged and aggravated bodily **Váyu.** 15—A.

**The Valá Taila :**—* An adequate quantity of sesamum oil should be cooked with eight times as much of the decoction of each of the following ; viz., *Valá* roots, *Das'a-mula* and the three combined drugs of *Yava, Kola* and *Kulattha* and with eight times as much of milk and (one-fourth as much of) a paste (Kalka) compound of the drugs included in the *Madhura* group as well as with *Saindhava*-salt, *Aguru, Sarja-rasa, Sarala-Káshtha, Deva-dáru, Manjishthá, Chandana, Kushtha,*

---

* Four seers of sesamun oil, thirty-two seers of the decoction of the Valá-roots, thirty-two seers of the decoction of Das'a-mula, thirty-two seers of the decoction of the drugs Yava, Kola and Kulattha taken together, thirty-two seers of milk and one seer of the paste compound (Kalka) should be taken in the preparation of the oil.

*Elá, Kálánusárivá, Mánsi, S'aileya, Teja-patra, Tagara, S'árivá, Vachá, S'atávari, As'va-gandhá, S'áta-pushpá* and *Punarnavá*. After the completion of its cooking the oil should be kept carefully in a golden, silver, or earthen pitcher with its mouth well-stoppered. This oil is known as the **Valá-Taila** and proves curative in all diseases due to the action of the deranged Váyu. A newly delivered woman should use this oil in adequate doses, according to her physical condition. Women wishing to be mothers and men seeking the blessings of fatherhood should use this Taila, which proves equally beneficial in cases of an emaciation of the body due to the action of the deranged Váyu, weariness of the body through hard labour, and also in cases of hurt or injury to any vital and vulnerable part of the body (Marma), in cases of fractured bones, convulsions, Váta-Vyádhi, hiccough, cough, Adhimantha, Gulma and dyspnœa. A case of hernia would likewise yield to the continuous use of this oil for six months. The essential and vital principles (Dhátus) of the organism of a man are strengthened through its use and his youth will suffer no decay. It should be used alike by kings, king-like and wealthy persons, as well as by those of a delicate and ease-loving temperament. 15—B.

**The Valá-Kalpa :**—Seeds of sesamum should be successively soaked a number of times in a decoction of *Valá* roots* and then dried (in the manner of a Bhávaná saturation). The oil pressed out of such sesamum should be successively cooked a hundred times with the decoction of *Valá*-roots. This being done, the oil should be poured into an earthen pitcher and the

---

* Valá wou'd be the Kalka in this oil, says Dallana. But he also says that some authorities hold that the Kalkas used in the Valá-Taila should be used as the Kalka in this oil as well.

patient, while taking it in adequate doses, should live in a lonely chamber protected from the wind. After its digestion, the patient should partake of milk and boiled Shashtika rice. A Drona measure of the oil, should in this way, be gradually taken and the regimen of diet (milk and Shashtika rice, etc.) should be observed for double that period. This oil is efficacious in improving one's strength and complexion and adds a century (of years) to the duration of one's life, and at the same time absolves him from all sins. It is said that the use of each succesive Drona measure of this oil adds a century to one's days on earth. 16.

Oils may similarly be prepared with each of *Ativishá, Guduchi, Áditya-parni, Saireyaka, Virataru, S'atávari, Tri-kantaka, Madhuka* and *Prasárani*, and may be prescribed by an experienced and erudite physician. 17.

*Nilotpala* and *S'atávari* should be cooked in milk. The milk thus prepared should be again cooked with sesamum oil successively a hundred times and a paste of all the drugs used as a paste in the **Valá Taila** should be added to it at the time of cooking. The therapeutic virtues of all these oils are the same as those of the Valá-Taila and the same regimen of diet and conduct should be observed in all such cases. 18.

Thus ends the fifteenth Chapter of the Chikitsita Sthánam in the Sus'ruta Samhitá which deals with the medical treatment of Mudha-garbha.

# CHAPTER XVI.

Now we shall discourse on the medical treatment of Abscesses and Tumours (**Vidradhi**). 1.

Of the six types of Vidradhis, the one of the Sánnipátika type should be regarded as incurable In all other types curative measures* should be speedily resorted to in their unsuppurated stage, as in the treatment of a case of Śopha (inflammatory swelling or boil). 2.

**Treatment of Vátaja-Vidradhi :**—In a case of Vátaja Vidradhi, a compact or thick plaster (Álepa) composed of pasted *Murangi*-roots,† mixed with clarified butter, oil and lard (Vasá), should be applied lukewarm. The flesh of the animals which frequent swamps and marshes as well as of aquatic animals boiled with the drugs of the *Kákolyádi* group, Kánjika, salt, barley-powder and Sneha (clarified butter, &c.), should be applied as a poultice (Upanáha), and the affected part should be constantly fomented with (warm) Veśavára, Kriśará, milk and Páyasa. Blood-letting should also be resorted to. 3.

If, in spite of the use of the preceding remedies, suppuration should begin to set in, suppurating measures should be resorted to and the abscess (finally) lanced

---

\* Commencing with Apatarpana up to purgative measures (Chikitsá, chapter.—1).

† Both Dallana and Chakrápani Datta read "Vátaghna" in place of "Murangi" of the text. Dallana explains the term "Vátaghna" as the "Bhadra-dárvádi group" and S'iva-dása, the commentator of Chakrapáni, explains it as the "Daś'a-mula". Both of them, however, say that he different reading is "Surangi" meaning "S'obhánjana." "Murangi" also means "S'obhánjana."—Ep.

with a knife. Cleansing measures should then be applied to the (incidental) ulcer. After incision, the ulcer should be washed with a decoction of the *Pancha-mula* ; and an oil cooked with the drugs of the *Bhadra-dárvádi* group and *Yashti-madhu*, and, mixed with an abundant quantity of salt, should be used in filling (healing up) the cavity of the wound. The cleansing of the ulcer should be effected with the powdered *Vairechanika* (purgative) drugs mixed with **Traivrita**\* and the healing should be effected with **Traivrita** cooked with the drugs of the *Prithak-parnyádi* group. 4–6.

**Treatment of Pittaja Vidradhi:**—In a case of Pittaja Vidradhi a plaster (Pradeha) composed of sugar, fried paddy, *Yashti-Madhu* and *Sárivá* pasted with milk should be applied. As an alternative, a plaster composed of *Payasyá*, *Us'ira* and (red) sandal wood pasted with milk should be used. Cold infusions of *Pákya* (Yava-kshára), sugarcane-juice and milk, and **jivaniya-Ghrita** mixed with sugar should be used in affusing the abscess. The patient should be advised to lick a lambative composed of powdered *Haritaki* and *Trivrit* saturated with honey ; and leeches should be applied (to an unsuppurated) abscess for letting out the blood. An intelligent surgeon should (lance a suppurated abscess and) wash the incidental ulcer with a decoction of *Kshira-Vriksha* or of aquatic bulbs. Poultices of sesamum and *Yashti-Madhu* mixed with honey and clarified butter should then be applied to it and bandaged with a piece of thin linen. Clarified butter cooked with *Prapaundarika*, *Manjishtha*, *Yashti-Madhu*, *Us'ira*, *Padmaka*, *Haridrá* and milk,

---

\* "**Traivrita**" is a technical term and means clarified butter mixed with the three other lardacious substances, viz., oil, lard and marrow, Vide Chikitsita Sthánam. Chapter—V.

should be used to heal up the cavity of a Pittaja ulcer by (inducing granulation). As an alternative, clarified butter cooked with *Kshira-S'uklá*, *Prithak-parni*, *Samangá*, *Rodhra*, Chandana and the tender leaves and bark of the drugs of the *Nyagrodhádi* group should be employed for the same end. 7-10.

**Karanjádya Ghrita :**—A Karsha measure of each of the following drugs, viz., the tender leaves and fruits of the *Naktamála*, the leaves of the *Sumana* (Játi flower), *Patola* and of *Arishta*, *Haridrá*, *Daru-Haridrá*, wax, *Yashti-Madhu*, *Tikta-Rohini*, *Priyangu*,* *Kus'a*-roots, *Nichula*-bark, *Manjishthá*, sandal wood, *Us'ira*, *Utpala*, *Sárivá* and *Trivrit* should be cooked with a Prastha measure of clarified butter. This medicated Ghrita is called the **Karanjádya Ghrita**, and it will cure malignant ulcers (Dushta-Vrana) and act as a purifier in sinus and recent ulcers, etc., burns and scalds, deep sores and even deep-seated sinuses. 11.

**Treatment of Kaphaja Vidradhi :**—In a case of Kaphaja Vidradhi, the seat of affection should be fomented with a heated brick, sand, iron, cow-dung, husks, ashes and cow's urine.† The Doshas involved in such a case should be curbed down by a constant use of medicinal decoctions, emetics, plasters (Álepa) and poultices (Upanáha). The vitiated blood of the locality should be cuffed out with an Alávu-yantra (gourd). The abscess when suppurated should be (lanced

---

\* Chakrapáni Datta in his compilation does not include Priyangu, Kus'a-roots add Nichula-bark in the list but he reads both the kinds of sárivá, i. e., Anantamula and S'yámá-latá.

† In Chakradatta, the reading is "मूत्रपिष्टे:" i.e., pasted in cow's urine, instead of "मूत्रेक्षणै:" । S'ivadása, the commentator, however, holds that this reading is not authoritative, though he says that some commentators have accepted it.

and) washed with a decoction of *Aragvadha*. The sore of such an ulcer should be filled up (healed) with a medicinal compound consisting of the paste of *Haridrá Trivrit, S'aktu,* sesamum and honey and bandaged in the manner described before. After that, a medicated oil properly cooked with a paste of *Kulatthiká, Danti, Trivrit S'yámá, Arka, Tilvaka,* cow's urine and rock-salt should be applied in such a case. 12-13.

**Treatment of Ágantuja and Raktaja Vidradhi :**—In a case of abscess of traumatic (Ágantuja) origin, or due to the vitiated condition of the blood (**Raktaja**), all the measures and remedies laid down in connection with those of the **Pittaja** type should be employed by a skilled surgeon. 14

**Treatment of internal Vidradhi :**—A case of an unsuppurated internal abscess yields to the use of a potion consisting of a decoction of the drugs of the *Varunádi* group saturated with the powders (Kalka) of those of the *Ushakádi* group. Clarified butter cooked with the decoction of the drugs of the two preceding groups, as well as clarified butter cooked with purgative drugs, taken every morning, will cure an internal abscess in a very short time. The decoctions of the above groups should be mixed with Sneha (oil or clarified butter) and speedily used as an Ásthápana as well as an Anuvásana measure. The bark of *Madhu-s'igru* mixed with the powders of the drugs antidotal to the Doshas involved in the case, being administered in food and drink and used as a plaster, proves curative in a case of an internal abscess in its **unsuppurated** stage. As an alternative, the said drug (i.e , Madhu-s'igru) should be taken with water, Dhányámla, cow's rine, or Surá (wine). Purified *S'ilájatu, Guggulu, S'unthi,* or *Devadáru,* dissolved in the decoction of the drugs antidotal to the aggravated Doshas involved in the case, should be administered. Applications of poultices, Sneha-Karma (emollient measures), as well as Anulomana (Váyu-subduing) measures should be frequently resorted to in such cases. 15-20.

The veins (S'irá) should be opened in a case of the Kaphaja type of abscess as directed before; while some authorities advise to open the veins at the arms in cases of Raktaja, Vátaja and Pittaja types. 21.

**Treatment of Suppurated internal Vidradhi :**—A suppurated internal Vidradhi having bulged up (above the surface of the body) should be opened with a knife and treated in the manner of an (incidental) ulcer. Whether the pus drains through the lower or the upper channel of the body (rectum or mouth) the patient should be made to take the drugs of the *Varunádi* group or *Madhu-s'igru* mixed with (a copious quantity of) *Maireya*, Surá, Ásava, or Kánjika. The diet should consist of rice boiled and cooked with white mustard seed in the decoction of *Madhu-s'igru* and taken with the soup of barley, *Kola* and *Kulalttha* pulse. The **Tilvaka Ghrita** (Chikitsá Sthána, ch. IV.), or clarified butter cooked with the decoction of the *Trivritádi* group, should be taken every morning in adequate doses for the purpose. Particular care should be taken by the phsyician to guard against the suppuration of an internal abscess, since suppuration in such cases leads but to a slender hope of success. 22-23.

**Treatment of Majja-játa Vidradhi :**—The medical treatment of a patient, afflicated with a Majja-játa abscess (abscess affecting the marrow), should be taken in hand without holding out any definite hope of recovery (as a proper course of treatment in such cases does not invariably prove successful). Sneha-karma (anointments, etc.) and fomentations should be first resorted to, after which blood-letting should be made ; and the remedial measures of the present chapter should be then employed When it reaches the suppurating stage, the bone should be operated upon, and after the full elimination of the pus and the putrid matter from the incised ulcer, purifying remedies should be employed. The incidental ulcer should be washed with the decoction of the bitter drugs and the **Tikta-Sarpis**\* should be used. An intelligent physician should apply the decoction of the drugs of the Samśodhaniya group, if the oozing out of the marrow is not arrested. A medicated oil cooked with *Priyangu, Dhátaki, Rodhra, Katphala, Nemi*† and *Saindhava* salt should be used in healing up an ulcer incidental to an opened up *Vidradhi*. 24-25.

Thus ends the sixteenth Chapter of the Chikitsita Sthánam in the Sus'ruta Samhitá which deals with the treatment of abscess.

---

\* This medicated Ghrita (Chikitsita Sthánam, Ch. IX) may be used both internally and externally with good results. Ed.

† Dallana reads "Tini" in place of "Nemi," both of which, however, mean "Tinis'a". Chakradatta does not include "Saindhava" in the list, but reads "Tinis'a-twacham" in place of "Nemi-Saindhavam". S'ivadása, however, adds another reading 'Tinis'am Dhavam" on the authority of Chandráta.

—:-o-:—

# CHAPTER XVII.

Now we shall discourse on the medical treatment of erysipelas, etc., **(Visarpa)**, sinus, etc., **(Nádi-Vrana)** and diseases of the mammary glands **(Stana-roga)**. 1.

Of the types of erysipelas (Visarpa) the first three (viz., the Vátaja, Pittaja and Kaphaja ones) are curable; the two remaining types, viz., those caused by the concerted action of the three Doshas (of the body) and those originating from wounds (Kshataja) should be considered as incurable. In cases of the curable types, medicated Ghritas, plasters (Upadehas) and affusions (Seka) prepared with the drugs (antidotal to the specific aggravated Dosha or Doshas (involved in the case) should be prescribed. 2.

**Treatment of Vátaja Visarpa :**—In cases of the **Vátaja** type of the disease, *Mustá, S'atáhvá, Sura-dáru, Kushtha, Váráhi, Kustumburu* (Dhanyáka) *Krishna-gandhá,* and the drugs of a heat-making potency (Ushna-gana)* should be used in preparing the medicinal washings (Seka), plasters and Ghritas. The drugs respectively included within the groups of the *Vrihat-Pancha-mula* and the *Svalpa-Pancha-mula,* the *Kantaka-Pancha-mula* and the *Valli-Pancha-mula* should be (separately) used to prepare the medicinal plasters, affusions, medicated Ghritas and as well as the necessary oils. 3.

---

* Chakradatta reads "Arka", Vams'á and Artagala instead of the drugs of a heat-making potency. Dallana explains the drugs of a heat-making potency to be the drugs of the Bhadra-dárvádi and the Pippalyádi groups.

**Treatment of Pittaja Visarpa :**—In cases of Pittaja Visarpa, a plaster consisting of *Kas'eruka, S'ringátaka, Padma, Gundrá* (Guduchi), *S'aivála, Utpala* and clay pasted together and mixed with clarified butter, should be wrapped* in a piece of linen, and applied cool to the affected part. A paste composed of *Hrivera, Lámajjaka* (Us'ira-mula), *Chandana, Srotoja* (Rasánjana), *Muktá, Máni* and *Gairika*, pasted together with milk and mixed with clarified butter should be applied thin and cool to the affected part to alleviate the pain. Pittaja erysipelas readily yields to the application of a medicinal plaster composed of *Prapaundarika, Yashti-madhu, Payasyá,† Manjishthá, Padmaka, Chandana* and *Sugandhiká* pasted together. Decoctions of the drugs of the *Nyagrodhádi* group should be used in washing (the affected part); or clarified butter should be cooked with the expressed juice of the above drugs and employed in the case. The part may be affused (Seka) with cold milk (or water), or with water mixed with honey or sugar, or with the expressed juice of the sugarcane. 4-5.

**Gauryádi Ghrita :**—A Prastha measure of clarified butter should be cooked with the Kalka of *Gauri,‡ Yashti-madhu, Aravinda, Rodhra, Ambu, Rájádana, Gairika, Rishabhaka, Padmaka, Sárivá, Kákoli, Medá, Kumuda, Utpala, Chandana, Madhu-S'arkará, Drákshá, Sthirá, Pris'ni-parni,* and *S'atáhvá* taken in equal parts (and weighing one seer § in all)

---

\* In order to facilitate its removal.

† It means "Kshira-vidári". Jejjata explains it as "Arka-pushpi".

‡ Some explain it as "Haridrá", while others explain it as "Gorochaná".

§ Dallana, however, says that these drugs will weigh four Palas i. e., half a seer in all.

and with the decoctions, weighing four times that of the Ghrita, of the drugs of the *Nyagrodhádi, Sthirádi* (minor Pancha-mula) and *Vilvádi* (major Pancha-mula) groups together with the same weight (sixteen seers) of milk. The washing (of the affected part) with this medicated Ghrita proves curative in Pittaja erysipelas and sinus. Visphota (boils), head diseases, malignant sores and inflammatory affections of the mouth, yield to the internal use of this Ghrita. It is called the **Gauryyádi Ghrita** and is highly efficacious in the derangements to which children are liable, (commonly) attributed to the malignant influences of evil stars, as well as in cases of emaciated ones. 6.

**Treatment of Kaphaja Visarpa :—** Cases of the **Kaphaja** type of Visarpa readily yield to a proper application of a medicinal plaster (Pradeha) composed of *Aja-gandhá, As'va-gandhá, Saralá,*\* *Kálá, Ekaishiká* † and *Aja-s'ringi* ‡ pasted with the urine of a cow. Drugs, such as *Kálánusáryá, Aguru, Chocha* (cardamom), *Gunjá, Rásná, Vachá, S'ita-s'iva, Indra-parni, Pálindi, Munjáta* and *Mahi-Kadamba* (applied similarly) are also efficacious in the present type. Drugs of the *Varunádi* group may be used in any form (such as plasters, washes, etc.), for erysipelas. Blood-letting (by means of leeches) and Samsodhana (purifying) measures are the principal remedies in all cases of this disease (Visarpa). Suppurated erysipelas should be first purified and then treated with the remedies described in the treatment of Vrana (ulcer). 7-8.

---

\* "Saralá" here means "Trivrit". Chakradatta reads "सरणा" which also means "Trivrit".

† 'Ekaishiká," according to Dallana, would mean S'atávari but S'ivadása explains it as Páthá.

‡ Gayadása explains it as Karkata-S'ringi.

**Treatment of Nádi-vrana :**—A Case of Nádi-Vrana (sinus) due to the concerted action of the three Doshas (Sannipátaja) baffles all cure, while the four remaining types are amenable to careful medical treatment. Poultices (Upanáha)* should be applied at the outset in the **Vátaja Nádi-Vrana** and then the course of the pus-channels should be (ascertained and) fully opened (with a knife) and bandaged with a paste of sesamum, *Apámárga*-seeds and *Saindhava* salt. A decoction of (the drugs of) the *Vrihat-Pancha-mula* group should be constantly used in washing the ulcer. Oil † duly cooked with the followiug drugs, viz , *Himsrá, Haridrá, Katuka, Valá, Gojihviká* and *Vilva*-roots should be used for the purification, filling up and healing of the sores of the sinus. 9-11.

**Treatment of Pittaja Nádi :**—In a case of **Pittaja** sinus, an intelligent surgeon should employ a porridge (Utkáriká) mixed with milk and clarified butter as a poultice. Then having opened the sinus with a knife, a plaster composed of *Tila, Nága-danti* and *Yashti-madhu* should be applied to heal it. A decoction of *Soma, Nimba* and *Haridrá* should be used by a skillful surgeon in washing the ulcer daily. A medicated Ghrita cooked with *S'yámá, Trivrit, Triphalá, Haridrá, Dáru-Haridrá, Rodhra* and *Kutaja* and with milk should be used to lubricate (Tarpana) the sinus. This Ghrita will even heal a sinus affecting the Koshtha. 12-13.

---

* Poulticing with the drugs which induce suppuration is not approved of by Gayadása.

† Four seers of oil, the (Kalka) drugs combindely weighing one seer and sixteen seers of water are to be taken in its preparation.— Dallana.

**Treatment of Kaphaja Nadi:**—In a case of the Kaphaja type of the Nádi, the sinus should be duly poulticed Upanáha) with *Kulattha*, white mustard seeds, *S'aktu* and *Kinva*. When softened by its application, the direction of the sinus (with the help of a director) should be first ascertained; and an expert surgeon should then open it fully with a knife and plaster it with a compound composed of *Nimba*, sesamum, *Saindhava* salt and *Saurashtra-mrittiká*. A decoction (Sva-rasa-lit.—expressed juice) of the *Karanja, Nimba, Játi, Aksha* and *Pilu* should be used in washing the incidental ulcer. Oil duly cooked with *Suvarchiká, Saindhava, Chitraka, Nikumbha, Táli,*\* *Nala, Rupiká* and *Apámárga*-seeds and with cow's urine should be used for healing purposes. 14.

**Treatment of S'alyaja Nadi :**—In a case of S'alyaja Nádi (incidental to any foreign matter into the body), the S'alya should be first extracted by an incision into the sinus. Then having fully cleansed the channel, the ulcer should be purified with a plaster of sesamum profusely saturated with honey and clarified butter. It should be then healed up. Oil cooked with the decoction of the tender fruits of the *Kumbhika, Kharjura, Kapittha, Vilva* and the *Vanaspatis* (Vata, etc.), and with the Kalkas of *Mustá, Saralá, Priyangu, Sugandhiká, Mocharasa,*† *Ahi-pushpa* (Nágesvara), *Rodhra* and *Dhátaki* flowers leads to a speedy healing up (granulation) of ulcers (Vrana) and traumatic sinuses. 15.

---

\* Dallana's reading evidently is "Táli-tala" and he explains it as the roots of "Bhumyámalaki". Chakradatta also prescribes this oil but he takes "Niliká" instead of "Táli". S'ivadása, again, in his commentary quotes from Sus'ruta but reads "Nili-Nala" in place of "Tála-Nala."

† "Mocha-rasa" is explained by Dallana to be "S'obhánjana," but it generally means "S'álmali-veshta," and S'ivadása explains it as such.—Ed.

**Treatment with Kshára-Sutra :**—An erudite surgeon should open a sinus, occurring in any of the Marmas, or in a weak, timid, or emaciated person with an alkalined string (**Kshára-Sutra**), and not with a surgical knife. The course of the sinus should be first ascertained with a director ; and a needle, threaded with a string of alkalined thread should be passed from one end of the sinus and quickly drawn out through the other. Then the two ends of the thread should be firmly fastened together. An intelligent surgeon should likewise pass another alkalined thread in the event of the alkali of the first thread being comparatively weak. This should be repeated till the sinus completely bursts out. The surgeon should know that the same procedure may be as well adopted in cases of fistula-in-ano. Similarly in cases of tumours (**Arvuda**), etc. they should be lifted up (with the hand) and tied round at their base with an alkalined thread, or it should be punctured around with a kind of needle with their mouth resembling a barley corn and then tied again at their base with an alkalined thread. After their bursting (and falling off), they should be treated as common ulcers (Vrana). 16.

The different kinds of **Plug-Stick** (Varti) described in the Dvi-Vraniya Chapter (Chikitsita—chap.-I.) may be similarly used with advantage in all cases of sinus. The use of a plug made of the following drugs, viz., the bark and fruit of the *Ghonta*, (the five officinal kinds of) salt,* *Láksha, Puga* and the leaves of the *Alavaná* †

---

\* According to Chakradatta's reading and S'ivadás's commentary thereon, only the Saindhava (instead of the five officinal kinds of salt) should be taken. We, however, follow Dallana's interpretation with good results.—*Ed.*

† "Alavaná" has been explained by Dallana as "Káka-mardaniká" and by S'ivadása as "Jyotishmati". S'ivadása is, however, followed in practice in this case.

pasted together with the milky juice of the *Snuhi* and *Arka* leads to the speedy healing up of a sinus. The powdered\* stones of *Vibhitaka*, mangoe fruits, *Vata*-sprouts, *Harenu, S'amkhini*-seed, *Váráhi-kanda* mixed with oil can also be used in a case of sinus. 17-19.

The seeds of the *Dhustura, Madana* and *Kodrava, Kos'átaki, S'uka-nasá, Mriga-bhojani* and the seeds and flowers of the *Amkota* should be pounded together and applied to a sinus (Nádi) after having washed it with a decoction of *Láksha*. Cases of sinus speedily yield to the curative efficacy of the application of these powders mixed with oil. The use of the oil cooked with cow's urine and with the preceding drugs (as Kalkas) brings about the healing up of a sinus in seven nights. 20-21.

The application of the oil cooked with the roots of the *Pinditaka* treated with the expressed juice of the *Varáha-kanda* in the manner of a Bhávaná saturation and with the bulbs of Suvahá brings about a speedy and effective remedy for a sinus. The same effect is produced by an application of the oil cooked with the bulbs of the the Vajra-kanda. 22.

**Bhallátakádya Taila:**—The use of the oil cooked with the paste (Kalka) of *Bhallátaka, Arka, Maricha, Saindhava* salt, *Vidanga, Haridrá, Dáru-Haridrá* and *Chitraka* and with the expressed juice of the *Bhringa-rája*, readily cures cases of sinus, Apachi and ulcer due to Váyu and Kapha. 23.

**Treatment of Stana-roga :**— In cases of a derangement of the milk (of the breast) a draught of clarified butter should be quickly given to the Dhátri

---

\* According to some different reading "burnt ashes" (instead of powders) of the drugs should be taken. In our humble opinion the reading in the text seems to be the correct one,

(mother or wet-nurse) by the physician; and in the evening a draught composed of the decoction of *Nimba*, mixed with honey and *Mágadhiká*, should be given to her for **emetic** purposes. Next day she should take a meal (of boiled rice) with the **soup** (Yusha) of *Mudga* pulse. The use of emetics should be continued for three, four, or six days; or she should be made to drink a potion of clarified butter (cooked) with *Triphalá*. A decoction of *Bhárgi*, *Ativishá*, *Vachá*, *Sura-dáru*, *Páthá*, the drugs of the *Mustádi Gana*, *Murvá* and *Katu-rohini*, or that of the drugs of the *Áragvadhádi* group mixed with honey, should be given to the Dhátri (wet-nurse) for the purification of her breast-milk. 26.

The above are the general remedial measures which are to be adopted in the affections of **breast-milk.** Any other defect in the breast-milk should be corrected specially with an eye to the nature of the Dosha involved in the case. In cases of inflammatory swellings of the breasts, the physician shou'd remedy them by means of any one of the various measures laid down under the head of **Vidradhi** with a due consideration to the requirements of each particular case. Medicinal remedies should only be internally employed and no poultices should be applied for the speedy suppuration of the swelling of the breast, even if found to have already commenced to suppurate; since the breasts are of an extremely soft and fleshy growth, any tight bandaging about those parts may be followed by local sloughing or even bursting. In a case where suppuration had already taken place, an operation should be made in the affected part, avoiding the milk-carrying veins as well as the nipple with its black surroundings. In all the cases of Stana-Vidradhi—whether non-suppurated, suppurating, or suppurated—the milk should be pressed out from the breast of the Dhátri* 27-29.

Thus ends the Seventeenth Chapter of the Chikitsita Sthánam in the Sus'ruta Samhitá which deals with the treatment of erysipelas, sinus and the diseases of the mammary glands.

* The milk should be pressed out of the Dhátri's breasts in the **non-suppurated** stage, to alleviate the burning sensation therein, in the **suppurating** stage for the avoidance of further suppuration, and in the **suppurated** stage for the prevention of sores, sinus, etc.

## CHAPTER XVIII.

Now we shall discourse on the medical treatment of Glandular Swellings, etc. **(Granthi),** Scurvy **(Apachi),** Tumour, etc. **(Arvuda)** and Goitre **(Gala-ganda).** 1.

**General treatment of Granthi :**—In the non-suppurated or acute (inflammatory) stage of **Granthi,** an experienced physician should prescribe the **measures** * laid down in connection with (inflammatory) swellings (Sopha) in general. As bodily strength arrests the progress of the disease, the strength of the patient should hence be always carefully guarded against suffering any diminution in that respect. The patient should be made to drink oil, or clarified butter, or both ; or he should be made to drink lard, oil and clarified butter, mixed together.† *Apehivátá* (Prasárani) and *Das'a-mula* cooked with the four kinds of lardacious or emollient substances (oil, clarified

---

\* Beginning with Apatarpana up to the purgative measures.

† Oil, clarified butter and lard mixed together is technically called the "**Trivrita** "—Dallana.

In the case of a Vátaja Granthi, a potion of oil cooked with the decoction and paste (Kalka) of the Váyu-subduing drugs should be prescribed for the patient ; in the case of a Pittaja Granthi, clarified butter cooked with the decoction and Kalka of the Pitta-subduing drugs should be administered in the same manner ; while in the case of a Kaphaja Granthi, oil cooked with the decoction and Kalka of the Kapha-subduing drugs should be taken by the patient. But in a case of Granthi due to the concerted action of the two, or three of the Doshas, any compound medicated oil, prepared by cooking any two, three, or four of the oily substances, *viz.*, oil, clarified butter, lard and marrow, with the decoction and Kalka of those drugs which are antidotes to the said Doshas, should be prescribed for the patient as drinks.

butter, lard and marrow), or with any two of them should be prescribed. 2-3.

**Treatment of Vátaja Granthi :**—A medicinal plaster composed of *Himsrá, Rohini, Amritá, Bhárgi, S'yonáka, Vilva, Aguru, Krishna-gandhá, Goji* and *Tála-patri* (Tála-parni—D. R ) pasted together, should be applied (to the inflamed gland) in the **Vátaja type** of Granthi. Different kinds of fomentation (Sveda), poulticing (Upanáha) and medicinal plasters (Lepa), possessed of the efficacy of subduing the deranged Váyu, should be likewise resorted to. A suppurated swelling should be opened and the pus drained. Then the incised wound should be washed with a decoction of *Vilva*,\* *Arka* and *Narendra* (Áragvadha) and purified (disinfected) with a plaster consisting of *sesamum* and the leaves of the *Panchnágula* (castor oil plants), together with Saindhava salt. After the purification, it should be healed up by applying a medicated oil, mixed with the powders of *Rásná* and *Saralá* ; or by a medicated oil prepared by cooking it with *Vidanga, Yashti-madhu* and *Amritá* and cow's milk. 4.

**Treatment of Pittaja Granthi :**—In a case of the **Pittaja** type of the disease, leeches should be applied to the affected part, which should be further affused with milk and water. The patient should be made to drink a cold decoction of the drugs of the *Kákolyádi* group with the addition of sugar ; or he should take the powders of *Haritaki* through the medium of grape-juice, or of the expressed juice of sugarcane. Hot plasters, prepared by pasting together the bark of the *Madhuka* (flower) tree, and of the *Jambu*

---

\* Some read "विल्वार्कगणादितोषैः" and explain that the decoctions of the Vilvádi and the Arkádi groups are to be taken for the purpose.

tree, *Arjuna* tree, and *Vetasa* creeper. As an alternative, hot plasters compounded of the roots of the *Trina-s'unya* (Ketaki), or *Muchukunda* mixed with sugar, should be constantly applied to the affected part. The Granthi should be opened when fully suppurated, and the pus let out; after which it should be washed with a decoction of the bark of the *Vanaspati*.* The incidental ulcer should then be purified with a plaster composed of sesamum and *Yashti-madhu*; and lastly it should be healed up with clarified butter cooked with the drugs of the *Madhura* (Kákolyádi group 5-6.

**Treatment of Kaphaja Granthi :**—In a case of the **Khaphaja** type of the disease, the Doshas should be first eliminated from the system with the regular and successive **measures**.† The affected part (Granthi) should then be fomented and firmly pressed (Vimlápana) and rubbed with either the thumb, or a piece of iron rod, or stone, or with a bamboo rod in order to bring about its resolution. A plaster composed of the roots of the *Vikamkata*, ‡ *Áragvadha, Kákananti* (Gunjá), *Kákádani* (Váyasa-tinduka), and *Tápasa-Vriksha* (Ingudi) and with *Pinda-phala* (Tiktálávu), *Arka*, § *Bhárgi, Karanja, Kálá* and *Madana*, pasted together, should be applied to it by an erudite physician. A glandular swelling (Kaphaja Granthi) on any part of the body other than a vital and vulnerable one (Marma) and

---

* The Vanaspati class consists of Vata, Plaksha, As'vattha and Udumbara trees.

† These are the applications of Sneha, fomentation, emetics, purgatives, Ásthápana, S'iro-virechana and blood-letting.

‡ Dallana explains "Vikamkata" as "Kanta-káriká," but it means Sruvá (called Vaincb in Bengal) and S'ivadása also explains it as such.—*Ed.*

§ Chakradatta does not read "Arka" in the list.

not (otherwise) resolved and absorbed should be cut open even in its non-suppurated stage and the glands removed. The expert surgeon should then cauterize the incidental wound after the cessation of the bleeding and treat it in the manner * of the **Sadyo-Vrana** treatment. These remedies should be employed by the experienced physician, where the swelling would be found to have assumed a large, stiff, elevated and fleshy aspect (bulging from the deeper tissues of the flesh). A Kaphaja Granthi should be opened with an incision as soon as it becomes fully suppurated and should then be washed with a decoction of appropriate medicinal drugs. The incidental ulcer should be purified (disinfected) with a purifying remedy prepared with a profuse quantity of *Yava-kshara*, honey and clarified butter; and finally it should be healed up by the application of an oil, cooked with *Vidanga, Páthá* and *Rohini*. 7-9.

**Treatment of Medoja Granthi :**—In a case of **Medoja** Granthi (originated from the vitiated condition of the bodily fat) a plaster of pasted sesamum, placed inside the folds of a piece of linen, should be applied to the seat of the affected part and fomentations with hot iron-rods should be frequently applied, inasmuch as application of heat (lit.—fire) is efficacious in such cases. As an alternative, the affected part should be fomented with a ladle, pasted with heated shellac (Lákshá). The Granthi (in its non-suppurated stage) should be opened by an incision and the fat removed; the incidental ulcer should then be (actually) cauterized. On the other hand, the Granthi, when fully suppurated, should be incised and washed with the urine (of a cow). Then a paste, composed of

* Applications of honey, clarified butter, etc.

sesamum, *Suvarchiká, Haritála* and rock-salt, pounded together and mixed with honey, clarified butter and an abundant quantity of Yava-kshára, should be applied to the incidental wound for purifying purposes. Oil, cooked with the two kinds of *Karanja, Gunjá,* the green scrapings of bamboo, *Ingudi* and the urine * of a cow, should be used to heal the ulcer. 10-11.

**Treatment of Apachi :**—Clarified butter cooked with the fruit of *Jimutaka* and *Kosha-vati,* and with (the roots of) *Danti, Dravanti* and *Trivrit,* is a very powerful and efficacious remedy.† Administered internally as well as externally, it leads to the cure of the advanced cases of **Apachi.** 12.

A strong emetic composed of *Nirgundi, Játi* (flower) and *Varihistha* (Válá) together with *Jimútaka,* profusely mixed with honey and *Saindhava,* should be given warm to the patient. It is a very powerful emetic, and leads to the recovery of even a malignant form of **Apachi.** An oil, cooked with the pastes (Kalka) of *Kaitaryya,*‡ *Vimbi* and *Karavira,* may be profitably used as an errhine (Śiro-virechana). Oil cooked with the expressed juice of *S'akhotaka* may also be used profitably as an errhine. § **Avapida** errhines (used in drops

---

* Cow's urine measuring four times the oil should be taken in the preparation of this medicated oil.

† In preparing this medicated Ghrita, the quantity of clarified butter should be taken four times as much as the combined weight of the Kalka (paste). These should be boiled with water, taken four times as much as the quantity of clarified butter. Some authorities, however, are of opinion that both the paste (Kalka) and the decoction of the drugs are to be taken in its preparation.

‡ Some read 'Nirgundi' after it.

§ This medicated oil should be cooked without any Kalka. But some are of opinion that both the decoction and the Kalka of S'ákhotaka should be used.

into the nostrils should be applied with *Madhuka-sára*, *S'igru*-seeds and *Apámárga*-seeds.* 13-15.

A glandular swelling (Granthi), occurring in any part of the body other than a Marma, should be opened in its non-suppurated stage and cauterized with fire ; † or it should be rubbed with an alkali ‡ after scarification as already advised. 16.

A length of twelve fingers should be measured (Mitvá) from and above the Párshni, *i.e.*, the posterior side of the ankle (and the space of **Indra-vasti** above this part should be ascertained). The Indra-vasti (occupying a space of half a finger, or, according to others, two fingers) having been carefully avoided, an excision (on the opposite side of the affection) should be made and the spawn-like glands having been removed (therefrom), the excisioned part should be cauterised with fire.

Others say that the excision should be made straight above the ankle (Ghoná) after carefully avoiding the space of **Indra-vasti**, measuring two fingers (and to make sure an additional space of half a finger should be left out), which would be found out by taking one-eighth part (of the Janghá, *i.e.*, the leg—excluding the foot and measuring twenty fingers) from the Khulaka (ankle-joint) of which the (two) Gulphas (ankles) look like the (two) ears. § 17-18.

* Madhuka-sára mixed with tepid water and the expressed juice of S'igru-seeds and of Apámárga-seeds should be used.

† In cases of the preponderance of Váyu and of Kapha.

‡ In cases of the preponderance of Pitta.

§ There is a good deal of difference as to the reading and explanation of this passage amongst the different commentators. The different explanations arise from the different interpretations put upon the word "प्रति" in the Text, "पार्ष्णिं प्रति द्वादश चाङ्गुलानि, etc." The words "पार्ष्णिं प्रति"

As an alternative, the region of the wrist (Manibandha) should be branded by a physician with three mark lines, one finger apart, for a radical cure of Apachi. 19.

may mean either of the following. (1) On the opposite side of the Párshni. Vágbhata subscribes to this view. (2) On the opposite (*i.e.*, the other) Párshni, that is to say, if the affection be on the right side of the body the operation should be made on the Párshni of the left leg and so on. Vriddha Vágbhata subscribes to this interpretation in the clearest language. (3) In the region of the Párshni, *i.e.*, on the dorsal side of the leg.

The different commentators, again, do not agree as to the seat and extent of the excision. Some say that the operation should be made **above** the Indra-Vasti and the extent should be two fingers in length. Vágbhata seems to subscribe to this view. Others hold that the operation should be made **below** the Indra-vasti and the extent should be two fingers' length : Dallana is of this opinion. A third class of commentators assert that the whole extent of the length from above the Párshni up to the Indra Vasti should be opened.

As to the extent of the Indra-Vasti, again, there is a difference. According to Dallana it occupies a space of two fingers. But Jejjata holds that it occupies a space of half a finger only. The Indra-Vasti (Marma) is situated twelve fingers above (*i.e.*, in the thirteenth finger of) the Párshni. The reading in the printed editions of the text is "भित्वा", whereas Vrinda and Chakradatta read "मित्वा". Dallana's reading also evidently is "मित्वा". "भित्वा" would be quite redundant and as "मित्वा" gives a better meaning, we accept this reading.

Now we come to the second stanza. Commentators differ more in the exposition of this stanza than of the former. By the expression "आगुल्फ-कर्णात्" is meant by some commentators "from the Gulpha to the Karna." Others, however, mean to take it as an adjective to "खुलकात्" and explain it as meaning "from above the Khulaka whereof the Gulphas look like the Karnas." As regards the expression "घोणाजुं वेध:", some are inclined to think that the excision should be made straight above the Ghoná (i.e., the posterior part and especially the big vein there which looks like the nose (Ghoná) of the ankle-joint).

Others, however, read it as "घोणाजंवेऽध:" and explain it (घोणाजंवे + अध:) as meaning "in a straight line with the Ghoná (which may mean

The ashes (Masi) of the skins of a peacock, cow, lizard (Godhá) and snake and of tortoise shells should be dusted (over an Apachi after lubricating it) with the (expressed) oil of the *Ingudi*. Medicated oils to be described under the treatment of **S'lipada** (elephantiasis) and Vairechanika fumes should also be applied in a case of **Apachi** and the diet should consist of cooked barley and Mudga pulse. 20-21.

**Treatment of Vátaja Arvuda :**—In a case of **Váta͏ja** Arvuda, a poultice composed of *Karkáruka, Erváruka,* cocoanut, *Piyála* and castor seeds, boiled with milk, water and clarified butter, and mixed with oil, should be applied lukewarm (to the tumour). As an alternative, a poultice made up of boiled meat or of Ves'a-vára, should be applied to it. Fomentation of the part in the manner of a **Nádi-sveda** (application of medicated fumes through a pipe) should be applied by an experienced physician and the (vitiated) blood (of the locality) should be repeatedly cuffed off with a horn. *S'atáhvá* or *Trivrit\**, boiled with the decoction of the Váyu-subduing drugs and with milk and Kánjika, should be given to the patient. 22-23.

**Treatment of Pittaja Arvuda :—** Applications of mild fomentations and poultices (to the

either the nose or the big Vein (Kandará) at the heel looking like the nose (Ghoná) of the ankle-joint and below the Indra-Vasti".

Dallana says that the part to be excisioned, according to the first stanza, is **below** the Indra-vasti and that, according to the second, is **above** the Indra-Vasti. We also think that the seat of the Indra-Vasti should be carefully avoided and an excision should be made both above and below the Indra-Vasti, according to the requirements in each case.

\* There is a different reading "श्वेताखंं चिव्रतं" in place of "शताख्वा चिव्रतं". In that case, roots of white Trivrit should be boiled with the decoction, etc.

affected part) and of purgatives are efficacious in **Pittaja** Arvuda. The tumour should be well rubbed with (the rough surface of) the leaves of the *Udumbara, S'áka,* or of the *Goji* and it should be plastered over with the fine powders of *Sarja-rasa, Priyangu, Pattanga* (red sandal wood), *Rodhra, Anjana* * and *Yashtimadhu,* mixed with honey. As an alternative, a plaster composed of *Aragvadha, Goji, Soma* and *S'yámá,* pasted together should be applied to it after the secretion Visráva Clarified butter, cooked with *Klitaka* (as a Kalka) and with the decoction of *S'yámá, Girihvá, Anjanaki, Drátshá* and *Saptaliká* should be prescribed for internal application in a case of Pittaja Arvuda and of abdominal dropsy (Jathara) of the Pittaja type. 24-26.

**Treatment of Kaphaja Arvuda :**—In cases of the **Kaphaja** type of Arvuda blood should be let out from the affected part after the system of the patient has been cleansed (by emetics and purgatives). Then a medicinal plaster composed of the drugs,† which are efficacious in correcting the Doshas, confined to the upper and lower parts of the organism, should be applied hot to the tumour. Or a plaster composed of *Kánsya-nila, S'uka, Lángalákhya* and *Kákádani* roots, and the dung of a *Kapota* and of *Párávata* pasted together with urine, or with alkaline water should be applied to it The Kalkas (pastes) of *Nishpáva* (S'imbi), *Pinyáka* (oil-cakes of sesamum) and *Kulattha* pulse, pasted with curd-cream and an abundunt quantity of flesh, should be used in plastering the affected part so that worms and parasites may be produced in the ulcer

---

* Chakradatta reads "Arjuna" in place of "Anjana".

† These are the drugs included in the emetic and purgative groups (see chap. XXXIX. Sutra Sthánam).

and flies attracted to it (and so consume the ulcer). A small portion of the ulcer, left unconsumed (un-eaten) by worms and parasites, etc., should be scarified and the ulcer should then be cauterised with fire. 27-28.

A comparatively superficial tumour (Arvuda) should be covered with thin leaves of zinc, copper, lead, or of iron, and cauterization with fire or with an alkali as well as surgical operations should be carefully and repeatedly resorted to, so as not to hurt, nor in any way injure the body. The incidental ulcer should be washed with the decoction of the leaves of the *Ásphota, Játi,* and *Karavira* for the purpose of purification. A medicated oil, cooked with *Bhárgi, Vidanga, Páthá,* and *Triphalá* should then be used as a healing remedy. An experienced physician should treat a tumour, spontaneously suppurating, in the manner of a suppurated ulcer. 29-31.

**Treatment of Medoja Arvuda :**—A **Medoja** Arvuda (fat origined tumour) should be first fomented and then incised. The blood in its inside having been cleansed it should be quickly sutured and then plastered over with a compound composed of *Haridrá, Griha-dhuma* (soot of a room), *Rodhra, Pattanga, Manah s'ilá* and *Haritála* pounded together and mixed with a proper quantity of honey After its purification, thus produced, it should be treated with the application of **Karanja-Taila** (prescribed before in cases of Vidradhi). Even the least particle of Doshas (pus, etc.) in a tumour, left unremoved, would lead to a fresh growth of the excrescence and bring on death just like the least particle of an unextinguished fire. Hence it should be destroyed in its entirety. 32-33.

**Treatment of Vátaja Gala-ganda :**—
A case of the **Vátaja** type of Gala-ganda (goitre) should

be treated with fomentations of the vapours of the decoctions of tender leaves of the Váyu-subduing drugs prepared by boiling them with Kánjika, various kinds of urine and milk as well as with minced meat and oil, and should be applied in the manner of a **Nádisveda.** After this fomentation, the contents should be carefully drained (from inside the goitre). Then after having duly purified (the incidental ulcer), it should be plastered with a medicinal compound composed of (the seeds of) the *S'ana, Atasi, Mulaka, S'igru* and sesamum and *Kinva* and the piths of the *Piyála,* or with that composed of *Kálá, Amritá, S'igru, Punarnavá, Arka, Gaja-pippali, Karahátá* (Madana) and *Kushtha,* or with that composed of *Ekaishiká, Vrikshaka* and *Tilvaka.* All of them should be pasted with Surá and Kánjika and applied hot to the affected part. The internal use of a medicated oil, cooked* with *Amritá, Nimba, Hamsáhvá, Vrikshaka, Pippali, Valá, Ati-valá,* and *Deva-dáru,* always proves efficacious in a case of goitre. 34–36.

**Treatment of Kaphaja Gala-ganda :** —A case of the **Kaphaja** type of goitre should be treated with applications of fomentation and poultice and should be duly drained (Visráva). Then a medicinal plaster composed of *Aja-gandhá, Ati-vishá, Vis'alyá, Vishániká, Kushtha, S'ukáhvayá, Gunjá* (taken in equal parts) and pasted with the alkaline water prepared from the ashes of the *Palás'a* wood should be applied hot to the affected part. A medicated oil cooked with the drugs of the *Pippalyádi* group and mixed with the five officinal kinds of salt should

---

\* Some say that the oil should be prepared with the decoction as well as with Kalka of the said drugs. Others, however, hold that water should be used in the preparation of the oil and the said drugs should be used only as a Kalka.

be taken by the patient. Emetics, errhines and inhalations of Vairechanika-dhuma are beneficial in such cases. In the **Va'taja** and the **Kaphaja** types of goitre (Gala-ganda), the skilful physician should employ suppurating measures in partially suppurated cases. The patient's diet should consist of rice, barley and *Mudga* soup and should be taken with honey, *Trikatu*, cow's urine, fresh ginger, *Patola* and *Nimba*. 37–39.

## Treatment of Medoja Gala-ganda :—

In a case of a **Medoja** goitre (due to the deranged fat), the patient should be first made to use oleaginous substances (internally and externally) and venesection should then be resorted to, as advised before (Sárira-Stháná, Ch VIII). A hot plaster composed of *S'yámá* (Trivrit), *Sudhá*, *Mandura*, *Danti* and *Rasánjana* pasted together should be applied to the seat of the disease. Powders of the essential parts (Sára) of a *S'ála* tree mixed with cow's urine may be given every morning with advantage

As an alternative, the Goitre (Gala-ganda) should be opened, its fatty contents fully removed and the wound then sutured. Or it should be cauterised with the application of heated animal marrow, clarified butter, lard, or honey ; after which it should be lubricated with clarified butter and honey (mixed together), and a pulverised compound of *Kásisa*, *Tuttha*, and *Gorochaná*, should be applied to it ; or after lubricating it with oil, it should be dusted with the ashes of cow-dung and of *S'ála-sára*. Daily washings with the decoction of *Triphalá*, hard bandaging and a diet of barley, prove efficacious (in cases of goitre). 40.

Thus ends the Eighteenth Chapter of the Chikitsita Sthánam in the Sus'ruta Samhitá, which deals with the medical treatment of Glands, Scrofula, Tumour and Goitre.

# CHAPTER XIX.

Now we shall discourse on the medical treatment of hernia, hydrocele, scrotal tumour, etc. **(Vriddhi)**, diseases of the genital organ **(Upadamsʹa)** and elephantiasis **(Ślipada)**. 1.

In the six types of **Vriddhi** other than the one known as the **Antra-Vriddhi** (Hernia), riding on horse back, etc., excessive physical labour, fastings, sitting in an unnatural position, constant walking, voluntary restraint of any natural urging (for stool and urine, etc.), sexual intercourse and eating of food difficult of digestion should be avoided. 2.

**Treatment of Vátaja Vriddhi :**—In the **Vátaja** type of Vriddhi, the patient should be first soothed (Snigdha) with the application of **Traivrita Ghrita** (vide, Chap. V. Chikitsita Sthána). He should then be duly fomented and subjected to a proper course of purgatives. As an alternative, he should be made to drink the expressed oil of the *Kosʹámra, Tilvaka*, or *Eranda* (castor) oil (as a purgative) with milk for a month. A decoction of the Váyu subduing drugs mixed with the powders of the same drugs should then be employed by an experienced physician at a proper time * in the manner of a Niruha Vasti. The patient should then be made to take a meal (of boiled rice) along with meat soup ; and oil cooked with *Yashti madhu* should be applied (in the manner of an Anuvásana measure).

* After a period of one week from the time of the application of purgatives and in case the patient is strong enough to undergo the Niruha Vasti measure.

Applications of Sneha (oil, etc.), poultices (Upanáha), and plasters (Pradeha) of the Váyu-subduing drugs should be applied to the affected part. If the tumour (Vriddhi) begins to suppurate, it should be made to do so fully. It should be then opened with an incision avoiding the median line (Sevani) of the perineum and the proper purifying (i.e., antiseptic and healing) measures should be resorted to in the usual way laid down (in the treatment of Dvi-vrana*). 3.

**Treatment of Pittaja Vriddhi :—** A case of the non-suppurated stage of Pittaja Vriddhi may be beneficially treated with the remedies laid down in connection with a case of the same type of glandular swelling (Pittaja Granthi). In the case of it being suppurated, the surgeon should open it with a knife and purify it with the application of honey and clarified butter. The incidental ulcer should then be healed up with oils and pastes of healing virtues. 4.

**Treatment of Raktaja Vriddhi :—** In a case of Raktaja Vriddhi (originated through the vitiated condition of the blood), the (vitiated) blood should be drawn out by the application of leeches. As an alternative, purgatives should be administered through the medium of honey and sugar Remedial measures described in connection with the Pittaja type of the disease should be employed both in the suppurated and the non-suppurated stages (of this type). 5.

**Treatment of Kaphaja Vriddhi :—** In a case of the Kaphaja type of the disease, poultices with the heat-making † drugs (i.e , Vachádi, Pippályadi

---

\* According to Gayadása, the measures to be adopted should be those laid down in the Mis'raka chapter (Chap. XXV).

† Some say that the heat-producing drugs are those comprised in the Aja-gandhádi group mentioned in the Mis'raka chapter, Sutra Sthánam.

and Mushkakádi groups, etc.) pasted with cow's urine should be applied. The patient should be made to drink a potion consisting of the decoction of *Dáru-Haridrá* mixed with the urine of a cow, and all the remedial measures with the exclusion of Vimlápana (resolution by pressure) laid down under the treatment of the Kaphaja Granthi should be employed. The tumour should be opened (with a knife) when suppurated, and the oil cooked with *Játi, Arushkara, Amkota* and *Sapta-parna* should be used for the purification (disinfection) of the incidental ulcer. 6.

**Treatment of Medoja Vriddhi :—**In a case of the Medoja (fat-originated) type of the disease, the affected part should be (lightly) fomented, * and plasters composed of drugs (of the roots) of the *Surasádi* group or of the *S'iro-virechana* group (Ch. XXXIX. Sutra Sthána) pasted with the urine of a cow should be applied to it in a lukewarm state. The inflamed and swollen scrotal tumour, (lightly) fomented as before, should be tightened round with a piece of cloth Then having encouraged the patient, the surgeon should open the tumour with a Vriddhipatra (knife) carefully avoiding the two **testes** (lying within the scrotal sac) and the **median line** of the perineum (Sevani). Then having carefully removed all morbid products (Medas) from its inside, Saindhava and sulphate of iron should be applied to the incised part, and the scrotum should be carefully bandaged (in the manner of a Gophaná bandage). After the proper purification (disinfection) of the ulcer, its healing should be effected with the application of an oil

---

* The fomentation should be applied according to S'ivadás'a, with balls of cow-dung, etc., slightly heated. It should be noted in this connection that strong fomentations should not, in any case, be applied to the testes.

cooked with *Manahs'ilá*, *Haritála* (yellow oxide of arsenic), rock-salt, and *Bhallátaka*. 7.

**Treatment of Mutraja Vriddhi:** — In a case of an enlargement of the scrotun (hydrocele) due to the derangement of urine, it should be first fomented and then a piece of cloth should be tightened rount it. A puncture should then be made in the bottom of the sac with a Vrihimukha instrument, on either side of the raphe of the perineum (Sevani). A tube open at both ends should be introduced (into the puncture) and the accumulated (morbid) fluid should be let out. The tube should then be taken off and the scrotum should be tied up with a bandage of the Sthagiká pattern and the incidental ulcer should be purified and healed up with appropriate medicinal applications. 8.

**Treatment of Antra-Vriddhi :** —A case of Antra-Vriddhi (hernia when strangulated) extending down to the scrotal sac (Kosha) should be given up as irremediable ; but, in the case of its not being so extended, it should be treated as a case of Vátaja-Vriddhi. If the colon be found to have descended down to inguinal region (Vamkshana), it should be cauterized with a heated crescent-mouthed rod (Arddha-Chandra S'aláká) to prevent its descending down into the scrotal sac. A case of hernia that, in spite of all these precautions, descends down into the scrotal sac (Kosha), should be given up as irremediable. The first finger of the hand opposite * the affected part (*i.e.*, the affected testes) should be incised at its middle and cauterized.

---

\* Incision and cauterization should be performed in the thumb of the right hand, if the left testis is affected, and in case the affection is in the right testis, incision and cauterization should be made in the thumb of the left hand.

In cases of hernia (Antra-Vriddhi) of the **Vátaja** and of the **Kaphaja** type the affected part should be carefully cauterized in the above manner ; but in these two cases, the Snáyu (ligaments) should be cut off in addition (before cauterization). In a case of Antra-Vriddhi the veins (S'irá) of the temples at the (upper) end of the ears on the opposite sides of the affection should be carefully opened avoiding the Sevani therein. 9-12.

**Treatment of Upadams'a** * :—In cases of the curable type of Upadams'a, Sneha (oleaginous substances) should be first applied, and the affected part should be fomented. Then the veins of the penis should be opened, or leeches should be applied (to the organ) for the elimination of the contaminated blood † (according as the affections are more or less severe). 13.

**General Treatments :**—The system of the patient should be cleansed with both emetics and purgatives in the event of an excessive aggravation of the Doshas inasmuch as the local pain and swelling would subside simultaneously with the elimination of the aggravated Doshas from the system Medicinal Vastis (enemas) should be injected (into the rectum) in the way of a Niruha-Vasti for the elimination of the aggravated Doshas, where the weakness of the patient would prohibit the application of purgatives. 14.

**Treatment of Vátaja Upadams'a :**—In a case of the Vátaja type of the disease, drugs such as, *Propaundarika, Yashti-madhu, Varshábhu, Kushtha, Deva-dáru, Sarálá, Aguru* and *Rásná*, should be used as a plaster (over the affected organ). Similarly

---

\* See note, Chapter XII., Nidána Sthánam.

† Jejjata holds that leeches should be applied in a case of superficial Upadams'a.

plasters composed of *Nichula*, castor-seeds, and pulverised wheat and barley grains pasted with Sneha (clarified butter, oil, etc.) should be applied lukewarm to the seat of the disease, which should also be affused with a decoction of the above-mentioned drugs, *viz.*, *Prapaundarika*, etc. 15.

**Treatment of Pittaja Upadams'a :—** In a case of the Pittaja type of the disease, a plaster composed of *Gairika, Anjana, Yashti-madhu, S'áriva, Us'ira, Padmaka,* (red) *Chandana* and *Utpala* mixed with a Sneha (clarified butter),* or that composed of *Padma, Mrinála, Sarjja, Arjuna, Vetasa,* and *Yashti-madhu* mixed with clarified butter should be applied to the affected organ which should be sprinkled with a solution of milk, clarified butter, sugar, sugar-cane juice and honey, or with a cold decoction of the drugs of *Vata*, etc. 16.

**Treatment of Kaphaja Upadams'a :—** In a case of the Kaphaja type of the disease, a plaster composed of the barks of *S'ála, As'va-karna, Aja-karna* and *Dhava* pasted with Surá and mixed with oil, should be applied hot to the affected part. As an alternative, the drugs such as, *Haridrá, Ativishá, Mustá, Saralá, Deva-dáru, Patra,* Páthá, and *Pattura* should be used for similar purposes and the affected organ should be affused with a decoction of the drugs of the *Surasádi* and *A'ragvadhádi* groups. 17.

The above remedial measures, *viz.*, plasters, sprinkling (Parisheka), blood-letting and Sams'odhana (*i.e.*, application of purgatives, emetics, etc.) as well as those

---

\* According to S'ivadása the Sneha to be used in the plaster should be clarified butter washed a hundred times.

described in the Sutra Sthánam (and the first Chapter of the Chikitsita Sthánam), should be resorted to in a case of (non suppurated) Upadams'a. The physician should try his best to arrest the setting in of suppuration (in a case of Upadamsa) inasmuch as suppuration in (and consequent putrefaction of) the (local) veins, ligaments, skin and flesh would lead to the destruction of the organ (Dhvaja). An incision should be made as soon as suppuration would set in, and the pus and other putrid matters being drawn out, the incised part should be plastered with the paste of sesamum mixed with honey and clarified butter. The incidental ulcer should be washed with a decoction * of the leaves of Karavira, of *Játi* and *A'ragvadha*, or of *Vaijayanti* and *Arka*. 18.

The use of a medicinal plaster composed of the fine powders of *Sauráshtra-mrittiká, Gairika, Tuttha, Pushpa-Kásisa, Saindhava, Rodhra, Rasánjana, Dáru-Haridrá, Haritála, Manahs'ilá, Harenuká* and *Elá*, mixed with honey is highly recommended in all cases of Upadams'a. 19.

A decoction of the tender leaves of *Jambu, A'mra, Sumanas, Nimba, S'vetá*, and of *Kámboji* † and the barks of *S'allaki, Vadara, Vilva, Palás'a, Tinis'a* and of the *Kshiri* trees, as well as *Triphalá* should be used by the physician for constantly washing the ulcer. Oil cooked with the preceding decoction, with the Kalkas of *Goji, Vidanga* and *Yashti-madhu*, as well as with the different spices (Eládi group) should be used as the best remedy for the purpose of the healing up (Ropana) of

---

* According to Chakradatta the five kinds of leaves should be separately used in the preparations of the decoctions for washing.

† "Máshaparni" according to Gayadása.

an Upadams'a-ulcer of whatsoever type. The use of a pulverised compound composed of *Svarjiká, Tuttha, Kásisa, S'aileya, Rasánjana,* and *Manahs'ilá* taken in equal parts arrests the extension of an ulcer and Visarpa. Cases of Upadams'a and Visarpa readily yield to the application of a pulverised compound of the ashes of *Gundrá, Haritála* and *Manahs'ilá.* An (external) application of *Bhrimgarája, Triphalá* and *Danti* mixed with the powders of copper and iron, destroys Upadams'a just as the thunder-bolt of Indra (completely) destroys a tree. 20.

**Treatment of Tridoshaja and Raktaja Upadams'a:**—The medical treatment of the two kinds of Upadams'a due to the concerted action of the three Doshas as well as that due to the vitiated blood (**Raktaja**) should be taken in hand without holding out any definite hope of recovery. The above-mentioned medicines specific to the different Doshas should be combinedly applied in these cases in consideration of the nature and intensity of the Doshas specifically involved in them. Now hear me discourse on the special treatment of **Tridoshaja** Upadams'a. It should be the same as in the case of a malignant ulcer (Dushta-Vrana). The putrid portion of the male organ should be cut off and the remaining portion should be fully cauterized (in the incised part) with a Jambvoshtha instrument, made red-hot in fire. Honey, and clarified butter should then be applied to the cauterized part, and medicinal plasters and oils possessed of healing properties should be applied to the incidental ulcer when it would be cleansed (disinfected). 21-22.

**Treatment of Slipada:**—In a case of Elephantiasis (Slipada) due to the action of the deranged and aggravated **Váyu**, the vein (Sirá) at a distance of four fingers above the instep (Gulpha) should be opened after an application of Sneha and Sveda * to the patient. Vastis should be employed when the patient has been (soothed and) restored to his former condition (with appropriate and nutritious diet, etc.). He should be made to take continuously for a month, a potion consisting of castor-oil mixed with (an adequate quantity of cow's) urine The patient should take rice as his diet with milk duly cooked with S'unthi. The use of the **Traivrita Ghrita** as well as cauterization of the affected part with fire is also recommended in such a case. 23

**Treatment of Pittaja Ślipada :** — In a case of Pittaja type of Elephantiasis, the vein (Sirá) below the instep (Gulpha) should be opened. Medicinal remedies mentioned in connection with the treatment of the Pittaja type of tumours (Arvuda) and of Erysipelas (Visarpa) as well as other Pitta-subduing remedies and measures should be employed†. 24.

**Treatment of Kaphaja Ślipada :** — In a case of the Kaphaja type of elephantiasis the principal vein (Sirá) of the first toe should be opened by an experienced surgeon and the patient should be made to take at intervals the decoction (of the Kapha-subduing drugs) with honey. As an alternative, the patient should be advised to take the powders (Kalka) of *Abhayá* mixed with any officinal kind of urine The affected locality should be constantly plastered with the paste

---

\* Chakradatta reads "स्वेदं दीपनाहांश्च" in place of "स्वेदं दीपपन्ने तु" meaning thereby that such Sveda and Upanáha should be applied before the incision of the Vein. Gayadása also supports this reading as is evident from Dallana's commentary.—Ed.

† The particle "च" in the text shows that Kapha-subduing remedies and measures should also be used in all these cases,

of *Katuka, Amritá, S'unthi, Vidanga, Deva-dáru* and *Chitraka*, or with *Chitraka* and *Deva-dáru*. An oil cooked with *Vidanga, Maricha, Arka, S'unthi, Chitraka, Deva-dáru, Elaká* and all the five officinal kinds of salt should be given him as a potion. Cooked barley is specially recommended as diet in the present case. 25.

As an alternative, the patient should be made to drink a potion of mustard oil* or of the expressed juice of the leaves of *Puti-Karanja* according to his capacity for the cure of S'lipada. In the same way† the juice of *Putranjivaka* should be prescribed by a physician after a due consideration as to the strength of the patient and of the time. The same juice (*i.e.*, of Putranjivaka) should be taken along with the juice of the bulbs of *Kechuka* with Pákima (vit) salt. 26.

**The Alkaline Remedies :**—An alkali should be prepared from the ashes of *Kákádani, Kákajanghá, Vrihati, Kantakáriká, Kadamba-pushpa, Mandári, Lambá Sukanasá* in the usual way by filtering them (twenty one times) after dissolving them in cow's urine. The expressed juice of *Kákodumbariká, Sukanasá* and the decoction of *Madana* fruit should be mixed with the above alkaline preparation (and duly cooked in the manner of Kshára-páka). Diseases, such as S'lipada

---

\* Chakradatta reads "पिवेत् सर्षप तैलेन" in place of "पिवेत् सर्षप तैल वा" which shows that the expressed juice of Puti-Karania leaves should be taken with mustard oil and not separately. Dallana evidently supports this in his commentary. That Chakradatta's reading is the correct one is also evident from the next copulet which says that the expressed juice of Putranjivaka should be taken in the preceding manner. This "preceding manner" evidently means "with mustard oil", and unless we accept Chakradatta's reading, the expression would be unmeaning.—Ed.

† It evidently means that the expressed juice of Putranjivaka should be taken with mustard oil—see last note.—Ed.

(Elephantiasis), Apachi (Scrofula), Gala-ganda (Goitre), Grahani (chronic diarrhœa), aversion to food and the affections of all kinds of poison, yield to the internal use of this alkaline preparation. An oil cooked with the aforesaid drugs, if used as errhines and anointments, will cure all the foregoing maladies as well as malignant ulcers (Dushta-vrana). 27.

The ashes of the *Dravanti, Trivrit, Danti. Nili, S'yamá, Saptalá* and *S'amkhini* should be filtered in the way of preparing alkalies after dissolving them in cow's urine. The solution, thus prepared, should be boiled with a decoction of **Triphala.** Taken internally it tends to act in the lower part of the body (*ie*, it moves the bowels). This medicine produces the same effect as the preceding ones. 28.

Thus ends the nineteenth Chapter of the Chikitsita Sthánam in the Sus'ruta Samhitá which deals with the medical treatment of Vriddhi, Upadams'a and S'lipada.

# CHAPTER XX.

Now we shall discourse on the medical treatment of the minor ailments or diseases (**Kshudra-roga**). 1.

**Treatment of Aja-gallika :**—Leeches * should be applied to the affected part in a case of non-suppurated **Aja-gallika**; it should be subsequently plastered with the alkalies (Kshára) of oyster-shells, *S'rughni* (Svarjiká), † and of *Yava*; as an alternative, it should be plastered with the paste compound (Kalka) of *S'yámá, Lángalaki* and *Páthá*. When suppurated it should be treated in the manner of an ulcer (Vrana). 2.

**Treatment of Yava-prakhyá, etc. :**— Fomentation (Sveda) should be the first remedy to be resorted to in cases of **Antrálaji, Yava-prakhyá, Panasi, Kachchhapi** and **Páshána-gardabha** (in their non-suppurated stages). They should then be plastered with the pastes (Kalka) of *Manahs'ilá, Haritála, Kushtha* and *Deva-dáru* An incision should be made as soon as suppuration would set in; and the treatment should be similar to that of an ulcer. 3-4.

**Treatment of Vivritá, etc. :**—The remedies mentioned in connection with the treatment of the Pittaja type of Erysipelas (Visarpa) should be employed in cases of **Vivritá, Indra-vriddhá, Gardabhi, Jála-gardabha, Irivelli, Kakshá, Gandha-námni** and **Visphotaka**. Clarified butter cooked with

---

* Gayadása explains that a non-suppurated **Aja-gallika** should be first plastered with Yava-kshára, oyster-shells and Sauráshtri. Leeches should be next applied to it.

† Chakradatta reads "शुक्तिसौराष्ट्रका क्षार &c." in place of "शुक्तियुक्त्री-यवक्षार &c.", evidently, after the commentary of Gayadása

the drugs of the *Madhura* (Kákolyádi) group should be applied in healing up the ulcers in the suppurated stages. 5.

**Treatment of Chipya, etc :**—In a case of **Chipya**, the affected part should be first washed* with hot water and (the incarcerated pus, etc.) drained (Visráva) by cutting it away (with a knife). Then after anointing it with (the oil known as) the **Chakra-taila** it should be dusted over with the powders of Sarja (resin) and duly bandaged. If this process of treatment fail, the affected part should be cauterised with fire and an oil cooked with (a decoction of) the drugs of the *Madhura* (Kákolyádi) group should be applied to heal (the incidental ulcer). The same course of treatment should also be adopted in a case of **Ku-nakha** (bad nail). 6-7.

**Treatment of Vidáriká :**—In a case of **Vidáriká**, the affected part should be first anointed (with oleaginous substances) and then fomented. It should then be rubbed (with the fingers) ; and a plaster composed of *Naga-Vriitika*, *Varshábhu* and *Vilva*-roots, well pasted together, should be applied to it. Purifying and disinfecting (Sams'odhana) remedies should be employed as soon as the affected part would be found to have been changed into the state of an ulcer (Vrana), and it should then be healed up with the application of an oil cooked with the decoction of (the drugs of the *Kasháya* (Nyagrodhádi) and *Madhura* (Kákolyádi) groups In the non suppurated stage of *Vidáriká*, the vitiated blood therein should be let out by means of Prachchhána (scarification), or by applying leeches. The affected part should then be plastered with

---

* Vrinda and Chakradatta prescribe fomentation (Sveda), and not washing, with hot water and they do not prescribe secretion (Visráva).

the roots of the *Aja-karna* and of the *Palása* pasted together. A case of fully suppurated **Vidárika** should be lanced and plastered with a paste compound of *Patola*, *Pichumarda* and sesamum, mixed with clarified butter and should then be duly bandaged. The incidental ulcer should then be washed with a decoction (of the barks) of the *Kshiri* trees and *Khadira*. Healing remedies should be applied after it has been properly purified (disinfected) 8-9.

**Treatment of Śarkarárvuda, etc.:**—A case of Sarkarárvuda should be treated like that of an Arvuda (tumour) of the fat-origined type. Cases of **Kachchhu, Vicharchiká** and **Pámá** should be treated in the manner of a Kushtha. A medicinal plaster composed of *Siktha* (wax), *S'atáhvá* and white mustard seeds, or of *Vachá*, *Dáru-haridrá* and mustard seeds, pasted together, should be applied (to the seat of the disease). As an alternative, *Naktamála* (Karanja) oil, or *Sára-taila* \* boiled with (the drugs of) the *Katuka* (Pippalyádi) group should be applied for anointing purposes. 10-11.

**Treatment of Páda-dári :**—In a case of Páda-dári, the prescribed vein should be opened, and the affected part should be treated with fomentations and unguents. † The affected part should be plastered with (an ointment composed of) wax, lard, marrow, powder of *Sarja* resin),‡ clarified butter, *Yava-Kshára* and *Gairika*. 12.

---

\* By "Sára-taila" is meant the oil pressed from the Sára (essential parts) of S'ims'apá, Aguru, Sarala, Deva-dáru and such other trees. Some, however, read "Sarala-taila" in place of "Sára-taila."—Dallana.

† According to Dallana and S'ivadása, fomentations and unguents should be first applied, and the Vein should be next opened.

‡ Chakradatta also prescribes a similar remedy, but there he does not read "Sarja" and "Gairika,"—Ed.

**Treatment of Alasa and Kadara :**—In a case of **Alasa**,.the legs should be sprinkled with *Árandla* (a kind of Kánjika); and a plaster composed of sesamum, *Nimba* leaves, sulphate of iron (*Kásisa*), Haritála and *Saindhava*, or of *Haritaki* pasted with the decoction of *Lákshá* (Lákshá-rasa)* should be applied to the affected parts. Blood-letting should also be resorted to. As an alternative, mustard oil boiled with the expressed juice of *Kantakári* should be applied to them or the affected localities should be rubbed or chafed (Piatisárana) with a pulverised compound of sulphate of iron (Kásisa), *Gorochaná* and *Manah-s'ilá*. In a case of **Kadara**, the seat of the disease should be scraped off (with the aid of a knife) and cauterised with (the application of) heated oil † 13-14.

**Treatment of Indra-lupta :**— In a case of **Indra-lupta** (baldness or Alopecia), the bald part or seat should be anointed and fomented, and then bleeding (by venesection) should be resorted to, after which a plaster composed of *Manah-s'ilá, Kásisá, Tuttha* and *Maricha*, or of *Kutannatá* and *Deva-dáru* pasted together, should be applied to it. As an alternative, it should be deeply scraped and constantly kept covered with a paste of *Gunjá*-seeds. As an alternative, **Rasáyana** medicines should be administered for its cure. An oil cooked with *Málati, Karavira, Chitraka* and *Naktamála* is highly efficacious in curing a case of Alopecia, if used as an unguent. 15.

**Treatment of Arumshiká :** - Blood-let-

---

* Chakrapáni reads ' लाचाभयारसालि प:' in place of "लाचारसोऽभया वारि". Sivadása explains "रस:" as ' गन्धरस: "—Ed.

† Chakradatta prescribes cauterisation with fire as well, in such a case.—Ed.

ting* from the affected part should be first resorted to in a case of **Arumshiká**; and it should then be affused with the decoction of *Nimba* Medicinal plasters prepared with the Rasa (liquid) pressed from horse-dung, mixed with *Saindhava,* should be applied to it. As an alternative, it should be plastered with the paste compound (Kalka) of *Haritála, Haridrá, Nimba* and *Patola,* or with that of *Yasthi-madhu, Nilotpala, Eranda,* and *Márkava.* 16.

**Treatment of Dárunaka, etc.:**—Anointment and fomentation of the diseased patches are the (preliminary) remedies in a case of **Dárunaka,** after which bleeding should be effected by opening the vein in the forehead Remedial measures such as, **Avapida-Sirovasti** and **Abhyanga** (anointment) should be employed as well ; and the affected parts should be washed with the alkaline solution of burnt *Kodrava* weeds. Measures for arresting the premature greyness of hair (**Palitá**) will be described later on (in the Mis'raka Chapter XXV). Curative plasters and remedies, etc , mentioned in connection with the treatment of Kushtha should be employed in cases of **Masuriká**; or those, laid down under the treatment of Erysipelas (Visarpa) originated through the concerted action of the deranged Pitta and Kapha should as well be used. 17-19.

**Treatment of Jatu-mani, etc. :**—The seats of affection should be scraped (with a knife) and gradually and judiciously cauterised† by applying an alkali or fire in cases of **Jatu mani** (congenital moles), **Mas'aka** and **Tila-kálaka**

---

\* According to Chakradatta blood-letting should be resorted to in such cases only by means of venesection, or with leeches.

† The cauterisation should be effected with an alkali, when the disease is superficial and with fire when it is deep-seated.

(freckles) An opening of the local veins in the temporal region, etc., should be effected in cases of **Nyachchha, Vyanga** and **Nilika**, in accordance with the prescribed rules. The affected parts should be rubbed (with Samudra-phena, etc.) and plastered with the barks of *Kshiri* trees, pasted with milk ; or with *Vala, Ati-vala, Yashti-madhu* and *Rajani*, pasted together. As an alternative, plasters composed of *Payasyá, Aguru* and *Káliya* pasted together with *Gairika*, or of a tooth of a boar pasted with clarified butter and honey, or of *Kapittha* and *Rájádana* pasted together, may also be used with benefit  20 21.

**Treatment of Yuvána-Pidaká, etc:.—** Emetics are specially efficacious in cases of **Yuvána-pidaká** (pimples) which disfigure the face in youth. The application of medicinal plasters composed of *Vachá, Lodhra, Saindhava* and (white mustard seeds or of *Kustumburu, Vachá, Lodhra* and *Kushtha* pasted together is also recommended. In a case of **Padmini-Kantaka**, a decoction of *Nimba* bark should be given as an emetic, and the patient should be made to drink a potion of clarified butter cooked with a decoction of *Nimba* and mixed with honey. A decoction * of *Nimba* and *Áragvadha* should be used for chafing (Utsádana) the diseased locality.  22-23.

**Treatment of Parivartiká, etc.:—**In a case of **Parivartiká** (retroflexion of the prepuce) the *glans penis* should be rubbed with clarified butter and duly fomented, and **Sálvana** and such other Váyu-subduing plasters (Upanáha) should be applied for three

---

\* Chakrapáni prescribes the powders (कल्क) in place of the decoction (क्वाथ) of Nimba and Áragvadha. He also reads "उद्वर्तन" in place of "उत्सादन", but here they mean the same thing.—Ed.

or five days. Then having lubricated the part (with Ghrita), the *glans penis* should be gently pressed and the prepuce should be smoothly drawn over the *glans penis*, so as to cover it entirely within its fold. The prepuce, being so drawn, should be fomented with warm poultices. Váyu-subduing Vastis (Clysters) should be employed and emollient diet should be prescribed (during the course of the treatment). A case of **Avapátiká** should be similarly treated, after a due consideration of the nature and intensity of the Doshas involved in the case. 24-25

**Treatment of Niruddha-Prakas'a :—** In a case of **Niruddha-Prakaśa** (constriction or stricture of the urethra), a tube (open at both ends) made of iron, wood, or shellac should be lubricated with clarified butter and gently introduced into the urethra. The marrow or lard of a boar, or of a porpoise, or the **Chakra-taila**, mixed with Váyu-subduing drugs should be sprinkled over the affected part. Thicker and thicker tubes should be duly introduced into the urethra every third day. The passage should be made to dilate in the aforesaid manner, and emollient food should be given to the patient. As an alternative, an incision should be made (into the lower part of the penis), avoiding the sevani (raphe of the perineum), and it should be treated as an incidental ulcer Sadyo-vrana). 26.

**Treatment of Sanniruddha-Guda, etc. :**—Cases of **Sanniruddha-Guda** (stricture of the anus), **Valmika** and **Agni-Rohini** should be duly treated with regard to the nature and intensity (of the Doshas engendering the disease), but without holding out any definite hope of recovery. The treatment of a case of **Agni-Rohini** should be like that of Visarpa (Erysipelas), while the remedial measures, mentioned in connection with Niruddha-prakaśa, should be employed in a case of Sanniruddha-Guda. 27.

**Treatment of Valmika :**—The diseased patches should be scraped off in a case of **Valmika** and cauterised with fire or with an alkali ; while the purification and healing up (of the incidental ulcer) should be effected as in the treatment of an Arvuda (tumour). A case of Valmika appearing in any part of the body other than a Marma, and not of a considerable growth should be duly treated with venesection after the application of Samśodhana measures (purgative, emetic, etc.). The affected part should be plastered (Pralepa) with a medicinal compound composed of the roots of (*Vana-*) *Kulattha, Arevata, Danti* and *S'yámá*, pasted together with *Guduchi*, rock-salt, Palala (pastes of sesamum) and powdered barley. It should be poulticed (Upanáha) with the same compound, well mixed with clarified butter and made lukewarm (in case suppuration be desired). When found to be fully suppurated, the course of the pus-channels should be ascertained by an experienced surgeon. The ulcer should then be opened (with a knife) and cauterised, and after being fully purified of the putrid flesh (in its cavity), it should be again cauterised with an alkali. Healing (Ropana) remedies should be applied to it after it has been found to be thoroughly cleansed **Nimba-oil** cooked with *Sumanas* (Játi leaves, *Granthi, Bhallátaka, Manah s'ilá, Kálánusári*, small *Elá, Aguru* and red *Chandana* should be applied with advantage to heal up the (incidental ulcer in a case of) Valmika. A patient suffering from an attack of Valmika appearing either on his hands or feet and attended with swelling and a large number of cavities should be abandoned by a wise physician. 28.

**Treatment of Ahi-putaná, etc.:**—In the treatment of an infant laid up with an attack of **Ahi putaná** the breast-milk of its mother or nurse should be first purified. Cases of Ahi-putaná yield to the use of a potion of clarified butter, cooked with *Triphalá, Rasánjana* and *Patola* leaves, and a decoction of *Triphalá, Kola* and *Khadira* should be used (as a wash) to heal the ulcer. Plasters composed of sulphate of iron, *Gorochaná,* sulphate of copper (*Tuttha*), *Haritála* and *Rasánjana,* pasted together with Kánjika, or of *Vadari* bark and rock-salt, should be applied (to the diseased locality). It should be dusted as well with the pulverised compound of a burnt earthen pot and sulphate of copper. The preceding measures should be adopted in cases of **Vrishana-Kachchhu** as well. 29-30.

**Treatment of Guda-Bhramśa:**—In a case of **Guda-Bhramśa,** the protruded part should be fomented and lubricated with Sneha.* It should then be gently re-introduced. The region of the anus should then be bandaged with a piece of hide in the manner of a Gophaná Bandha, with an opening in it (lying immediately below the anus), so that it may not in any way interfere with the emission of Váyu. The affected part should then be constantly fomented. A quantity of milk, *Mahá-pancha-mula* and the body (flesh) of a mouse, bereft of its entrails should be first boiled together (with water). An oil cooked with the milk thus prepared (with water) and the Váyu–subduing drugs should be administered as drink and unguents. By these measures the most difficult cases of **prolapsus ani** would be cured. 31-32.

---

* According to S'iva-dása, cow's fat only should be used.

Thus ends the twentieth Chapter of the Chikitsita Sthánam in the Sus'ruta Samhitá which deals with the treatment of minor ailments.

# CHAPTER XXI.

Now we shall discourse on the medical treatment of the Sores on the penis produced by the Śuka, a kind of poisonous insect (**Śuka-Roga**). 1.

**Treatment of Sarshapi, etc.**:—In a case of the **Sarshapi** type of the disease, the affected (ulcerated) part should be scarified and dusted with the (powdered) drugs of an astringent taste (as described in the Miśraka chapter), and an oil, cooked with (the Kalka and decoction of) the same drugs, should be applied for healing purposes. In a case of the **Ashthiliká** type of the disease, the skilful physician should apply leeches to the seat of affection. In case the swelling does not still subside, it should be removed and treated as a Kaphaja Granthi (glandular swelling). A **Granthi** type of the disease should be constantly fomented in the manner of **Nádi-Sveda**, and should be poulticed with a lukewarm medicinal compound mixed with a profuse quantity of Sneha (oil). 2-4.

**Treatment of Kumbhiká, etc.**:—An incision should be made into the suppurated seat of affection in a case of the **Kumbhiká** type of the disease, and the incidental ulcer should be purified (disinfected) and healed up with the application of the oil, cooked with *Triphalá, Lodhra, Tinduka* and *Ámrátaka*.* In the **Alaji** type of the disease, the affected part should be bled by applying leeches to it and should then be affused with a decoction of the astringent drugs. An

---

\* Śiva-dása in his commentary on Chakra-datta quotes this couplet from Suśruta, but there he reads आम्रकृतेन in place of आम्रातकेन; that is to say, he says that Ámra should be used in place of Ámrátaka. He further adds that the stones of Ámra and Tinduka fruits should be taken.

oil, cooked with the decoction of the same drugs, should be used to heal up the (incidental) ulcer. 5-6.

**Treatment of Mridita, etc. :**—In the **Mridita** type of the disease, the affected part should be affused with tepid **Valá** oil and poulticed with a lukewarm plaster (Upanáha) of the drugs of the *Madhura* (Kákolyádi) group, pasted and mixed with clarified butter. Leeches should be speedily applied to the condylomatous growths (**Pidaká**) in a case of **Sammudha-Pidaká**. In cases of suppuration, they should be opened and plastered with honey and clarified butter. In a case of **Avamantha**, the growths (Pidaká) should be opened, when suppurated, and healed up with the application of an oil, cooked with *Dhava, As'va-Karna, Pattanga, S'allaki* and *Tinduka.* 7—9

**Treatment of Pushkariká, etc. :**—In a case of **Pushkariká**, all kinds of cooling measures should be applied and the vitiated blood should be extracted by applying leeches. The affected part should be subsequently affused with clarified butter. In a case of the **Sparśa-háni** type of the disease, blood should be let out and plasters (Pradeha) of *Madhura* (Kákolyádi) drugs should be applied. The affected part should be affused with a very cold compound of milk, clarified butter and the expressed juice of sugar cane. In the type of the disease known as **Uttamá**, the Pidakás (condylomatous growths) should be removed with the help of a Vadisa instrument, and powders of astringent drugs with honey should be applied to the seat of affection. 10—12.

**Treatment of S'ata-ponaka, etc.:**—In a case of the **S'ata-ponaka** type of the disease, the affected part should be scarified and the measures laid down in connection with Rasa-Kriyá should be resorted to,

After this, an oil, cooked with the *Prithak-parnyádi* drugs,* should be likewise applied to the seat of the disease. The medicinal treatment, in a case of **Tvak-páka,** should be the same as described in connection with Erysipelas (Visarpa). The remedial measures, laid down under the head of Rakta-vidradhi, should be employed in a case of the **Śonitárvuda** type of the disease. 13-14.

**General Treatment :**—Remedies such as medicinal decoctions, pastes (Kalka), medicated clarified butter, powders, Rasa-Kriyá, etc., and the measures for purifying and healing (incidental sores or ulcers), should be employed with due consideration to the nature and intensity of the aggravated Doshas involved in the case The application of specifically prepared medicated clarified butter, purgatives, blood-letting and light diet should be similarly prescribed.† 15.

**Prognosis :**—The medical treatment of the patient affected with any of the following types of the disease, viz., Arvuda, Mámsa-páka, Vidradhi and Tila-Kálaka should be undertaken without holding out any definite prospect of recovery. 16.

Thus ends the twenty-first Chapter of the Chikitsita Sthánam in the Susruta Samhitá which deals with the treatment of S'uka-Roga.

* For Rasa-kriyá and the Prithak-parnyádi drugs, see Chapter XXXVI—Sutra-sthána.

† This seems to be the general treatment of all the types of S uka-Roga.

## CHAPTER XXII.

Now we shall discourse on the medical treatment of the affections of the mouth (**Mukha-Roga**). 1.

**Treatment of Vátaja Oshtha-kopa:**— In a case of inflammation of the lips (Oshtha-Kopa) due to the action of the deranged **Váyu**, the affected part should be rubbed with (an ointment composed of) the four kinds of lardacious (Sneha) substances mixed with wax. Fomentations in the manner of **Nádi-Sveda** should also be resorted to by an intelligent physician Applications of the **Sálvana** poultices and those of the medicated oils, possessed of the virtue of subduing the deranged Váyu, as errhines and **Mastikya** (S'iro-vasti) are also recommended. The lips should be treated with the powder composed of S'ri-veshtaka,* Sarja rasa, Sura-dáru, Guggulu and Yashti-madhu. 2-4.

**Treatment of Pittaja Oshtha-kopa, etc.:**— In a case of Oshtha-kopa of traumatic origin, (**Abhigha'taja**) or one due to the deranged action of the blood (**Raktaja**) or of the Pitta, bleeding of the affected part should be effected by the application of leeches and all the measures and remedies (Sams'odhana and Sams'amana) mentioned in connection with the treatment of the Pitta-Vidradhi should be likewise employed. 5.

**Treatment of Kaphaja Oshthakopa:** —The use of medicated S'iro-virechana (errhines), fumigations, (Vairechanika Dhuma), fomentation and (Sveda) Kavala (gurgles), prepared from the Kapha-subduing drugs should be recommended after blood-letting in the **Kaphaja** type of Oshtha-kopa. The swollen and inflamed lips should be treated (Prati-sárana) with a compound con-

* Vágbhata reads " मधूच्छिष्टं " i. e., wax, in place of श्रीवेष्टकम् ।

sisting of *Trikatu, Sarjiká-kshára, Yava-Kshára* and *Vid-lavana* (black-salt) * pounded together and made into a thin paste with the admixture of honey. 6

**Treatment of Medoja Oshtha-kopa :** —In a case of the **fatty** type of Oshtha-kopa, the affected part should be fomented and opened (when suppurated) ; and should then be purified and cauterised with fire. A paste compound of *Priyangu, Triphalá, Lodhra* and honey should be rubbed over the affected part (Prati-sárana). These are the remedies for the curable types of Oshtha-kopa. 7-8.

**Treatment of the Diseases of Danta -Mula :** —Now we shall describe the treatment of the affection of the roots of the teeth (Gingivitis). In a case of the **Sitáda** type of the disease, the gums should be first bled and a decoction of *Sarshapa, Nágara, Triphalá* and *Musta* † mixed with *Rasánjana* should then be used as gurgles. The gums should be plastered (Pralepa) with *Priyangu, Musta* and *Triphalá* and (clarified butter, cooked with) the decoction of *Triphalá, Madhuka, Utpala* and *Padmaka* should be used as an errhine. In an acute case of **Danta-Pupputaka**, the gums should be first bled and then rubbed (Prati-sárana) with the five officinal kinds of salt and *Yava-Kshára* mixed with honey. The use of errhines (Siro-virechana), medicated snuffs (Nasya) and demulcent food is recommended. 9-10.

**Treatment of Danta-Veshta, etc. :—** In a case of **Danta-Veshta**, the swelling should be first bled and then rubbed with a pulverised compound of *Rodhra, Pattanga, Yashti-madhu* and *Láksha* mixed with a profuse quantity of honey. A decoction of (the bark

---

\* Vrinda and Chakrapáni do not read Vid-laVana.

† Vrinda and Chakra-datta do not read Musta, nor Rasánjana.

of) the *Kshiri* trees, mixed with sugar, honey and clarified butter (as an after-throw) should be used as gurgles (Gandusha). Clarified butter, cooked with the drugs of the *Kákolyádi* group with ten times its own weight of milk, should be used as snuff (Nasya). In a case of **Saushira**, the affected parts, after being properly bled, should be plastered (Lepa) with *Lodhra, Musta* and *Rasánjana*, pounded together and mixed with honey. A decoction of the *Kshiri* trees should be used as gurgles (Gandusha), and clarified butter cooked with the paste-compound of *Sárivá, Utpala, Yashti-madhu, Sávara* (Lodhra), *Aguru,* (red) *Chandana* and ten times its own weight of milk should be recommended as an errhine. 11-12.

**Treatment of Pari-dara, etc. :**—In a case of **Pari-dara** the treatment should consist of the remedies described in connection with Sítáda. In a case of **Upa kusá** as well,[*] the system of the patient should be cleansed both ways (by means of emetics and purgatives), and his head should be cleansed with Siro-virechana. The affected part (in a case of Upa-kusá) should, in addition, be bled (by rubbing it over) with the leaves of the *Kákodumbariká*, or of the *Goji,* or with the application of a medicinal compound composed of the five officinal kinds of salt and *Trikatu* mixed with honey. Tepid watery solutions[†] of *Pippali,* (white) *Sarshapa, Nágara,* and *Nichula* fruits should also be used as gurgles (Kavala). The use of clarified butter cooked with the drugs of the *Madhura* (Kákolyádi)

---

[*] This shows that cleansing the system by means of emetics and purgatives, as well as with S'iro-virechana should be resorted to in a case of Pari-dara as well.

[†] The solution may be prepared with the drugs taken together or separately.

group as errhine (Nasya) and gurgle (Kavala) is also recommended. 13-14.

**Treatment of Danta-Vaidarbha, etc.:** —In a case of **Danta-Vaidarbha**, the regions about the roots of the teeth should be cleansed by opening them with a (Mandalágra) instrument and subsequently treated with alkaline applications. Cooling measures should also be resorted to (during the treatment of this disease). In a case of **Adhika-danta,** the additional tooth should be uprooted and removed; then (in order to arrest the bleeding, if any), the part should be cauterised with fire, and then an experienced physician should apply the remedies mentioned under the head of worm-eaten teeth (Krimi-dantaka). 15-16

**Treatment of Adhi-mámsa :**—In a case of **Adhi-mámsa,** the additional fleshy growth about the roots of a tooth should be removed (with a knife) and treated with a compound of *Vachá, Tejovati, Páthá, Sarjiká* and *Yava-kshára,* pasted together with honey. Powdered *Pippali,* mixed with honey, should be used as a gurgle (Kavala); and a decoction of *Patola, Triphalá* and *Nimba* for washing the affected part. Errhines (Śiro-virechana) and inhalation of Vairechana smoke, (that lead to the secretion of mucus from the head), would likewise prove efficacious in such cases. 17.

**Treatment of Danta-Nádi :**—In a case of **Danta-Nadi,** the treatment of Nádi (Sinus) about the teeth is identical with that of sinus in general. The specific remedial measure, however, is that the gum of the affected tooth should be incised, and the tooth should be extracted, if it be not in the upper jaw The affected part should then be purified and cauterised with an alkali or fire Hence in a case of Sinus (Nádi), a complete extraction of any fragment of the broken bone, or tooth, is essentially necessary (for its cure), inasmuch as, if left unextracted, it may cause the sinus to affect (run below) the jaw-bone. If the affected tooth be in the upper jaw, and if it be found to be firm and steady at its roots, though attended with tooth-ache,* it should not be extracted, inasmuch as it might produce an excessive hæmorrhage from its roots, and usher in blindness, facial paralysis, or other dangerous affections (such as convulsion, etc.) due to the excessive loss of blood. Hence in the case of a looseness of such a tooth in the upper jaw, it should not be extracted A decoction † of *Játi*, *Madana*, *Svádu-Kantaka* and *Khadira* should be used to wash the mouth. An oil cooked with *Játi*, *Madana*, *Katuka*, *Svádu-Kantaka*, *Yashti-madhu*, *Rodhra*, *Manjishthá* and *Khadira* should be used to cleanse and heal a sinus invading the roots of a tooth. The remedial measures to be employed in the diseases affecting the roots of the teeth have thus been described above.

---

\* Both Vrinda and Chakradatta quote this passage from the text, but both of them read "शोणितं सम्प्रसिच्यते" (excessive bleeding takes place) in place of "सम्यूले स्थिरबन्धने" (if it be found to be firm and steady at its roots, though attended with tooth-ache). S'ri-kantha Datta, again, in his commentary quotes another reading "समूलेऽस्थिरबन्धने" (if it be loose in its sockets and be extracted with its roots). In our humble opinion, however, the current reading of the text seems to be the correct one, inasmuch as both the readings quoted above seem to be redundant in the presence of the two following sentences "रक्तातियोगात्......" and "चलमप्युत्तरं दन्तं..."—Ed.

† According to S'rikantha and S'ivadása, it appears that the application of this decoction as a wash is not to be found in all editions of the Sus'ruta Samhitá, but they say that it is found only in Jejjatá's reading. Jejjatá's reading and explanation seem to be correct and have been followed by us in the translation.—Ed.

We shall now proceed to describe the medicinal remedies to be employed in the diseases which confine themselves exclusively to the teeth. 18-21.

**Treatment of the diseases of Tooth proper :**—A case of Danta-harsha yields to the use of any lukewarm Sneha,* or the **Traivrita-ghrita** (mentioned in Chapter V), or of the decoction of the Váyu-subduing drugs as gurgles (Kavala). An application of **Snaihika Dhuma** (emulsive fumes) and the use of snuff (Nasya), emulsive articles of food, meat soups, gruel prepared with meat (Rasa-Yavágu), milk, milk-cream, clarified butter, Śiro-vasti and the other Váyu-subduing measures generally prove efficacious. 22.

In a case of **Danta Sarkará** (Tartar-calcareous deposits on the teeth), the deposit should be removed in such a way as not to hurt the roots of the tooth, after which the part should be dusted (Prati-sárana) with powdered *Lákshá* with honey. All the remedies mentioned in connection with the treatment of Danta-harsha may as well be employed in this disease. 23

**Treatment of Kapáliká, etc. :**—These remedies are also efficacious in a case of **Kapáliká** (caries of the tooth) which is extremely hard to cure. In a case of **Krimi-Danta** (worm-eaten tooth) found to be firm and unloosed (in its socket), the affected tooth should be fomented, and the accumulation (*i. e.*, the pus, blood, etc.) should be removed. It should then be treated with some Váyu-subduing errhines of the **Ava-pida** form and with emollient gurgles (Gandusha), as well as with plasters, prepared with *Varshábhu* and the drugs of the *Bhadra-Dárvádi* group and with a diet of emulsive articles of food. In the case, however, where

* All the four kinds of Sneha should be used separately or combinedly.

the tooth is found to be loose (in the socket), the loose tooth should be extracted, and the cavity cauterised with fire or an alkali (for the purpose of arresting the bleeding). An oil cooked with the pastes (Kalka) of *Vidári, Yashti-madhu, S'ringátaka,* and *Kas'eruka* and with ten times its own weight of milk should be administered as an errhine (in such cases). The course of treatment in a case of **Hanu-moksha** is the same as in one of facial paralysis. 24-27.

A person suffering from any affection of the teeth should refrain from taking acid fruits, cold water, dry (Ruksha) food, excessively hard articles of food and from brushing his teeth (with a twig). The treatment of the curable types of tooth-diseases has been thus described above, we shall now (proceed to) describe the treatment of the curable types of **tongue**-diseases. 28 29.

**Treatment of Tongue-diseases :—**In the **Vátaja** type of **Jihvá-kantaka** (Papilla), the treatment should be the same as in the case of Vátaja Oshtha-kopa. In the **Pittaja** type (of Jihvá kantaka), the vitiated blood should be made to secrete from the affected organ by rubbing it with any article of rough surface (such as the leaves of *S'ákhotaka*, etc.), and the drugs of the *Madhura* (Kákolyádi) group should be used for gurgles and errhines, as well as for being rubbed over (Prati-sárana) the affected organ. In the **Kaphaja** type (of Jihvá-kantaka), the organ should be bled by scarifying it (with a Mandala patra and such other instrument) ; it should then be rubbed with the powders of the drugs of the *Pippalyádi* group mixed with honey. A compound of powdered white mustard-seed and Saindhava should be administered as gurgles (Kavala), and the patient should be made to take his food with the soup of *Patola, Nimba,* and *Vártáku* mixed with (a liberal quantity of) *Yava-Kshára* 30.

**Treatment of Upa-Jihvá:**—In a case of Upa-jihvá (Ranula), the affected part should be scarified and rubbed with an alkali, and the patient should be treated with errhines (S'iro-vireka), gurgles (Gandusha) and inhalations of smokes (Dhuma). The treatment of the tongue diseases has been thus described above. We shall now describe the medical treatment of the affections of the palate (Tálu-gata Roga). 31-32.

**Treatment of the Tálu-gata diseases:** —In a case of Gala-s'undiká, the Sundiká (protuberance) should be drawn out along the tongue with the help of the thumb and the second finger of the hand, or with a Samdams'a (forceps) and then cut off with a Mandalágra instrument. But it should be severed neither more nor less than three-quarters of the appendage, inasmuch as profuse hæmorrhage might follow an excessive incision, and death might result therefrom; whereas, a case of lesser severance is usually found to be attended with swelling, excessive salivation, somnolence,* vertigo, darkness of vision, etc. Hence a surgeon, well-versed in the science of surgery and well-skilled in practical operations, should carefully operate a Gala-s'undiká (with a knife) and subsequently adopt the following measures The incidental ulcer should be treated with the pulverised compound of *Maricha, Ati-vishá, Páthá, Vachá, Kushtha* and *Kutannata*, mixed with honey and rock-salt. A decoction of *Vachá, Ati-vishá, Páthá, Rásná, Katuka-rohini* and *Pichu-marda* should be used as gurgle (Kavala). The five drugs, viz.,

---

* S'rikantha Datta, in his commentary on Vrinda's compilation, quotes this passage from the text, but does not include "somnolence" therein. He reads "लालासावी भमस्तम:" in place of "लाला निद्रा भमस्तम: " ।

*Ingudi, Apámárga, Danti, Saralá* and *Deva-dáru* should be pasted together and made into **Vartis** (sticks), well flavoured by the addition of perfuming drugs. Twice every day (once in the morning and again in the evening), should the patient be made to inhale the fumes of these burning Vartis (sticks) which have the property of subduing the (deranged) Kapha, and should be made to take the soup of *Mudga* boiled in alkaline water.* In cases of **Tundikeri, Adhrusha, Kurma, Mámsa samgháta** and **Tálu pupputa**, the preceding measures should be adopted, but the surgical operation should vary with the nature of the particular disease under treatment. 33-34.

**Treatment of Tálu-páka, etc. :—** Remedies which destroy the deranged Pitta should be employed in **Tálu-páka** (suppuration of the palate); while applications of Sneha (oil, etc.) and Sveda (fomentations), as well as Váyu-subduing measures should be the remedies in a case of a **Tálu-Sopha** (swelling of the palate). The remedies to be employed in the diseases affecting the palate have been thus described above. Now hear me discourse on the remedial measures in **Kantha-Roga** (diseases of the throat). 35-36.

**Treatment of Throat-diseases :—** In a curable type of **Rohini**, blood-letting and the applications of emetics, gurgles, inhalations (of medicated fumes) and errhines (Nasya) are efficacious. In cases of **Vátaja Rohini**, blood-letting should be first effected, and the affected part should then be

* The alkaline water to be used in the Mudga-soup should be prepared from Yava-kshára according to Dallana. But according to Śivadása, alkaline water prepared from the ashes of Mushkaka, Apámárga, etc., should be used.

rubbed with salts. Gurgles (Gandusha) of tepid Sneha (oil, clarified butter, etc.) should be constantly resorted to In cases of the **Pittaja Rohini**, the powdered *Pattanga*, honey and sugar should be rubbed (Prati-sárana) over (the affected part), and the decoctions* of *Drákshá* and of *Parushaka*, should be used as gurgles (Kavala). In the **Kaphaja** type of **Rohini**, the affected part should be rubbed with *Katuka* and *Ágára-dhuma* (soot of a house—chimney-soot). An oil properly cooked with *S'vetá Vidanga*, *Danti* and *Saindhava* should be employed as (Nasya) and employed as gurgles (Kavala). In a case of **Raktaja Rohini**, a physician shall employ the same measures of treatment as in the Pittaja type of the disease. 37.

**Treatment of Kantha-Sáluka, etc.:**—In a case of **Kantha-Sáluka**, it should be bled and treated as a case of Tundikeri, and the patient should be enjoined to take a single meal in the day consisting only of a small quantity of *Yavánna* (barley-rice) with clarified butter. The treatment of a case of **Adhi-jihviká** should be the same as that of Upa-jihviká. In a case of **Eka-vrinda**, blood-letting of the affected part should be resorted to (by the application of leeches), and Śodhana† (purifying) remedies should be employed. The medical treatment of a case of **Giláyu** (Siláyu.-D.R.) consists of a surgical operation (on the seat of the disease). Incision should be made into a

---

* According to Chakra-páni, Dráksha and Parushaka should be combinedly used in preparing the decoction.

† The "purifying remedies" here means S'iro-virechana, fumigation, plasters and applications of alkali, etc., for purifying the Doshas in the throat.

Gala-Vidradhi (throat-abscess) in its suppurated stage and appearing at a part other than a Marma (vulnerable part). 38-42.

**Treatment of Sarva-sara Mukha-Roga :**—The affected part should be rubbed with powdered salts* in a case of **Sarva-sara Mukha-roga** (invading the entire cavity of the mouth) due to the aggravated **Váyu.** Oil cooked with the (decoction and the pastes of) Váyu-subduing drugs (such as, the Bhadra-dárvádi group, etc.) and used as errhines (Nasya) and gurgles (Kavala) is efficacious in this disease. After the application of this oil, the patient should be treated with the **Snaihika** form of fumigation (Dhuma) in the following manner. *Tuntuka* leaves smeared with honey should be plastered with a compound of the Sára of *S'ála*, *Piyála* and castor wood, the marrow of *Ingudi* and *Madhuka*, *Guggulu*, *Dhyámaka* (Gandha-trina), *Mámsi*, *Kálánu-sárivá*, *S'ri* (Lavanga), *Sarja-rasa*, *S'áileya* and wax pounded together and mixed with an adequate quantity of clarified butter or oil. It should then be burnt, and the patient made to inhale the fumes. This medicinal fumigation (Dhuma) proves remedial in the disease. It destroys the deranged **Váyu and Kapha,** and proves curative in all affections of the mouth. In the **Pittaja type** of the Sarva-sara Mukha-roga, all the morbific principles (Doshas) should be eliminated from the patient's body (with emetics and purgatives),

---

* Dallana and Nis'chala explain the term "चूर्णलेवणै." as the powders of the five official kinds of salt. S'iva-dása, however, holds that powdered Saindhava salt only should be used. Vrinda reads " चूर्णलावणै :" and the commentator S'ri-kantha Datta explains it to mean either the powders of "लवणा", *i.e.*, Jyotishmati or those of "लवण", *i.e*, the five official kinds of salt.—Ed.

and all kinds of sweet, soothing and Pitta subduing drugs should be administered. Medicated gurgles (Gandusha), fumigation (Dhuma), Pratisárana (rubbings) and purifying (S'odhana) measures as well as the Kapha-subduing remedies should be employed in the **Kaphaja type** of the Sarva-sara-Mukha-roga, and the patient should be made to take one Dharana measure (Twenty-four Ratis) of powdered *Ati-vishá Páthá, Musta, Deva dáru, Katuka* and *Kutaja* seeds, with an adequate quantity of cow's urine. This medicine acts as a potent remedy for all the Kaphaja disorders of the body. Gurgles (Kavala) with milk, sugarcane juice, cow's urine, curd-cream, Kánjika, oil, or clarified butter (Sneha) should be prescribed according to the nature of the aggravated Doshas involved in each case (of the Sarva-sara-Mukha-roga). We have described above the medical treatment of the affections of mouth which yield to medical remedies. 43-45.

**incurable Types :**—Now we shall enumerate the different incurable types of mouth-diseases. Of the types of **Oshtha-páka**, those due to the vitiated condition of the flesh, or of blood, and those due to the concerted action of the aggravated Doshas (Sannipáta) should be deemed as incurable. Of the diseases peculiar to the roots of the teeth, the affections known as the Sánnipátika **Danta-nádi** (Sinus in the gums) and the Sánnipátika **Saushira** (Mahá-Saushira) should be also deemed as incurable Of the affections of the teeth, those known as the **Syáva-dantaka, Dálana** and **Bhanjana**, and of the diseases which restrict themselves to the tongue, the one known as the **Alása** should be looked upon as incurable. Similarly, of the affections of the palate, the **Arvuda** should be deemed as incurable. Of those of the throat, the **Svara-**

ghna, Valaya, Brinda, Balása, Bidáriká, Galaugha, Mámsa-tána, Sataghni and Rohini should be regarded as beyond the pale of medicine. The nineteen kinds of the disease mentioned above are incurable, and the medical treatment of these diseases should be taken in hand without holding out any definite hope of recovery. 46—49.

Thus ends the Twenty-second Chapter of the Chikitsita-Sthánam in the Sus'ruta Samhitá which deals with the medical treatment of the diseases of the mouth.

# CHAPTER XXIII.

Now we shall discourse on the (symptoms and) medical treatment of swellings (**Sopha**). 1.

The six kinds of swelling (Sopha) appearing in the particular parts of the body have already been described* with the variations in their symptoms and the medical treatment to be pursued in each case. But the swelling known as the **Sarva-sara** Sopha (general Anasarca) may be divided into five subheads. They are as follows, namely, the **Vátaja, Pittaja, Kapahja Sannipátaja** and **Vishaja** (*i.e*, the one due to the introduction of any extraneous poison into the system). 2.

**Their causes :**—The Doshas (morbific principles) become aggravated and give rise to swellings (Sopha) of the body, by such causes, as by undertaking a journey immediately after a meal, or by the use of *Harita-sákas* (potherbs), cakes and salts in inordinate quantities, or by the excessive use of acids by weak and emaciated persons, or by the use of clay, baked or unbaked, of lime-stones, or of the flesh of aquatic animals, or of those frequenting swampy places, excessive sexual intercourse, use of fares consisting of incompatible articles and lastly by the joltings when riding on elephants, horses, camels, in vehicles, etc., or on persons on the part of dyspeptic patients. 3.

**Specific Symptoms :**—A swelling (Sopha) of the **Vátajá** type is vermilion or black-coloured and is attended with softness and a pricking pain in the swelling which disappears at intervals. A swelling of the **Pittaja** type assumes a blood-red or yellow colour, swiftly expands and is attended with a burning and

---

* See Sutra-sthána, Chapter XVII.

drawing pain (Chosha). A swelling of the **Kaphaja** type assumes a white or greyish colour, becomes hard, cold to the touch and glossy, is slow in its growth, and is attended with itching, pain, etc  A swelling of the **Sánnipátika** type (due to the concerted action of all the three Doshas of the body) exhibits all the symptoms which specifically belong to each of the three abovesaid types. 4-7.

**Symptoms of Vishaja-Sopha :** —A swelling (Sopha) which results from the contact or introduction of a (weakened) chemical poison (**Gara**) with or into the body, or from the use of polluted water, or by bathing in a foul and stagnant pool or tank, or by dusting the body with the powders of substances poisoned by any poisonous animal, or from the contact with weeds and plants, which have become poisoned by the urine, fœcal matter, or semen of poisonous animals, is called a **Vishaja** swelling  The swelling is soft, pendent and persistent, expands rapidly and moves gradually (from one part of the body to the other) and is attended with a burning sensation and suppuration. 8.

**Memorable Verse :**—The aggravated Doshas of the body confined in the stomach (Ámásaya) give rise to a swelling in the upper part of the body. Confined in the intestines (Pakvásaya), they give rise to a swelling in the middle part of the body. If they are confined in the receptacle of the fœces (Malásaya), the lower part of the body becomes swollen. The swelling extends all over the body in the event of their (Doshas) being diffused throughout the organism. 9.

**Prognosis :**—An œdematous swelling (Sopha) occurring in the middle part (trunk) of the body or extending all over it may be cured with difficulty as well as the one which first occurs at either (the upper or lower) half of the body and tends to extend upward. A case of swelling attended with dyspnœa, thirst, weakness, fever, vomiting, hiccough, dysentery, colic (S'ula,, and a want of relish for food is extremely hard to cure and soon proves fatal. 10-11.

We shall now proceed to describe their **general** and **specific** remedies. The use of acids, salts, milk, curd, treacle, lard, water, oil, clarified butter, cakes and all kinds of heavy (in digestion) edibles should be refrained from in all the types of œdema (S'opha). 12-13.

**The Special Treatment of Śopha :—** Traivrita (Ghrita) or castor oil should be administered for a month or a fortnight to the patient suffering from the **Vátaja** type of œdema (Śopha). Clarified butter cooked with the decoction of the drugs of the *Nyagrodhádi* and the *A'ragvadhádi* groups should be respectively prescribed in the **Pittaja and Kaphaja** types. In the **Sannipátaja** type, the patient should be made to drink a potion of clarified butter cooked with a Pátra* measure of the milky exudation of the *Snuhi* plant and twelve Pátra measures of fermented rice gruel (Kánjika) with an adequate quantity of *Danti* as a Kalka. The remedy in regard to a swelling due to the action of poison (**Vishaja**) imbibed into the system will be duly described in the Kalpa Sthánam. 14.

**The general remedies :—**Now we shall describe the general remedies (which are applicable in cases of Śotha). Any of the four Ghritas ending with the Tilvaka Ghrita which have already been mentioned under the treatment of **Udara** would prove remedial in a case of Śvayathu (Œdematous Swelling). The use of (the officinal) urine and the applications of the

---

* A Pàtra measure is equal to eight seers

(medicated) Vartis are likewise recommended. The patient should be made to take every day the medicine known as the **Naváyasa*** through the medium of honey. He should be made to take a Dharana weight of the compound of powdered *Vidanga, Ativishá, Kutaja*-fruit, *Bhadra-dáru, Nágara* and *Maricka* in tepid water. *Trikatu, Yava-kshára* and powdered iron should be mixed together and administered through the medium of the decoction of *Triphalá*; or, cow's milk and cow's urine, in equal proportions should be taken. As an alternative, treacle and *Haritaki* mixed in equal proportions should be administered. *Deva-dáru* and *S'unthi*† may be given; or Gugguluǂ dissolved in cow's urine or in the decoction of *Varshábhu*. Equal parts of treacle and *S'ringavera* § may as well be prescribed; or the roots of the *Varshábhu* pasted with the decoction of the same drug and mixed with powdered *S'unthi* dissolved in milk should be given to the patient every day for a month. He should take *Mudga* pulse fried with the clarified butter prepared by cooking it with the decoction of *Trikatu* and *Varshábhu*. Milk boiled with *Pippali, Pippali*-roots, *Chavya, Chitraka, Mayura* (Apámárga) and *Varshábhu*, or with *Sunthi* and *Surangi*-roots, or with *Trikatu, Eranda*-roots and *S'yámá*-roots, or with *Varshábhu, S'unthi, Sahá* and *Deva-dáru* should be given to the patient. A paste of *Alávu* and

---

\* See Chapter XXII, para. 10, Chikitsita-sthánam.

† Some commentators explain that the compound of Deva-dáru and S'unthi also should be taken through the medium of cow's urine or the decoction of Varshábhu.

ǂ According to Chakradatta's reading, DeVa-dáru, S'unthi and Guggulu should be taken together with cow's urine.

§ The S'ringavera in this compound may be either fresh or dried.—Ed.

*Vibhitaka* dissolved in the washings of rice, should likewise be administered. 15.

The diet of the patient should consist of cooked barley or wheat saturated with the unsalted soup of *Mudga* pulse, cooked with *Yava-kshára, Pippali, Maricha* and *S'ringavera,* and prepared with only a small quantity of oil or clarified butter. A decoction of *Vrikshaka, Arka, Naktamála, Nimba* and *Varshábhu* should be used in effusing (**Parisheka**) the affected part. It should be plastered with a compound consisting of *Sarshapa, Suvarchalá, Saindhava* and *S'árngashtá,* pasted together. Strong purgatives, Ásthápana measures and applications of **Sneha, Sveda** and **Upanáha** should be constantly employed according to the nature and instensity of the aggravated Doshas involved in the case. In a case of Śotha, other than what is the outcome or supervening symptom (**Upadrava**) of any other disease, the patient should be frequently bled by opening a vein of the locality. 16.

**Memorable Verse :**—A patient wishing to get rid of an attack of Śopha (œdematous swelling) should refrain from taking all sorts of cakes, acid substances, liquor, clay, **salts**, oil, clarified butter,* **water**, heavy and indigestible articles of food, sleep in the day time, the flesh of animals other than that of the animals of the Jángala group and from visiting the bed of any woman. 17.

Thus ends the Twenty-third Chapter in the Chikitsita Sthánam of the Sus ruta Samhitá which deals with the medical treatment of S'opha.

* Some read " गुड़म्," .e., treacle in place of " घृतम्," i.e., clarified butter. This reading seems to be the correct one, inasmuch as it is supported by all other authoritative works on Áyurveda —Ed.

# CHAPTER XXIV.

Now we shall discourse on the rules of hygiene and the prophilactic measures in general (**Anágatá-vádha-Prati-shedhaniya**). 1.

**Metrical Texts :**—Now we shall describe the rules of conduct to be daily observed by an intelligent man (after leaving his bed) seeking perfect health and a sound body. 2.

**Tooth-brushing :**—A man should leave his bed early in the morning and brush his teeth. The tooth-brush (Danta-Káshtha) should be made of a fresh twig of a tree or a plant grown on a commendable tract and it should be straight, not worm-eaten, devoid of any knot or at most with one knot only (on one side), and should be twelve fingers in length and like the small finger in girth The potency and taste of the twig (tooth-brush) should be determined by or vary according to the season of the year and the preponderance of any particular Dosha in the physical temperament of its user.* The twig of a plant possessed of any of the four tastes as sweet, bitter, astringent and pungent should be alone collected and used. *Nimba* is the best of all the bitter trees ; *Khadira* of the astringent ones ; *Madhuka* of the sweet ; and *Karanja* of the pungent ones. 3

---

* A man of a **Kaphaja** temperament should use a twig of a plant possessed of a **pungent** taste (Tikta) in brushing his teeth. A man of a **Pittaja** temperament should brush his teeth with a twig possessed of a **sweet** taste (Madhura), while a man of a **Vátika** temperament (nervous) should use that with an **astringent** (Kasáya) taste. This rule should be observed even in respect of the preponderant Doshas of the body, in a disease.

The teeth should be daily cleansed with (a compound consisting of) honey, powdered *Tri-katu*, *Tri-varga\**, *Tejovati*, *Saindhava* and oil Each tooth should be separately cleansed with the preceding cleansing paste applied on (the top of the twig bitten into the form of) a soft brush, and care should be taken not to hurt the gum anywise during the rubbing. This tends to cleanse and remove the bad smell (from the mouth) and the uncleanliness (of the teeth) as well as to subdue the Kapha (of the body). It cleanses the mouth and also produces a good relish for food and a cheerfulness of mind†. 4.

**Cases where tooth-brushing is forbidden** :—Tooth-brushing is forbidden to the persons suffering from affections of the teeth, lips, throat, palate, or tongue, or from stomatitis, cough, asthma, hiccough and vomiting, weakness, indigestion, epilepsy, head-disease, thirst, fatigue, alcoholism, facial paralysis, ear-ache, and to persons tired with over-drinking. 5.

---

\* The term "**Tri-varga**" generally means Tri-katu, Tri-phalá and Tri-mada. Dallana explains it as meaning Tri-sugandhi, *i.e.*, Tvak, Elá and Patra.—Ed.

† **Additional Texts** :—It brings on a relish for food, imparts a cleanliness, lightness and sense of freedom to the teeth, tongue, lips and palate. It protects the mouth, throat, palate, lips and tongue from being affected by any disease. It arrests salivation, imparts an agreeable aroma to the mouth and relieves nausea and water-brush. It strengthens the religious inclination and gives a lightness to the organs. Hence one should every day use the tooth-twig, but its use is prohibited in respect of persons suffering from diseases of the palate, lips or tongue as well as from Mukha-páka (stomatitis), dyspnœa, hiccough, parchedness of the mouth and nausea. The last two lines of the additional text, however, occur in the text in a slightly different form. See the next two lines of the text.

The use of a thin, smooth and flexible foil of gold, silver, or wood, ten fingers in length, is commended for the purpose of cleansing the tongue by scraping. It gives relief and removes the bad taste, fœtor, swelling and numbness of the mouth. Sneha (oil) should be used as a gurgle (Gandusha) every day (after the cleansing of the teeth), as it makes them firm, and brings on a natural relish for food. 6-7.

**Eye and Mouth-washes :**—The mouth and the eyes of a person of sound health should be washed with the decoction of the barks of *Kshira* trees mixed with milk, or with that of Bhillodaka, or of *Ámalaka*, or with (a copious quantity of) cold water.\* This procedure would soon prove efficacious in destroying such affections of the body, as Niliká, dryness in the mouth, pustules or eruptions, Vyanga and the diseases due to the (concerted) action of the Rakta and Pitta, and by such washings the face becomes lighter and the sight stronger. 8.

**Collyrium :**—Srotonjana, produced in the river Indus, is the best and purest of **Collyriums.** It alleviates the burning and itching sensations in the eyes, removes all local pains, secretions and impurities, increases the range of vision, enables the eyes to bear

---

\* Gayadása interprets that the mouth should be washed with the decoction of Bhillodaka and the eyes with that of A′malaka. He also interprets that the eyes and the mouth may both, however, be washed with cold water.

Perhaps Gayadása was of opinion that the decoction of Ámalaka, being astringent, might arrest the dilatation of the pupils due to age, and so help to keep the eye-sight unimpaired. Others explain that the mouth should be washed with the decoctions of Bhillodaka and of Ámalaka, and the eyes with cold water. The decoctions, however, if used as an eye-wash, should be used in a cold state.—Ed.

the blasts of the wind and the glare of the sun and guards against the inroads of occular affections. Hence the application of collyrium (along the eye-lids) is highly recommended ; but its use is forbidden just after taking one's meal or bath (washing the head) and after the fatigue of vomiting, or riding, etc., nor after keeping late hours and also not during an attack of fever. 9-11.

A **betel-leaf** prepared with cloves, camphor, nutmeg (Játi), lime, araca-nut, *Kakkola* and *Katukáhva* (Latá-kasturi), etc., should be taken (chewed after meals), as it tends to cleanse the mouth, impart a sweet aroma to it, enhance its beauty and cleanse and strengthen the voice, the tongue, the teeth, the jaws and the sense-organs. It checks excessive salivation, soothes the body (Hridya), and acts as a general safeguard against throat disease. A **betel-leaf** (prepared as before) proves wholesome after a bath, after meals, after anointing as well as after rising from sleep. A person suffering from Rakta-Pitta, Kshata-Kshina, thirst, or parchedness of the mouth should refrain from taking betel-leaf, the use of which is equally forbidden in such diseases as anæmia, internal dryness of the organism and epilepsy. 12.

**Śirobhyanga :**—Anointing (Abhyanga) the head with oil is a good cure for the affections of the head. It makes the hair grow luxuriantly, and imparts thickness, softness and a dark gloss to them. It soothes and invigorates the head and the sense-organs and removes the wrinkles of the face. The medicinal oil known as the **Chakra-Taila** should be cooked with the paste (Kalka) and the decoction of *Madhuka, Kshira-s'uklá, Sarala, Deva-dáru* and the minor *Pancha-mula* taken in equal parts (in each case). The head should be constantly anointed with this cooling oil. 13-14.

**Combing** the hair improves its growth, removes dandriff and dirt, and destroys the parasites of the scalp. Pouring oil (Karna-purana) into the cavities of the ears is highly efficacious in pains of the jaws (Hanu) and of the Manyá, and acts as a good cure for head-ache and ear-ache. **Anointing** (Abhyanga) the body (with oil, etc ) imparts a glossy softness to the skin, guards against the aggravation of the Váyu and the Kapha, improves the colour and strength and gives a tone to the root-principles (Dhátus) of the body. * 15-17.

**Parisheka :**—Affusing the body (Parisheka) removes the sense of fatigue, and brings about the adhesion of broken joints. It alleviates the pain which usually attends burns, scalds, bruises and lacerations, and subdues the actions of the deranged Váyu. Sneha (oil) affused on the human organism imparts a tone and vigour to its root-principles (Dhátus), in the same manner as water furnishes the roots of a tree or a plant with the necessary nutritive elements, and fosters its growth, when poured into the soil where it grows. The use of **Sneha** (oil, etc.) at a bath causes the Sneha to penetrate into the system through the mouths of the veins (Sirás) and the ducts (Dhamanis) of the body, as also through

---

* Rubbed on the body and allowed to stand or kept unwiped, the Sneha (oil) reaches down the skin, through the hair-follicles in the course of time necessary to utter four hundred Mátrás. It reaches the principle of blood in the course of that necessary to utter five hundred Mátrás, and to the principle of flesh in the course of that necessary to utter six hundred Mátrás. It penetrates further to the principle of fat in the course of that necessary to utter seven hundred Mátrás, and to the principle of bone in the course of that necessary to utter eight hundred Mátrás, and lastly to the principle of marrow in the course of that necessary to utter nine hundred Mátrás. It successively cures the diseases respectively located in those principles.—Dallana.

the roots of the hair, and thus soothes and invigorates the body with its own essence. 18—20.

Under the circumstances, **affusions** and **anointments** of the body with oil or clarified butter should be prescribed by an intelligent person with due regard to one's habit, congeniality and temperament and to the climate and the season of the year as well as to the preponderance of the deranged Dosha or Doshas in one's physical constitution. 21.

**Prohibitions of anointments, etc.:—** Anointments of the body simply with (unmedicated) Sneha are strictly forbidden in cases of undigested (Áma) Doshas (as long as the aggravated Doshas of the body continue in an unassimilated or undigested state and in their full virulence and intensity). Anointment should not be resorted to in cases of acute fever and indigestion, nor after the exhibition of emetics and purgatives, nor after an application of a Nirudha-Vasti. Anointment in the first two cases (acute fever and indigestion) serves to make the diseases curable with difficulty and even incurable, while that made on the same day after the application of purgatives, emetics, or a Nirudha-Vasti, tends to impair the digestive capacity, etc. Anointment is similarly prohibited in diseases due to Samtarpana (repletion, etc). 22—24.

**Physical Exercise :**—What is (popularly) known as physical exercise is (nothing but) a sense of weariness from bodily labour, and it should be taken every day. After taking physical exercise, the whole body should be shampooed, until it gives rise to a comfortable sensation in the limbs. It makes the body stout and strong, helps the symmetrical growth of the limbs and muscles, improves the complexion and the digestive powers, prevents laziness and makes the body light and glossy, firm and compact. The power of enduring fatigue and weariness and the variations of temperature, thirst, etc., are the virtues which are invariably found to follow in its train. It leads to an undiseased existence and is the best means of reducing corpulency. The enemies of a man habituated to regular physical exercises, dare not molest him through fear (for his strength—D. R.). Imbecility and senile decay never approach him, and the muscles of his body become firm and steady. Diseases fly from the presence of a person, habituated\* to regular physical exercise and (subsequent) shampooing, just as small beasts do on seeing a lion. It makes an aged and deformed man (young and) good-looking. Food consisting of articles incompatible in their potency, and indigested and decomposed food are easily digested in a man who takes regular physical exercise (and cannot produce any bad effect). Regular physical exercise is (particularly) beneficial to a strong man accustomed to the use of emollient food (abounding in proteid matter), in all seasons of the year; but in the winter and the spring, it is highly (indispensably) necessary for him. A man seeking his own good should take physical exercise every day only to the half extent of his capacity (Valárdha), as otherwise it may prove fatal. That amount of exercise which makes the Prána-Váyu come out through the mouth† (*i.e.*, as soon as

---

\* Dallana's reading here evidently is "व्यायामखिन्नगात्रस्य" in place of "व्यायामहृष्टगात्रस्य" । This would mean "of one taking so much exercise as produces sweat."

† According to several authorities, the appearance of perspiration on the nose, the axilla, the forehead and in the joints of the hands and the legs and dryness of the mouth are the symptoms which indicate that one has taken **Valárdha** physical exercise (*i.e.*, to the half extent of his capacity).—Dallana.

hard-breathing would set in), is known as the **Valárdha** exercise. One's own age, strength, physique and food as well as the season of the year and the physical nature of the country are the factors which should be considered before one began to take physical exercise, as otherwise it might bring on some disease 25.

Consumption, hæmorrhage (Rakta-pitta), thirst phthisis, aversion to food, vomiting, illusiveness, weariness, fever, cough and asthma are the diseases, which are likely to originate from **excessive** physical exercise, and is, therefore, forbidden after a meal and the fatigues of sexual intercourse, in a fit of vertigo and in respect of persons suffering from hæmorrhage, phthisis, cachexia, cough, asthma and ulcer. 26-27.

The deranged Váyu of the body is restored to its normal condition by the help of **Udvartana** (massage). It reduces the fat and the aggravated Kapha of the system, smoothes and cleanses the skin and imparts a firmness to the limbs. 28.

**Utsádana** (rubbing) **and Udgharshana**\* (friction) tend to dilate the orifice of the (superficial) ducts and increase the temperature of the skin. Utsádana specifically improves the complexion of females and gives a lovely appearance, cleanliness, beauty and suppleness to the female form. Udgharshana (friction) pacifies the bodily Váyu, cures itches, rashes and eruptions (Kotha). **Phenaka** † imparts lightness and steadiness to the thighs, cures itches, eruptions, Váta-stambha and excretal diseases. Friction of the body with brickbat powders excites the heat of skin, brings

---

\* Utsádana and Udgharshana are the two kinds of rubbing the body with medicinal powders with and without a Sneha respectively.

† **Phenaka** is a kind of friction of the body with small wooden rollers.

on the dilation of the orifices of the bodily ducts, and cures itches and Kotha. 29-32

**Bathing :**—Bathing removes somnolence, (inordinate) bodily heat and a sense of fatigue. It allays thirst and checks itching and perspiration, brings on a fresh relish for food, removes all bodily impurities, clears the sense-organs, gladdens the mind, purifies the blood, increases the appetising power, destroys drowsiness and sin, and increases semen. The sight of a man is invigorated by applying **cold water** to the head at the time of bathing, while the pouring of **warm water** on the head tends to injure the eye-sight. In cases of an aggravation of the deranged Váyu and Kapha, the head may be washed with warm water, as a medicine, after a careful consideration of the intensity of the disease. 33-35

**Prohibition of Bathing :**—Bathing in extremely cold water in winter tends to enrage the bodily Váyu and the Kapha, while bathing in hot water in summer agitates the blood and the Pitta. Bathing is not beneficial in fever, diarrhœa, ear-ache, tympanites, Ádhmána, aversion to food and indigestion, and in the disorders or diseases due to the actions of the deranged Váyu. It should not also be taken just after a meal. 36-38.

**Anulepana :**—Anointing (Anulepana) the body (with scented pastes) removes a sense of fatigue and fœtor and perspiration. It produces a sense of pleasure and improves the Ojas, the strength and the complexion of the body enhances the beauty and glow of the frame and gives it a lovely appearance Anulepana is forbidden in those cases in which bathing is prohibited. 39.

The wearing of gems, flowers and clean clothes is beneficial in a variety of ways, as it acts as a good prophylactic against the influences of monsters and malignant spirits, enhances the Ojas and the beauty of the body and keeps the mind in a cheerful mood and proves highly auspicious. 40.

**Álepa :**—B-smearing (Álepa the face (with scented pastes, etc.) imparts steadiness to the eyes, brings on a broad and graceful contour of the cheeks and mouth, produces their healthful glow like that of a lotus flower and prevents its disfigurement by pimples, moles and such like growths and eruptions (Vyanga). The use of collyrium (**Anjana**) furthers the growth of large and beautiful eye lashes, cleanses the eyes by removing the unhealthy secretions, makes the eyes more wide and graceful and also imparts a brilliant lustre to the pupils. 41-42.

Devotion to the gods and Bráhmanas and hospitality towards guests (Atithi) add to one's good name, piety, wealth, progeny and duration of life. Food (**Áhára**) nourishes and gladdens the heart and directly contributes to one's bodily strength. It improves the memory, appetising power, energy and the natural strength of the mind (Tejas), and increases the Ojas and the duration of one's life. 43-44.

Washing the feet increases the semen (Vrishya), removes the sense of fatigue, gladdens the heart, makes the soles free from all adhering dirt and local diseases, acts as a prophylactic against evil spirits (Rakshoghna) and clears up* the vision. Anointing (**Abhyanga**) the feet (with oil, etc) brings on sleep. It is refreshing and invigorating to the body and the sight, removes all

---

\* Dallana explains that washing the feet keeps the nerve (Nádi) joining the soles with the eyes cool and thus helps to clear up the vision. There is a custom of frequently washing the feet amongst the Hindus most probably on this account.—Ed.

drowsiness and sense of fatigue and softens the skin of the soles of the feet. 45-46.

The use of shoes is efficacious in curing the diseases of the feet and is conducive to pleasure and verile potency. It acts as a prophylactic against the influences of evil spirits, makes walking easy and pleasant, and improves the Ojas in the body. Walking without shoes is perilous to life and health, and is attended with the danger of impaired vision. 47-48.

The shaving of hair and the paring of nails lead to the expiation of one's sins, make a man cheerful, tend to appease his fate, increase his energy and impart a lightness to the frame. The putting on of armour (**Vánavára**) improves one's strength, energy and complexion and gives a lustre to the body. The wearing of a turban (**Ushnisha**) acts as a protection against wind, dust, sun and light, helps the luxurious growth of hair and tends to improve the purity of the mind. 49-51.

The use of an umbrella is a protection against rain, wind, dust, dew and sun. It improves one's energy, Ojas, eye-sight and complexion, and is an auspicious thing in itself. The use of a stick (**Danda**) dispels the fear of dogs, snakes, beasts of prey, (tigers, etc.) and horned animals. It considerably alleviates the toil of a journey, lessens the probability of making a false step and is specially commended to the weak and imbecile. It increases one's energy, strength and patience, makes the mind firm and bold, acts as a proper support and makes one fearless. 52 53.

Sitting idle (**Ásyá**) gives pleasure. It improves the glow of one's complexion, increases the Kapha and corpulency and makes the body delicate, while an active pedestrian habit (**Adhva**) is detrimental to the complexion. It reduces the fat and Kapha of the body, and removes the delicateness of the frame. Contrary results (to those produced by sitting idle) are produced by excessive walking which further brings on weakness and emaciation of the body. A gentle walk or stroll, which is not very fatiguing to the body, tends, on the contrary, to improve his memory, strength, digestive capacity (Agni) and the functions of the sense-organs. It increases also the duration of life. 54-57.

Lying down in an easy posture on a soft bed removes the sense of fatigue, pacifies or soothes the bodily Váyu, brings on sleep and lost recollections to the mind, is spermatopoetic and is conducive to the growth of the body; while lying down in a contrary manner is attended with contrary results. Fanning with Chowries (**Vála-vyajana**) is refreshing and keeps off flies and mosquitoes; while fanning (with ordinary fans) arrests perspiration, removes the sense of fatigue and fainting fits, and alleviates the burning, scorching and parched sensations. Shampooing (**Samváhana**) is pleasant, refreshing, soporific, and spermatopoetic (Vrishya). It destroys the bodily Váyu and Kapha, removes the sense of fatigue and is soothing to the blood, skin and the muscles. 58-60.

A strong wind (**Pravata**) is parchifying in its effect and injurious to the complexion. It destroys the burning sensation (if any) in the body, allays thirst, removes fainting fits and stops perspiration, but (at the same time) produces numbness of the body and destroys the digestive powers; whereas the contrary results are produced by a gentle wind. The gentle breeze of summer and of autumn should be breathed (as it is attended with beneficial results to the health). A seeker after health and a long life should reside in a chamber, not exposed to strong blasts of wind (**Niváta**). An undue exposure to the sun (**Átapa**) aggravates the Pitta, but increases the power of digestion. It agitates the blood and begets thirst, perspiration, faintness (sun stroke), vertigo and a burning sensation in the body attended with a discolouring of the complexion, etc.; whereas the contrary results are produced by a (cool) shade (**Chháyá**). A basking in the glare of fire (**Agni**) remedies the (wrong) coursing of the Váyu and Kapha, removes cold and shivering, digests the slimy secretions in the channels; but aggravates the blood and Pitta. A good sleep (**Nidrá**) enjoyed at the proper time (and for the proper period) tends to improve the growth, strength, vigour and complexion of the body. It increases the power of digestion, removes drowsiness, and restores the natural equilibrium among the different fundamental principles (Dhátus) of the organism. 61 65.

**General rules of conduct :**—The first rule is that one should keep his nails and hair short, always put on clean and white clothes, wear a light turban and a pair of shoes and carry an umbrella and a stick in his hand. One should discourse, when necessary, with another in a sweet and gentle voice and his speech should be laconic and pleasing. He should first accost his elders and acquaintances in cases of meeting before they speak. He should be kind and compassionate to all creatures, and be approved of by his elders and superiors. He should be in full possession of resources and in an undisturbed state of the mind. One should not stir out at night nor walk about in the grounds of public executions, undulated places, dens and rocks.* He should not go (at night) to where roads cross nor to places covered with heaps of husks, ashes, bones,

---

* The text has Indra-kila which means a hilly country inhabited by barbarous people.

hair, stones, baked earth and charcoal, nor to places commonly considered as unholy. 66.

Men should never deride a king, nor use harsh and impolite words to, nor act meanly and treacherously towards him. One should not speak ill of the king, the gods, the Bráhmanas and the Pitris (departed Manes), and he should never use harsh and slanderous words. He should not tell a lie nor associate with king-haters nor with the insane, degraded, mean and narrow-hearted persons. 67.

Climbing up trees, mountains, ant-hills and undulating grounds, etc, and going up to a waterfall as well as riding on a wild and unbroken horse or elephant are strictly prohibited. One should not descend into an unknown tank, den as well as into the sea or into a river at flood times. Old haunted and deserted houses, cremation grounds and solitary forests should be strictly shunned. One should not come into actual contact with fire, wild beasts, snakes and venomous insects. The site infested with wild beasts, snakes, venomous insects, lizards and horned animals as well as where virulent epidemics would be raging should be avoided, nor should the sites of actual affrays and battles be resorted to, nor the scene of a violent conflagration of fire. 68.

Passing between two rows of fire, between cows, elders, Bráhmanas, moving cradles and a married couple is forbidden. One should not (unnecessarily) follow a corpse. Even the shadow of a fallen, degraded and sick person as well as of a cow, Bráhmana, divine image, banner or of a Chaitya (tree growing on a cremation ground) should not be trodden upon. One should not gaze at the rising or the setting sun. One should not report to another the fact of a milch cow sucking her own calf, nor of her traversing or freely grazing in another's field nor the fact of witnessing a rainbow or a meteor fall. One should not blow up a fire with one's breath, nor hit the ground or water with one's hands and feet. 69.

A man should never repress any natural urging of his body, nor should he pass water or evacuate excrements in an open or public place, within the confines of a town or village, close to a cremation ground or any place of worship, at the crossing of roads, in reservoirs of water or on the high road nor should he do so facing a fire, in the presence of his superiors, cows, the sun and the moon nor facing against the wind. 70.

Scratching (unnecessarily) the ground with one's nails, etc., should not be done, and one should not yawn nor sneeze, nor raise any eructations nor breathe hard in an assembly (of gentlemen) without previously covering his face. Sitting in an unseemly raised-up position on a couch as well as with extended feet in front of one's superiors should be renounced. 71.

The hair, nostrils, ear holes, teeth or any channel of the body should not be fingered. The hair, face, fingernails, clothes and the body should not be shaken. Never keep time with music by beating the body or the cheeks with the hands or by striking the finger nails against each other. Never (wantonly) strike or break or cleave a piece of wood or stone or weed, etc. 72.

Never expose yourself to the rays of the sun, or to the gusts of wind blowing in your face. Basking before a fire immediately after a meal or sitting on one's legs on a narrow wooden stool should not be indulged in. Never hold the neck in a contrary (contorted) posture. Neither do nor eat anything by keeping the body in a contrary posture. Never look steadfastly towards any object and particularly towards the sun or any luminous body* or towards any extremely attenuated, revolving or moving object. Never carry a load on the head. Sleeping, waking, sitting, lying down, walking, jumping, running fast, plunging in water, swimming, riding on a horse or in a vehicle, talking, laughing, sexual intercourse and taking (any other) physical exercise though accustomed and recommended should not be inordinately indulged in. 73.

A bad habit should be gradually discontinued and a good one even when (beneficial to health) should similarly be gradually inculcated by a quarter only and not all at once. 74.

It is improper to lie down with one's head downward. One should not drink water from a broken vessel nor with the help of blended palms. Food, which is wholesome and approved of by one's physician and which abounds in articles of sweet and emollient properties† should be taken at the proper (and regular) time (every day) in a moderate quantity. It is forbidden to take any food in the house of a trader (*i.e.*, of a (hotel-keeper) or a courtesan, nor in the house of a wily, degenerate or inimical person, nor at a village-assembly. The refuse of another's dishes, as well as articles of food infested with flies, insects, etc., or possessed of an objectionable colour, taste, smell, touch or

---

\* Some explain "Jyotish" as a blaze of fire and others explain it as stars.

† The framers of the ÁyurVeda were aware of the fact that the human system is incapable of directly assimilating starchy substances without converting them into sugar. This has been emphasised in the Sutra-Sthána, where Sus'ruta insists that a food stuff, in order to be worthy of the epithet, must be Madhura (*i e*, of sweet flavour) and contain a large quantity of proteid matter such as is found in milk, butter, meat, etc.—Ed.

sound or those which produce an unpleasant impression in the mind, or food of like nature as well as those served (handled) by many persons should not be partaken of (in spite of repeated requests in that behalf). It is not advisable to sit down to a meal without washing one's hands and feet. One should never take anything by repressing a natural urging for stool and urine, nor sit down to a meal just at the break or the close of day, nor in an unprotected situation (*i.e.* without any shade, or without something to sit upon). One should not take his meal after the expiry of the (daily) appointed time nor in an insufficient or inordinate quantity, nor partake of food whose Sneha (oleaginous substance) has been removed. 75.

**Metrical Text :**—It is forbidden to see one's image reflected in water, nor is it advisable to plunge naked into water. Curd should never be taken at night, nor should it be taken (at all) without sugar * or clarified butter, nor without saturating it with *Mudga*-soup or the admixture of honey, nor without (the expressed juice of) the *A'malaka*, nor with any hot substance † or article, as otherwise it may bring on Kushtha (cutaneous affections), erysipelas, etc. 76-77.

Exercise, addiction to wine, gambling and music are bad. One should not bear witness to any fact (before a

---

\* Dallana adds that curd should not be taken without an addition of water and salt as well. This is also the practice in general.

† All the existing editions of the Sus'ruta Samhitá read "नोषा:" (*i e.*, curd should not be taken with any "hot" substance). Here it should be noted that the term "hot" may also include the substances which are heat-making in their potency. Here, however, the reading seems to be incorrect. The lines are found *verbatim* in the work of Charaka, where he reads "नोषां," *i.e.*, hot curd should not be taken, since it produces, as he himself tells us later on, an aggravation of the blood and the Pitta.—Ed.

law court), nor stand surety for any body. One should not use the shoe, umbrella, garland (of flowers), ornaments or ragged clothes previously used by another. Never defile a Bráhmana, or a fire, or a cow by touching them before washing (your hands and mouth) after eating. 78.

**Memorable Verses :**—The general rules of (good) conduct are described above. Health, wealth and longevity never fall to the lot of those who do not follow these rules of conduct. A wise man should take food of such tastes (Rasa) in any particular season of the year as is antidotal to the bodily **Dosha** which is naturally aggravated in that season. 79-80.

**Rules of drinking water, etc. :**—Water should not be taken during the rainy season and only in moderate quantities in autumn. Water may be sparingly taken during the first four months of the rainy season if found to be indispensably necessary). Hot water should be taken in winter and spring (Vasanta), but cold water to one's fill in summer Sidhu and Arishta should be taken in winter and spring. Water boiled and subsequently cooled should be drunk in summer and meat-juice in Právrit. Yusha (Mudga-soup, etc.,) should be taken in the rainy season and cold water after the expiry of the rains These rules should be observed only by persons in sound health, whereas the rules regarding persons suffering from any disease should be regulated by the prescription of any diet according to the particular Doshas involved in each case. 81-82.

Any Sneha (such as oil or clarified butter) saturated with powdered Saindhava salt and *Pippali* should be regularly taken for the purpose of improving the digestive capacity. The natural urging of the body should never be repressed (as a repressed physical propulsion is sure to usher in a physical distemper). A Sneha (oleaginous substance) should be freely and largely used during the Právrit and the spring seasons as well as in antumn (Sarat) as such a proceeding would act as a good appetising measure and a cure for diseases. Emetics, purgatives and applications of Vastis are respectively beneficial in diseases due to the actions of the deranged Kapha, Pitta and Váyu, whereas a regular course of physical exercise tends (equally) to curb an aggravation of all the three preceding Doshas of the body, so much so that their aggravation can never be detected in persons in the habit of taking it regularly every day, though otherwise addicted to an incompatible diet, etc. 83-86.

The attention should not be diverted to any other subject at the time of urination, defecation, sexual intercourse, taking of food, as well as at the time of taking emetics and purgatives, etc. It is not wise to anticipate and indulge in the gloomy thoughts of a future and probable invasion of a disease, and to suffer any physical privation on that account. 87-88.

All sexual excesses should be studiously abstained inasmuch as they are sure to produce Śula (colic), cough, asthma, fever, emaciation, phthisis, jaundice, epilepsy, convulsions, etc. A person, who is moderate in sexual intercourse, lives a long life, becomes good-looking, healthy, strong and firm in his nerves and muscles, and becomes capable of averting (untimely) decay. One may visit his wife (lit. a woman) on each fourth night in all the seasons of the year except in summer when he may see her once a fortnight. 89-A.

**Women unfit to visit :**—A woman in her menses, not amorously disposed, uncleanly in her habits, not sufficiently endeared and endearing and belonging to a higher social order,* older than one's self, affected with any disease, wanting in any limbs, inimically disposed to one's self, in her period of gestation, suffering from any uterine disorder, belonging to his own blood (Gotra), or leading the life of an anchorite, or who is his preceptor's wife, should not be gone unto by a man (seeking health and longevity). A woman should not be gone unto in the Sandhyás (morning and evening), as well as on the Parva days† (prescribed in the S'ástras), early in the morning, at mid-day, or in the dead of night. Going unto a woman at an infamous, unwholesome, or exposed place is similarly forbidden. Sexual intercourse by a man who is hungry, or thirsty, or who may be suffering from any disease, or may be angry, or in a cheerless spirit, is strictly forbidden. A man should not go unto a woman by repressing a natural urging for Váta (flátus), stool or urine, or if he is in a weak state of health, (as it would be highly injurious to his health). Incest with lower animals, unnatural sexual intercourse, obstruction of semen in its passage, as well as sexual intercourse with a woman having any vaginal disease are strictly forbidden even in respect of a strong person. 89-B.

It is highly injurious for a man to indulge excessively in sexual intercourse, or to enjoy it while standing, or while lying on his back, or to shake his head at the time ; these should not be indulged in by an intelligent

---

\* The text has "Varna-Vriddha" which literally means superior to the man in respect of Varna or the magnetic vibrations of the body, which are determined by one's birth in a certain family. It means several castes of the Hindus.—Ed.

† The Parva days are the 8th, the 14th and 15th days of either fortnights and the last days of the solar months.—Ed.

and judicious person even (occasionally for pleasure's sake. 89-C.

### Evil effects of the foregoing abuses :

—Visiting a woman in her menses results in the loss of sight, longevity and vital power, and should be accordingly considered as a sinful act The duration of a man's life is diminished by going unto a woman, older in age or higher in social status (Varna), or unto the wife of his preceptor or superior, in the morning or the evening, or on the Parva days (the interdicted days), or unto a woman belonging to the same blood as he. A visit to a woman big with child is extremely painful and injurious to the fœtus confined in the womb. A visit to a diseased woman results in the loss of the man's vital power. A going unto a deformed, uncleanly, spiteful, non amorous, or sterile woman, or at an unclean, infamous, or exposed place is detrimental to the semen and intellect of the visitor. 89-D.

Similarly, sexual intercourse enjoyed by a man at noon time, or by one who is in an enfeebled, thirsty, or hungry state of the body, in a standing up posture, or in a cheerless mood, brings on an excessive loss of semen and aggravation of the bodily Váyu. Phthisis due to the loss of semen is the result of over-intemperance in sexual matters. Pain, enlargement of the spleen, epilepsy and even death may follow from sexual gratifications in a diseased state of health. The Váyu and the Pitta become aggravated by the sexual intercourse enjoyed early in the morning or at midnight. An incest with lower animals, unnatural sexual intercourse, or that with a woman having a diseased vagina is attended with an excessive loss of semen and an aggravation of the bodily Váyu, and is the cause of Upadamśa (syphilitic virus). An act of coition enjoyed by holding the woman on one's bosom or by repressing the natural urgings towards urination or defecation, as well as a repressing of seminal discharge would help the early formation of seminal concretions (in the bladder). 89-E.

Hence these (injurious and harmful) practices should be shunned by a man for his welfare in this life as well as for that in the next On the contrary, repression of a natural and (legitimate) sexual desire, from a sense of unwise delicacy or shame, is a physical sin.* Hence a healthy and passionate man possessed of the necessary fecundating element, under the course of a proper Vájikarana (aphrodisiac) remedy, should cheerfully go unto and duly enjoy the pleasures of company with a girl, beautiful in looks, tender in years, modest, virtuous, equally passionate, cheerful, kindred to him both in physical and mental temperaments, and well-decked with ornaments. Fatigue after coition should be removed by the enjoyment of a bath †, a cool breeze, or a

---

* It should be always borne in mind that God has implanted this desire in the mind of man and provided him with the necessary organic appendages only for the propagation of his species and not for the gratification of any diseased or morbid sexual propensity which is found nowhere else in Nature save and except in debauched human subjects and which lowers them even below the level of brutes. Hence love should be the essence of the bond which binds a couple and converts them into a kind of human centaur, the man and the wife, and union sexually considered, should be effected only under the promptings of that sacred instinct in Nature which makes the lilies blow and causes the pollens to unite their fecundating principles with one another and which a healthy unsophisticated human heart can instinctively read as the **seed time** of youthful exuberance.

† A bath is recommended for a man of strong Virile power, in case of sexual intercourse in the day time or it may be possible to take a bath early in summer nights.—Dallana.

sound sleep. Food or milk, saturated with sugar, and meat-juice, prove very refreshing after the act. 89.

Thus ends the Twenty-fourth Chapter in the Chikitsita Sthánam of the Sus'ruta Samhitá which deals with the rules of Hygiene and the prophylactic measures in general.

# CHAPTER XXV.

Now we shall discourse on the medical treatment of a variety of diseases (**Miśraka-Chikitsita**). 1.

It has been stated before that blood-letting is the remedy in diseases of the **Páli** (ear-lobes). Now hear me describe in detail the treatment of those affections which are confined to the lobes of the ears. They are five in number and are called the **Paripota, Utpáta, Unmantha, Duhkha-Vardhana** and the **Parilehi.** 2-3.

**Causes and Symptoms :**—If the lobe of an ear be suddenly pulled and kept in that position for a long time, a numbed and painful swelling of a blackish red colour is produced on the lobe, owing to its soft and delicate nature. This is found to spontaneously burst or crack, and is called the **Paripota,** which should be ascribed to the action of the deranged **Váyu** (of the system). 4.

A painful swelling attended with a burning sensation and suppuration, appearing in the lobe of the ear, owing to the friction and movements of a heavy ornament worn in the lobe, is originated from the vitiated condition of the **blood** and the **Pitta.** Its colour is either brown or red and is called the **Utpáta.** 5.

Pulling the ear-lobes down by force tends to enrage the Váyu (of the localities) which in union with (the deranged) Kapha gives rise to a painful swelling in those regions, attended with itching and tinged with the specific colours\* and symptoms of the Doshas involved. The disease is called the **Unmantha,** and is

---

\* Mádhava in his compilation reads "सअमवेदनम्" (that the swelling is attended with a numbness and no pain) in place of "तद्वर्णवेदनम्." Vágbhata also supports this.—Ed.

originated through the concerted action of the deranged **Vâyu** and the **Kapha**. 6.

A swelling in an ear-lobe attended with pain, burning and itching sensations owing to its being (pulled down and) lengthened, when found to suppurate (in the end) is called the **Duhkha-vardhana** ; it* restricts itself only to the skin (of the affected part. 7.

Small exuding pustules resembling mustard-seeds (in size) and attended with pain, burning and itching sensations, appear in the lobes of the ears owing to the action of the vitiated blood, or the deranged **Kapha**, or to the presence of parasites (in those localities). The disease soon spreads itself (and assumes an erysipelatious character). It is called the **Parilehi** from the fact of its eating away the affected lobe with the entire helix. 8.

**General Treatment :**—These dreadful diseases (which invade the lobes of the ears) are highly dangerous and tend to destroy and eat away the affected appendages, if not properly attended to at the outset and specially when the patient is addicted to unwholesome food and drink and to an injudicious conduct of life. Hence a physician should speedily remedy these complaints with applications of medicated **Sneha**, **Sveda**, etc., ointments, washes, plasters, poultices and blood-letting.† This is the general treatment of those diseases. 9.

---

* Madhava adds "an unsuccessful perforation (in the ear lobe)" to be an additional cause of this disease. He also reads "त्रिदोष", i.e., "due to the concerted action of the three Doshas" in place of "लक्ष्योऽसी". Madhava has Vagbhata's support in this.—Ed.

† In cases of the predominance of the **Vâyu**, anointment, Anuvâsana and poultices should be resorted to. In cases of **Pitta**-predominance, purgatives should be applied. Emetics should be applied in cases of **Kapha**-predominance and lastly blood-letting, purgatives and washes,

**Specific Treatment:**—Now we shall describe the medical remedies which should be specially used in anointing (the affected parts in these diseases). Drugs, such as *Khara-Manjari, Yashti-madhu, Saindhava, Deva-dáru, As'va-gandhá* and the seeds of *Mulaka* and of *Avalguja* should be pasted together and cooked with a compound of milk, oil, clarified butter, lard, marrow and wax. This preparation should be applied lukewarm to the affected lobe in a case of the **Paripotaka** type. 10-11.

*Manjishthá*, Sesamum, *Yashti-madhu*, *Sárivá*, *Utpala*, *Padma-káshtha*, *Rodhra*, *Kadamba* and the tender leaves of the *Valá*, *Jambu* and *Ámra* (mango) should be cooked together with (an adequate quantity of) oil and Dhányámla (Kánjika). This oil proves curative in a case of **Utpáta**. 12.

Similarly (a medicated) oil cooked with *Tála patri*, *As'va-gandhá*, *Arka*, *Vákuchi*-seeds, *Saindhava*, *Saralá*,* *Lángali*, lard of a Karkata (crab) and of a Godhá (a kind of lizard), proves beneficial in cases of **Unmantha**. The affected lobes should be washed (Sechana) with a decoction of the leaves of the *As'mantaka, Jambu* and *Ámra* (in such cases). 13.

In a case of **Parilehi**, the affected lobe (Páli) should be dusted with powdered *Prapaundarika*, *Yashti-madhu*, *Manjishthá* and the two kinds of *Haridrá* after lubricating it with the oil cooked with the Kalkas of *Láksá* and *Vidanga*. It should be as well fomented with heated cow-dung and plastered with the lukewarm pastes of *Vidanga* alone, or in combination with *Trivrit*,

---

etc, should be resorted to in cases of the affection being due to the concerted action of the vitiated **blood** and the **Pitta**.

\* Saralá here means Dhupa-káshtha, according to Dallana.

*S'yámá* and *Arka* pasted together (with cow's urine), or with the pastes of *Karanja*-seed, *Ingudi* seed, *Kutaja* and *Áragvadha* (pasted with cow's urine). Mustard oil cooked* with the admixture of all the foregoing drugs and with *Maricha*, *Nimba*-leaves and wax, proves efficacious as unguents (in such cases). 14-15.

In cases where the ear-lobes are affected and have become either thin, or hard, an ointment should be applied to them in order respectively to increase their growth, or to soften them. 16

The marrow of a jackal and of an animal frequenting and living in swampy grounds (Ánupa, such as a buffalo, etc.), together with lard, oil and fresh clarified butter, should be cooked with a quantity of milk weighing ten times their combined weight and with the drugs of the *Madhura* (Kákolyádi) group, *As'va-gandhá* and *Apámárga* and *Lákshá-Rasa* (decoction or infusion of Lákshá). The oil thus prepared should be filtered and preserved carefully in an earthen pitcher. The affected ear-lobes should be constantly fomented and well-lubricated with it. The use of this medicated oil helps the growth of the ear-lobes and makes them healthy, soft, smooth, painless, evenly developed and capable of bearing the weight of ear-pendants. 17.

**Treatment of Palita :**—The expressed juice of the *Bhringa-rája* and (the decoction of) *Triphalá*, powders of indigo leaves, *Arjuna*-bark, *Bhringa-rája*, *Pinditaka*, black-iron, flowers of the *Vija* and of *Sahachara*, *Haritaki*, *Vibhitaka* and *Ámalaka* mixed together and pasted with a quantity of mud found adherent to lotus-bulbs weighing as much as the combined

---

* Dallana says that this oil should be cooked with cow's urine weighing four times as much as the oil.

weight of the aforesaid drugs should be kept in an iron-pitcher well covered and preserved inside a room for a fortnight. After this period it should be cooked with (an adequate quantity of) oil and with the expressed juice* of the *Bhringa rája* and (a decoction of) *Triphalá*. For the purpose of ascertaining the proper cooking of the oil, a (white) feather of a Valáká (crane) should be dipped into it, and satisfactory preparation should be judged from the deep blue colour imparted to the feather. The oil should be then preserved in a black-iron pitcher for a month. Used as anointments, this oil arrests a premature greyness of the hair. 18.

The flowers of the *S'airiya, Jambu, Arjuna* and of the *Kás'mari*, sesamum, *Bhringa-rája*-seeds, mango-stones, *Punarnavá*, † mud, *Kantakári, Kásisa*, marrow of the seeds of *Madana, Triphalá*, powdered iron, *Rosánjana, Yashti-madhu, Nilotpala, Sárivá*, and *Madayanti*‡ should be pasted together with the decoction of the Sára (pith) of the *Vijaka*. It should then be mixed with seven Prastha measures of the decoction of the Sára of Vijaka and preserved for ten days in a covered iron vessel. This compound should then be carefully cooked with an A'dhaka measure of **Vibhitaka**-oil and again preserved in a new iron-pitcher for a month. Then after cleansing the system of the patient, the oil thus prepared

---

\* In the cases of cooking an oil, the liquid substance to be used, should be, as a general rule, four times as much as the oil; but in this case, the expressed juice of *Bhringa-rája* and (the decoction of) *Triphalá* should be continued to be added, so long as the feather does not become deep blue.

† According to Dallana, the reading would have been "पुनर्नवे," *i.e.*, the two kinds of Punarnavá.

‡ One Karsha measure of each of the aforesaid drugs should be taken.

should be used as errhines (Nasya) and in anointing the head, and the patient should be advised to live on diet consisting of *Másha-pulse*, or of *Kris'ará*. In the course of a month, it imparts a (deep black) gloss like that of a black bee, or that of *Rasánjana* to the hair and makes it grow thick and curly. It cures baldness, arrests the susceptibility of the system to an attack of premature decay, removes the wrinkles of the face, and invigorates the sense-organs in the performance of their proper and respective functions. This oil should not be given to a man who does not wish to use it, nor to an indigent person, to an ungrateful wretch, nor to an enemy. 19.

**Treatment of Vyanga, etc. :**—*Lákshá, Rodhra*, the two kinds of *Haridrá, Manah s'ilá, Haritála, Kushtha, Nága* (lead), *Gairika, Varnaka, Manjishthá, Vacha, Saurástra-mrittiká, Pattanga, Gorochaná, Rasánjana*, bark of *Hemánga* (Champaka), the tender leaves of *Vata, Káliya-Káshtha, Padma-káshtha*, the filaments of a lotus, both red and white *chandana*, Mercury* and the drugs of the *Kákolyádi* group should be pasted together with milk. The paste, thus prepared, as well as lard, marrow, wax, clarified butter, milk, and a decoction of the drugs of the *Kshira* trees should be cooked together. This medicated clarified butter, is the best of all the unguents that may be applied to the face. It cures the most difficult cases of Vyanga and Niliká, and removes all tans, specks, marks, moles, eruptions, etc., from the face. It imparts smoothness to the wrinkled skin, gives a healthy plumpness and bloom to the cheeks, and makes the face as beautiful as a lotus.

---

\* This is the first time that we come across the mention and use of "Párada" (**Mercury**) in the Sus'ruta Samhitá.—Ed.

It should be recommended to kings and to the ladies of the royal court, as well as to persons of the same rank. It acts as a good remedy for cutaneous affections (Kushtha), and may be as well applied in cases of Vipádiká. The use of a cosmetic compound consisting of powdered *Haritaki,* leaves of *Nimba,* the bark of *mango,* stems of the pomegranate, and the flowers and leaves of *Madyantiká* pasted together, imparts a god-like effulgence to the complexion of a man. 20-21.

Thus ends the Twenty-fifth Chapter of the Chikitsita Sthánam in the Sus'ruta Samhitá which deals with the treatment of a variety of diseases.

# CHAPTER XXVI.

Now we shall discourse on the medical treatment for increasing the strength and virile power of weak persons **(Kshina-Valiyam Váji-Karana).** 1.

A youth in sound health taking regularly some sort of **Váji-Karana** (aphrodisiac) remedy may enjoy the pleasures of youth every night during all the seasons of the year. Old men, those wishing to enjoy sexual pleasures or to secure the affections of women, as well as those suffering from senile decay or sexual incapacity, and persons weakened with sexual excesses, should do well to submit themselves to a course of Váji-karana remedies. They are highly beneficial to gay, handsome and opulent youths and to persons who have got many wives. 2-A.

**Definition of Váji-Karana :**—If duly taken, the Váji-karana\* remedies make a man sexually as strong as a horse (Váji), and enable him to cheerfully satisfy the heat and amorous ardours of young maidens, a fact which has determined the nomenclature of this class of (medicinal) remedies. 2-B

**Means of Váji-Karana :**—Various kinds of (nutritious and palatable) food and (sweet, luscious and refreshing) liquid cordials, speech that gladdens the ears, and touch which seems delicious to the skin, clear nights mellowed by the beams of the full moon and damsels young, beautiful and gay, dulcet songs that charm the soul and captivate the mind, use of betel-leaves, wine and wreaths of (sweet-scented) flowers,

---

\* The **Váji-Karana** remedies are of three kinds, *viz.,* (1) those producing the semen, (2) those secreting the semen, and (3) those producing as well as secreting the semen.

and a merry careless heart, these are the best aphrodisiacs in life. 2.

**Causes of Sexual Incapacity :**—A cessation of the sexual desire owing to the rising of bitter thoughts of recollection in the mind of a man, or a forced intercourse with a disagreeable woman (who fails to sufficiently rouse up the sexual desire in the heart of her mate) illustrates an instance of **mental impotency.** Excessive use of articles of pungent, acid, or saline taste, or of heat-making articles of fare leads to the loss of the Saumya Dhátu (watery principle) of the organism. This is another kind of impotency. Virile impotency resulting from the loss of **semen** in persons addicted to excessive sexual pleasure without using any aphrodisiac remedy is the merit form of virile impotency. A long-standing disease of the male generative organ (syphilis, etc.), or the destruction of a local Marma (such as the spermatic cord) destroys the powers of coition altogether. This is the fourth form of impotency. Sexual incapacity from the very birth is called the congenital (**Sahaja**) impotency. Voluntary suppression of the sexual desire by a strong man observing perfect continence, or through utter apathy produces a hardness of the spermatic fluid, and is the cause of the sixth form of virile impotency Of the six foregoing types of impotency, the congenital form as well as the one due to the destruction of any local Marma (spermatic cord) should be regarded as incurable, the rest being curable and amenable to the measures and remedies antidotal to their respective originating causes. 3.

**Their Remedies :**—Now we shall describe the different **Váji-Karana** (aphrodisiac) remedies. Powders of sesamum, *Másha*-pulse, *Vidári*, or *S'áli*-rice should be mixed with *Saindhava* salt and pasted with a copious quantity of the expressed juice of the sugarcane of the *Paundarika* species. It should then be mixed with hog's lard, and Utkáriká should be prepared by cooking it with clarified butter. By using this (medicinal) **Utkáriká**, a man would be able to visit a hundred women. 4.

The testes of a he-goat should be boiled in milk. Sesamum seeds should then be successively treated with this milk in the manner of a Bhávaná saturation Cakes should be made of these sesamum seeds with the lard of a porpoise. This medicine exerts the same action as the preceding one without producing any exertion whatever. By eating the testes of a he-goat with (an adequate quantity of) salt and powdered long-pepper (Pippali), fried in clarified butter prepared from churning milk (and not from curd), a man is enabled to visit a hundred women. 5.

Powders of *Pippali*, *Másha*-pulse, *S'áli*-rice wheat and barley, should be taken in equal parts. Cakes (**Pupáliká**) should be prepared with this compound and fried in clarified butter. By taking these **cakes** and a potion of milk sweetened with (a copious quantity of) sugar, a man becomes potent enough, to enjoy the pleasures of love like a sparrow (Chataka). 6.

Powdered *Vidári* successively soaked in the expressed juice of the same and dried, should be licked with honey and clarified butter, whereby a man would be able to visit ten women successively (at a time). Similarly powders of (dried) *Ámalaka* successively soaked in its own expressed juice should be licked with honey, sugar* and clarified butter, after which a quantity of

* According to S'ivadása it may also be taken with honey and clarified butter only.

milk should be taken. This compound would make even an old man of eighty sexually as vigorous as a youth. 7-8

The testes of a he-goat or of a porpoise mixed with salt and powdered long-pepper, and fried in clarified butter should be taken for speedy and effective aphrodisiac purposes The eggs of a tortoise, of an alligator, or of a crab,* or the semen† of a male buffalo, of a he-ass, or of a he-goat should be similarly taken for the same purpose. 9.

Milk boiled and cooked with the sprouts, bark, roots and fruit of an *As'vattha* tree, should be sweetened with sugar and honey, and taken; this enables a man to enjoy sexual pleasures like a sparrow. The powdered bulbs of *Vidári,* weighing an *Udumbara* (one Tolá) in measure, and taken with milk and clarified butter,‡ would make an old man young again A Pala measure of the pulverised *Másha* pulse, mixed with honey and clarified butter should be licked and a potion of milk should then be taken; this would make a man sexually as strong as a horse. Wheat and *Átma-guptá* seeds should be boiled in milk, and taken, when cold, with clarified butter, and a potion of milk should then be taken for the same purpose. 10-13.

Clarified butter should be boiled with eggs or the testes (as the case might be) of alligators, mice, frogs and sparrows. By lubricating the soles of the feet with this Ghrita, a man would be able to visit a woman with undiminished vigour so long as he would not touch the ground with his feet. 14.

* Some explain "कुलीर" as house-sparrows.

† Here semen would mean the testes, the receptacle of the semen.

‡ Some read "घृतेन" (boiled) in place of 'घृतेन'. In that case the boiled milk only should be taken and no clarified butter should be added thereto.

65

The use of pulverised *Átmaguptá* and *Ikshuraka* (Kokiláksha) seeds mixed with sugar and taken with milk just milched enables a man to indulge in the pleasures of youth for the whole night without any sense of fatigue. The powders of the *Uchchatá* should also be taken similarly (with milk and sugar). S'atávari and *Uchchatá* roots should also be similarly taken by a man wishing to have (sexual) vigour. A soup of *Átmaguptá* seeds and *Másha*-pulse (boiled together) should be taken. *Átmaguptá*-seeds, *Gokshura* seeds and *Uchchatá* should be boiled with milk and constantly stirred with a ladle. The use of this preparation (with an adequate quantity of sugar) enables a man to enjoy the pleasures of love all the night long. Likewise the milk boiled with *Másha-pulse*, *Vidári*, or *Uchchatá* should be taken with honey, clarified butter and sugar. By using this a man may indulge in the pleasures of the bed for the whole night like a sparrow. 15-19.

The use of the milk of a **Grishti** (a cow delivered only once) with a grown up calf (one year old) and exclusively fed on the (fresh) leaves of the *Máshaparna*, is recommended as a sexual tonic. All kinds of meat and milk, as well as the drugs of the *Kákolyádi* group should be regarded as being highly possessed of the virtue of imparting tone and vigour (to the male productive organs). They should, therefore, be used (for that purpose). The medicinal remedies and compounds described in the present chapter should be taken in sound health and proper seasons, as they are exhilarating and invigorating, and help the procreation of children. 20-21.

Thus ends the Twenty-sixth Chapter of the Chikitsita Sthánam in the Sus'ruta Samhitá which deals with the treatment of the Virile impotency.

# CHAPTER XXVII.

Now we shall discourse on the recipes and modes of using elixirs and rejuvinators of the human organism which will make it invulnerable to the inroads of any disease or of decay **(Sarvopaghāta-Śamaniya-Rasāyanam).** 1.

**Metrical Texts :**—A wise physician should (invariably) prescribe some sort of **tonic** (Rasáyana) for his patients in their youth and middle age after having their systems (properly) cleansed by the applications of a Sneha and purifying remedies (emetics and purgatives). A person whose system has not been (previously) cleansed (Śodhana) with the proper purifying remedies (emetics and purgatives) should not, in any case, have recourse to such tonics inasmuch as they would fail to produce the wished-for result, just as the application of a dye to a piece of dirty cloth will prove non-effective. 2.

Now we shall describe the remedial measures and agents for the maladies due to the aggravated **Doshas**[*], both mental and physical, which have already been described (in several places). Old age and senile decay would be arrested (lit. perpetual or life-long youth would be secured) by drinking milk, cold water, honey and clarified butter, either severally or jointly (*i.e*, in any combination[†] taken one, two, three or four at a time), in early life (just on or

---

[*] The mental Doshas are Rajas and Tamas, whereas the physical Doshas are Váyu, Pitta and Kapha.

[†] There would be four combinations of one each, six of two each, four of three each and one of four jointly ; thus there would be fifteen combinations in all.

just before the completion of the process of organic development) 3-4.

**Vidanga-Rasáyana :**—The powdered seeds of the *Vidanga* (Tandula) and pulverised *Yashti-madhu* should be mixed together and taken in cold water in an adequate dose (according to the strength of the patient), and a potion of cold water should then be taken. This medicine should be regularly continued for a month. The same pulverised *Vidanga* seeds should be similarly taken for a month through the vehicle of the decoction of *Bhallátaka* mixed with honey; or of the decoction of grapes mixed with honey; or with the expressed juice of *Ámalaka* sweetened with honey; or through the vehicle of the decoction of *Guduchi*. Thus there are these five ways (of taking pulverised *Vidanga* seeds (Tandula) as an elixir. A meal of boiled rice with a copious quantity of clarified butter should be taken with the soup of Ámalaka and *Mudga* pulse unseasoned with salt and cooked with only a small quantity of Sneha (clarified butter) after the medicine has been well digested. These (Rasáyana) remedies prove curative in cases of hæmorrhoids and in complaints of worms. They improve memory and the power of comprehension and their use for every month increases the life-time of the user by one hundred years. 5.

**Vidanga-Kalpa :**—One Drona measure of **Vidanga** (seeds) should be boiled in the way of preparing cakes in an Indian cake-pan. When the watery portion (of the cakes) have been removed (evaporated) and the *Vidanga*-grains well boiled, they should be taken down and well pasted on a stone-slab. They should then be kept in a strong iron pitcher after having been mixed with a copious quantity of the decoction* of *Yashti-madhu*. The pitcher should be buried in a heap of ashes inside a closed room during the rainy season and preserved there during the four months of rain ; after that period the pitcher should be taken out (of the ashes). Its contents should then be consecrated with (appropriate) Mantras by uttering them a thousand times and should be taken every morning in suitable quantities after the system has been thoroughly cleansed (by appropriate emetics and purgatives, etc.). The diet should consist of cooked rice and clarified butter mixed with a copious quantity of the soup of *Mudga* pulse and *Ámalaka* cooked with a small quantity of Sneha and salt ; and should be taken after the digestion of the medicine. The patient should lie on the ground (and not on a bedding). **Worms** would be found to have been issuing out of the body after the regular and continuous use of the medicine for a month, which should be extracted with the aid of a pair of bamboo tongs or forceps after the body had been anointed with the **Anu-taila** (described before) **Ants** would be coming out of the body during the second, and vermins (**Yuka**) in the third month of the use of the medicine which should also be removed as in the preceding manner. The hair, nails and teeth begin to fall off and become dilapidated in the fourth month of its use. In the fifth month the body beams with a divine glow, becomes resplendent as the midday sun, and exhibits features which specifically belong to the etherial being. The ears become capable of hearing the faintest and remotest sound (under its use), and the vision extends far into space and beholds objects at a great range

---

* Dallana explains the term *Madhukodakottara* to mean a large quantity of Madhuka and water, (and by water he means the decoction of *Vidanga*).

(which is not usually given to mortal eyes to descry). The mind, shorn of the qualities of Rajas (action) and Tamas (nescience), becomes possessed of Sattva (illuminating principles or true knowledge). Things are permanently and indelibly impressed upon his (user's) memory at a single hearing and the faculty of invention wonderfully expands Old age and decay permanently vanish and youth returns to stay in him for good, bringing with it an elephantine strength and a horse-like speed, and he is enabled to live for eight hundred springs. The medicated oil known as **Anu-taila** should be used in anointing (the body at this stage of treatment); a decoction of *Aja-karna* for Utsádana (washing) purposes, well-water saturated with *Us'ira* for bathing purposes, sandal paste in anointing (Anulepana) the body, and the regimen of diet and conduct as described in connection with the **Bhallátaka** treatment (Vidhána) should be observed. 6.

**Kásmarya Kalpa :**—The use of huskless **Kásmaryaja** seeds for rejuvinating purposes, is similar to the preceding one, except that it requires a separate kind of diet and does not require the use to lie on the ground. Under this treatment, the diet should consist of (boiled) rice and well-boiled milk and the beneficial effects that would result from its use, are identical with those of the foregoing one. These remedies should be employed in diseases originating through the vitiated blood and Pitta of the system. 7.

**Valá-Kalpa :**—A Pala or half a Pala weight of the (powdered) roots of the **Valá** should be well-stirred in cow's milk and taken (every day), and the patient or the user should not be allowed to stir out of his room as prescribed before (during the entire course of taking the medicine). He should be advised to take a meal consisting of boiled rice, milk and clarified butter after the medicine had been fully digested. Premature old age and senile decay would be arrested for a period of twelve years by taking this elixir continuously for twelve days in the foregoing manner, whereas an extension of its course to a hundred days would add a hundred summers to the duration of his youthful age. **Ati-valá, Nága-valá, Vidári, Śatávari** may be similarly taken for the same purposes, with this distinction that the (powders of) the *Ati-valá* should be taken with water, those of the *Nága-valá*, with honey, whereas *Vidári* and the *S'atávari* powders should be taken with milk. The regimen of diet and conduct as well as the beneficial results produced therefrom should be the same (as from the use of Valá). The present remedies are recommended to persons seeking strength or suffering from an attack of Hœmatemesis or Hœmatochezia.* 8.

**Várahi Kalpa :**—A Tulá measure of the powders of **Várahi**-bulbs should be taken in an adequate dose (everyday) by mixing it with honey and stirring it with milk A meal of boiled rice with clarified butter and milk should be taken after it had been digested and the patient should be advised to observe a regimen of diet and conduct (Pratishedha) as laid down before (in connection with the foregoing elixirs). By using it a man is enabled to witness a hundred summers and does not feel any fatigue after sexual excesses. A quantity of this powder should be mixed with milk and boiled (according to the rules of Kshirapáka). When sufficiently cooled, the milk should be churned and the clarified butter produced therefrom should be taken after the medicine had been digested. A

---

* Suffering from consumption and hœmoptysis.—D. R.

continuous use of the medicine for a month enables a man to live up to a good hundred years. 9.

A decoction should be made by boiling together the pith of the *Vijaka*\* (Pita Sála) and the roots of the *Agni-mantha* with which a Prastha measure of *Másha*-pulse should be duly cooked. When the Másha-pulse is sufficiently boiled, an Aksha measure of powdered *Chitraka* roots and the expressed juice of the *Ámalaka* weighing a fourth part of the *Másha*-pulse should be added to it, and the whole compound should be removed (from the oven) at the close of the cooking. When cooled down this compound should be taken in adequate doses with honey and clarified butter after consecrating it a thousand times with appropriate Mantras. Persons seeking longevity and a stronger or improved range of vision should take this and they should be advised to take their meals without any salt. The meal, after the digestion of the medicine, should consist of boiled rice and a copious quantity of clarified butter and should be taken with unsalted *Mudga*, and *Ámalaka* soup or with milk alone. A continuous use of either of these two medicines for three consecutive months would make a man's eye-sight as keen and foresighted as that of a Suparna† and enable him to witness a hundred summers in the full vigour of health, strength and manhood.‡ 10.

---

\* Dallana recommends one Pala weight of Vijaka Sára and Agnimantha to be boiled in an Ádhaka measure of water which should be reduced to one half for the preparation of the decoction.

† Suparna is the king of birds and is said to be the most keen-sighted.

‡ Dallana says that some commentators do not read this, since they do not consider it to be a part of the original text. Jejjata also has not read this.

**Memorable Verse :**—The use of Śana (seeds) boiled with milk and taken also with milk guards against the loss of flesh and prevents the body from suffering any decay. 11.

Thus ends the Twenty-seventh Chapter of the Chikitsita Sthánam in the Sus'ruta Samhitá which deals with elixirs and rejuvenators.

# CHAPTER XXVIII.

Now we shall discourse on the elixirs and remedial agents which tend to improve the memory and invigorate the mental faculties as well as to increase the duration of human life **(Medháyushkámiyam Rasáyanam).** 1.

**Svetávalguja-Rasáyana :**—The fruit (seeds) of the white **Avalguja** should be dried in the sun and then reduced to a fine powder. This powder should be stirred with (an adequate quantity of) treacle and placed in an earthen pitcher which previously contained clarified butter (Sneha-kumbha). The pitcher should then be kept buried in a heap of paddy for seven days after which it should be taken out and its contents given in convenient doses every morning before sunrise to a person, seeking improvement of memory and longevity, after his system has been thoroughly cleansed (with proper emetics and purgatives, etc.). Hot water should then be drunk. After taking the medicine, the patient should enter his room in accordance with the rules laid down in connection with the Bhallátaka-Vidhána. After the digestion of the medicine, the patient should be advised to take a cold bath and to partake in the evening of a meal of well-cooked *S'áli* or *Shashtika* rice with (boiled) milk sweetened with sugar. This medicine continuously taken in this manner for six months would make the life of its user sinless, and extend it in the full glow of health and vigour and in the sound enjoyment of a vigorous memory and of all his intellectual faculties to a hundred green summers. 2.

In cases of Kushtha, jaundice and abdominal dropsy (Udara), the medicine should be prepared by stirring (the powdered seeds of) the Krishná* (black **Avalguja**) with the urine of a cow (instead of with treacle) and given to the patient in doses of half a Pala weight every morning after the sun has ceased to look red.† In the afternoon the patient should be made to partake of a meal of boiled rice with clarified butter and unsalted *A'malaka* soup. A continuous use of this medicine in the aforesaid manner for a month would improve the memory and intellectual faculties of the user, and enable him to witness a hundred summers on earth in the full enjoyment of sound health. **Chitraka** roots‡ and **Rajan**i (turmeric) may be used in the same manner and for similar purposes with this distinction that the dose of the *Chitraka*-root preparation should be two Pala measures (instead of half a Pala as laid down in regard to the foregoing compounds). The rest are identical with the above. 3.

**Manduka-parni Rasáyana:**—The Doshas of the system of a person should be first thoroughly cleansed (with the help of proper emetics and purgatives, etc.), and he should be advised to undergo the prescribed diet of (Peyá, Yavágu, etc , in their proper order) He should be further advised to enter his chamber in the prescribed manner (and to remain there during the entire

---

* Jejjata explains "Krishná" to mean Pippali. But both Gayi and Dallana explain it to mean the black Avalguja. It should be mentioned, here, that Dallana recommends the roots of black Avalguja, but we think that its seeds should be taken.—Ed.

† Before sunrise.—D. R.

‡ The roots of the Chitraka with black flowers should be taken.— Dallana.

course of the treatment). An adequate dose of the expressed juice of the **Manduka-parni** should then be stirred with milk, and should be taken after consecrating it by reciting the proper Mantras a thousand times. A potion of milk may then be taken immediately after. After it had been fully digested a meal of cooked barley grains with milk should then be partaken of; or (the expressed juice of *Manduka-parni*) with an admixture of sesamum seeds followed by a potion of milk. A meal of boiled rice with milk and clarified butter should then be taken after the digestion of the medicine and should be continued for three months in succession. This would ensure a long life of a hundred years in the full vigour of retentive memory and intellectual faculties, and would impart a god-like effulgence to the complexion. As an alternative, the patient should fast three days and take only the expressed juice of **Manduka-parni** for these three days After this period he should live on milk and clarified butter only, or he should be made to take a Vilva measure (of the paste of Manduka-parni) stirred with milk for ten consecutive days which would ensure a life of a hundred years in the full enjoyment of his intellectual faculties. 4.

**Bráhmi Rasáyana :**—Having had the Doshas of the system duly cleansed (with proper emetics and purgatives, etc.), a person (wishing to undergo a treatment of Rasáyana) should be advised to take the prescribed diet of (Peyá, Yavágu, etc , in their proper order), and should be made to enter his room (Agára). He should then take the expressed juice of the **Bráhmi** in an adequate dose after consecrating the juice a thousand times with the proper Mantras. After the medicine had been fully digested he should be advised to take in the evening Yavágu (gruel) without any salt; or with boiled milk in the event of his being habituated to its use. A continuous use of the medicine for a week improves the memory, leads to the expansion of the intellectual faculties and imparts a celestical glow to the complexion. In the second week of its course it revives old and forgotten memories in the user and adds to his proficiency in the writing out of any book to be written. In the third week it enables a man to reproduce from memory as many as one hundred words if twice heard or read (at a single sitting'. In the same manner a (further) use of the drug for twenty-one days removes all inauspicious features whether of the body or of the mind, the goddess of learning appears in an embodied form to the (mind of the) user, and all kinds of knowledge come rushing into his memory. A single hearing is enough to make him reproduce (*verbatim* from memory a discourse however lengthy), and he is enabled to live for five hundred years. 5

**Bráhmi Ghrita :**—Two Prastha measures of the expressed juice of the **Bráhmi** and one Prastha measure of clarified butter should be cooked with one Kudava measure of *Vidanga* seeds, two Pala weight of each of *Vacha* and *Trivrit*, and twelve (in number) of each of *Haritaki*, *Ámalaka* and *Vibhitaka* well pounded and mixed together. When properly cooked, the (prepared) Ghrita should be carefully preserved in a covered pitcher. It should then be taken in adequate doses as in the preceding manner. The patient should be advised to take meals of boiled rice, clarified butter and milk, after the medicine had been fully digested. Under its use worms and vermin would be expelled (from their unsuspected seats in the organism) and creep out of the upper, lower and lateral parts of the body.

This preparation would give a favourable turn to one's fortune, impart a lotus-like bloom (to the cheeks) with perpetual youth, unparalleled intellectual faculties and a life that would cover a period of three centuries of song and sunshine. This elixir or **Rasáyana** covers within its therapeutic range such affections of the body as cutaneous diseases (Kushtha), chronic fever, epilepsy, insanity, and the diseases due to the effect of poisons and to the evil influences of ghosts and malignant spirits, as well as of all other dangerous diseases. 6.

**Vachá Rasáyana:**—A paste of white **Vachá** to the size of an *Ámalaka* should be taken with (an adequate quantity of) milk, after consecrating it (in the proper manner). The medicine should be taken after cleansing the system (with emetics and purgatives, etc.) and after entering the Agára (room). After the medicine had been digested, a meal of boiled rice with milk and clarified butter should be partaken of. A continuous use of this elixir for twelve days improves the power of hearing. It increases the power of memory if taken for the next twelve days. It enables the user to remember a hundred words at a time by a thrice repetition of the same (*i.e.*, by taking it for a period of thirty-six days). A repetition of a twelve days' (*i.e*, forty-eight days) use of the medicine leads to the expiation of all sins; it imparts a keenness of sight like that of Garuda and enables the user to witness a hundred summers on earth. A decoction prepared with two Pala weight of any other species of **Vachá** should be taken with milk.* The benefits which would result from its use and the rules of diet and conduct to be

---

* According to Dallana, this preparation of Vachá should be prepared by boiling it in the manner of Kshira-páka Vidhi.

observed (during its course) are identical with those of the preceding one. 7.

**Śata-páka Vachá-Ghrita :**—Clarified butter should be cooked a hundred times in succession with an adequate quantity of **Vachá** The use of a Drona measure of this medicated Ghrita (taken every day in an adequate dose) extends the earthly career of its user to five centuries, and proves beneficial in cases of scrofula, goitre, elephantiasis and hoarseness. 8.

**Measures for prolonging life—M. T. :**
—Now we shall discourse on life-prolonging measures and remedies. The powders of **Vilva** (roots) should be consecrated a thousand times with *Vilva* flowers by reciting the **Sree-Sukta** (as mentioned in the Rig-Veda). They should then be mixed with (powdered) gold, honey and clarified butter (in the form of an electuary), and licked every morning. It is thus a combination of medicine and Mantra, and, if used continuously for a year, would remove all inauspicious features (both of the body and of the mind). 9-10.

Every morning after a bath, a man should offer ten thousand oblations in fire and take the powders and decoction of the roots and bark of the **Vilva** with milk in a spirit of self-control, whereby he would be able to acquire longevity. This remedy should be considered as a good Rasáyana. Similarly a decoction of **Mrinála** mixed with honey and fried paddy and duly consecrated a hundred thousand times with oblations in fire would be considered an infallible Rasáyana. 11-12.

The use (of a compound consisting of gold, **Padma-seed**, **Priyangu** and fried paddy mixed with honey and taken in (an adequate quantity of) cow's milk gives a favourable turn to one's fortune. A potion of milk cooked with the decoction of the petals (Dala) of *Nilotpala* (in the manner of Kshira-páka Vidhi) and mixed with gold and sesamum seeds, is attended with similar results. 13-14.

Cow's milk with **gold,** wax and Mákshika (honey), if (regularly) taken after having performed a Homa ceremony a hundred thousand times, should be considered the best Rasáyana. The use of the pulverised compound of the three things *viz.,* *Vachá,* **gold** and *Vilva,* if taken with clarified butter, tends to improve the health, memory, intellectual powers and physical growth. It increases the duration of one's life and brings good luck in its train. 15-16.

A (medicated) oil prepared by duly cooking it with the decoction of a Tulá weight of *Vásá*-roots should be taken by a man after having performed a Homa ceremony with a thousand libations for the expansion of his intellectual faculty and the increase of the duration of his life on earth A Tulá weight of barley grains should be powdered. The preparations of this barley powder (gradually) taken with honey and powdered *Pippali* increases one's capacity for study. 17-18.

The use of pulverised *Ámalaka* and **gold** with honey imparts vitality to a dying man. A regular use of the **Sátávari-ghrita** mixed with honey and pulverised gold enables a man to subjugate even his king. A compound consisting of *Go-chandaná, Mohaniká,* honey and **gold** should be taken by a man wishing a good turn to his destiny 19-21.

Clarified butter cooked with an admixture of the pasted *Yashti-madhu* and with the decoction of *Padma* and *Nilotpala* should be regularly taken with gold, and then a potion of milk cooked with the foregoing drugs should be taken. It invariably removes the evil features (of both mind and body), and gives a good turn to fortune. It increases longevity and makes the user (fortunate like) a king. 22-A.

The Tri-padi (lit. three-footed) Gáyatri should be recited in connection with the use of any of these elixirs where no Mantra would be found to be specifically mentioned. The use of the foregoing medicinal compounds improves one's beauty, surrounds a man with the majesty and effulgence of the gods and makes him as strong as an elephant. Constant study, disquisitions (on philosophical and scientific topics), discussions in other subjects, and residence with professors or men learned in the respective branches of knowledge, are the best means for improving memory and expanding one's intellect. Eating after the digestion of a previous meal, non-repression of any natural urgings of the body, annihilation of all killing propensities, perfect continence, self-control and refraining from rash and hazardous undertakings, should be deemed the keys to a long life. 22.

Thus ends the Twenty-eighth Chapter of the Chikitsita-Sthánam in the Sus'ruta Samhitá which deals with elixirs and remedial agents for improving the memory and intellect and increasing longevity.

# CHAPTER XXIX.

Now we shall discourse on the restorative and on the constructive agents (Rasáyana) which arrest innate morbific tendencies and decay* **(Svábhávika-Vyádhi Pratishedhaniya Rasáyana).** 1.

**Metrical Text:** —In the days of yore the gods such as Brahmá, etc created a kind of **Amrita** (ambrosia) which is known by the epithet of **Soma**, for the prevention of death† and decay of the body. We shall now deal with the mode of using this (ambrosia). 2.

The one and the same divine Soma plant may be classified into twenty-four species according to the difference of their habitats, structures, epithets and potencies. They are as follows:—*Ams'umán, Munjaván, Chandramáh, Rajataprabha, Durvd-Soma, Kaniyán, S'vetáksha, Kanakaprabha, Pratánaván, Tála vrinta, Karavira, Ams'aván, Svayam-prabha, Mahá-soma, Garudáhrita, Gáya trya, Traishtubha, Pámkta, Jágata, S'ámkara, Agnishtoma, Raivata, Yathokta* and *Udupati*. All these kinds of Soma secure for the user a mastery of the Gáyatri (and hence in the Vedas), and are known by the above auspicious names mentioned in the Vedas ‡

---

\* These are decrepitude, death, hunger, thirst, sleep, etc.

† Here death may mean, according to some authorities, the death of tissues as well.

‡ The whole of the hymns in the 9th Book of the Rig-Veda, besides a few in other places, are dedicated to the honour of **Soma**, but these twenty-four names do not occur there. The plant is there represented as a god, and his worship must at one time have attained a remarkable popularity. The extraordinary properties of the exhilarating juice of the Soma are frequently mentioned in the Rig-Veda and the language throughout in which it is behymned could not be more eulogistic. As an instance of

Their virtues and methods of using them are identical with each other and are described below. 3 4.

**Mode of using the Soma :**—A room or an inner chamber (Ágára) in a commendable site protected with three walls on each side and provided with all kinds of accessories and attendants, should be first secured before taking (the expressed juice of) any of the aforesaid **Soma** plants. Then at an auspicious hour on an auspicious day marked by favourable astral combinations and lunar phase, the person desirous of using the Soma should enter the inner or central **Chamber** after having had his system cleansed (with the proper emetics, purgatives, etc ) and having had his diet in the proper order (of Peyá, etc.). A (whole) plant of the *Ams'umán* (or of any other kind of) Soma should be procured in the manner to be observed at the time of collecting the Soma for an (Agni-shtoma) sacrifice and (all) the (preliminary) rites of Homa should be performed (in the usual orthodox way). After that the bulb (of the Soma plant) should be pricked with a golden needle and a quantity of the secreted milky exudation should be collected in a golden vessel. The patient (with the auspicious rites of protection,

---

this we might refer to Rig-Veda VIII. 48.3 which has been metrically translated by Muir as follows :—

> We've quaffed the Soma bright,
> And are immortal grown ;
> We've entered into light,
> And all the gods have known.
> What mortal now can harm,
> Or foeman vex us more ?
> Through thee, beyond alarm,
> Immortal god, we soar.

It should be mentioned, however, that as far as our knowledge goes, this Soma is now-a-days not within our reach.—Ed.

etc., done unto him) should drink off an Anjali (Kudava) measure of the secreted juice at a draught without tasting it, and the remainder, if any, should be cast into water. He should then wash and rinse his mouth with water in the manner of Áchamana. Then having controlled his mind and speech with the vows of Yama (paramount duties,\* and Niyama (minor duties)† should stay in the protected inner chamber surrounded by his friends. 5.

**Metrical Text :**—After having drunk the Rasáyana (Elixir) one should reside in a windless (prescribed) chamber, spend his time in perfect control over his senses, sitting, standing or walking about in his chamber in a holy spirit and by no means indulging in sleep (which is injurious under the circumstances). 6.

Or the patient may, after taking his meal in the evening and hearing the benedictory words, lie down on a mattress of Kus'a-grass covered with black-deer skin and thus pass the night among his friends and may take cold water when thirsty. Then having got out of his bed in the morning he should hear the benedictory words recited and have the benedictory rites performed unto him. He should then touch the body of a cow and sit down in the same manner (in his chamber). Vomitings mark the digestion of the Soma-juice and after vomiting the blood-streaked worm-infested matter,

---

\*Patanjali, the propounder of the Yoga system of Philosophy, enumerates the Yamas as follows :—"अहिंसा" (harmlessness), "सत्य" (truthfulness), "अस्तेय" (abstinence from stealing), "ब्रह्मचर्य्य" (continence) and "अपरिग्रह" (non-acceptance of offerings except in prescribed cases).

†The Niyamas, according to the same authority, are :— "शौच" (purity—external or internal), "सन्तोष" (contentment) "तप:" (penance), "स्वाध्याय" (religious study) and "ईश्वर-प्रणिधान" (meditation of the Divine Being).

milk boiled and cooled should be given him in the evening. Worm-infested stools follow on the third day (of its use) which help the system in purging off all filth and obnoxious matter (accumulated in the organism) through errors in diet and conduct, etc. The patient should in that case bathe in the evening and take cold boiled milk as before and lie down on a piece of Kshauma cloth stretched over (the aforesaid mattress). Swellings appear on the body on the fourth day (of its use) and worms are found to creep out from all parts of the body. The patient should lie down that day on a bed strewn over with dust and in the evening, he should be made to drink a potion of milk as before. He should pass the fifth and sixth day in the same manner, but milk should be given him in the morning and in the evening (instead of only in the evening). The muscles become withered by this time and on the seventh day the patient is found to be a mere skeleton covered with a skin only and left with bare animation, the vital spark being retained by the potency of **Soma**. The body should be washed with tepid milk on that day and plastered with a paste of sesamum, *Yashti-madhu* and sandal wood, and milk (only) should be given him to drink. 7-A.

On the morning of the eighth day, the body should be washed with milk, and plastered with sandal paste, and potions of milk should be prescribed for him after which the patient should be advised to leave his bed of dust and lie down on one covered with a piece of Kshauma cloth. From now the muscles of the body begin to show signs of fresh and vigorous growth, the skin becomes cracked, and the teeth, nails and hair begin to fall off. On and from the ninth day the medicinal oil known as **Anu-Taila** should be used to anoint (the body) and the decoction of *Soma-valka* for bathing (Pari sheka). The same should be prescribed on the tenth day, and from thence the skin becomes firm. The eleventh and twelfth day should be passed in the same way. From the thirteenth till the sixteenth day (both the days inclusive) the body should be washed with the decoction of *Soma-valka*. New teeth well-formed, symmetrical, strong, hard and as clear as a diamond or crystal or ruby would appear on the seventeenth and eighteenth days. Gruels (Yavágu) prepared with old *S'áli-rice* and milk should form his diet till the twenty-fifth day. After that period well boiled *S'áli* rice should be taken in the morning and evening with milk. Fixed, glossy and coral coloured finger-nails resembling the new rising sun in lusture and possessed of auspicious marks would be found to be growing after the lapse of that period and hair begin to grow, the skin would assume the soft hue of a blue lotus (Nilotpala), *Atasi* flower or of a ruby stone. After a month the hair should be shaved and a plaster composed of *Us'ira, Chandana* and black sesamum applied to the scalp, and the patient should take a milk-bath. This would lead to the growth of deep bee-black curls of hair in the course of a week. 7-B.

Then the patient should be allowed to stir out from the inmost chamber only to re-enter it again after a stay of a Muhurta (forty-eight minutes) in the outer chamber. Thenceforth **Valá taila** (described before) should be used in anointing (Abhyanga) his body; pasted barley in rubbing (Udvartana); tepid milk in washing (Parisheka) it; and a decoction of *Aja-karna* in rubbing (Utsádana) the dirt of. Similarly well water (scented) with *Us'ira* should be used for the purpose of bathing (Snána); Sandal pastes as unguents (Anulepana) and the expressed juice of the *A'malaka* should be invariably mixed with any kind of Yusha or supa (he may take). Soup and black sesamum seeds boiled with milk and *Yashtimadhu* should be used (in the preparation of the food). These rules of diet and conduct should be observed for ten consecutive days. 7 C.

The patient should stay in the second (outer) chamber for a second ten days. Then he should be made to come out and enter the third (outmost) chamber (veranda) and to remain there for ten days with a quiet control over the mind and should be allowed to take a short exposure to the sun and wind during this period (of ten days). He should then be made to re-enter again the inner compartment. 7·D.

The patient should not contemplate himself in a mirror during this time owing to his enhanced personal beauty and renounce all passions and anger for a further period of ten days. This rule holds good in respect of all kinds of **Soma**; but there is this distinction that the Soma plants which are found to trail upon the ground or grow as small shrubs or in bushes should (themselves) be taken (instead of their expressed juice being drunk) and a dose of these would be four Mushtis* and a half. 7.

The expressed juice of the *Ams'umán* (Soma) should be pressed and taken in a golden pot and that of the *Chandramáh* (Soma) in a silver one. By its use a man is sure to develop the eight godly powers † and is thus able to imitate the god Is'ána. The expressed juice of a Soma plant belonging to any other species should be

* A Mushti measure is equal to eight Tolás.
† The eight godly powers, according to some authorities, are :—
अणिमा लघिमा व्याप्ति: प्राकाम्यं महिमा तथा ।
ईशित्वञ्च वशित्वञ्च तथा कामावसायिता ॥

taken in a copper or an earthen pot or in a (pot prepared of a) piece of red-coloured and stretched skin. A member of any of the three twice-born castes but none of the S'udra class is privileged to drink this ambrosial elixir (Soma). In the fourth month (of taking it) and under the auspices of a full moon a Soma-drinker should be allowed to stir out of his chamber with the auspicious rites done unto him and to resume the daily avocations of his life after he had worshipped the Bráhmanas in a holy place. 8.

**Metrical Texts :**—The use of the (expressed juice of a) **Soma** plant, the lord of all medicinal herbs is followed by rejuvenation of the system of its user and enables him to witness ten thousand summers on earth in the full enjoyment of a new (youthful) body. Such a person bears a charmed life against fire, water, poison and weapon and develops a muscular energy in his limbs which would be in no way inferior to the combined strength of a thousand excited (rutted) elephants, of the Bhadrá class (which are the most ferocious and irresistible) in their sixtieth year. Equipped with such an excellent physique, he can easily and without any opposition cross the Kshiroda (ocean) and go up to the abode of S'akra (the king of the gods) and roam to the extreme confines of Uttara (northern) Kuru or to any other place he likes. He is invested with a beauty of frame which belongs to Kandarpa (the god of love) and his complexion (lustre) vies with the beams of the full moon. The presence of such a beautiful man gladdens the hearts of all, and the entire Veda with all their allied branches* of knowledge

---

\* The allied branches of the study of the Vedas are six in num
They are :—शिक्षा काल्पो व्याकरणं निरुक्तं कन्दसां चयः ।
ज्योतिषामयनञ्चैव बेदाङ्गानि षड़ेव तु ॥

instinctively dawn upon his consciousness. Like the gods, he knows no failure in life and roams about in the world in the full glory of divine majesty. 9.

**Distinctive features of the Soma Plants :**—A Soma plant of whatever species is furnished with fifteen leaves which wax and wane with the waxing and the waning of the moon. Thus one leaf grows every day in the lighted fortnight attaining the greatest number (fifteen) in the night of the full moon and then the leaves begin to decrease in number dropping one by one every day till the bare stem of the creeper is left on the night of the new moon. 10.

**Their description :**—The Amsumán species of the Soma is characterised by a smell like that of clarified butter and has a bulb, while the Rajata-prabhá is possessed of a bulb resembling a plantain in shape. The Munjaván puts forth leaves like those of a garlic while the Chandramáh species is possessed of a golden colour and is aquatic in its habitat. The Garudáhrita and S'vetáksha species are yellowish (Pándura) and look like the cast-off skins of a snake and are usually found to be pendent from the boughs of trees 11.

All other species are marked with parti-coloured circular rings. Possession of fifteen leaves of variegated colours, a bulb, a creeper-like appearance, and secretion of milky juice are the general characteristics of all the Soma plants. 12-A.

**Their habitats :**—The Himálayas, the Arvuda, the Sahya, the Mahendra, the Malaya, the S'ri-Parvata, the Deva-giri, the Deva-saha, the Páripátra, the Vindhya mountains and lake Devasunda are the habitats of the Soma plants. Somas, of the Chandramáh species are often found to be floating here and there on the mighty stream of the river Sindhu (Indus) which flows down at the foot of the five large mountains lying to the north bank beyond the Vitastá (river). The Munjaván and the Amsumán species may also be likewise found in the same locality while those known as the Gáyatri, Traishtubha Pámkta, Jágata, S'ámkara, and others looking as beautiful as the moon are found to float on the surface of the divine lake known as the little Mánasa in Kashmir. 12-B.

The Soma plants are invisible to the impious or to the ungrateful as well to the unbeliever in the curative virtues of medicine and to those spiteful to the Bráhmanas. 12.

Thus ends the Twenty-ninth Chapter of the Chikitsita Sthánam in the Sus'ruta Samhitá which deals with the Prophylactic elixirs for the innate maladies.

# CHAPTER XXX.

Now we shall discourse on the tonic remedies which remove mental and physical distress (**Nivritta-samtápiya-Rasáyana**). 1.

**Metrical Text :**—Even in this world mortals may live happily, free from disease and care like the gods in heaven if they (mortals) can secure the after-mentioned drugs (of all-healing potency). 2.

**Persons unfit for the use of Rasáyana :**—The (following) seven classes of persons, viz., the intemperate, the lazy, the indigent, the unwise, the immoral (Vyasani),* the sinful and the triflers of medicine, are unfit to take these ambrosial (Rasáyana) drugs on account of their respective ignorance, inactivity, poverty, vascillation, intemperance, impiety and inability to secure the genuine medicines. 3.

**Names of all-healing drugs :**—Now we shall discourse on these drugs. They are *S'vetakápoti, Krishna-kápoti, Gonasi, Várdhi, Kanyá, Chhatrá, Ati-chchatrá, Karenu, Ajá, Chakraká, Adityaparnini, Suvarchalá, Brahma-suvarchalá, S'rávani, Mahá-s'rávani, Golomi, Aja-lomi* and *Mahá-Vegavati*. These are the names of the eighteen different kinds of drugs of mighty potency. The mode of their use, their

---

* व्यसन is a technical term and is divided into two classes, viz., कामज (*i.e.*, produced by passion or desire) and क्रोधज (*i.e.*, originated from anger). The first group comprises hunting, dice-playing, day-sleep, censuring, addiction to woman, intoxication, singing, dancing, playing on musical instruments and idle wanderings. The second class comprises wickedness, violence, malice, jealousy, envy, extravagance, roughness in language and assault. See Manu, Ch. 7. 47, 48.

therapeutical effects and the religious rites to be observed in their connection, have been described in the Sástras and are identical with those of the **Soma** plants. In order to use them a man should enter the (prescribed) chamber (Agára) and perform the (prescribed) Homa ceremonies. A Kudava measure of the milky juice of the secreting species of the plants should be taken once for all after entering the chamber. 4.

Three twigs or branches, however, to the length of a span of those of the non-secreting species having roots should be taken for a single dose. The (whole of) *S'veta-kápoti* with its leaves and roots should be used. A quantity of the severed pieces of either of the *Gonasi*, *Ajagari* (Suvarchalá) or *Krishna-kápoti* species including their thorns, and weighing a Musti (Sanakha-mushtika)* should be boiled with (an adequate quantity of) milk (and water). The milk thus cooked and prepared should be passed through a piece of cloth and taken only once duly consecrated. The milk cooked and prepared with one of the *Chakraká*† species also should be taken with milk only once, whereas (that of one of) the *Brahma-suvarchalá* species should be taken for seven days in succession. 5.

Five Palas of any of the remaining species should be boiled with an A'dhaka measure of milk and taken down with one quarter left. This should then be strained and the milk thus cooked should be taken in a single

---

\* Some explain "Sanakha mustika" as what would be contained in the hollow of a palm, with the finger nails (*i.e.*, the fingers) extended. But "Nakha" seems to refer to the thorns of the plants and "Mushti" a Pala weight (*i.e.*, eight Tolás).

† Gayi reads "कन्यकायाः पायसम्" in place of "चक्रकायाः पयः" and explains it as a preparation of one part of the powders of the fruit of Kanyaká and two parts of rice cooked with milk.

dose and once only. The regimen of diet and conduct is the same as in the case of **Soma,** until the patient comes out of his prescribed chamber, with this difference that his body should be anointed with butter (Navanita). 6.

**Memorable Verses:**—The use of any of the aforesaid drugs rejuvenates the system, fills it with the strength of a lion, invests it with a beautiful shape, blesses the user with such powerful memory that he can commit to memory anything once heard, and ultimately extends his career to two thousand earthly years. Crowned with diadems of celestial beauty, decorated, as if, with Angadas (bracelets), Kundalas (earrings), crowns and heavenly wreathes (of flowers), Sandal paste and dress, the users are enabled to traverse, like the gods, the cloud-spangled high ways of heaven, unflinchingly in their pursuits. Persons whose systems have been fortified with these medicinal herbs (Oshadhis), like the users of Soma go not by the roads on earth but scale those inaccessible heights of heaven from whence the pendent rain-clouds look down upon the soil below and where the feathered wingers of the ethereal blue frequently soar up to. 7.

**Differentiating Traits:**—Now we shall describe the different traits of these (all-healing) Oshadhis. The **Ajagari*** Oshadhi is found to put forth five leaves which have a brown colour and are marked with variegated ring-like patches. It looks like a snake and measures five Aratnis (a cubit of the middle length from the elbow to the tip of the little finger) in length. The

---

* There is no mention of "Ajagari" in the list (para. 2) and there is no mention of "Suvarchalá" in this descriptive list. It seems, therefore, probable that "Ajagari" and "Suvarchalá" are identical.

S'veta-kápoti is a leafless, gold-coloured, snake-shaped plant with a root two fingers in length and is red at the extremities. The **Gonasi** is a bulbous plant possessed of two leaflets, red-coloured and is marked with black rings. It measures two Aratnis in height and resembles a Gonasa (boa) snake in shape. The **Krishna-kápoti** is a soft, hairy, milk-secreting plant and its juice is possessed of a colour and a taste like that of sugar-cane juice. The **Várahi** is bulbous and puts forth a single leaflet; it is resplendent like broken pieces of black antimony. It resembles a black lance-hooded Kobrá (Krishna Sarpa) in shape and is possessed of mighty potency. 8.

The **Chratrá** and the **Ati-chchhatrá** are bulbous in their origin and are found to be attached to a plant of the Sveta-kápoti species Both of them are possessed of the virtue of arresting death and decay and act as prophylactic against the Rakshas as (malignant spirits). A plant of the **Kanyá** species is found to put forth a dozen leaflets beautifully coloured like the breast-feathers of a peacock. It is bulbous in its origin and exudes a gold-coloured juice. An Oshadhi plant of the **Karenu** species abounds in milky juice and its bulb resembles an elephant. It puts forth two leaves which look like those of a *Hasti-karna-palása* tree. An Oshadhi plant of the **Ajá** species abounds in milky juice, grows like a Kshupa or bushy plant and is white-coloured like the moon, a conch shell, or a *Kunda* flower ; its bulb resembles the udder of a she-goat. An Oshadhi plant of the **Chakraká** species is white-coloured, puts forth flowers of variegated colours, grows in bushes, resembles a *Kákádani* plant in shape and size and is possessed of the efficacy in warding off death and decay. An Oshadhi plant of the **A'ditya-parnini** species grows from roots (and has no bulb) and is furnished with five red-coloured leaflets as soft as a piece of linen and which always point towards the sun (change their direction with the progress of that luminary in heavens) An Oshadhi plant of the **Brahma-Suvarchalá** species, is gold-coloured, abounds in milky juice, resembles a lotus plant in appearance, grows by the side of water (*i.e.*, in marshy lands) and spreads in all directions. An Oshadhi plant of the **Mahá-S'rávani** species bears flowers like a *Nilotpala* and collyrium-coloured fruit. The stem of the Kshupa (bushy) plant measures an Aratni and the leaf two fingers in length. It is gold-coloured and abounds in milky juice. An Oshadhi plant of the **S'rávani** species, possesses all the preceding features, (of the Mahá-s'rávani) but is tinged with a yellow colour. The Oshadhi known as the **Golomi** and the **Ajalomi** are hairy and bulbous (in their origin). A **Vegavati** Oshadhi plant puts forth leaves from its roots; its leaves are severed like those of a *Hamsapádi* creeper, and move about violently (even in the absence of any wind), or it resembles a Samkha-pushpi creeper in all its features, looks like the cast-off skin of a snake and grows at the end of the rainy season (*i.e.*, in autumn). 9.

**Mode of culling the above drugs :—** The first seven of the all-healing Oshadi plants enumerated above should be culled by reciting the following Mantra :—"We appease thee with the holy energy and dignity of Mahendra, Ráma, Krishna and of the Bráhmanas and of cows. Exert your beneficial virtues for the good of mankind". The intelligent one should consecrate all these Oshadhis with this Mantra. The lazy, the impious, the ungrateful and the unbelieving invariably fail to see and secure the Soma plants, or the drugs possessed of similar virtues. The gods after having drunk the celestial ambrosia to their fill cast the residue to the Somas and kindred plants as well as to the moon, the lord of the Oshadhis. 10-A.

**Their habitats :**—The *Brahma-suvarchalá* species (of the Oshadhis) is found to grow in and about the waters of the great river Indus and the lake Devasunda. The *Áditya parnini* species may be had in those two regions at the end of winter, and *Gonasi* and *Ajagari* at the beginning of the rains The *Karenu*, the *Kanyá*, the *Chhatrá*, the *Ati-chchhatrá*, the *Golomi*, the *Aja-lomi*, and the *Mahá-s'rávani* varieties of the Oshadhis are found (in spring) in the lake of Kshudraka-Mánasa in Kashmir. The *Krishna-sarpákhyá* and the *Gonasi* species also are found in that locality during the spring. The *S'veta-kápoti* species is white coloured and is found to grow on the ant-hills which cover a space of three Yojanas on the other (viz, the western) side of the river Kaus'iki and to the east of the Sanjayanti. The Oshadhi of the *Vegavati* species grows on the Malaya hills and on the Nala-setu. 10-B.

Any one of these Oshadhis should be taken after a fast under the auspices of the full-moon in the month of Kártika. The regimen of diet and conduct is the same as laid down in connection with **Soma-Rasáyana** and the results have been already described to be the same. 10 C.

**The common habitats of all the Oshadhis :**—The Soma as well all the other Oshadhi plants may be had on (the summits of) the Arvuda mountains whose cloud-rending summits are the favourite haunts of the gods and which abound in holy pools and fountains frequented by the gods, the Siddhas and the holy Rishis, and whose large hollow caves are reverberated with the thundering roars of lion and which are moated on all sides by swift coursing rivers, whose waters are perpetually tossed by sportive elephants of the forests and whose brows are effulgent with the lustres of various brilliant metals imbedded in their hearts. 10.

These ambrosial plants (as well as other drugs) are to be sought in the rivers, the holy forests and hermitages, as well as in lakes and on hills, since this world is a bed of gems and is known to hold priceless treasures in all places 11.

Thus ends the Thirtieth Chapter of the Chikitsita Sthánam in the Sus'ruta Samhitá which deals with the tonic remedies which have the power of removing the mental and physical distresses.

# CHAPTER XXXI.

Now we shall discourse on the medicinal uses (both internal and external) of the Snehas\*, *i.e.*, oleaginous substances (**Snehaupayogika-Chikitsita**). 1.

A **Sneha** or an oleaginous substance forms the essential factor of the physical organism, and the self-conscious animated element (which contributes directly to its vitality and makes life possible) abounds in oleaginous principles; both are consequently in constant want of a Sneha. Snehas or oleaginous substances are enjoined to be administered in food and drinks as well as in Anuvásana, Mastikya-s'iro-vasti and Uttara-vasti (urethral or vaginal enemas), errhines (Nasya), ear-drops (Karna-purana) and unguents (Abhyanga). 2.

There are four kinds of Snehas which, however, are divided into two classes according to their origin : viz., vegetable and animal. **Clarified butter** prepared from cow's milk is the best of the animal Snehas, while **Sesamum oil** is the best of the vegetable ones. 3

Now we shall describe the ends for which the different vegetable oils should be used as well as the modes in which they should be prepared and employed. 4.

The expressed oils prepared from (the seeds of) *Lodhra, Eranda, Kos'ámra, Danti, Dravanti, Saptalá, S'amkhini, Palás'a, Vishániká, Gavákshi, Kampillaka, Sampáka* and of *Nilini* act as **purgatives**. The oils prepared from (the seeds of) *Jimutaka, Kutaja, Kritavedhana, Ikshváku* (bitter gourd), *Dhámárgava* and of *Madana* act as **emetics**. The expressed oils prepared from (the seeds of) *Vidanga, Khara manjari, Madhu-*

---

\* The **Sneha** is of four kinds, viz., clarified butter, oil, lard and marrow, of which clarified butter and oil are generally used.

*S'igru, Surya-valli, Pilu, Siddhárthaka* and of *Jyotishmati* act as **errhines** (S'iro-virechana). 5.

The expressed oils prepared from (the seeds of) *Karanja, Putika, Kritamála, Mátulunga, Ingudi* and of *Kiráta-tikta* are used in cases of **Dushta-vrana** (malignant ulcers). The expressed oils of *Tuvaraka, Kapittha, Kampillaka, Bhallátaka* and of *Patola* are used in cases of **Mahá-vyádhi** (Kushtha, etc.). The expressed oils of *Trapusha, Erváruka, Karkáruka, Tumbi* and of *Kushmánda* are used in cases of **Mutra-sanga** (for diuretic purposes). The expressed oils of *Kapota-vamka, Avalguja* and of *Haritaki* are used in cases of **Sarkara-s'mari** (gravels, stones, etc). The expressed oils of *Kusumbha, Sarshapa, Atasi, Pichu-marda, Atimuktaka Bhándi, Katu-tumbi* and of *Katabhi* are used in cases of **Prameha** (urinary complaints). The expressed oils of the fruits of *Tála, Nárikela, Panasa, Mocha, Piyála, Vilva, Madhuka, S'leshmátaka* and of *Ámrátaka* are used in diseases due to the deranged **Váyu** acting in concert with the deranged Pitta. The expressed oils of *Vibhitaka, Bhallátaka* and of *Pinditaka* are used in **Krishna-karma** (blackening the cicatrix of a healed ulcer, etc.). The expressed oils of *S'ravana, Kanguka* and of *Tuntuka* are used in imparting a yellow colour (to a cicatrix). The expressed oils of the pith of *S'ims'apá* and of the *Aguru* are used in cases of Kushtha known as **Dadru** (ring-worm) and **Kitima**. 6-7

The primary action of all kinds of Sneha (oil, clarified butter, etc.) is to subdue the aggravation of the deranged Váyu of the body, and the general virtues of all kinds of (vegetable) oil have been described above. 8.

Now we shall describe the process of preparing drug-decoctions and of medicating oils (therewith). According to several authorities, the bark, roots and leaves, etc., of the drugs to be used should be boiled with water weighing four times their combined weight, and should be taken down with three-fourths of the original water evaporated by boiling. This is the rule of preparing **drug-decoctions** (Kasháya). Six Prasrita (one Prasrita being equal to sixteen Tolás) weight of oil, twenty-four Prasrita weights of the liquid (decoction prepared before) and four Aksha measures (one Aksha being equal two to Tolás) of pasted drugs (as **Kalka**) are the proportions to be observed in cooking a medicated oil. But this is not correct. Why? Because it is not in conformity with the injunctions of the Scriptures (officinal standard). We shall now proceed to explain the different measures of Pala, Kudava, etc. 9-10.

**Measures of Drugs :**—The weight of twelve middle-sized Dhánya-máshas (corns of paddy) make one Suvarna-máshaka. Sixteen Suvarna-máshakas make one Suvarna. The weight of nineteen middle-sized *Nishpávas* (pulse) make one Dharana. Three Dharanas and a half make one Karsha. Four Karshas make one Kudava. Four Kudavas make one Prastha.* Four Prasthas make one Ádhaka. Four Ádhakas make one Drona. Hundred Palas make one Tulá. Twenty Tulás make one Bhára. This is the measure in respect of dried substances. The quantity should be doubled in cases of fresh vegetables and fluids † 11.

---

* Thirty-two Palas make one Prastha in respect of water; but in respect of non-oily substances a Prastha is equal to twenty Palas, whereas in respect of fresh drugs it is equal to only sixteen Palas.

† Some drugs, viz :—Vásá, Kutaja, Kushmánda, Prasa'rani Valá, Amrita and Nimba, etc., are invariably employed in their fresh state and the practice is not to take them in double measures in spite of their freshness. Two different kinds of measure have been adopted in the Áyurvedic Pharmacopœia. One is called the **Kálinga** and the

**The Kasháya-Páka Kalpa :**—The bark, roots and leaves, etc., of medicinal drugs should be dried in the sun and taken in any of the aforesaid measures, should be cut in small pieces, or pounded, as the case may be, and soaked in a quantity of water* weighing eight or sixteen times their combined weight. They should then be boiled over a fire and the decoction should be taken down from the oven with only a quarter part of the water left. This is the **general rule** for preparing a decoction (**Kasháya**). 12.

**The Sneha-Páka Kalpa :**—One part of the **Sneha** (oil, clarified butter, etc.), four parts of (any one or more) liquid† substances, a fourth part of the medicinal pastes (**Kalka**) should be boiled together. This is the **general rule** for the preparation of a medicated Sneha (oil, clarified butter, etc.). 13.

**Alternative Methods :**—As an alternative, a Tulá measure of the bark, roots and leaves, etc. (as the case may be) of the drugs to be decocted, should be boiled with a Drona measure of water. The water in the preparation should be boiled down to a quarter part of its original quantity and then considered as cooked and

---

other the **Magadha** measure. Maharshi Charaka has adopted the first, but that adopted by Sus'ruta is the second one.

* Water weighing four times as much as the drugs when the drugs are of a soft consistency and eight times as much when they are hard and sixteen times as much when they are very hard.

† When there are more liquids to be used than one, the general rule is that the total weight of all the liquids would be four times that of the **Sneha,** if not otherwise directed. All this liquid part should, however, be boiled away and the Sneha part should be left before the Sneha is removed from the fire and before it can be fit for use. It should be noted that the cooking of a Sneha should not be completed in one day.—Ed.

prepared. A Kudava measure of oil should be boiled and cooked with four times as much of the liquid and a Pala measure of pasted drugs (Kalka). This is another process of cooking medicated Snehas (oil, etc.). 14.

**Memorable Verses :**—The foregoing rules should be adopted where no measures would be found to have been specifically given of the Sneha, the liquid and of the drugs, whereas in cases of specification, the specific quantities should be taken. Water should be used as the liquid, where no other liquid would be mentioned by name (in connection with medicating a Sneha, viz., oil, clarified butter, etc, by cooking). Both for the decoction and paste (Kalka), the drugs mentioned in the respective list should be used in preparing a medicated Sneha in the absence of any explicit and specific injunction to that effect. 15.

Now we shall discuss the degrees of medically cooking a Sneha (oil or Ghrita). Mild (**Mridu**), middling or intermediate (**Madhyama**) and hard (**Khara**) are the three degrees which the boiling process undergoes in medically cooking a Sneha. A cooking is said to be mild (Mridu-Páka) when the oil is found to drop off entirely from its drug-paste (Kalka) leaving it dry and sapless; whereas in an act of middle-cooking (Madhyama-Páka) the paste would be found to have become pellucid and non-sticky like wax ; a cooking done until the paste (in the Sneha) assumes a little clear, glossy, frothless, black colour is termed strong (Khara-Páka). A Sneha cooked beyond the last-named degree is called a burnt Sneha. A Sneha should, therefore, be properly cooked. A mildly cooked Sneha should be administered in food and drinks. A middling-cooked one for the purposes of errhines and anointments, while a strongly cooked one should be used for the purposes of Vasti-Karma and as ear-drops.* 16.

**Memorable Verses :**—The cooking of a Ghrita should be considered medically complete as soon as the froth and the sound would vanish and the peculiar smell, colour and taste of preparation would be manifest. The medically cooking of an oil resembles in all respects that of a Ghrita with this exception that an abundance of froth appears on the surface of the oil at the completion of the cooking. 17.

**The process of taking a Sneha internally :**—Now we shall describe the process of taking a Sneha internally. A man with an empty stomach should be made to take a draught of a medicinal or medicated oil or Ghrita, just as the god of day (sun) would appear on the summit of the hill at dawn and lighten up the horizon with the first shoots of his vermilion-tinted golden rays. Rites of benediction should be first done unto the patient before administering to him the oil or the Ghrita in an adequate dose. After that he should wash his mouth with warm water and quietly stroll about with his shoes on. 18.

**Metrical Texts :**—The use of a potion of a (medicated) Ghrita is recommended to patients suffering from an extremely parched or dry condition of the organism, or from ulcers, or from the effects of a poison, or from those due to the actions of the deranged **Vâyu** and **Pitta**, as well as to persons of weak memory and intellect. Potions of (medicated) oils should be prescribed in aggravations of the **Kapha** and

---

\* Charaka, on the contrary, holds that a Khara (strongly cooked) Sneha should be used in anointing the body, a middling-cooked one for the purposes of drinks and Vasti-karma and a mildly cooked (Mridu) one for the purposes of errhines.

of **fat**, as well as in cases of worms (in the intestines) and incarcerated flatus (wind in the abdomen), or when the patient is found to be habituated to the internal use of any oil, or seeks the firmness of his body (muscles). The use of lard is recommended to persons emaciated with over-fatiguing physical labour, or to persons whose blood and semen are greatly diminished or to those suffering from an attack of Mahá-vyádhi (due to the vitiated condition of the blood), or to persons of a voracious appetite (Mahágni), or of Vátaja (nervous) temperament, as well as to those possessed of great physical strength. The use of marrow or of medicated Ghritas mixed with appropriate drugs is beneficial to men of strong digestive capacity (Dipta-vahni), or to those afflicted with a deranged Váyu, or to those whose bowels are not easily moved, or who are capable of undergoing a large amount of physical hardship. Clarified butter, without any other thing added thereto, should be administered in the affections of the deranged Pitta ; whereas it should be mixed with salt before use in the diseases due to the action of the deranged Váyu and with the admixture of Yava-kshára and powdered *Trikatu* in the affections of the aggravated and deranged Kapha. Oil or clarified butter should be administered through the medium of one, two or more of the sixty three different combinations\* of the (six different) Rasas (flavour) according to the nature and intensity of the aggravated Dosha or Doshas involved in each case. 19-A.

**Clear** (filtered) oil, clarified butter, etc., should be taken by a man habituated to its use and capable of undergoing physical hardships during the months of

---

\* *Vide* Uttara-Tantra, Chapter LXIII.

the year which are neither too hot nor too cold\* inasmuch as the use of clear or transparent oil or Ghrita is above being commendable. A Sneha should be taken in the morning (lit. day-time) during the cold months of the year and in case of the joint aggravation of the bodily Váyu and Kapha ; whereas it should be taken in the evening (lit. night) during summer and in cases of the joint aggravation of the bodily Váyu and Pitta. Potions of oil or clarified butter taken in summer by a person suffering from an aggravation of the bodily Váyu and Pitta may bring on thirst, epileptic fits and insanity. In the same manner draughts of oil or clarified butter taken in winter by a person suffering from an aggravation of the bodily Váyu or Kapha may be followed by a heaviness of the limbs, aversion to food and colic (Śula). If a patient feels thirsty after taking a Sneha, he should take warm water, and be made to vomit the Sneha with (further) draughts of hot water in the event of the thirst still not subsiding. Cooling plasters should be applied to his head and a cold water bath should be prescribed. 19-B.

**The Dosage :**—The Dosage of a Sneha which requires the quarter part of a day (*i.e.*, three hours) to be digested, should be deemed appetising and beneficial in slight aggravations of the bodily Doshas ; that which requires half a day to be digested should be regarded as invigorating, spermatopoietic, constructive and beneficial in moderate aggravations of the

---

\* Both Vrinda and Chakrapáni read this but with little difference. Both of them read "काले च शीतले," *i.e.*, in the cold season. But their commentators accept the reading "काले नात्युष्णशीतले," as in the text, to be a Variant. We have the authority of Charaka, however, to accept the reading of the text.

bodily Doshas. The dosage of a Sneha which takes three-quarter parts of a day to be digested, acts as a bodily emollient and should be prescribed in cases of extreme aggravation of the bodily Doshas, while the quantity which can only be digested in the course of an entire day (twelve hours) should be considered efficacious in all affections of the body and does not produce physical lassitude, fainting fits and delirious conditions. The measure or quantity of a Sneha which takes a whole day and night to be digested without undergoing any kind of vitiation (reactionary acidity) in the stomach, proves curative even in cases of Kushtha (cutaneous affections), insanity, poisoning (effects of poison) and Apasmára (hysteric convulsions), ascribed to the baneful influences of the malignant stars. 19-C.

**The evil effects of Over-dosage :**—A patient should be made to take as much of the Sneha as he would be able to easily digest inasmuch as an excessive over-dose may prove fatal. The patient should be made to vomit with draughts of hot water in a case of over-dose or abuse of a Sneha and in the event of its continuing in an undigested or partially digested state in the stomach. In cases of doubtful digestion, similar potions of hot water should be administered which would produce good eructations and bring on a fresh relish for food. 19-D.

When the Sneha begins to be digested, it is attended with thirst, vertigo, lassitude, weariness, a disturbed state of the mind and a burning sensation. When the Sneha appears to have been fully digested the patient should be affused with hot water. A gruel prepared with only a small quantity of rice should be given lukewarm to the patient (at this stage). As an alternative, a wellaromated soup (of Mudga, etc.) or meat-juice cooked without the addition of any Sneha (oil or Ghrita) or with only a small admixture of clarified butter should be given, or he may take Yavágu (pure and simple). 19-E.

A Sneha should be taken three, four, five or six days consecutively ; used (continually) for more than a week it becomes habituated to the user. A Sneha should be taken with food (at the time of mid-day meal) by a weak, or an old man or an infant, or a thirsty person, or one of a delicate constitution, or one averse to its use in summer. 19-F.

**Sadyah-Snehana :**—The administration of a potion composed of powdered *Pippali* and (Saindhava) salt mixed with curd-cream and the four kinds of oleaginous substances (Sneha) constitute what is known as the **Sadyah-Snehana** (*i.e.*, it produces the effects of the Sneha within a very short time). The use of a Yavágu well-cooked* with the soup of half-fried meat (instead of water) and a Sneha (clarified butter), and mixed with honey acts as a Sadyah-snehana. A Yavágu prepared with milk† and a small quantity of rice and taken lukewarm with clarified butter produces the same result. The use of cow's milk milched into a pot containing clarified butter and sugar produces an instantaneous emulsive effect (Sadyah-snehana), if taken by a man with a parched state of the organism. Clarified butter cooked with three parts of the decoction of *Yava, Kola* and

---

* In place of "सूपकल्पिता" (well-cooked), Chakradatta reads 'खल्व-तण्डुला' (prepared with a small quantity of rice).

† In place of "पयःसिद्ध" (prepared with milk), Chakradatta reads 'बहुतिला' (prepared with an abundance of sesamum which, according to S'ivadása, would constitute three parts with only one part of rice).

*Kulattha* pulse (taken together) and one part each of milk, curd, wine and clarified butter churned from *milk* acts as an instantaneous demulcent (Sadyah-snehana) and is hence recommended to kings and king like personages. This potent emulsive measure (Sadyah-snehana) should be prescribed for the old, the imbecile, to females and to persons of sluggish appetite, as well as to sensitive persons and in diseases due to a slight aggravation of the bodily Doshas. 19-G.

**Forbidden cases of Sneha-pána :—** The internal use of a Sneha is forbidden to persons suffering from ascites, fever, delirium, alcoholism, aversion to food and vomiting, as well as to weak, corpulent, thirsty, fatigued, or intoxicated persons. It is forbidden on a cloudy day, in an improper season of the year, after the application of Vasti-measures, purgatives and emetics and after premature parturition. The internal use of a Sneha (oil or Ghrita) gives rise to a host of maladies in the foregoing cases, or the diseases become more serious or may even become incurable. In cases of premature parturition, there remains a quantity of mucus and vitiated lochia in the womb; therefore, stomachic (Páchana) and parching (Ruksha) drugs should be administered to females after child-birth. After a period of ten days, however, draughts of oil or clarified butter should be given according to requirements. 19.

A dry or parched condition of the organism should be inferred from a general dryness of the body, the hard and knotty character of the fœcal matter (stools), a sluggish digestion with a burning sensation on the epigastrium (Uras) and an upward coursing of the Váyu from the abdomen (Koshtha) as well as from the weakness and discoloration of the body. Lassitude, a sense of heaviness in the limbs, the oozing out of the Sneha through the lower orifices of the body and an aversion to any kind of oleaginous substance are the indications which mark the satisfactory action of an emulsive remedy in a human organism, while its abrupt excess or abuse is followed by aversion to food, salivation, a burning sensation about the anus, dysentery and diarrhœa and such like symptoms. A condition of dryness in the organism should be remedied with a Sneha, while an excess of the latter should be corrected with meals of *S'yámáka* or *Koradusha* grains, as well as with milk-curd (Takra), levigated sesamum paste (Pinyáka) and powdered barley (S'aktu). 20-23.

### The good effects of Sneha-pána :—

The blessings which attend a person who has duly taken a Sneha are improved digestive capacity, regular and satisfactory motions of the bowels, a growth of all the vital principles of the body, strength and firmness of the organs, improvement of complexion, a delayed old age and the enjoyment of a hundred summers on earth. The application of a Sneha is potent enough to increase the strength and the digestive capacity of a weak person suffering from impaired digestion, and a person having his health and digestive capacity recouped (by the use of a Sneha) does not yield to the evil effects of errors of diet. 54-55.

Thus ends the Thirty-first Chapter in the Chikitsita Sthánam of the Sus'ruta Samhitá which deals with the treatment of the diseases where oleaginous medicines are useful.

# CHAPTER XXXII.

Now we shall discourse on the medical treatment by measures of fomentations, diaphoretic measures, etc. **(Svedá-vacharaniya)**. 1.

**Sveda*** (calorification, fomentation, diaphoretic measures, etc.) may be divided into four groups such as, the application of direct heat (Tápa-sveda), fomentation (Ushma-sveda), poulticing (Upanáha sveda) and the application of heated fluids (Drava-sveda). All kinds of diaphoretic measures (Sveda) belong to one or the other of these groups. 2.

**Tápa-sveda:**—Of these the Tápa-sveda consists in repeatedly applying heat to (any affected part of the body of) a patient made to lie down (on a bed) with the help of the palm of the hand, a piece of brass, an Indian saucer, a piece of baked clay or sand, or a piece of cloth after heating them over a fire of Khadira wood, etc. 3.

**Ushma-sveda :**—A piece of stone, brick, iron, or baked clay should be made red-hot and sprinkled over with water or with sour gruel (Kánjika). The affected part of the body should be covered with (cotton plugs soaked in) Alaktaka† and then fomented with

---

\* The Sanskrit term "**Sveda**" is not properly rendered by the terms fomentations, diaphoretic measures or any other such word or phrase. Sveda is used to mean the application of heat in any possible way—it may be to cause or not to cause perspiration. Vapour baths, hot water baths, applications of warm poultices, etc., are also included in the meaning of the term Sveda. We have, however, for convenience sake, used the term fomentation as a synonym of Sveda in general.

† Jejjata reads "तैराद्रैर्लक्तकपरिवेष्टितं" instead of "तैराद्रीलक्तकपरिवेष्टितं" and explains that the cotton plug soaked in Alaktaka should be made wet and placed over the affected part before applying the fomentation.

the above-named (heated) articles. As an alternative, a metal saucer containing milk, curd, Dhányámla, meat-soup and a decoction of the tender leaves of the Váyu-subduing plants (jointly or separately) should be heated over a fire. The mouth of the saucer should be covered (with a piece of blanket or such other cloth)* and the affected part of the body should be fomented with the vapours rising therefrom. As an alternative, another pitcher should be placed with its mouth downward over the mouth of the above pitcher (containing the above-named heated articles). Then an aperture should be made in the side of the upper pitcher and a pipe to the shape of an elephant's trunk should be inserted into it. The affected part of the body should then be fomented with the **vapour** escaping through that pipe. 4.

**Metrical Texts :**—The mode of applying heat to a patient suffering from any disease or affection of the bodily Váyu (disease of the nervous system, etc.,) is as follows :—He should be first anointed with oil, etc., and wrapped up in a thick cloth. He should then be made to sit in an easy posture. Heat should then be applied through a pipe shaped as an elephant's trunk. The advantage of this mode of fomentation is that the entire body of the patient may be easily fomented without causing him any serious trouble. The pipe should be made half a Vyáma† in length with three bends or turns‡ in its body to resemble

---

\* The mouth of the pitcher should be covered only to mitigate and regulate the heat.

† A Vyáma is the length measured by the outstretched hands of a man.

‡ The reasons for bending the tube are to make the fomentation delightful, in consequence of the vapour not passing in a straight course.

the trunk of an elephant.* The use of a pipe made of the materials (such as *Kus'a, Kás'a,* etc.) used in the making of a Kilinji (basket) and resembling the trunk of an elephant in shape is only recommended for the purposes of Sveda (heat-application). 5.

A plot of ground commensurate with the length of the patient's body should be dug and heated with fire of *Khadira* wood and then sprinkled over with milk, water and Dhányámla. The heated ground should be then covered with a layer of leaves (of the Váyu-subduing plants) and the patient should be made to lie down full stretched upon the (bed of) leaves and thereby fomented.† As an alternative, a stone slab should be heated and the fomentation (Sveda) should be applied similarly to the patient by making him lie down upon it after the ashes and cinders have been removed ‡. As an alternative, the patient should be seated inside a chamber with four doors (one on each side) and fomented by lighting up a good blazing fire (of Khadira wood) at all the doors (simultaneously §. Another alternative is that the patient should be laid on a mattress (made of Kus'a, Kás'a, etc.) or on a similar bed as before and fomented with the fumes of duly boiled paddy (and Másha-pulse, etc.) kept under the same mattress. In the same manner, Sveda (fomentation) might be applied with the help of heated cow-dung, ashes, husks of paddy, weeds, etc. 7.

**Upanáha-Sveda** (Poulticing) :—The roots of the Váyu-subduing drugs should be pasted together

---
\* This is called the " **Nádi-sveda** ".
† This is called the " **Karshu-sveda** ".
‡ This is called the " **As'ma-ghana-sveda** ".
§ This is called the " **Kuti-Sveda**".

with Amla (Kánjika) and mixed with an abundant quantity of rock-salt and of Sneha (clarified butter, etc.). The paste should be heated and applied lukewarm to the affected part. The pastes of the drugs included within the *Kákolyádi*, the *Eládi* or the *Surasádi* groups as well as a paste of mustard seed, sesamum or linseed, or **Kriśará, Páyasa** (porridge) **Utkáriká**, or **Veśavára**, or the drugs of S'álvana\* (as described under the treatment of Váta-Vyádhi) should be similarly applied (lukewarm to the affected locality) folded in a piece of thin linen. This is what is called the **Upanáha-Sveda**. 8.

**Drava-Sveda** (Diaphoresis with fluids):—A jar or a cauldron should be filled with a lukewarm decoction of any of the Váyu-subduing drugs and the patient should be immersed therein. In the same way, the patient might be immersed in a tubful of warm milk, meat-soup, soup (of Mudga or Másha pulse), oil, Dhányámla (fermented or sour gruel), clarified butter, lard, cow's urine, etc.† The patient may also be sprinkled over or washed with a tepid decoction (of the above-mentioned drugs).‡ This is what is called the **Drava-Sveda**. 9.

Of the four forms of Sveda described above those known as the Tápa-Sveda and Ushma-Sveda pre-eminently destroy the deranged **Kapha**, while the Upanáha-Sveda subdues the deranged **Váyu** of the body ;

\* Drugs of the Kákolyádi group should be used in cases of the dominant deranged Pitta acting in concert with the deranged Váyu ; those of Eládi group in cases of the dominant deranged Kapha acting in concert with the deranegd Váyu and the S'álvana, or sesamum, linseed, etc., in cases of a simple or complicated deranged Váyu.

† This is called the **Avagáha-Sveda**.
‡ This is called the **"Parisheka-Sveda."**

the Drava-Sveda, however, is beneficial in cases due to the concerted action of the deranged **Pitta** with either of the other two Doshas (*viz.*, **Váyu and Kapha**). 10-A.

The patient should be diaphorised by making him put on warm clothing or exposing himself to the sun or by becoming fatigued after a long walk, or by wrestling, or some other physical exercise, load-carrying, etc., or by arousing his anger in a case where the deranged **Váyu** would be found to be subcharged with the deranged **fat** or **Kapha**. 10.

**Memorable Verses :**—The four forms of Sveda mentioned above may be employed in two ways, *viz.* :—either to the whole body or to any particular part of it. Sveda should be first employed in cases of patients fit to be treated with errhines (Nasya), purgatives, emetics or with Vasti-measures. It should be applied to the enciente in cases of obstructed fœtus (Mudha-garbha) unattended with any other supervening distresses (*i.e.*, excessive discharge of blood, etc.) after the extraction of the S'alya (the obstructed fœtus) from the womb, and after parturition, and in cases where pregnancy runs to its full and natural term. Sveda should similarly be applied both before and after the surgical operation in cases of fistula-in-ano and stones, gravel, etc., (in the bladder) and of hæmorrhoids. Specific modes of applying Sveda in other diseases should be duly described under their respective heads. 11.

Men conversant with the rules of **Sveda** (fomentations, etc.) should, under no circumstances, employ it before rubbing or softening the body or the limb with a Sneha (oil, etc.) inasmuch as a piece of wood is found to break or burst immediately under the application of heat if not previously rubbed with a Sneha. 12—A.

**Effects of Sveda :**—Improved digestive capacity (Agni-dipti), softness of the limbs, smoothness and clearness of the skin, relish for food, clearness of the bodily ducts or channels, absence of somnolence and drowsiness and restored functions (free movements) of the numbed bone-joints are the benefits which result from an application of Sveda. The Doshas (morbific principles) having been moistened with a Sneha and lying inherent in the root principles (Dhátus) of the body or imbedded in its ducts or channels or located in their specific seats within the system, become liquefied and carried down into the bowels (Koshtha) by and after an application of Sveda and are eventually totally eliminated from the system (by means of correcting measures—D. R.). 12-B.

A **perfect** or satisfactory application of Sveda is marked by a copious flow of perspiration, an abatement or amelioration of the disease, a lightness of the body and a desire for cool things and the softening of the patient's limbs, while the contrary effects result from an **imperfect** or unsatisfactory application of the same. An **excessive** application of Sveda would produce pain in the joints, and a burning sensation (in the body). It produces blisters, an aggravation of the Pitta, an excited condition of the blood, epileptic fits, vertigo, thirst, and fatigue. In such a case the evils should be speedily remedied with cooling measures. 12.

**Prohibited cases of Sveda :**—Applications of Sveda should not be resorted to in cases of persons suffering from jaundice, urinary complaints, hæmorrhage, pulmonary consumption (Kshaya), emaciation, indigestion, ascites (Udara),* thirst, vomit-

---

\* Vrinda evidently quotes this verse from Sus'ruta Sambitá but by a little change in the versification he excludes cases of Vomiting and poisoning from the list and mentions only the cases of Dakodara

ing, dysentery, and from diseases due to the effects of poison. It is also prohibited in respect of pregnant women and intoxicated persons, inasmuch as an application of Sveda proves fatal in these cases or tends to impart an incurable character to the disease (inflicting an irreparable injury to the whole organism). 13.

Mild Sveda may be applied (and that only in cases of emergency) to the aforesaid persons suffering from diseases amenable only to an application of Sveda, as well as to the regions of the eyes, the heart (Hridaya) and the scrotum. 14.

Sveda should be applied unto a patient in a covered and windless place and after the complete digestion of his ingested food, and after having anointed his body with a Sneha. During the application of Sveda (to the eyes and to the heart) the eyes of the patient should be (first) covered with something cold (*e g.*, lotus leaves, etc.) and the heart should be constantly touched with something cold (*e.g.*, cold palms of the hand, etc.). 15.

After a full and complete application of Sveda, the (body of the) patient should be well rubbed with a Sneha (oil, etc.) and a hot bath should be prescribed. The patient should then be made to keep his body well covered (with warm clothes) and be removed to a windless chamber (immediately afterwards). The diet should consist of such articles as would not produce any internal secretion (in the channels of the system) and he should observe, if necessary, the other rules of conduct (enjoined in such cases). 16.

(instead of Udara in general) as unfit for Sveda and this is consistent with the treatment prescribed by Sus'ruta himself in Chapter XIV, Chikitsita Sthána.

Thus ends the Thirty-second Chapter in the Chikitsita Sthánam of the Sus'ruta Samhitá which treats of the applications of Sveda.

# CHAPTER XXXIII.

Now we shall discourse on the treatment of the distresses which prove amenable to the use of purgatives and emetics **(Vamana-Virechana-Sádhyopadrava). 1.**

The principal maxims to be followed are to augment the loss or deficiency, to pacify the aggravation and reduce the increment of the Doshas and maintain them in a state of healthy equilibrium. Emetics and purgatives are the principal remedies in cleansing the system of all the Doshas (morbific principles). Now hear me, therefore, discourse on the mode of their administration. 2.

The body of the patient should be first anointed with a Sneha (oil, etc.) and Sveda should then be applied thereto. He should then be made to partake of meals which would produce internal secretions from the system, so that all the Doshas (morbific diathesis, etc.) accumulated in the organism would be loosened and dislodged from their seats. Thus having observed the liquefaction and dislodgment of the Doshas (morbific diathesis) from their locations, the physician should feed the patient to his satisfaction, if he be found to be sufficiently strong with a strong digestive capacity and habituated to the use of emetics, but troubled with a plethora of Doshas and subject to serious diseases (Mahá-vyádhi), telling him at the same time that an **emetic** medicine will be given to him on the day following. 3.

**Memorable Verse :**—An emetic medicine does its fullest action, when given to a man after having applied a Sneha and Sveda (to him) and after having stirred up the Doshas of his body with the help of a soft mucilaginous (Kapha-producing)* fluid and emollient food so as to accelerate their easy expulsion from the system 4.

On the next morning, when it is neither too hot nor too cold† the patient should be made to vomit with an adequate dose of an emetic in any of the following forms, viz., powder, paste, decoction, (medicated) oil or Ghrita as the case may be. Such things as have a fetid or an obnoxious smell or sight should be used for emetic purposes having regard to the characteristic nature of the patient's stomach (Koshtha), the contrary being the rule in respect of the use of purgatives. 5.

Infants, old men, weak and timid persons as well as those who are of a delicate constitution should be first made to drink their full of milk, curd, milk-curd (Takra) or a gruel (Yavágu)‡ in diseases amenable to emetics and in such quantities that the patient feels it rising up to the throat. After the emetic has been administred, the body of the patient should be (gently) fomented for a short time with the heated palms of the hands and the effect (of the emetic, observed.) The dislodgment and passing of the Doshas from their respective seats into the Kukshi (stomach ?) should

---

\* Vrinda reads "श्रेष्मले:" in place of "पेश्मले:" but they would ultimately mean almost the same thing

† Dallana says that some explains "साधारणे काले" to mean "in the proper seasons, viz., the rainy season, the Autumn and the Spring."

‡ The milk, the curd, the milk-curd and the gruel prescribed to be taken in this case should, according to Dallana, be either medicated with emetic drugs or should be taken alone as an after-potion.

be inferred from the flow of perspiration (Sveda) that would ensue. The patient should then be made to sit on a seat as high as his knees and as soon as he would feel the least tendency to vomit, the attendants should be told to catch hold of his waist, sides, back, throat and forehead. Then a finger or the stem of (a leaf of) a castor plant or of a lotus should be inserted down his throat and the patient should be made to fully eject the contents of his stomach until the symptoms of satisfactory vomiting would fully appear. 6.

**Memorable Verses :**—The symptoms of an imperfect emesis are water-brash (Kaphapraseka), sticking secretion or sensation of impurity in the regions of the Hridaya (heart) and itching sensations. An excessive discharge of the Pitta, the loss of consciousness, pains in the throat and in the region of the heart are the features which mark excessive or over-vomiting. The indications which characterise the perfect and satisfactory action of an emetic remedy are the free emission of Pitta after that of Kapha, a light and pleasing sensation in the heart, the throat and the head, a lightness of the body and the complete cessation of the emission of Kapha (mucus). 7.

Thus having observed the symptoms of a satisfactory emesis, the patient should be advised to inhale the fumes (Dhuma) of a (burning) drug of either the Snehana, Vairechana or Sámana (soothing) virtues in such doses as he could conveniently take and to observe the proper regimen of diet and conduct. 8.

**Memorable Verses :**—Then having washed his body with tepid water and having perceived him to be in a pure state of mind and body the patient should be advised to take his evening meal with the soup of *Kulattha* or of *Mudga* or of *Ádhaki* or with the soup of the flesh of any Jángala animal.* A person treated with emetics (at regular intervals) by cough, accumulation of Kapha in the throat, loss of voice, somnolence, drowsiness, fetid smell in the mouth, evil effects of poisoning (other supervening distresses of Kapha—D. R.), water-brash and lienteric diarrhœa (Grahani). The (accumulated) Kapha of the system having been ejected by vomiting under a course of emetic treatment, the possibility of all Kapha-origined affections is removed, just as a felled tree soon dries up together with all its twigs, fruits and flowers. 9-10.

### Cases where emesis is forbidden :—

Emesis or the exhibition of emetics is forbidden in cases of Timira (cataract), upward determination of the Váyu in the body (Urdhva-váta), Gulma, Udávarta, abdominal dropsy, enlargement of the spleen, worms (in the intestines) and urinary complaints, as well as in respect of fatigued, corpulent, thirsty, hungry, emaciated and too old persons and of infants, Kshata-kshina patients and those suffering from a loss of voice, and in respect of those also who are of studious habits or are capable of being treated with a strong emetic and that only with the greatest difficulty. It should be never resorted to in cases of Hœmoptysis and obstinate constipation of the bowels and in the case of an enciente and after the application of a Niruha-vasti. It should not be applied in an extremely dry or parched condition of the organism† as well as in simple diseases due to the Váyu. 11.

* The diet of the patient who has taken an emetic should be very carefully prescribed inasmuch as his digestive capacity is liable to become very weak in such cases.

† Persons afflicted with cataract or blindness, Gulma, facial paralysis, convulsion (Ákshepaka), jaundice, ascites, hæmorrhoids and corpulency

To induce vomiting with an emetic medicine in the (aforesaid) diseases in which it ought not to have been resorted to is likely to give an irrecoverable turn to those diseases. Emetics should not, therefore, be applied in such cases. To induce vomiting, however, with the help of the decoction of *Madhuka* (Yashti-madhu)* is not forbidden even in these cases, if the patient be suffering from indigestion or from an extremely aggravated condition of the deranged Kapha as well as from poisoning symptoms. 11-12.

**Cases where emesis is recommended :**—On the other hand, vomiting or the exhibition of an emetic is recommended in cases of poisoning, in wasting diseases (S'osha), in the derangements of the breast-milk, in precarious or sluggish (Vishama) appetite, in insanity, in Apasmára (hysteric convulsions), in Elephantiasis (S'lipada), in Vidáriká, in tumours (Arvuda), in obesity, in Meha (urinary complaints), in cases of slow chemical poisoning (Gara-dosha) in the system, in fever, in aversion to food, in scropfula (Apachi), in mucous dysentery, in heart-disease, in distraction of the mind, in erysipelas, in inflammatory abscesses (Vidradhi), in indigestion, in water-brash, in nausea, in asthma, in cough, in Pinasa (catarrh), in fetid smell of the nostrils (Puti-nása), in inflammations of the lips, throat and mouth,† in (fetid) discharges from the ears, in Adhi-jihviká, Upa-jihviká and Gala-s'undiká

---

as well as extremely old men and Kshata-kshina patients should not be treated with emetics (lit. should not be caused to vomit).—D. R.

* Jejjata explains Madhuka to mean honey. He means to say that Vomiting should be induced with honey and water.

† Some read here "Kushtha, Galaganda, Prameha and S'opha (swelling)" but as Meha is mentioned above separately it seems to us that that reading is not a good one.—Ed.

(affections of the glottis and the thorax), in hæmorrhage from the lower channels, in the derangements due to the bodily Kapha and in all affections of the location of Kapha*. 13.

**Mode of administering purgatives :**—Purgatives should also be administered to a patient after the due application of Sneha (oil, etc.) and Sveda (for a second time) after the administration of an emetic. On the day before the administration of the purgative, the patient should be told that a purgative should be given to him the next morning. He should at this time be provided with a light repast followed by potions of hot water and (the expressed juice of) acid fruits. On the next morning an adequate dose of the (purgative) medicine should be administered after clearly ascertaining that the patient's body has been cleansed of all mucous (Sleshmá) accumulations and in the manner laid down in the Áturopakramaniya chapter (Chapter XXXV. of tho Sutra-sthána). 14.

**Classification of Koshtha :**—Koshtha (bowels) may be grouped under three heads as mild or easily movable (**Mridu**), middling or moderately constipated (**Madhya**) and hard or constipated (**Krura**). The first kind (Mridu) of the Koshtha should be ascribed to the abundance of **Pitta** therein and can be moved even with milk only ; the last (Krura) is ascribable to the action of an abundance of **Váyu** and **Kapha** and can be moved only with the greatest difficulty ; while the second, Madhayama, should be held as the product of a condition of equilibrium among the (three) Doshas and this is the most general type. Purgatives

---

\* Dallana says that some commentators do not read this part, but they say that the necessity of applying emetics is mentioned in each particular case where required.

should be administered in small doses to persons of lax bowels (Mridu Koshtha), in moderate doses to those of moderately constipated bowels (Madhayama Koshtha), and in large doses to persons of extremely constipated bowels (Krura Koshtha). After having taken a purgative the patient should think of nothing else but purging and when passing his stool he should not go far from his bed-side. 15.

**Metrical Texts :**—He should at this time lie in a windless chamber, foregoing the use of cold water and exposure to cold wind, and should not repress any urging (towards stool) nor should he strain. Emission of urine, stool, Pitta, the (purgative) medicine and lastly of Kapha consecutively follow under a course of purgative, in the same manner as an emission of saliva, the (emetic) drug, Kapha, Pitta and lastly of Váyu are consecutively ejected under the course of an emetic. 16-17.

**Memorable Verses :**—An aggravation of the Kapha and Pitta, a burning sensation in the body, an aversion to food, heaviness of the limbs and impaired digestion (lassitude—D. R.) are the effects of an improper application of a purgative. Heaviness of the Kukshi and of the heart, itching and burning sensation, and the retention of stool and urine are the symptoms which follow in the wake of a purgative medicine which has failed to satisfactorily open and cleanse the bowels. Loss of consciousness, prolapsus of the anus, aggravation of the bodily Kapha and Śula colic pain in the intestines) result from an act of over-purging. A sense of lightness about the region of the umbilicus\* and hilarity of the wind due to the discharge of the dis-

\* In place of "नाभ्या लघुत्वे" some read "म्लान्यां लघुत्वे" which means "a sense of lightness and lassitude".

tempers connected with the Kapha (mucus, stool, etc.) and restoration of the bodily Váyu to its normal condition due to the discharge of the (deranged) Váyu (from the system) are the symptoms which mark the satisfactory action of a purgative medicine. 18-A.

**Diet :**—No liquid food or Peyá should be given to the patient on the day in the event of his not being properly purged and not being feebled (with purging) and in the event of his impaired digestion (after the use of a purgative). A light and lukewarm Peyá should, however, be given to him in small doses, whenever he would feel weak and thirsty after the proper exhibition of a purgative medicine. 18-B.

**Benefits of proper purgation :**—Clearness and expansion (Prasáda) of the intellect, firmness of the organs and of the Dhátus (root-principles) of the body, increase of energy (Bala)*, improved digestive capacity and a late or delayed old age are the blessings which follow a proper administration of purgative remedies. The deranged Pitta of the system, having been fully removed (with the help of a purgative), precludes the possibility of the existence of any Pitta-origined complaint, just as the waters of a tank or any other reservoir of water, having been fully baled out, bar against the possibility of the existence of all aquatic animals and plants living therein. 18.

**Persons who should not be purged :** —Exhibition of purgatives are prohibited in respect of persons of impaired digestion, or of those treated with an excessive application of any emulsive remedy (Sneha-Karma), or of those who are exceedingly corpulent, too old, fatigued, thirsty or intoxicated, or of those suffering from any ulcer. They are similarly prohibited in

---

* Vrinda does not include "Bala" (energy) in the list.

respect of frightened persons and Kshata-kshina patients or of those afflicted with hæmorrhage from the downward orifices of the body or of persons with any dart or foreign matter (śalya) lying imbedded in the organism as well as in respect of infants and enciente. A purgative medicine should not be administered before the digestion of a meal previously taken, neither in the diseases due to an abuse of wine, nor in acute catarrh and acute fever or to a newly parturient woman and persons not previously treated with a Sneha (oil or Ghrita). A mild purgative may, however, be administered (in cases of emergency) to a person of extremely Pitta-predominant temperament. Purgatives administered by ignorant physicians to persons who ought not to be purged (often) prove fatal. 19.

**Persons who should be purged :—** The distempers of the body in which a purgative should be exhibited with good results are : —fever, effects of slow chemical poison (retained in the system), an aversion to food, hæmorrhoids, tumours (Arvuda), ascites (Udara), glandular swellings (Granthi), abscess (Vidradhi), jaundice, hysteric convulsions (Apasmára), heart-disease, Váta-rakta, vaginal or uterine diseases, fistula-in-ano, vomiting, erysipelas (Visarpa), Gulma, pain in the Pakváśaya (intestines), retention of stool, Visuchiká, Alasaka, strangury (Mutrágháta), cutaneous affections (Kushtha), Visphotaka (carbuncle, etc.), Prameha, distension of the abdomen with the suppression of stool and urine (Ánáha), enlargement of the spleen, œdematous swellings (Śopha), Vriddhi (enlargement of the scrotum, etc.) and kindred complaints, ulcers inflicted by weapons, alkaline scalds and burns, malignant ulcers, (Dushta-vrana), inflammation of the eyes (Akshi-páka), Kácha, Timira, conjunctivitis (Abhishyanda), burning sensations in the head, ears, eyes, nose, mouths, anus and the penis, hæmorrhage from the upper channels (Urdhva-Rakta-pitta), worms, diseases of the Pittás'aya (bowels?) *i.e.*, the diseases which are peculiar to the seats of the Pitta in the organism as well as any other disease due to an aggravation of the Pitta. 20.

**Metrical Texts :**—Emetic and purgative remedies, in spite of their possessing in common the powers of motion (Saratva), subtlety, keenness, expansiveness and heat-making properties, tend to remove the injurious and deranged morbific principles (Doshas) of the body in (two) different ways by virtue of their respective inherent qualities (Prakriti)*. A purgative, in the course of its digestion, carries down with it all the Doshas from the system (loosened and dislodged by virtue of its own specific properties). An emetic, on the other hand, is not digested, owing to (its lightness due to) its inherent extraordinary qualities†, but it soon forces its way up with the Doshas (to be) removed. 21-22.

A strong purgative given to a man of loose or lax bowels (Mridu-Koshtha) or of strong digestive capacity, cannot remove all the Doshas fully owing to their being suddenly and forcibly purged off. 23.

A purgative medicine, which is capable of being digested and of expelling the Doshas from the body in the time which a morning meal ordinarily takes to be digested, should be regarded as pre-eminently the best. 24.

---

* Dallana quotes a different reading which means that emetic and purgative remedies produce the wished-for result, if properly administered, otherwise not.

† The extraordinary qualities of an emetic are those of the Váyu and of the Agni.

The (aggravated) Doshas accumulated in a large quantity in the organism of a weak patient and found to be dislodged from their seats should be gradually expelled from the system, while soothing (S'amana) remedies should be used in cases of the Doshas being very slight, even if they be found to have been dislodged from their seats. The aggravated Doshas matured and spontaneously dislodged (from their seat or place of accumulation in the system) should be purged off, whether the patient be strong or weak, inasmuch as, if neglected (and not expelled from the system), they (Doshas) tend to produce lasting troubles. 25-26.

A purgative should be administred to a patient of impaired digestive capacity and extreme habitual constipation of the bowels (Krura-koshtha) after having improved his digestion with the admixture of rock-salt, *Yava-kshára* and clarified butter and after applying Sneha and Sveda (as usual). A purgative remedy used after a due application of Sneha and Sveda to the body, leads to the looseness and dislodgment per force of the aggravated Doshas from their seats, since they do not adhere to the internal channels and passages just as a drop of water does not adhere to a pot or vessel saturated with a Sneha. An oleaginous purgative should not be given to persons who have already taken internally* an abundant quantity of Sneha, as it would tend to make the aggravated Doshas of the body dislodge from their seats and again adhere to the internal channels and passages. 27-28.

An excessive quantity of Sneha should be used in cases of poisoning, hurt, pustular eruptions (Pidaká),

---

* Vrinda reads "अतिस्निग्धकायस्य" in place of "अतिस्नेहपीतस्य". This means that the Sneha might have been used both internally and externally.

œdema and cutaneous affections before the application of purgatives or emetics. The body of a patient, habituated to the use of oleaginous articles (Sneha), should be first made dry (Ruksha). Sneha should then be used again as usual and purgatives or emetics applied. The aggravated Doshas would be thereby expelled from the system and the patient would grow stronger*. 29-30.

Mild emetics and purgatives should be given at the outset to a person to be treated with such medicines; who had never taken any purgative or emetic before. Emetics and purgatives should then again be administered to him, after thus finding out the state and nature of his Koshtha (bowels). An emetic or purgative medicine of tested efficacy and which is pleasant, aromatic, agreeable and small in dose but of mighty potency should be given to a king; (in addition to these qualities) the medicine should be such as would not produce any serious injury. 31-32.

The body (health) of a patient to whom a purgative or emetic medicine is administered without first applying Sneha and Sveda thereto breaks up like a piece of sapless wood at the time of bending it. The aggravated Doshas dislodged from their seats in the organism through the effects of Sneha and Sveda and stirred by emollient food† are easily expelled by emetics and purgatives. 33.

Thus ends the Thirty-third Chapter of the Chikitsita Sthánam in the Sus'ruta Samhitá which deals with the treatment of diseases amenable to the use of emetics and purgatives.

\* Vrinda reads "स्नेहबस्मना" in place of "बलवर्द्धना". This means that the Doshas, so long obstructed by Sneha, are thereby expelled.

† Some explain "रसै: स्निग्धै:" to mean "with emollient meat-soup".

# CHAPTER XXXIV.

Now we shall discourse on the treatment of the disorders resulting from an injudicious use of emetics or purgatives (**Vamana-Virechana-Vyápach-Chikitsitam**). 1.

**Their Classes :**—Fifteen different kinds of disorders may result from an injudicious use of emetics and purgatives owing to the ignorance of the physician or of the patient. Of these (fifteen), the upward coursing in cases of purgatives and the downward coursing in cases of emetics are peculiar to each of them respectively. The fourteen other remaining disorders (Vyápat) are common to both They are **Sávaseshaushadhatva** (continuance of the drug in the stomach), **Jirnaushadhatva** (complete digestion of the medicine), **Hinadoshápahritatva** (insufficient elimination of the Doshas from the system) **Adhika-doshápahritatva** (excessive elimination of the Doshas from the system), **Váta-śula** (Vátaja colic), **Ayoga** (insufficient dosage), **Ati-yoga** (over dosage), **Jivádána** (hæmorrhage), **Ádhmána** (tympanites), **Pari-kartiká** (cutting pain in the anus, etc.), **Parisráva** (oozing out of stools), **Praváhiká** (diarrhœa), **Hridayopasarana** (rising of the Doshas towards the heart) and **Vibandha** (suppression of stool and urine). 2.

**Causes and Treatment :**—An emetic taken by a hungry or a weak person or by one possessed of a very keen digestive capacity (Tikshnágni) or of lax bowels (Mridu koshtha), naturally drops down into the intestines in virtue of the identical nature and intensity of their attributes, in the event of its being retained in the stomach, even for a short while. A failure of the medicine to produce the wished-for result and a further stirred or agitated condition of the aggravated Doshas are the effects thereof. In such a case Sneha (and Sveda) should be again applied and a stronger emetic administered. 3.

An obnoxious and large-dosed purgative taken by a person with a residue of a previous meal remaining undigested (in the stomach) or with an aggravated Kapha or with a disordered stomach (Ámás'aya), is forced upward and is ejected through the mouth. In a person of disordered stomach the accumulations (Kapha) in the stomach should be first speedily ejected with an emetic and a stronger purgative should then be administered. A case where the food remains still undigested (in the intestines) should be treated (with fastings and digestants) as in a case of mucous diarrhœa. A pleasant or tasteful purgative should be given in a moderate dose in the event of a previous one having been ejected on account of its obnoxious taste and abnormal dosage. A third dose should not be given in the event of the second also being not retained in the stomach. At this stage, purging should be effected with the help of a lambative (Leha) prepared with honey, clarified butter and treacle. 4.

**Sávas'eshaudhatva** (Evils of an unpurged residue of a purgative or emetic) :—A small dose of medicine, whether an emetic or a purgative, if it is absorbed by the deranged Doshas of the body and retained in the system, cannot produce the wished-for result of cleansing the system. In such a case, it gives rise to thirst, pain in the sides, vomiting, epileptic fits, nausea, piercing or breaking pain in the joints, aversion to food, impure eructations, and such like symptoms. The patient in such a case should be made to vomit the contents of his stomach with draughts of hot water. When a least residue of a purgative medicine previously administered would be found to have been retained in the stomach of a strong patient and with extremely aggravated Doshas of the body, the patient, if there be an insufficient purging, should be similarly made to vomit. 5.

**Jirnaushadhatvam** (Evils of a digested purgative, etc.) :—A mild purgative or emetic or a medicine administered in a small dose to a man of extremely constipated bowels (Krura-koshtha) or of an extremely keen digestive capacity (Tikshnágni), is like food easily digested in the stomach (and therefore fails to produce the wished-for results). The aggravated Doshas, being thus unexpelled by the (purgative or emetic) medicine from the body, brings on fresh distempers and loss of strength (**Bala**)* of the body. Under the circumstances a stronger medicine or a larger dose of the same should be administered to the patient. A mild medicine as well as a medicine administered without a previous application of Sneha and Sveda subdues only a slight aggravation of the Doshas. 6.

**Evils of insufficient or excessive expulsion of the Doshas:**—A nausea, a sense of heaviness in the limbs, a sticky sensation in the chest and aggravation of the (existing) disease are the evils which attend an insufficient ejection of any bodily Dosha from the system after the administration of an **emetic**. More satisfactory vomitings should be induced in such cases with the help of an appropriate (and stronger) medicine. Tympanites, heaviness of the head, suppression or incarceration of Váyu (flatus), a cutting pain (Pari-kartana) in the anus and aggravation of the (existing) disease, are the evils which result from an imper-

* For the meaning of "**Bala**" here see Chapter XV., Sutra-Sthána.

fect or partial expulsion of the Doshas from the system under the administration of a purgative remedy. The remedy in such cases should consist in inducing stronger purgings after a further application of Sneha and Sveda to the patient. A mild medicine should be administered on the third day to a strong-limbed patient, if there be a large quantity of dislodged agitated Dosha in his system. 7.

**Váta-s'ula** (Flatulent colic) :—The bodily Váyu become enraged or agitated by the use of parching (Ruksha) medicines by a person who has not been treated with a previous application of Sneha and Sveda or by one who does not observe a total abstinence in sexual matters. The Váyu thus enraged tends to produce a kind of pain (S'ula) in the sides, waist (S'roni), back, tendons and the (principal) Marma (heart) and brings on vertigo, epileptic fits and loss of consciousness. The remedy under such circumstances consists in anointing the patient's body with oil or clarified butter, fomenting it with (hot and half-boiled) paddy (Dhánya-Sveda) An oil cooked with *Yashti-madhu* should then be employed as an Anuvásana-Vasti. 8-A.

**Ayoga** (Partial and deficient medication):—A mild or an insufficient dose of an emetic or purgative, administered without a previous application of Sneha and Sveda to the patient, fails to find an outlet either through the upper or the lower fissures of the body and hence brings about an aggravation of the Doshas incarcerated in the organism and produces a loss of strength (Bala), as well as tympanites with a catching pain in the chest (Hridaya-graha), thirst, epileptic fits and a burning sensation in the body This is called **Ayoga**. The remedy in such cases should consist in inducing, without any delay, vomiting with powered *Madana* fruit dissolved in a saline solution, or in moving the bowels with a stronger purgative in the shape of decoctions. 8–B.

The bodily Doshas are aggravated through deficient or scanty vomitings under the action of an emetic drug and expands through the entire organism, giving rise to itching, swelling, cutaneous affections, pustular eruptions, fever, aching of the limbs, piercing pain and such-like symptoms. The remaining or uneliminated Doshas should then be expelled with (adequate) medicines of strong potency (Mahaushadhi). Similarly, insufficient purgings under the action of a mild purgative, administered without a previous application of Sneha and Sveda to the patient, produce a numbed and drum-like distension of the abdomen below the umbilicus, causing a retention of the stool and flatus, and produce (colic) pain (S'ula), itching and urticarious eruptions (Mandala). The remedy under these circumstances should consist in employing emulsive measures (Sneha) and a stronger purgative after having employed an Ásthápana-Vasti. Draughts of hot water should be given to the patient and the abdomen and the sides should be fomented with the heated palms of the hands for exciting or inducing purging in the event of an unsatisfactory purging and of obnoxious matter not being expelled from the system. The purging (of Dosha) would thus be induced. A second dose of a purgative should be again administered in the evening with a due consideration to the strength of the patient when the first would be found to have been digested before producing a sufficient purging if the system of the patient be still full of Doshas and morbid matter. In case of failure of this also to remove the Doshas (excreta), the system of the patient should be first treated with

Sneha and Sveda after the lapse of ten days and should then be again cleansed with a further dose of a purgative*. Patients in whom purging can be induced only with the greatest difficulty should be first treated with Ásthápana. Sneha should again be applied and a strong purgative should then be administered. 8.

**Ati-yoga** (Over-drugging with purgatives, etc.) :— Women, merchants, persons attending a king and pious Bráhmanas learned in the Vedas (S'rotriya) are often subjected to the necessity of repressing their natural urgings of the body towards micturition, etc., out of a sense of delicacy, fear or greed. The Váyu in their systems remains consequently aggravated and accordingly purgatives fail to easily produce any effect in their organism. Hence their system should be cleansed with purgatives preceded by Sveda (fomentations) and a copious application of Sneha. An over-dose of a purgative or a strong one administered to a person copiously treated with Sneha and Sveda or to one whose bowels are easily moved would exhibit the symptoms of an over-dosage (**Ati-yoga**) of purgatives.

Excessive emission of Pitta (bile), loss of strength (Bala) and an aggravation and augmentation of the deranged Váyu follow from the over dosage (**Ati-yoga**) of an emetic medicine. In such cases, the body of the patient should be anointed with clarified butter and he should be bathed in cold water and made to take a lambative† with sugar and honey with a due consideration of the nature and intensity of the Doshas involved. An over-dose of a purgative may bring on excessive

---

\* Dallana says that the system of the patient, in this case, should be cleansed with an emetic or a purgative as the case may be.

† A different reading says that the patient should be fomented with washings of rice mixed with honey.

emission of Kapha (mucus) mixed even with blood in the end. In this case, too, loss of strength (Bala) and enragement of the bodily Váyu would be the consequence. The patient in such a case should be sprinkled over with or bathed in very cold water and vomiting should be induced with potions of cold washings of rice mixed with honey. Applications of Pichchhá-vasti and of Anuvásana enemetas with milk and clarified butter are recommended. The patient should also be made to drink potions of the washings of rice mixed with the drugs of the *Priyangvddi* group The diet should consist of boiled rice with milk or meat-soup. 9-10.

**Jivádána** (Hæmorrhage) due to excessive vomiting :—In the event of an excessive use of an emetic the patient may spit or vomit blood. In such a case the tongue hangs out (of the mouth) and the eyes seem to expand, and numbness of the jaws, thirst, hiccough, fever and faintness are found to supervene. A potion of goat's blood, red Chandana, Us'ira, Anjana and the powders of fried paddy mixed with water and sugar, should be administered in these cases. As an alternative, the patient should be made to take his food in the Peyá form with the expressed juice of fruits (such as the *Dadimba, etc.,*) and with clarified butter, honey and sugar, or a Peyá prepared with the sprouts of Vata, etc. with honey, or one cooked with any drug having the power of producing costiveness ; or he should be made to take his food with milk or with the soup of the meat of a Jángala animal. Measures laid down in respect of excessive bleeding or hæmorrhage should also be resorted to 11.

In a case of excessive protrusion or hanging down of the tongue, the organ should be rubbed with powdered *Trikatu* and rock-salt or pasted with a plaster of sesamum and grapes (Drákshá and re-introduced into its proper place and position after which some other men should be made to taste any acid article in the sight of the patient. In a case of the expansion of the eyes they should be rubbed with clarified butter and (gently) pressed. Errhines and fomentations (of the part with drugs) antidotal to the deranged Váyu and Kapha, are recommended in a case of a numbness or catching pain of the jaw-bones in such cases. The other supervening distresses such as thirst etc, should be treated with appropriate medicinal remedies A faintness (under the circumstances) should be broken with the (sweet) sounds of a lute or a lyre 12.

**Jivádána** (Hæmorrhage) due to excessive purging : — An excess (Ati-yoga) of purging is marked, at the outset, by a flow of watery mucus through the rectum, resembling the crest of a peacock's plume in colour This is followed by an emission of shreddy and blood-streaked mucus resembling the washings of meat, succeeded by an oozing out of actual red **blood** attended with a shivering, protrusion of the anus and all the supervening distresses of emetics. The treatment in such cases should be as in those of hæmorrhage. The protruded anus should be first lubricated (with a Sneha) and subsequently fomented and re-introduced into its proper place or it should be treated according to the directions laid down in the chapter of Kshudra-Roga\*. The shivering should be treated with remedies laid down in connection with Váta-vyadhi. Remedies in cases of a protrusion of the tongue, etc., have been already described. Milk boiled (according to the Kshira-páka-vidhi) with *Kás'mari* fruit, *Vadari* fruit, *Us'ira*

---

\* The remedial measures for the treatment of Guda-bhrams'a, etc., under the Kshudra-Roga, should be employed in such cases.

and *Durvá* grass subsequently cooled and mixed with the cream of clarified butter and Anjana, should be syringed into the rectum in the manner of an Ástha-pana-Vasti in the case of an excessive flow of red blood (lit. life-blood) from the bowels. Vasti should be employed in such cases, with a decoction of the drugs of the *Nyagrodhádi* group mixed with milk, clarified butter, expressed juice of sugar-cane and (goat's) blood. Remedies mentioned under hæmoptysis (Rakta-pitta) and bloody dysentery should be employed in cases marked by spitting of life-blood (Jiva-s'onita). Decoctions of the drugs of the *Nyagrodhádi* group should be given with food and drink. 13.

**Jiva-S'onita, how to be known :**—A piece of a linen or cotton should be soaked in (and dyed with) the emitted blood where any doubt would arise whether it is a case of arterial blood (Jiva-s'onita) or one of Rakta pitta. The continuance of the dye or red stain on the linen even after being washed with hot water would conclusively establish its identity with the arterial blood or Jiva-s'onita. As an alternative, the discharged blood mixed with barley-powder or any other kind of food should be given to a dog to eat. If it is eaten by the dog, it would at once establish the identity of the emitted blood with the healthy arterial blood of the organism. 14.

**Ádhmána** (flatulent distention of the abdomen):— If a person who is suffering from a plethora of the Doshas in his system and who has not previously been treated with a Sneha and whose bowels still contain the undigested residue of a previous meal and (consequently) an abundance of Váyu therein, takes a (purgative or an emetic) which is neither emollient nor hot, the medicine is likely to produce a flatulent distention of his abdomen (Ádhmána) It arrests the emission of flatus (Váyu), stool and urine, makes the abdomen distended, produces a breaking pain in the sides, a pricking pain in the anus (Guda) and in the urinary bladder (Vasti) as well as a disrelish for food. This is called **Ádhmána** The patient, in such a case, should be treated with Ánába-varti, appetising medicines and with Vasti measures. 15.

**Parikartiká** (cutting pain in the anus, etc.) — The Váyu and Pitta in the organism of an enfeebled person or of a person whose bowels can be easily moved or of one of a dry and arid temperament or afflicted with impaired digestive capacity, are deranged and aggravated by the use of any extremely sharp, hot, saline or dry (emetic or purgative) which give rise to a sort of cutting, sawing pain (Parikartiká) in the anus, penis, umbilical region and the neck of the bladder (Vasti). The emission of flatus is arrested, the Váyu (wind) lies incarcerated in the abdomen and relish for food vanishes. The remedy consists in employing a **Pichchhá-Vasti** with *Yashti-madhu* and black sesamum pasted together and dissolved in clarified butter and honey. The patient should be laved in cold water and be given his food with milk. Anuvásana-Vasti\* with the cream of clarified butter or with oil cooked with *Yashti-madhu* should be employed. 16.

**Parisráva** (Dysenteric stools) :—The Doshas and the morbid matter accumulated in the system of a man of extremely constipated bowels and almost saturated with a plethora of Doshas (morbific diathesis) are stirred up but are not fully emitted under the action of a mild

---

\* In cases of a **Pitta**-predominance, the Vasti should be employed with the cream of clarified butter and in cases of a **Váyu** predominance, with oil.

(emetic or purgative) medicine. The Doshas (consequently) try to pass out of the body constantly but in small quantities and bring on weakness, numbness and rigidity of the abdomen, aversion to food and lassitude of the limbs. The deranged Pitta (bile) and Kapha (mucus) are constantly emitted with pain (through the anus) in such a case, and the disease is called **Parisráva**. Ásthápana-vasti with a decoction of *Aja-karna*, *Dhava*, *Tinis'a* and *Palás'a* saturated with honey is recommended in such cases. After the subsidence of the bodily Doshas involved in the case, the patient should be treated with Sneha and Samsodhana * (emetic or purgative) remedies should again be employed. 17.

**Praváhiká** (Diarrhœa) :—A medicine (purgative or emetic) administered to a person who has been excessively treated with Sveda or with Sneha produces **Praváhiká** in him by making him pass his stool and flatus without any straining or by restraining altogether those natural urgings respectively. Constant passing of slimy, black, white or red-coloured mucus (Kapha) with cramps, loud flatus and burning sensation form the chief characteristics of this disease. Its medical treatment should be similar to that of a case of Parisráva. 18.

**Hridayopasarana** (Overwhelming the heart):—Urgings towards vomiting or purging being injudiciously checked by a person from ignorance, causes a downward or upward coursing of the Doshas of the body to and in the heart, thus pressing the greatest of the Marmas and giving rise to an excruciating pain in that locality. The patient, in such a case, drops down unconscious in a swoon with upturned eyes, violently

---

* Dallana recommends that a strong purgative or emetic should be employed.

gushing his teeth and biting his tongue. An inexperienced physician usually abandons such a patient as lost, whereas the remedy in such cases consists in anointing his body with a Sneha (oil or clarified butter) and fomenting it with half-boiled and unhusked paddy (Dhánya-Sveda). Oil cooked with *Yashti-madhu* should be employed in the manner of an Anuvásana Vasti, and strong errhines (Nasya) should also be administered. After that the patient should be made to vomit with draughts of the washings of rice mixed with *Yashti-madhu* and Vastis\* should be employed in consideration of the preponderance of the Dosha or Doshas involved in the case. 19.

**Vibandha** (retention of flatus, stool and urine):— Use of cold water, exposure to cold winds and resorting to cool places and such other conduct during the action of an emetic or a purgative remedy in a person tend to thicken the Doshas loosened and dislodged from their seats by virtue of its potency, arrest their out-flow, make them adhere to the internal passages through which they pass and, by affecting the excretions, give rise to a suppression of stool, urine and Váyu (flatus), attended with rumbling in the intestines, fever, burning sensation and excruciating pain. The patient should in such a case † be made to speedily vomit the contents of his stomach, and the concomitant symptoms (such as fever, etc.) should be treated with appropriate medicinal remedies (as in the case of their actual and respective attacks). Drugs efficacious in subduing the Doshas confined in the lower cavity (abdomen) of the body (*Adhobhága-hara*) ‡ should be employed for purgative purposes with the admixture of

---

\* Dallana recommends both Niruha and Snaihika Vastis in such cases.

† This evidently refers to the case of an abuse of an emetic.

‡ See Chapter XXXIX., Sutra-Sthanam.

*Saindhava, Kánjika* and cow's urine in cases of the retention of the stool, etc., due to an abuse of a purgative. Proper Ásthápana and Anuvásana Vastis should be prescribed in consideration of the nature and intensity of the Doshas involved in the case. The nature of the diet should be judiciously determined according to the nature of the Doshas The supervening distresses in both the cases should be remedied with due consideration of the nature of the Doshas originating them. 20.

The cutting pain in the anus in connection with purging corresponds to the digging in the throat in a case of vomiting. The oozing out of the fæcal matter downward (Parisráva) in connection with a purgative corresponds to the water-brash in the case of an emetic. What diarrhœa (Praváhiká) is to purging, a dry eructation is to vomiting. 21.

**Memorable Verse :**—The fifteen kinds of distempers (Vyápat) described in the present chapter originate through an excessive, injudicious or insufficient use of purgatives or emetics. 22.

Thus ends the Thirty-fourth Chapter of the Chikitsita Sthánam in the Sus'ruta Samhitá which deals with the treatment of the disorders resulting from an injudicious use of purgatives and emetics.

# CHAPTER XXXV.

Now we shall discourse on the dimensions and classifications of a Netra and a Vasti (pipes, nozzles and apparatus) with their therapeutic applications (**Netra-Vasti-Pramána-Pravibhága-Chikitsitam**). 1.

Sages of authority hold an application of the Vasti to be the best of all measures such as, the application of a Sneha, etc.; and why ? Because on account of its varied functions and of its being composed of the various kinds of medicinal drugs a Vasti helps to restrain (Samgraha), pacify (Sams'amana) and cleanse (Sams'odhana) the different Doshas (morbific principles) of the body. It helps the recreation and growth of fresh semen, contributes to the building up of an emaciated frame, reduces corpulency, invigorates eyesight, arrests premature old age and tends to rejuvenate. A regular and proper use of a Vasti tends to improve one's complexion and bodily strength, imparts longevity, contributes to the growth of the body, ensures the enjoyment of sound health and guards against the inroad of any disease whatever. Applications of Vastis are highly efficacious in cases of fever, dysentery, cataract, catarrh, diseases of the head, Adhimantha, vomiting, facial paralysis, epileptic fits, convulsions, (Ákshepaka), hemiplegia, locomotor ataxy (Ekánga) and paraplegia (Sarvánga-Roga), tympanites, ascites or abdominal dropsy, S′arkará (gravels or urinary concretions), gastralgia (S′ula), scrotal tumours (including hydrocele, hernia, etc.), Upadams'a, retention of stool and urine (Ánáha), strangury (Mutra-krichchhra), Gulma, Váta-rakta, upward coursing of urine, stool and Váyu, loss of semen, breast-milk and of catamanial fluid, Hrid-graha (catching pain in the chest), Manyágraha (wryneck), Hanu-graha (numbness of the jaws), hæmorrhoids, Aśmari (stone) and Mudha-garbha (false presentation and difficult labour). 2.

**Memorable Verse :**—Applications of Vasti are always efficacious in diseases due to the action of the deranged Váyu, Pitta and Kapha, in those due to the vitiated condition of blood and in those brought on by the concerted action of any two or all of them. 3.

**Dimensions of the pipe :**—The length of the pipe of a Vasti should be made six fingers in respect of an infant of one year and eight and ten fingers in respect of a boy of eight and an adult of sixteen years respectively, the girth of its calibre being respectively equal to those of the small finger, the ring finger and the middle finger respectively in the three afore-named instances. The pipe should have Karnikás * or bulb-like protrusions attached to it at one of the ends above a space of one finger and a half, two fingers, and two fingers and a half respectively in the three afore-said forms of the apparatus. The girth of their mouths (to be introduced into the rectum) should be respectively made to equal those of the calibres of feathers of a crow, a falcon and a peacock, and the girth of the channels of the main body of the pipes should respectively be such as to let a *Mudga* pulse, a *Másha* pulse and a *Kaláya* pulse to pass through them. The quantity of the fluid with which an Ásthápana-Vasti should be charged is equal respectively to two, four, and eight Prasritas †

---

\* The Karnikás are attached to the pipes for guarding against their being thrust into the rectum

† A Prasrita measure is generally equal to two Palas, *i e.*, sixteen Tolás. But here it has the particular meaning as given in the text.

(in volume). A Prasrita measure being here equal to what can be contained in the hollow of the patient's own palms (in each particular case). 4.

**Memorable Verse :**—The length of the pipe and the quantity of the fluid to charge with should be gradually increased with the progress of the patient's age and in consideration of his strength and bodily capacity. 5.

The pipe of a Vasti in respect of an adult above twenty-five years of age, should be made twelve fingers in length having a girth equal to that of his thumb at its base and a girth equal to that of the small finger at its mouth. At a distance of three fingers from above the mouth the Karnikás should be fixed. The bore should be such as to allow a feather of a vulture to pass through it, while the fissure at the mouth would have a girth to allow the stone of a *Kola* fruit or of a boiled *Kaláya* pulse. The pipe should in all cases be supplied with two Karnikás at its root, for the purpose of firmly securing it to the mouth of the Vasti (bladder). The quantity of the fluid to charge with in the case of an **Ásthápana** Vasti is twelve Prasritas. The length of the pipe in respect of persons above seventy years of age should be like that in the preceding case but the quantity of the fluid to charge with should be made as in the case of a youth of sixteen. 6.

**Materials of the pipes :**—The pipe should be made either of gold, silver, copper, iron, brass, ivory, horn, gems or wood. It should be straight, smooth and firm, tapering at the top like the tuft of hair in the tail of a cow, and bulbular (*i.e*, not pointed) at its mouth. The **Vasti** * should be (prepared with) the

---

\* The Vasti is so called from its being prepared with the bladder (Vasti) of an animal. Dallana notes in this connection that the bladder

bladder (Vasti) either of a full-grown ox, buffalo or a sheep nor should it be soft (flexible) and firm, neither too thick nor too thin and of adequate dimensions. 7.

**Metrical Text :**—In the absence of a pipe, a reed, bamboo, or horn might serve the purpose. In the absence of the bladder of any of the foregoing animals, the Vasti should be made of skin or of thick linen. 8.

**Construction of the Vasti:**—The bladder (of which a Vasti should be made) should be cleansed, tanned and dyed (disinfected). It should be softened and repeatedly lubricated with a Sneha. It has generally a wide mouth which should be bent and lightly fitted to the butt end of the pipe (Netra). The mouth of the bladder should then be tied above the (Karniká). The whole bladder should be heated with a piece of hot iron (in order to polish the surface and remove the pores therein, if any). The mouth of the bladder should then be folded and again tied (below the Karniká). The whole should then be carefully preserved. The Ásthápana or the oily (Snaihika) Vasti should be applied, as the case may be, with the help of such a Vasti. A mild Vasti should be applied specially to infants and old men, since a strong one is likely to injure their health and strength. 9.

Vastis may be grouped under two heads—**Nairuhika** (dry or oilless) and **Snaihika** (oleaginous). The term Ásthápana is synonymous with Niruha. The Vasti known as the Madhu-Tailika is only an alternative of a Niruha-vasti. The terms Yápana, Yukta-ratha, and Siddha-vasti convey also the same meaning. A **Niruha-vasti** is so called from the fact of its expelling the Doshas (morbific

of an ox, buffalo, or a hog, should be used in the Ásthápana and Anuvásana measures, and the bladder of a goat or a sheep should be used in the Uttara-Vasti.

diatheses) from the system and from its curing the diseases of the body ; while **Asthápana** is so named from its virtue of rejuvenating the organism or producing longevity. The process of **Madhu-tailika** would be described in connection with the mode of applying a Niruha-vasti. 10.

The **Anuvásana** is only an alternative of a Sneha-Vasti, but (with this difference that) the quantity of the fluid to charge with should be three-fourths, and the amount of the good effect therefrom would also be three-fourths. An **Anuvásana-vasti** is so called from the fact of its not injuring the system even in the event of its being retained in the bowels a whole day, or from the fact of its being adapted to daily application. The **Mátrá-vasti** again which is applicable in all cases, is an alternative to an Anuvásana-vasti, but should be charged with only a half part of the fluid of that used in an Anuvásana-vasti. 11.

**Metrical Texts :**—A Niruha-vasti acts as a cleanser of the system (Śodhana). It is anti-fat (Lekhana), emulsive (Snehana) and constructive (Vrimhana). Oleaginous matter (Sneha) may freely enter into the organism when all its ducts and channels have been previously cleansed by the application of a Niruha-vasti. As water will freely run through channels previously cleansed of all refuse matter, so does an Anuvásana tend to cleanse the organism of all Doshas (morbific diatheses) and to increase the vitality of the organism. A **Sneha-vasti** should, therefore, be applied to a person previously purged of all Doshas by the application of a Niruha-vasti. 12.

Both the Anuvásana and the Ásthapána Vastis should be regarded as forbidden in cases of insanity, in the mental conditions of terror and grief, of a thirsty state of the body, of aversion to food and of indigestion, jaundice

(Pándu), giddiness, delirium, epilepsy, vomiting, Kushtha, Meha, ascites, obesity, asthma, cough, dryness of the throat and œdema as well as in respect of a Kshata-Kshina patient and a pregnant woman in (and before) the third or the fourth month of her gestation, in the case of a person suffering from dulness of appetite, impatient and incapable of bearing the least pain as well as in respect of infants, old men and persons emaciated by a bodily distemper other than one due to Váyu   13.

**Metrical Text :**—The Ásthápana-vasti should be exclusively applied in cases of ascites, urinary complaints (Meha), **Kushtha** and obesity. The application of an Anuvásna-vasti is entirely forbidden in those cases inasmuch as it might make the disease run into an incurable type, and a great amount of lassitude of the organism would be the consequence.   14.

Medicine duly injected (through the rectum) with the help of a Vasti remains in the intestines (Pakvás'aya), in the region of the pelvis and below the umbilical region. The potency of the Vasti (medicine) spreads over the whole organism from the intestines (Pakvás'aya), just as the potency of the water poured at the root of a tree tends to permeate the whole tree (through its minutest cells and fibres). The liquid part of the Vasti is emitted out through the rectum either by itself or with the **fœcal** matter, etc.*, but its potency acts over the whole organism through the intervention of the Apána and the other Váyus. The potency of the Vasti in the Pakvás'aya acts on the whole organism from top to toe, like the sun in the heavens acting on the humidity (Rasa)

---

* Srikantha Dutta in his commentary quotes this sloka, but he reads there "सकफ" (with Kapha) in the place of "समल" (with the fœcal matter, etc.). The reading in the text, however, is preferable inasmuch as Kapha is included in *Mala*.

of the earth below. The Vasti, if duly applied, tends to eliminate completely from the system all the Doshas (morbific diatheses) accumulated in the regions of the back, waist and the abdomen (Koshtha). 15-A.

As the aggravation of all the Doshas (morbific principles) of the body is principally dependent on the derangement of the bodily Váyu ; an aggravated condition of the latter may hence lead to the dissolution of the body, and consequently the application of a Vasti, and nothing else, is the only means of coping with the aggravation of the Váyu (by subduing and restoring it to its normal condition), just as the sea-coast is the only barrier to the swollen and wind-agitated surf of the sea. A well-applied Vasti contributes to the growth, health, strength and longevity of the body and to the improvement in its complexion. 15

**The different defects of a Vasti :**—Now we shall deal with the defects and the evil effects which are consequent upon the wrong and injudicious application of a Vasti. The defects of wrongly handling a Vasti (**Pranidhána-dosha**) are six in number, viz., the pipe may shake or revolve ; it may also be pressed sidewise or thrown upwards ; and it may sink down or may be pressed slantingly. Excessive thickness, coarseness, bending down, narrowness, cleavage, nearness or distance of the tying bands (Karniká), narrowness or excessive width of its internal aperture, excessive length or extreme shortness are the eleven defects which the pipe of a Vasti (**Netra-dosha**) may have. The five objectionable features in the bladder (**Vasti-dosha**) are an excessive flabbiness, narrowness, width of its internal aperture, leakiness and an imperfect bending at its mouth (neck). Variation in pressures put upon a Vasti (Enema syringe) during its application may be attended with any of the four objectionable features (**Pidana-dosha**), viz., over-pressure (pressing the injection into the rectum with an injuriously excessive force), under-pressure, repeated pressures and pressure at long intervals. The eleven defects in the ingredients of the Vasti (**Dravya-dosha**) are insufficient cooking, excessive or insufficient quantity, extreme coldness, excessive heat, extreme keenness of potency, excessive mildness, excess or want of oiliness (Sneha), extreme thickness of consistency and over-fluidity. Lying with the head raised up or hung down or in a bent or sitting posture or resting on one's back or in a contracted posture or on one's right side are the seven defective postures (**Sayyá-dosha**) in which a patient should never be laid during the application of a Vasti. These are the twenty-four defects which attend the wrong application of a Vasti owing to the ignorance or inexperience of a physician, while those which are the effects of the injudiciousness of a patient are fifteen in number and would be described in the chapter on Áturopadrava-Chikitsita (Chapter XXXIX, Chikitsita-sthána). 16.

The Sneha injected into the bowels by a Vasti is obstructed in its passage and cannot consequently leave the system but is retained in it through any of the following eight causes, *viz.*, obstruction of the food by the three Doshas, its admixture with the fœcal matter (accumulated in the bowels), its being injected too high up into the intestines, an omission to foment (the patient's body), using the Sneha in a cold state or in a small quantity and lastly use of no meals or of scanty meals by the patient previous to the application of a Vasti. These (retentive conditions) are due to the indiscretion of both the physician and the patient. Nine distressing symptoms (Vyápad) namely as a defective application of either the Anuvásana or the Ásthápana Vastis, distension of the abdomen, (Ádhmána), a cutting pain in the region of the anus, (Parikartiká) Dysenteric stools (Parisráva), diarrhœa (Praváhiká), affecting the heart (Hridayaopasarana), catching pain in the limbs, over-dosage, hæmorrhage manifest themselves in consequence of any act of indiscretion of the physician in attendance. 17.

**Memorable Verse :**—The seventy-six kinds of the distressing symptoms (Vyápad) have been briefly described above. Their symptoms and treatment would be described in the following chapter. 18.

Thus ends the Thirty-fifth Chapter in the Chikitsita Sthánam in the Sus'ruta Samhitá which deals with the dimensions, classifications and therapeutical applications of a Netra and a Vasti.

# CHAPTER XXXVI.

Now we shall discourse on the medical treatment of the mishaps which are consequent on an injudicious application of the pipe and of the vasti (**Netravasti-Váypach-Chikitsitam**). 1.

**Metrical Text :**—A displacement or retroversion of the pipe during the application of a Vasti produces a painful and bleeding ulcer in the rectum, which should be treated as a recent or incidental ulcer. An extremely up-turned or down-turned posture of the pipe at the time gives rise to a pain in the rectum which should be treated with Pitta-subduing remedies and sprinkled with Snehas (oil, clarified butter, etc.). A slanting or one-sided posture of the pipe after its introduction into the rectum causes its mouth to be closed and thus prevents a complete and satisfactory injection of the fluid (into the bowels). Hence its mouth should be held straight (and steady) by an experienced physician. The use of an excessively thick or rough pipe or of one with a down-turned or bent mouth, produces a bleeding and painful ulcer in the rectum which should be remedied in the manner mentioned above. The injection of a Vasti proves abortive in the event of the Karniká (attached to the pipe) being too near the end of the pipe or itself being broken or too small. These defects should, therefore, be carefully avoided In a case of the Karniká (attached to the pipe) being at a greater distance from the mouth of the pipe, it would hurt the Guda marma (marma at the anus) and produce a considerable bleeding therefrom. Pitta-subduing remedies and

Pichchhila-Vastis should be employed in such a case. The application of a Vasti with a pipe of small length or narrow calibre produces pain, and the injected fluid dribbles out (without entering into the rectum), thus occasioning all the maladies* which attend an insufficient or abortive use of a Vasti†. In the event of the pipe being large and wide-calibred one, the result would be that a large quantity of the fluid would be at once injected into the bowels just as in a case of Avapida-dosha (constant pressing). 2.

**Disorders resulting from a defective bladder :**—The effects which result from the use of a bladder (Vasti) too large or too thick are identical with those which follow from an imperfect fitting of its neck with the pipe. A (proportionately) smaller efficacy is obtained from the use of a small bladder capable (necessarily) of injecting a smaller quantity of the medicinal fluid. An imperfectly fixed bladder or the one with small pores therein produces effects similar to those resulting from the use of a cracked pipe. 3.

An injection made with considerable force by a Vasti (Enema-syringe) enters the stomach (Ámáśaya) which being forced higher up by the up-coursing Váyu in the organism is emitted through the mouth and the nostrils. ‡ Under the circumstances, the

---

\* These are strangury (Mutra-krichchhra), suppression of urine (Mutrághata), etc.

† According to Dallana the remedy in this case would be that applicable in a case of Mutrágháta, etc. ; but Jejjata holds that the remedy lies in applying a Pichchhila Vasti as in the preceding case.

‡ An additional reading says that it causes Vomiting, nausea, epileptic fits and a burning sensation of the body. Vrinda supports this additional reading.

patient should be immediately pressed by the neck and (his body) shaken. Strong purgatives and errhines should be administered, and sprinkling him with cold water should be prescribed. If a Vasti be applied with lesser force, the medicinal fluid of the Vasti cannot reach the intestines (Pakváśaya) and (consequently) fails to produce the desired effect Hence it should be duly pressed. If it be pressed at intervals, the wind (Váyu) in the abdomen becomes enraged, and gives rise to tympanites (Ádhmána) and excruciating pain therein. The medicinal treatment in such a case should be the applications of proper Vastis in consideration of the nature of the aggravated Doshas involved therein If the pipe be retained for an (unnecessarily) long time in the rectum during the application of a Vasti, it tends to increase the pain, and bring about an aggravation of the disease. This should be remedied by a second application of the Vasti charged with proper antidotal solutions sufficient to cope with the intensity of the disease. 4.

The use of an insufficiently cooked Sneha (in a Vasti) leaves a slimy sticky deposit on the inner lining of the rectum accompanied by a local swelling which should be remedied by the application of a Samśodhana-vasti and the exhibition of purgatives.* The application of a Vasti of either kind (Ásthápana and Anuvásana) charged with a deficient or inadequate quantity of a medicinal solution, proves abortive in all instances; whereas diarrhœa (Atisára), fatigue and Ánáha (distension of the abdomen with the retention of stool, urine, etc.) result from the application of one charged with an excessive quantity of the fluid. The application of a Vasti charged with an extremely warm or

---

* Gayadása reads and recommends that the purgatives to be used in such a case should be devoid of any oleaginous substances (Sneha).

strong solution produces epileptic fits, a burning sensation, diarrhœa and (an aggravated condition of the) Pitta. The use of any extremely cold or mild medicine for the purpose of a Vasti arrests the emission of the flatus (Váyu), and produces Ádhmána (distension of the abdomen).* Antidotal measures should be adopted in cases of the deficient or excessive quantity, etc The fluid to be used in charging a Vasti should be thickened in the event of its extremely attenuated consistency and *vice versa.* The application of a Vasti charged with a fluid consisting of an excessive quantity of Sneha would produce a general inertness of the organism, (dullness of organic functions), while one entirely bereft of any Sneha would produce numbness of the organism and a distension of the abdomen. The remedy in either case consists in employing a Vasti of the opposite kind (*viz.*, an oily or non-oily Vasti respectively). 5.

The application of a Vasti to a patient with his head downward is attended with symptoms peculiar to an act of over-pressing (the bladder of the Vasti), and the remedy also would be similar. The application of a Vasti to a patient with his head held up high and erect would block the urethra, *i.e.*, would suppress the urine, in which case the patient should be treated first with Sveda and then with an Uttara-vasti (urethral syringe,† which would give the patient much relief. The injected fluid goes astray (within the abdomen)

* An additional reading says that a dry (thickend ?) Niruha-vasti produces a slimy deposit in the rectum and in the pelvic region, while one with its fluid of an extremely thin consistency would produce only a little effect and might produce diarrhœa.

† Jejjata's reading of this passage does not include the application of Sveda but means that the Uttara-vasti should be applied with a Sneha.

and fails to enter into the intestines (Pakvás'aya) in the event of the patient lying in a stooping posture during the application of a Vasti. The Váyu in such a case becomes aggravated and gives rise to pain in the regions of the heart, abdomen and rectum. The injected fluid fails to penetrate into the bowels in the event of the patient lying on his back during the application of a Vasti owing to the consequent obstruction of the passage. The bodily Váyu becomes in this case agitated and enraged by the (introduction of the) pipe (of the Vasti). A contracted position of the body or of both the thighs, during the application of a Vasti prevents the full outflow of the injected medicine from the intestines, owing to its being acted upon by the bodily Váyu. In a case of the application of a Vasti to a patient in a sitting posture, the fluid rolls down without entering into the bowels; it cannot consequently soothe the Ás'aya and thus proves abortive. The injected medicine cannot fully enter into the Pakvás'aya (intestines), when the Vasti is applied to a patient lying on his right side, since the Pakvás'aya is situated on the left side (of the abdomen). The application of a Vasti is not recommended when the patient lies on his face or in such other posture since it is followed by an aggravation of the bodily Váyu, which should be remedied by medicines chosen according to the exigencies of each case. 6.

We shall describe hereafter (in the next chapter) the dangers (**Vyápat**) which attend the misapplication of a **Sneha-vasti** and the course of the medical treatment to be adopted in each. The dangers (**Vyápat**) attending a deficient application (**Ayoga**) of a (Niruha) Vasti with their respective treatment are described here in this chapter. 7.

**Ayoga :**—Cramps or colic pains (Śula) in the intestines, and heaviness and distension of the abdomen result from the application of a Vasti charged with a medicinal solution either cold, inadequate in quantity, or deficient in its therapeutic virtues. All these symptoms are included within the term **Ayoga** or deficient application of a Vasti which should be remedied by a strong Vasti and a strong purgative. 8.

Distension of the abdomen and consequently an excruciating pain (Śula) in the regions of the sides, back, waist and the heart result from the applications of a Vasti to a person who has taken a second meal before the digestion of a previous one, or in the event of the presence of a large accumulation of Doshas (in his body). If the Vasti be applied in a tepid state and in a large quantity just after a heavy meal, the results would be the same. Similar results would follow injections of cold medicinal solutions in large doses saturated with only a small quantity of salt and Sneha (oil or clarified butter as well as from those in a person with a large accumulation of fœcal matter (in his bowels. The remedy in all these cases should consist in the application of a Vasti charged with stronger medicinal solutions as well as of an Anuvásana-vasti. 9.

The Pitta and the Váyu of the body are conjointly aggravated by the application of a Vasti charged with extremely parching, hot and saline solutions which give rise to the distress, known as Parikartiká, attended with a sort of cutting pain in the pelvis and about the anus and the region of the umbilicus. Applications of the **Pichchhila-vasti** of a medicated Sneha cooked with the drugs of the *Madhura* group should be the remedies in these cases 10.

The distress known as **Parisráva** attended with loss of strength, and bodily lassitude results from the application of a Vasti charged with solutions of extremely strong, acid and saline substances. Pitta begins to secrete at this stage, and produces a consequent burning sensation in the anus. Applications of a Pichchhila-vasti as well as a Vasti of clarified butter churned from *milk* should be the remedy in these cases. 11.

The distress known as **Praváhiká** or the passing of bloody stools or painful motions, attended with colic (Śula) and a burning sensation, is the effect of an excessively strong Asthápana or Anuvásana Vasti. This disorder should be remedied by the application of a Pichchhila-vasti, a diet of boiled rice saturated with milk and with injections into the bowels, in the manner of an Anuvásana Vasti, of a medicated Sneha (oil or clarified butter) cooked with the drugs of the *Madhura* group. 12.

The distress known as **Hridayopasarana**, accompanied with such symptoms as, aching pains in the limbs, epilepsy, delirium, heaviness of the body and all other discomforts peculiar to the action of the deranged Váyu, originates from the application of a Niruha-vasti charged with extremely parching solutions as well as from those of an Anuvásana-vasti in the complicated diseases of the deranged bodily Váyu. The remedy in these cases consists in applying the Śodhana Vasti charged with solutions efficacious in subduing the actions of all the Doshas of the body. 13.

A breaking pain in the joints and the limbs, numbness (Anga-graha), yawning, shivering and lassitude are the symptoms which follow the applications of a Vasti inadequately charged, or charged with medicinal solutions which are either too mild or too Ruksha (dry) in their potency, or applied in the case of a patient having lain in any of the objectionable postures at the time of the application, or possessed of a dry or Váyu-predominating temperament. The remedy in these cases should consist in applying Sveda, anointments and appropriate Vastis. 14.

Symptoms which are known as **Atiyoga,** following applications of Vastis charged with an inordinate quantity of medicinal fluid or with extremely hot or strong solutions as well as the application of Vastis after an excessive application of Sveda (fomentation) and in slight derangements of the bodily Doshas should be treated identically as in cases laid down in connection with an Atiyoga (excessive use) of purgatives. The use of a Pichchhila vasti in a cold state is also recommended, as it would give the patient much relief. 15.

Measures and remedies mentioned in respect of Jivádána (hæmorrhage of the bowels) in connection with an excessive use of purgatives should be employed in the case of similar symptoms (**Jivádána**) following the excessive use of a Vasti. Applications of Pichchhila-vasti charged with blood are likewise recommended in these cases. 16.

The foregoing nine kinds of distressing symptoms (**Vyápat**) resulting from an injudicious application of a Niruha-vasti are also found to result from the injudicious application of a Sneha-vasti. All the distresses (of the injudicious applications of a Vasti) with their symptoms and the course of medical treatment to be adopted (in each case) have thus been described. A discrete and experienced physician should so act as not to induce these distresses (Vyápat) in connection with the applications of a Vasti. 17-18.

A purgative should be given after the lapse of a fortnight from the date of the exhibition of an emetic drug. An Ásthápana-vasti should be applied a week after the date of purging. An Anuvásana-vasti should also be applied on the very same day. 19.

Thus ends the Thirty-sixth Chapter of the Chikitsita Sthánam in the Sus'ruta Samhitá which treats of the medical treatment of the diseases consequent on the injudicious applications of a Vasti.

# CHAPTER XXXVII.

Now we shall discourse on the treatment of an Anuvásana vasti and an Uttara vasti **(Anuvásan-ottara-Vasti-Chikitsita).** 1.

**Metrical Texts:**—An Anuvásana-vasti should be applied to a patient fit to be treated therewith, seven days after the administration of a purgative and after he has regained his strength and taken his meal of rice. Three-quarter parts of the medicinal solution enjoined to be used in connection with a Niruha-vasti (dry or oilless) in consideration of the age and temperament of the patient form the (full) dose of a Sneha vasti An enema (Vasti) should be applied after the emission of stool, flatus and urine from the system, since they resist the penetration of the Sneha into the bowels. A Sneha-vasti (emulsive or oleaginous enema) should not be applied to a person whose organism has not been previously cleansed (by an appropriate emetic and purgative). The potency of the Sneha would be able to easily infiltrate into a system previously cleansed in the manner before indicated. 2.

Now we shall describe (the process of preparing) the several medicated oils in due order with reference to the different Doshas which should be used as drink and errhines and in charging a Sneha-vasti and which have the power of destroying a variety of diseases (if so used). 3-A.

**First Taila :**—Drugs such as *S'athi, Pushkara, Krishná, Madana, Deva-dáru, S'atáhvá, Kushtha, Yashti-madhu, Vacha, Vilva* and *Chitraka* should be pounded together, made into a paste and duly cooked with oil (of four times their combined (weight) and milk weighing twice and water, four times as much as the oil. The use of this medicated oil as a Vasti-measure proves curative in pacifying the incarcerated Váyu and in cases of hæmorrhoids, lienteric diarrhœa (Grahani), tympanites with retention of stool aud urine, Vishama-jvara and the affections of Váyu (nervous disorders) in the waist (lumbago), the thighs (sciatica), the back and the abdomen. 3.

**Second Taila:**—*Vachá, Pushkara, Kushtha, Elá, Madana, Deva-dáru, Saindhava, Kákoli, Kshira-Kákoli, Yashti-madhu, Medá, Mahá-medá, Narádhipa* (Áragvadha), *Páthá, Jivaka, Jivanti, Bhárgi, Chandana, Katphala, Saralá* (white Trivrit), *Aguru, Vilva, Válaka, As'vagandhá, Chitraka, Vriddhi, Vidanga, Áragvadha, S'yámá Trivrit, Pippali* and *Riddhi* should be pasted together and cooked with the proper quantity of oil, milk and the decoction of the drugs of the (major) Pancha-mula group. Anuvásana-vastis of this kind are highly efficacious in cases of Gulma, tympanites with suppressed stool and urine, impaired digestion, hæmorrhoids, lienteric diarrhœa (Grahani), retentions of urine and diseases due to the action of the deranged Váyu. 4.

**Third Taila :**—*Chitraká, Ativishá, Páthá, Danti, Vilva, Vacha, Ámisha* (*Guggulu*), *Saralá* (white Trivrit), *Ams'umati* (Sálaparni), *Rásná, Nilini, Chaturangula* (Áragvadha), *Chavya, Ajamodá, Kákoli,* the two kinds of *Medá, Deva-dáru, Jivaka, Rishavaka, Varsklábhu, Aja-gandhá, S'atáhva, Harenu, As'va-gandhá, Manjishthá S'athi, Pushkara* and *Taskara* (Choraka) should be pasted together and cooked with the proper quantity of milk and oil. The oil thus prepared is highly efficacious in the disorders of the deranged Váyu. Injected into the bowels in the manner of (an Anuvásana-vasti), it speedily cures Gridhrasi (sciatica), lameness, haunch-back, Ádhya váta, urinary diseases, obstinate constipation of the bowels (Udá-varta), impaired digestion and weakness of the body. 5.

**Fourth Taila :**—A decoction of the drugs *Bhutika, Eranda, Varshábhu, Rásná, Vásaka, Rohisha,* the drugs of the *Das'a-mula* group, *Sahá* (Mudga-parni), *Bhárgi, Shad-granthi* (Vacha), *Deva-dáru, Valá, Nága-valá, Murvá, As'va-gandhá,* the two *Amritá* (Guduchi and Haritaki), *Saháchara, Vari* (Satá-vari), *S'unthi, Káka-násá, Vidári Yava, Másha, Atasi, Kola* and *Kuláttha* should be cooked in an adequate quantity of oil with (a Kalka of) the drugs of the *Jivaniya* group and a quantity of milk weighing four times as much as the oil. The oil, if employed in the manner of a Vasti, would prove beneficial in cases of diseases due to the action of the deranged Váyu localised in the regions of the thighs, legs, coxcy (Trika), sides (Pársva), balls of the shoulders (Amsa) and in the hands, the head and Manyá (nerves of the neck). 6.

**Fifth Taila** (with clarified butter) :—The drugs *Jivanti, Ativalá, Medá,* the two kinds of *Kákoli, Jivaka, Rishavaka, Ativishá, Krishná, Káka-násá, Vacha, Deva-dáru, Rásná, Madana, Yashti-madhu, Saralá* (white Trivrit), *S'atávari, Chandana, Svayam-guptá* with an adequate quantity of oil and clarified butter (in equal parts) with a quantity of milk weighing eight times as much as the combined weight of the oil and clarified butter. This oil should be employed in the manner of an Anuvásana-vasti in cases of Gulma and retentions of stool and urine with a distension of the abdomen. It conquers the deranged Váyu and Pitta of the body, acts as an invigorating and constructive tonic, improves digestion, increases strength and creates fresh semen. Used as an errhine or as a drink it tends to alleviate all affections confined to the regions above the clavicles. 7.

**Sixth Sneha :**—*Yashti-madhu, Us'ira, Kás'm-arya, Katuka, Utpala, Chandana, S'yámá,\* Padma-Káshtha, Jimuta, Indra-yava, Ativishá* and *Válá* (in equal parts) should be pasted together and cooked with an adequate quantity of clarified butter and oil, the oil weighing a fourth part of the whole quantity of Sneha to which should be added a quantity of milk weighing eight times as much as the Sneha (oil and clarified butter added together) with a decoction of the drugs of the *Nyagrodhádi* group. This (medicated Ghrita), used as a Vasti proves efficacious in cases of Asrig-dara (menorrhagia), erysipelas (Visarpa), Váta-Rakta, abscess (Vidradhi), fever, burning sensations in the body and all other disorders due to the action of the deranged Pitta. 8.

**Seventh Sneha :**—A paste of *Mrinála, Utpala, S'áluka,* the two kinds of *Sárivá,* (Ananta-mula and Śyamalatá), *Nága-kes'ara,* the two kinds of *Chandana* (red and white), *Bhu-nimba, Padma-vija, Kas'eruka, Patola, Katuka, Raktá* (Manjishthá), *Gundrá, Parpataka* and *Vásaka* (weighing one seer in all) should be cooked with (sixteen seers of) the decoction of *Trina-mula*† with (four seers of) oil and with milk twice as much as the oil. A variety of Pittaja diseases yields to the curative efficacy of this medicated oil, used as a Vasti, or as errhines, drink unguent. 9.

**Eighth Sneha :**—A paste composed of *Triphalá, Ativishá, Murvá, Trivrit, Chitraka, Vásaka,*

---

\* Dallana explains " S'yámá " as " Priyangu " and " Jimuta " as "Mustaka."

† Dallana explains "Trina mula" as "Trina-pancha-mula" for which see Ch. XXXVIII, Sutra-Sthánam.

*Nimba, Áragvadha, Shad-granthá* (Vacha), *Sapta-parna,* the two kinds of *Haridrá,* (Haridrá and Dáru-haridrá), *Guduchi, Indra-sura,* (Indra-varuni), *Pippali, Kushtha, Sarshapa* and *Nágara* in equal parts (weighing one seer in all), should be cooked with an adequate quantity (four seers) of oil and (sixteen seers of) the decoction of the drugs of the *Surasádi* group. Obesity, a feeling of physical languor, itches, etc., as well as diseases due to the deranged condition of Kapha, readily yield to the use of this (medicated oil) employed as a medicinal snuff (Nasya), a gargle (Gandusha), a drink, or anointment, or as a Vasti. 10.

**Ninth Sneha :**—A paste (weighing one seer in all) composed of *Páthá, Ajamoda, S'árṁgashtá, Pippali, Gaja-pippali, S'unthi, Saralá* (D. R.—Saptalá) *Aguru,* Káliya, *Bhárgi, Chavya, Deva-dáru, Maricha, Elá, Haritaki, Katuka, Pippali-mula, Katphala* pounded together and mixed with a decoction of the *Valli* * and the *Kantaka* each weighing twice as much as the weight of the oil, should be cooked with an adequate quantity of sesamum or castor oil (weighing four seers). All kinds of diseases due to a deranged condition of the bodily Kapha readily yield to the use of this (medicated) oil when employed in the manner of an Anuvâsana enema (Vasti). 11.

**Tenth Sneha :**—A pasted compound of *Vidanga, Udichya, Saindhava* salt, *S'athi, Pushkara, Chitraka, Katphala, Ativishá, Bhárgi, Vacha, Kushtha, Deva-dáru, Medá, Madana, Yashti-madhu, S'yámá* †,

---

* The "Valli" and the "Kantaka" here evidently mean the "Valli-pancha-mula" and the 'Kantaka-Pancha-mula" respectively for which see chapter XXXVIII. Sutra-Sthánam.

† Dallana explains "S'yámá" as "Vriddha-dáraka" and "Renu' as "Parpataka".

*Nichula* (Jala-Vetasa), *Nágara, S'atáahvá, Nilini, Rásná, Kadali, Vásaka, Renu, Vilva, Ajamoda, Pippali, Danti, Chavya, Naradhipa* (Áragvadha) with the decoction of the drugs of the *Mushkakádi* group, should be cooked with an adequate quantity of sesamum or castor oil. The use of this oil in the manner of an Anuvásana-vasti (enema) speedily proves curative in cases of Plihodara (enlargement of the spleen), obstinate constipation of the bowels, Váta-Rakta, Gulma, retentions of stool and urine with a flatulent distention of the abdomen, in diseases due to the action of the deranged Kapha, in urinary complaints, gravels in the bladder (S'arkarâ) and in hæmorrhoids. 12.

An Anuvásna-vasti may be applied in all parts of the day and night and even (if necessary) without any previous exhibition of emetics and purgatives, in the case of a patient in whose system the Váyu has been incarcerated and extremely aggravated. The application of a Nirudha-vasti (enema) should, however, be made in respect of a person of an extremely dry temperament, or in whose system the deranged and aggravated Váyu extremely predominates, only after his system had been made sufficiently emulcent (Snigdha) by two or three injections with an Anuvásana-vasti. But if his system be agitated only with an extremely aggravated condition of his bodily Váyu, a Nirudha-vasti (enema), charged with a medicinal solution and with a profuse quantity of Sneha added therewith, may be applied even before applying a Sneha (Vasti). On finding that the Nirudha-vasti has fully acted, the physician should treat the patient with medicinal solutions of oils prepared with *Yashti-madhu* and *Madana* fruit respectively in the manner of an Anuvásana-vasti in cases of the aggravations of Váyu, etc. 13.

A Vasti should not be applied in the night since the Doshas of the system are (generally) aggravated at this time and since the Sneha (of the Vasti) owing to its potency is likely to give rise to a distention of the abdomen attended with fever and heaviness of the limbs. The mouths of the internal ducts of the body remain dilated and the Doshas remain in their proper places (*i.e.*, are not generally agitated), and the digestive fire remains surcharged with the essence of the digestive food during the day time, hence the **potency** (Ojas) of a Sneha-vasti employed during the day time easily spreads through the ducts of the body. An Anuvásana-vasti may be applied during (the early part of) the night in summer in a case marked by a preponderance of the deranged Pitta and a (consequent) weakness of the Kapha, and an extremely parched condition of the organism, as well as in cases of the affections of Váyu (Váta-roga). Unfavourable symptoms such as a burning sensation in the body, etc., arise from the application of a Vasti in the day time during a preponderance of the Pitta, or in summer. The physician should, therefore, make such applications in the evening (Pradosha) in such instances. 14.

**Proper time for the application of the Sneha-vasti:**—A Sneha-vasti should be employed during the day in spring and winter and in the evening during summer and the rainy season, with a view to ward off the dangers due to the misapplication in the internal use of a Sneha.\* It may, however, be applied at any time during the day, or in the night in a case marked by a preponderance of the deranged bodily Váyu. 15.

In the serious stage of a disease an Anuvásana-enema should be applied after the patient has partaken

---

\* See Chapter XXXI., Chikitsita-Sthánam.

of a second meal, having already digested his previous one. The use of a Sneha-vasti is forbidden in an empty stomach as it might otherwise send the injected fluid higher up into the intestines owing to the emptiness and cleansed * (unencumbered) state of the stomach. An application of the Anuvàsana-vasti should be made just after a meal, since the application of a Vasti made during the continuance of a partially digested or undigested meal in the stomach brings on fever. An Anuvàsana enema should not, however, be applied after the patient had taken his meal, richly saturated or cooked with a Sneha (oil or clarified butter), since the double introduction of the Sneha into the system through the medium of food and the Vasti brings on vertigo and epilepsy. The strength and complexion of the patient suffer much by the application of an Anuvàsana-vasti after he has taken a dry (Ruksha) meal containing no Sneha. A patient should, therefore, be first fed with a diet saturated with a moderate quantity of an oleaginous substance before being treated with an Anuvàsana-vasti. The patient before being treated with an Anuvàsana vasti should be fed with *Mudga-*soup †, cow's milk and meat-essence to a quarter part ‡ less than the quantity he can ordinarily take   16.

* Gayadâsa reads " सूच्मवात् " in place of "शुद्धवात्" and explains it to mean " owing to the potency of the Sneha in traversing through the minutest channels of the body."

† Dallána explains that the Mudga soup should be taken without being mixed with any Sneha. He further says that the patient should be given Mudga-soup, cow's milk and meat-essence in accordance with the aggravation of the deranged Kapha, Pitta and Vâyu respectively.

‡ Dallana, on the authority of the older Commentators explains that the patient should not be fed to his fill but only to three-fourths, half and one-fourth of what he can ordinarily take according to his digestive capacity.

**The mode of applying a Sneha-vasti :**—The body of the patient to be treated with an Anuvàsana-vasti should be first anointed (with a Sneha) and gently fomented with hot water. Then he should be advised to take his meal in the prescribed way and made to take a short walk. Then having passed stools and urine, he should be treated with the Sneha-vasti. The mode of applying (the apparatus) is described under that of Niruha-vasti. He should be kept silently lying on his back as long as it would take to count a hundred words (Vâk). The potency (Virja) of the injected Sneha spreads through the entire organism in the event of one's lying with outstretched limbs in the above manner after the application of a Sneha-vasti. The patient should be gently struck* three times on each of the soles and the palms of his hands and on the buttocks†. The (patient with his) bedding should be thrice raised (and shaken with gentle jerks). After that he should be laid on a bed stretched out at full length and be advised to speak and exert himself as little as possible and conform to a strict regimen of diet and conduct. 17-19.

A quantity of *S'atâhvâ* and *Saindhava* should be mixed with the Sneha (to be used in the Vasti) and (the whole compound) applied lukewarm, inasmuch as the injected Sneha would thereby easily flow back (without producing any pain and burning sensation, etc.) and dribble

---

* Dallana explains that the patient should be caught hold of by his wrists and ankles and given the gentle jerks so as to allow the potency of the Sneha spread through the organism.

† Some explain that the buttocks of the patient should be raised up with his bedding and his couch. At any rate his buttocks should be raised up in order to enable the injected Sneha to remain inside the intestines and not to come out instantly.

down in due time after the application. If at any time a quantity of the Sneha injected into the bowels in the manner of an Anuvásana enema (Vasti) is instantly driven back by the pressure of the incarcerated abdominal Vâyu, or the Vâyu (air) of the bladder (Vasti), or by an excessive heat, keenness (in potency), or an over-dose of the injected fluid itself, or by the over dose of the medicines (subsequently) added thereto, a Snehavasti charged with a smaller dose of the Sneha should be again applied, since a Sneha un-retained in the abdomen fails to produce any emulsive effect. 20-21.

Retention of stool, urine and Vâyu (flatus) is produced by using an insufficient quantity of Sneha in an Anuvásana-vasti. A burning sensation in the body, diarrhœa (Pravâha) and fatigue accompanied with pain set in as the natural resultants of an excessive Anuvásana enema. The satisfactory nature of the application of an Anuvásana-vasti should be inferred from the timely discharge of the injected Sneha with flatus and fœcal matter* out of the bowels of a patient without giving rise to any distressing symptoms such as burning and sucking † sensations, etc. 22.

The patient may be given a light ‡ meal or diet in the evening, in case he is possessed of a keen digestive capacity§, subsequent to the digestion of a previous meal and (should he feel hungry) after the discharging of the injected Sneha. Tepid water boiled with *Dhanyáka*

---

\* It should be noted that the particle "च" in the text means that on the satisfactory action of an Anuvásana-Vasti, the injected Sneha may come out with urine as well.

† Dallana explains "चोष" to mean thirst.

‡ "Light" means both light in quantity as well as in quality.

§ Some commentators explain this couplet to mean that a patient of ordinary digestive capacity should be given a light food, whereas a patient of keen digestive capacity may take a full one.

and *S'unthi* should be given hot to the patient on the (following) morning as it would sharpen his appetite and produce a fresh relish for food. 23.

This is the procedure of applying a **Sneha-vasti.** Six, seven, eight or nine applications of Sneha-vastis should in this manner be made in succession alternately with those of a Nirudha-vasti. 24-A.

**The Successive actions of the Vastis :**—The first application of the Vasti permeates the pelvic and the inguinal regions with the emulcent essence of the injected Sneha. The second tends to restore the Vâyu in the cephalic part of the body to its normal condition. The third contributes to the improvement of bodily strength and complexion. The fourth permeates the Rasa (lymph chyle) with its own oily essence In this way the fifth application of a Vasti permeates the blood, the sixth the flesh, the seventh the fat, the eighth the bones, and the ninth the marrow with the oily essence. This series of Vasti-applications repeated twice tends to purify the semen from all its impure or unhealthy constituents. 24.

A person treated with eighteen series (three hundred and twenty-four in number) of such Sneha-vastis and Niruha-vastis in the above mentioned way and observing the prescribed rules of diet and conduct is enabled to develop a muscular strength in no way inferior to that of an elephant, and to live a sinless life a thousand years, in the full enjoyment of his intellectual faculties, god-like beauty and horse-like swiftness. 25.

An excessive application of only one kind of Vasti, either of a Sneha-vasti, or of a Niruha vasti, should be avoided, since an excess of the first (Sneha-vasti) tends to impair the digestive capacity* and to bring on an aggravation of the deranged Kapha, while an excess of the second (Niruha-vasti) tends to aggravate the bodily Vâyu. Hence an application of the Sneha-vasti should be followed by one of the Niruha-vasti and *vice versa*, in order to avoid all apprehension of an aggravation of Pitta, Kapha and Vâyu. Daily applications of a Sneha-vasti are not forbidden in respect of a person of parched or dry (Ruksha) and Vâyu-predominating temperament, while in other instances they should be made on each fourth day, so that the digestive capacity might not be thereby impaired. The application of a moderate quantity of Sneha with a Sneha-vasti is always beneficial to persons of parched or dry temperament. Similarly, an application of the Niruha vasti in a small quantity always proves beneficial to the persons who have been already treated with a Sneha (Vasti). 26.

**Distresses from Sneha-vasti :**—Now we shall describe the distresses which are found to attend (an abuse or excess of) a **Sneha vasti.** Various kinds of distressing symptoms are produced by the application of a Sneha-vasti of a mild or weak potency in the case of a patient whose stomach is filled with the aggravated Doshas so that the Sneha cannot flow back, being overwhelmed, as it would be, by the aggravated Doshas. 27.

**Specific Symptoms :**—An astringent taste in the mouth, yawning, shivering and Vishama-Jvara with the peculiar Vâyu-origined distempers such as, pain (in the limbs) are the symptoms which mark the retention of the injected Sneha in the bowels over-whelmed

\* Vrinda reads " स्वेद्यात् पित्तकफोत्क्लेशौ " in place of ' स्वेद्याग्नि-वधोत्क्लेशौ ". This means that the Pitta and the Kapha would be aggravated by an excessive use of a Sneha-Vasti. The next couplet in the text would better support Vrinda's reading.—Ed.

by the action of the deranged **Váyu**. Fever, a burning sensation (of the body), thirst, perspiration, a pungent taste in the mouth and yellowness of the complexion, urine and the eyes are the features which are due to the retention of the injected Sneha in the bowels overwhelmed by the action of the deranged **Pitta**. Waterbrash, a sweet taste in the mouth, heaviness of the limbs, vomiting, difficult breathing, catarrhal fever (Sita-Jvara) and an aversion to food are the indications due to the retention of the injected Sneha in the bowels overpowered by the action of the deranged **Kapha**. In these cases, applications of (Sneha) Vastis and such other remedial measures as are soothing to the Dosha or Doshas (giving rise to the retention of the Sneha in the bowels) should be adopted with due regard to the nature and intensity of each. 28-29.

Cramps (Sula) and heaviness in the stomach (Ámásaya), suppression of the Váyu (flatus), affection of the heart, a bad taste in the mouth, difficult respiration, epileptic fits, vertigo and an aversion to food are the symptoms which attend a retention of the Sneha in the bowels owing to the pressure of food matter carried down into the abdomen of a person who has been so treated after a heavy meal, and they should be remedied first by fasting and then by appetising measures. 30.

A languid feeling in the limbs attended with a distension of the abdomen, colic (S'ula), difficult breathing and a sense of heaviness in the intestines mark the retention of the injected Sneha surcharged with the fœcal matter of a person previously uncleansed by proper remedies. The remedy in such cases consists in the application of Niruha-vastis as well as Snehavastis with the admixture of keen-potencied drugs. 31.

A scent of the Sneha in the mouth, cough, difficult breathing, an aversion to food and dullness of all sense-organs which become internally charged with a coating of oil and a glossy appearance of the skin (mouth—D. R.) mark an undesirably higher introduction of the Sneha injected into the system previously cleansed (with proper emetics and purgatives). Such a case should be treated as a case of *Ati-pidita* (over-pressure on the bladder of the) enema and with the applications of Ásthápana-vastis as well. 32.

An inadequate quantity of Sneha of a mild or weak potency, injected cold with the help of an enema, is not retained in the system, if not duly fomented and cleansed before, but gives rise to scanty stools, cramps (S'ula), heaviness and distention in the region of the intestines (Pakvás'aya) and (ultimate) suppression of stool, etc. Such cases should be speedily remedied by the application of an Ásthápana as well as by that of an Anuvásana-vasti. 33.

A small quantity of Sneha of mild potency, injected into the bowels of a patient taking only a small quantity of food, fails to flow therefrom and gives rise to a dullness of spirit, a tendency to vomit and a sense of lassitude which should be remedied by the application of Asthâpana-vastis charged with (the decoction of) S'odhaniya (cleansing) drugs and by the application of Anuvásana enemas charged with Sneha boiled and cooked with those (S'odhaniya) drugs. 34.

The Sneha of a Vasti, if found to dribble down (from the system) after the lapse of even a whole day and night from the time of its application, without giving rise to any physical discomfort, does no mischief but exerts all the good effects of the application of the Vasti.

Whereas, if digested, it produces but very little benefit to the patient. The retention of the whole or of any portion of the Sneha injected into the bowels of a patient without producing any special physical discomfort should be ascribed to an extremely parched or dry condition of his organism, and would not require any special medical treatment. 35-36.

In case of a Sneha not flowing out from the bowels within a period of twenty-four hours of its introduction (and in case of its producing any supervening symptoms), corrective (S'odhana) remedies should be employed and all subsequent applications of Sneha should be stopped. Thus we have finished describing the diseases (Vyâpat' and symptoms which result from the injudicious use of Sneha (-Vastis) together with the nature of the medical treatment to be employed in each of them. 37.

**Uttara-vastis:**—Now we shall describe the mode of applying an **Uttara-vasti** (injection into the urethra of a male or of a female patient). The pipe to be used for the purpose (in the case of a male patient) should be made to measure fourteen fingers in length, measured by the patient's own fingers. It should be shaped like the stem of a *Mâlati* flower (in girth) at its top-end and provided with an aperture admitting the passage of a mustard seed. Several authorities hold that the length of the pipe should be equal to that of the penis (of the patient). The largest dose of a Sneha to be used in connection with an urethral injection (Uttara-vasti) is only one Kuncha (Pala); and this should be determined with discretion in respect of patients below twenty-five years of age. There should be (two) Karnikâs (protrusions) in the middle part of the pipe (Netra) in the case of a male.

In the case of a female patient, however, the Karnikás should be placed above a space of four fingers (from its end). The whole pipe should be ten fingers in length and should be made to suit the urethral channel (of the patient) with an aperture sufficient to allow a *Mudga-* pulse to pass through it. 38.

In the case of a vaginal douche or injection (Vasti), the pipe of the **Uttara-vasti** should be introduced to the extent of four fingers only into the vaginal canal. Two fingers only of the entire length of the pipe should be inserted into the channel of the urethra in the case of an adult woman, whereas, in the case of a young girl of tender years, the pipe should be introduced to the length of one finger only. Here it should be noted that these measures are to be determined by the standard of the patient's own fingers. A *Prasrita* measure of the Sneha by which is meant a quantity that would be contained in the hollow of the palms of the patient's hand extending to the roots of the phalanx is the largest dose to be used in both these instances. In the case of patients of tender years the dosage should be determined with discretion in each case. 39.

The Vasti (bladder of the enema) should be made of the bladder of a hog, lamb, or, a goat, or in its absence, of the skin of the neck of a bird, or of the leg of a *Driti* (a leathern bag for holding water), or of any other soft skin. 40.

**Mode of application :**—The body of the patient should be first treated with a Sneha and with fomentation (Sveda), and his bowels (Ás'aya) should be cleansed. He should then be made to partake of a gruel (Yavágu) mixed with milk and clarified butter according to his digestive capacity. He should be made to sit on a cushion placed on even ground and as high as his knee-joints. Lukewarm oil should be rubbed over the region of the neck of the bladder, and the penis should be (artificially) excited and made steady and straight. The orifice or the channel of the urethra should be first (dilated and) searched with the help of an indicator (S'aláká), and then the pipe of the Uttara-vasti, lubricated with clarified butter, should be gently and gradually inserted therein to the extent of six fingers. The Sneha should be injected into the urethra by gently pressing the bladder of the Uttara-vasti, and the pipe should then be gradually withdrawn from the urethra. The patient should be made to partake of a moderate quantity of boiled rice with milk, Yusha (Mudga-soup, etc.), or meat-soup* in the evening after the dribbling out of the injected Sneha. Three or four injections should be thus made with the help of an urethral enema (Uttara-vasti). 41.

**Vaginal Uttara-vasti :**—A grown up female patient, (under the circumstances), should be laid on her back with arched and up-drawn knees, and an injection should be made into her vaginal canal (Yoni) by an experienced physician (D. R.—carefully). The pipe should be most gently pressed in the case of a girl before menstruation. For the purpose of purifying the uterus (Garbhás'aya), double the ordinary (one Prasrita) quantity of Sneha should be injected into the vaginal canal (by means of a Vasti) with a pipe having three Karnikás (protuberance) attached to it. 42-43.

In case the injected fluid does not come back (within the prescribed time), a fresh Vasti (enema) should be

---

* Milk, Yusha and meat-soup should be prescribed in cases of the predominance of Kapha, Pitta and Váyu respectively.—Dallana.

again applied with (the decoctions of) the S'odhana*
(purifying) drugs, or a Varti (plug) prepared with the
Sodhana drugs should be injected into the rectum.
As an alternative, an indicator (Eshani) should be
inserted into the mouth of the bladder, or the region
of the abdomen below the umbilicus, and be firmly
pressed with a close fist, or medicinal plugs or sticks
(Varti) of the size of a *Mudga*-pulse, cardamom-seed
(Elá), or mustard-seed should be made up of Saindhava
and the leaves of the *Áragvadha* pasted with the expressed juice of *Nirgundi* and cow's urine, and these
plugs (Varti) should, according to the age of the
patient, be inserted (into the mouth of the bladder) with
(the top-end of) a rod or an indicator (Saláká) for the
out-flow of the injected fluid. Another alternative is to
use a stick (Varti) made up of the pendant soot of a room
(Agára-dhuma), *Vrihati, Pippali, Madana* fruit, Saindhava salt and *S'unthi* pasted with S'ukta (a sort of
Kânjika) and cow's urine (in the preceding manner).
Other (similar) measures should be adopted for the
successful action of an Anuvásana enema (Vasti).
44-A.

A cold decoction of *Yashti-madhu* saturated with
honey and sugar† or a decoction of the (bark of the)
milk-exuding trees (Kshiri-Vriksha), or cold milk, should
again be injected into the bladder, in the event of there
being a burning sensation in that organ. 44.

Diseases such as derangements of the semen, or of
ovum, or difficult menstruation, excess or suppression

---

\* The S'odhana drugs here are the Trina-pancha-mula and such other drugs.—Dallana.

† According to Dallana a quantity of sugar and honey should be added in each of the three cases, viz., (1) the decoction of Yashti-madhu, (2) that of the Kshiri-trees, and (3) milk.

of the monthly flow, diseases of the uterus and of the vaginal canal, non-falling of the placenta, strangury and other diseases of the urine, gravel, stones (As'mari), spermatorrhea (S'ukrotseka), cramps in the bladder, in the groins and in the urethra and all other severe diseases of the bladder other than Meha, will all yield to the application of an **Uttara-vasti** (urethral enema). Symptoms which mark, or dangers which attend, a judicious or an injudicious application of an Uttara-vasti are respectively identical with those which characterise or attend those of a Sneha-vasti. 45-46.

Thus ends the Thirty-seventh Chapter of the Chikitsita Sthánam in the Sus'ruta Samhitá which deals with the Anuwásana-Vasti and the Uttara-vasti.

# CHAPTER XXXVIII.

Now, we shall discourse on the mode of applying as well as on the treatment with a Nirudha-vasti **(Nirudhopakrama-Chikitsitam).** 1.

**The mode of preparing a Vasti :**—The application of an Anuvásana-vasti (enema) should be followed by that of one of the Ásthápana class. The body of the patient should be first anointed (with a Sneha) and fomented. Previous to the application of a vasti, the bowels and bladder should be relieved of all (fœcal) accumulations (flatus and urine). The clyster (Vasti) should be applied at noon in a well-cleansed chamber, devoid of any gust of wind, and the patient should be laid on his left side on a spacious bed not furnished with any pillows, but a little raised up there where his buttocks would rest, and there should be attendants at his feet. The patient should continue in a cheerful mood with his left thigh held in an outstretched posture and the right one flexed, and should refrain from speaking to any body. The digestion of the ingested food taken by the patient is necessary (before the application of the Vasti). The physician having placed the pipe of the enema (Vasti) upon his left foot should firmly press its Karniká with the first and the second toes of his right foot. One half of the mouth of the Vasti should be kept contracted by pressing it with the small and ring finger of his left hand and the (other) half should be stretched with the aid of his thumb, index and middle fingers, and thus the medicinal solution should be poured into the bladder (Vasti). The pipe should be held with the middle and the index finger of the right hand. Care should be taken not to let the medicinal solution overflow from the surface of the pipe, nor to admit of even a bubble of air into the bladder (of the enema), nor to produce its over-contraction nor dilatation during the process (of pouring the medicine). The bladder filled with the proper quantity of medicinal solution should then be held in the left hand, and washed with the right hand. It should then be firmly tied (at the neck) just over the (surface of the) medicinal solution with ligatures of two or three rounds of thread. 2-A.

**The mode of applying a Vasti :**—The Vasti should then be held up on the palm of the right hand, its pipe gripped with the middle and index fingers of the left hand, and the orifice closed with the thumb of the same hand. The neck of the pipe should be previously lubricated with clarified butter, and gently introduced into the rectum of the patient up to its *Karniká* (protuberance) along the line of spinal column and with its mouth up-turned. The patient should be asked to take the same with care. 2.

**Metrical Text :**—The physician should then hold the enema (Vasti) with his left hand and press its bladder with his right. The injection (of the medicinal solution contained in the enema) should be made at once, neither too slowly nor too hurriedly. 3.

The pipe should then be withdrawn and removed, and the patient should be asked to remain in the same position for a period sufficient to utter thirty Mátrás*

---

\* According to Agnives'a the time necessary for the tips of the fingers to fall down upon the right thighs, *i.e.*, the time required for a twinkling of the eye (Nimesha) is called a **Mátrá**. Parás'ara says that the time necessary to close and open the eye-lids (Nimesha and Unmesha) once, while throwing the arm around the right thigh is called a Mátrá. He has prescribed one hundred such Mátrás in respect of a patient of constipated bowels, and thirty-seven in respect of a patient of lax

from the time of injection. The patient should then be asked to get up and sit on his legs for the full outflow of the injected solution. The period of a Muhurta (about forty-eight minutes) is usually required for a complete outflow of the Niruha-vasti (from the bowels). 4.

**Metrical Texts :**—This method of applying the Vasti should be continued three or four times as required in each case by the physician, experienced in the application of the same. It should be discontinued after certain characteristic symptoms had been fully developed and manifested (in the system of the patient). Less is better than excess (in respect of Vasti-applications' and more so particularly in the case of a patient of a delicate constitution. 5.

**Symptoms of an inadequate and excessive application of a Vasti :**—The emission of only a small quantity of flatus (Váyu), fœcal matter and (of the medicinal solution applied in) the Vasti, as also the appearance of the supervening distresses of urinary disorders, an aversion to food and physical lassitude indicate the inadequacy of the application of the Vasti. Symptoms which have been described before* as marking an excessive use of purgatives are also said to result from an excessive application of a Niruha-vasti. 6-A.

**Symptoms of a satisfactory application of a Vasti :**—A lightness of the body, experienced in consequence of the successive and satisfactory evacuations of stool,† Pitta (bilious matters),

bowels.—Dallana. The period of a Mátrá has elsewhere been defined as that required to utter a short Vowel. —*Ed.*

\* See Chapter XXXIII, Para. 18, Chikitsita Sthánam.

† Satisfactory urination should also be understood as one of the symptoms of the satisfactory application of a Niruha-Vasti.—*Ed*

Kapha (mucus) and Váyu (flatus) from the bowels, are the salient features of a satisfactory application of a Niruha-vasti (Su-nirudha). After the manifestation of the foregoing symptoms the patient should be advised to bathe (in hot water) and to take meat-soup (Rasa), milk and pulse-soup (Yusha) in diseases due to the action of the deranged Váyu, Pitta and Kapha respectively. The essence (Rasa) of the meat of any Jángala animal may, however, be prescribed in all cases under the circumstances, since it would produce no harm. Only a quarter, a half or three-quarter part of the usual diet should be prescribed according to the digestive capacity of the patient, and the nature and intensity of the Doshas involved in each case. 6-B.

The subsequent treatment should consist in applying a Sneha-vasti (oleaginous enema) according to the nature and intensity of the underlying Doshas in each case. A lightness of the body, sprightliness of the mind, amelioration or abatement of the disease, an emulsive condition of the organism, are the features which mark the satisfactory application of an Ásthápana as well as of an Anuvásana-vasti. 6-C.

The patient should be made to partake of his meal with meat-soup on the day of his being treated with a (Niruha) Vasti ; since there is an apprehension of the Váyu being greatly deranged and aggravated (by the application of the Vasti). He should then be treated with an Anuvásana (Vasti) on the same day. Thereafter the application of the Sneha-vasti should be regulated* with a regard to the state of the appetite and the intensity of the deranged Váyu, and in the

* A second application of the Sneha-vasti should be made, if necessary, on the 2nd, 3rd, or 5th day with a due regard to the symptoms mentioned in the text.

event of the *Koshtha* (stomach) being found to have been stuffed with food. 6

A fresh and stronger Nirudha injection (Vasti), composed of *Yava-kshára*, cow's urine, *Kánjika* and the *S'odhana* (purifying) drugs, should be applied (into the bowels) in the event of the previous one not passing out within a *Muhurta*, since a Nirudha injection (Vasti) long retained in the bowels by the enraged and aggravated Váyu causes S'ula (colic), an aversion to food, fever and Anáha\* (distension of the abdomen with suppression of stool and urine), or may ultimately have a fatal termination. 7.

The application of an Ásthápana enema is forbidden after a meal as it may bring on an attack of Visuchiká\* (D. R.—Áma), or of vomiting, or may tend to aggravate the Doshas of the body. Hence an Ásthápana-vasti (enema) should be applied only on an empty stomach. The Doshas (in the system) of a person lie in a free and potent state at the close of the process of digestion, and are easily and spontaneously eliminated from the system (by the application of the Ásthápana-vasti), when the stomach (Ás'aya) is not further oppressed or stuffed with food. The digestive fire (*Játharágni*) can not digest the food, if scattered or diffused by the application of an Ásthápana-vasti (into the bowels). Hence it is that an Ásthápana injection should be made on an empty stomach. The application of a Niruha-vasti (which is not applicable in all cases) should, however, be determined with a regard to the exigencies of the case, since the strength of the aggravated Doshas of the body abate with the evacua-

---

\* Both Vrinda and Chakradatta read "*A'topa*" (rumbling sounds in the intestines) in place of "*A'náha*."

tions of the bowels (as well as with the elimination of all filthy matters from the system). 8.

**Drugs to be used in a Niruha-vasti :**—The following drugs and articles, or as many of them as would be available, such as, all kinds of milk, acid group (Kánjika, etc.), urine, Sneha (oleaginous substances), the drug decoctions (Kasháya), meat-soup (Rasa), salts, *Phala* (Triphalá), honey, *S'atákvá*, *Sarshapa, Vacha, Elá, Trikatu, Rásná, Sarala, Devadáru, Rajani, Yashti-madhu, Hingu, Kushtha,* the drugs of the *Sams'odhana* (corrective) group (Trivrit, etc.), *Katuka, Sugar, Musta, Us'ira, Chandana, S'athi, Manjishthá, Madana, Chandá Tráyamáná, Rasánjana,* (dried) *Vilva* fruit, *Yamáni, Phalini, Indra-yava, Yava, Kákoli, Kshira-kákoli', Jivaka, Rishabhaka, Medá, Mahámedá, Riddhi, Vriddhi* and *Madhuliká,* should be used in charging a **Nirudha-vasti.** 9.

**Formula of the Niruha-vasti :**—In the case of a healthy person (marked by an equilibrium of Váyu, Pitta and Kapha), the solution to be injected should be composed of four parts of the decoction of drugs* and one part (a fifth part of the entire compound) of the Sneha (any oleaginous substance) In any case marked by a preponderance of the deranged **Váyu,** the Sneha should measure a quarter part of the whole, one-sixth in a case of a preponderance of the deranged **Pitta** and an eighth part in a case of the deranged **Kapha.** In a case of aggravation of all the (three) Doshas, the Kalka should measure an eighth part (of the entire quantity of the medicinal solution to be injected), and the following drugs or articles,

---

* Dallana means to say that of the whole compound weighing **twelve Prasrita** measures (twenty-four Palas), there should be four Prasrita weights (8 Palas) of the decoction, and so on.

*viz.*, salt, honey, cow's urine, Phala (Madana), milk, acid group (Kánjika, etc.) and extract of meat, in charging a Nirudha-Vasti should, as regards *dosage*, be determined by a due consideration of the requirements in each case. When the Kalka, the Sneha, and the decoction would be well mixed together, the solution for injection should be considered to have been well prepared The application of such a solution would be supposed to produce the wished-for results. 10-A.

**The process of preparation :—**An Aksha measure (two Tolás) of Saindhava salt should be first mixed with the palms of the hand on a plate with two Prasrita (thirty-two Tolás) measures of honey, to which Sneha (oil, etc.) should be gradually added. When well dissolved, the pastes of (Madana) Phala should be added thereto. The drugs to be used as the Kalka in proportion to the prescribed parts should then be finely powdered and mixed with the preceding compound. The whole should then be well stirred in a deep vessel with a ladle (Khaja) * so as not to make it too thick, nor too thin. The compound thus prepared should be mixed with five Prasrita measures of the well-filtered drug decoction (prescribed in each case) and with cow's urine, meat-essence, milk and acid articles (Kánjika, etc.) according to the nature of the Doshas involved in the case. 10

**Dvá-dasá Prasriti :—**Now we shall describe the (recipe and preparation of) Vastis (technically) called the "Dvá-dasá-Prasrita" (weighing twelve Prasritas). An Aksha measure (two Tolás) of Saindhava salt should be rubbed with two Prasritas (thirty-two Tolás) of honey to which should be added three Prasritas

---

* The hand would serve the purpose of a ladle best in this case.

of a Sneha (oleaginous substance). The whole should then be stirred and when the Sneha would be well mixed, a Prasrita measure of a medicinal Kalka, four Prasritas of a decoction, and two Prasritas of medicinal after-throws (powdered drugs thrown to or cast in a medicinal compound at the close of its decoction) should be added to it. In this way an enema solution should be made to measure twelve Prasritas in all and is hence called "**Dvá-daśa-Prasrita**". This should be regarded as the rule in respect of a full dose and the physician may reduce the numbers of Prasritas (if required). This kind of variation according to the age of the patient, in the quantity of each drug of a Niruha-Vasti which commences with the Saindhava salt and ends with the liquid (*viz.*, Kasháya) has always been observed by the physician aspiring after success (in prescribing a Vasti). 11.

**Classification of Vastis according to the range of their therapeutic applications :** – Now we shall deal with the classification of (Nirudha) enemas (according to the difference in their therapeutic ranges) which, when applied with due consideration of the aggravated Doshas (acting as the exciting factors), will conquer many a disease. 12.

A decoction should be prepared with one Pala of each of *Sampáka, Ruvu, Varshábhu, Aśva-gandhá, Niśá-chchhada* (Śathi), *Pancha-mula, Valá, Rásná, Guduchi* and *Deva-dáru* and *Madana* fruit eight (two Palas) in number (boiled together and reduced to a quarter part of the original quantity of water). After that a paste (Kalka) composed of *Mágadhiká, Ambhoda,* (Mustá), *Havushá, Misi* (anisi), *Saindhava, Vatsáhva, Priyangu, Ugrá* (**Vacha**), *Yashtyáhva,* and *Rasánjana* being mixed with honey, etc.,* should be dissolved in the preceding medicinal decoction and injected lukewarm (into the bowels) in the manner of an Ásthápana-Vasti. Pain in the back, the thighs and in the regions of the sacrum (Trika), stone, retention of stool, urine and flatus, diarrhœa (Grahani), Hæmorrhoids and diseases due to the action of the deranged Váyu, readily yield to the curative efficacy of such injections, by which also, the blood, muscles and the strength are improved. 13.

A decoction duly prepared with *Guduchi, Triphalá, Rásná, Das'a-mula* and *Valá* weighing one Pala † each, and a pulverised compound consisting of *Priyangu, Rasánjana, Saindhava, S'ata-pushpá, Vachá, Krishná, Yamáni, Kushtha, Vilva* fruit and treacle each weighing an Aksha (two Tolás) and half a Pala of pulverised *Madana* fruit, should be injected into the bowels (in the manner of an Ásthápana enema injection), stirred and mixed with an adequate quantity of honey, oil, clarified butter, milk, S'ukta, Kánjika, Mastu (curd-cream) and cow's urine‡. Strength, energy, vigour, complexion, digestive capacity, verility and vital duration of the user would be increased by its application, and all derangements of the bodily Váyu would yield to its curative efficacy. It is one of the best rejuvenating agents. 14.

A decoction should be made by boiling together the drugs of the *Kshudra-Pancha-mula* group, *Musta*,

---

* Honey, Sneha, milk, Kánjika, cow's urine, meat-juice, etc., should be taken.

† Dallana takes Pala in the sense of meat मांसम् (Mámsam).

‡ The quantity of honey, oil, and clarified butter, should be as before, that of S'ukta, Kánjika, Mastu and urine half a Pala each, and that of milk two Palas.—*Dallana*.

*Tri-phalá, Utpala, Vásaka, Sárivá, Manjishthá, Rásná, Renu,* and *Parushaka* each weighing one Pala. A compound of *S'ringátaka, Átma-guptá, Gaja-pippali, Kes'ara, Aguru, Chandana, Vidári, Misi* (anisi), *Manjishthá, S'yámá, Indra-yava, Saindhava-salt, Madana-Phala, Yashti-madhu, Padma-káshtha* pasted together, should be dissolved in the preceding decoction which should be mixed and stirred with milk, honey and clarified butter and injected cold without the addition of any acid substance, in the manner of an Ásthápana enema (Vasti). It should be applied in liquid form. A burning sensation of the body, menorrhœa (Asrig-dara), Hæmorrhage, Pittaja-gulma, Pittaja-fever, yield to the curative efficacy of such a medicinal injection (Vasti). 15.

A decoction should be duly prepared with *Lodhra, Rakta-chandana, Manjishthá, Rásná, Anantá, Valá, Riddhi, Sárivá, Vrisha, Kás'maryya, Medá, Madhuka* (Yashti-madhu), *Padmaka,* the drugs included in the Sthirádi (minor Pancha-mula) and the *Trina-Pancha-mula* groups, each weighing three Karshas (six Tolás). Then a paste composed of *Jivaka, Rishabhaka Kákoli, Kshira-Kákoli, Riddhi, Yashti-madhu, Utpala, Prapaundarika, Jivanti, Medá, Renu* (Parpataka), *Parushaka, Abhiru* (S'atávari), *Misi, Saindhava, Vatsaka, Us'ira, Padmaka, Kas'eru* and sugar pasted together should be mixed with the preceding decoction made into a fluid solution with an adequate quantity of milk, honey, and clarified butter and other fluid substances\* other than

---

\* Dallana recommends the use of meat-juice (one Pala) and sugar-cane juice (two Palas) as the liquefacient agents in this preparation. It should also be noted that coldness and non-addition of any acid substances are recommended as the injection is to be applied in cases of diseases due to the derangement of **Pitta.**

strong acid ones (Kánjika, etc.). It should then be injected well cooled in the manner of an Ásthápana-Vasti. It would undoubtedly prove curative in cases of Gulma, menorrhœgia (Asrig-dara), heart diseases, Jaundice, Vishama-jvara, Hæmorrhage (Rakta-pitta), dysentery, and other Pittaja ailments. 16.

A compound of *Valá, Madana* fruit, *Sarshapa, Saindhava, Deva-dáru, Kushtha, Elá, Pippali, Vilva* and *S'unthi* (weighing three Palas in all) pounded together and mixed with the decoction of *Bhadrá, Nimba, Kulattha* pulse, *Arka, Kos'átaki, Amrita,* (Guduchi), *Deva-dáru, Sárivá, Vrihati, Páthá, Murvá, Áragvadha* and *Kutaja*-seeds (weighing sixteen Palas in all) cooked with water (one hundred and twenty-eight Palas) should be injected in the manner of an Ásthápana-Vasti, with the addition of an adequate quantity of mustard oil, honey, alkali, cow's urine, sesamum oil and water (three Palas). This would speedily conquer an attack of Chlorosis (Kámalá), Jaundice, Meha, obesity, impaired digestion, aversion to food, goitre, slow poisoning, (Gara visha), elephantiasis, Udara, or of any disorders due to the deranged Kapha. 17.

*Musta, Saindhava, Deva-dáru, Páthá, Pippali* and *Indra-yava,* pounded together, and made into a paste with the admixture of the decoction prepared with such drugs as *Das'a-mula, Haridrá, Vilva, Patola, Triphalá,* and *Deva-dáru,* should be stirred and saturated with oil, *Yava-kshára* and honey and reduced to a soluble fluidity by adding (an adequate quantity of) cow's urine, *Madana-phala* and *Kánjika.* The solution thus prepared should be injected (into the rectum of the patient) in the manner of an Ásthâpana enema-injection and this would prove curative in cases of Jaundice, deranged Kapha, alcoholism, lassitude, suppression of flatus (Váyu) and of urine, in cases of there being any rumbling sounds in the intestines (Átopa), and Gulma and in diseases due to worms. 18.

*Madana-phala, Yashti-madhu, Vacha, Deva-dáru, Sarshapa, Pippali-mula, Saindhava* salt (Sindhuttha), *Yamáni, Misi* and *Indra-yava* should be pounded together and made into a paste with the admixture of the decoction prepared with a Pala measure each of *Vásaka, As'ma bheda, Varshábhu, Dhánya, Eranda-mula, Das'a-mula, Valá, Murvá, Yava, Kola, Nis'a-chchhada* (Sathi), *Kulattha, Vilva,* and *Bhu-nimba* and dissolved in an adequate quantity of honey and the expressed juice of sugar-cane, milk, oil, clarified butter, meat-essence, and the urine (of a cow) by stirring them together. The solution thus prepared should be speedily injected in the manner of an Ásthápana injection into the rectum of a patient suffering from a disease marked by the concerted action of two or more of the deranged Doshas. Diseases such as Gridhrasi, S'arkará, Ashthilá Tuni and Gulma may be rapidly cured with this injection (Vasti) 19.

*Madana* fruit, *Yashti-madhu, Misi* (anisi), *Saindhava, Priyangu* and *Indra-yava* pounded together and made into a paste with the decoction of the drugs, one Pala each of *Rásná, Áragvadha, Varshábhu, Kaluka, Us'ira, Mustaka, Tráyamáná, Amrita* (Guduchi), *Raktá* (Manjishthá), *Pancha-mula, Vibhitaka* and *Valá* should be duly mixed with (an adequate quantity) of *Rasánjana,* extract of meat (Rasa), honey, Sauvira and the expressed juice of the *Drákshá*. The solution thus prepared should be injected lukewarm into the bowels of the patient in the manner of an Ásthápana-Vasti. It adds to the growth of flesh, creates fresh semen and Ojas, improves the digestive capacity and the strength of the body, imparts longevity and cures and conquers the following diseases, *viz.*, Gulma, Menorrhagia, Erysipelas (Visarpa), Strangury, *Kshata-kshaya*, Vishama-jvara, Hæmorrhoids, Diarrhœa (Grahani), Váta-kundali, catching pain due to the incarceration of the Váyu in the regions of the thighs, knee-joints, head and bladder (Vasti), obstinate constipation of the bowels, (Udávarta) and the other distempers of the bodily Váyu, Vata-rakta, Śarkará (gravels in the bladder), Ashthilá, cramp in the groins, Udara, aversion to food, Rakta-pitta (Hæmorrhage), affections of the deranged Kapha, Insanity, Prameha, distension of the abdomen (Ádhmána), catching pain at the heart (Hrid-graha). 20.

A Vasti composed of the decoction of the Váyu-subduing drugs mixed with *Trivrit**, *Saindhava* and *Kánjika* (or the expressed juice of acid fruits) should be applied lukewarm in cases due to the aggravation of the bodily **Váyu**. Similarly, a Vasti composed of the decoctions of the drugs included within the *Nyagrodhádi* group mixed with sugar, clarified butter, powders of those included within the *Kákolyádi* group should be applied in diseases due to the aggravation of the **Pitta.** A Vasti composed of the decoction of the drugs of the *Áragvadhádi* group saturated with the pulverised compound of those included within the *Pippalyádi* group, should be employed with (an adequate quantity of) cow's urine, added thereto in a case of the aggravation of **Kapha.** A Vasti composed of a copious quantity of the decoction of *Kshira-Vrikshas* mixed with (an adequate quantity of) the expressed juice of the sugar-cane, milk,

---

* According to Dallana, "Trivrit" should be understood to mean the same as "Traivrita" mentioned in the treatment of Mahá-Váta-vyádhi (see Chapter V., Para. 25, Chikitsita Sthánam).

sugar, and clarified butter should be applied in a cold state in cases marked by a vitiated condition of the blood of the system. 21—24.

**Śodhana (corrective) Vastis :**—The drugs of the *S'odhana* group (possessed of corrective therapeutic properties) should be pounded together and mixed with an admixture of their own decoction. The solution thus formed should be mixed with *Saindhava* and Sneha and stirred with ladle. It should then be injected into the bowels of the patient. This is called the S'odhana-Vasti*. 25.

**Lekhana-Vasti :**—The powders of the drugs of the *Ushakádi* group should be mixed with the decoction of *Triphalá* and with cow's urine, honey and *Yava-kshára*. The whole solution should be applied as a Vasti and is called the **Lekhana-Vasti**. 26.

**Vrimhana-Vasti :**—A paste composed of the drugs of the *Madhura* (Kákolyádi) group mixed with the decoction of the drugs possessed of tonic and constructive properties (Vrimhana drugs) should be injected into the bowels with clarified butter and the extract of meat added thereto. It is called the Vrimhana-Vasti. 27.

**Váji-karana-Vasti :**—The seeds of the *Átmaguptá* should be pounded and mixed with the decoction of (the roots of) the *Uchchatá* together with (the contents of) the egg of a sparrow (Chataka) and an adequate quantity of milk, clarified butter and sugar. The solution should be injected into the bowels in the manner of a Vasti and is called the **Váji-karana-Vasti** (aphrodisiac). 28.

---

\* According to Dallana, four Pala weights of honey, one Pala of milk, one Pala and a half of cow's urine, and four Pala and a half of Kánjika, should be added to this solution.

**Pichchhila-Vasti :**—Milk cooked with *Vidári,*\* *Airávati, S'elu, S'álmali* and the tender sprouts of *Dhanvana* should be used as a Vasti with the blood and honey (added to it) ;† it is called the **Pichchhila-Vasti**. The fresh blood of a buffalo, hog, sheep, or of a cat, or the contents of a newly laid (hen's) egg‡ may be used for the purpose. 29-30.

**Gráhi-Vasti :**—A paste of the drugs of the *Ambashthádi* group, dissolved in a decoction of those of the *Priyangvádi* group and mixed with honey and clarified butter, may be used as a Vasti and is called the **Gráhi-Vasti**. 31.

**Sneha-Vasti :**—A Sneha-Vasti should be prepared by duly cooking the drugs of one or two of the above groups with a Sneha. 32.

Sterile women should be treated with a Vasti consisting of the S'ata-páka-Valá-Taila or the Traivrita-Ghrita (as described before)§ after being cleansed (S'odhana) in due succession. 33.

**Strong** enemas (possessed of keen medicinal potency) should be employed in respect of extremely strong

---

\* Both Vrinda and Chakrapáni read "Vadari" in place of "Vidári", and their annotators mean to say that the tender sprouts of all trees, *viz.*, Vadari, etc., should be used.

† Vrinda does not recommend the addition of honey; he reads "सुशीताः स्युः" (*i.e.*, the Vasti should be in a cold state), in place of "चौद्रयुता:". But it is evident from the reading of Dallana's commentary, as quoted by S'rikantha Datta, that honey should be added.

‡ Both Vrinda and Chakrapáni read "आज" in place of "अरुडं" which means that the newly spilt blood of a goat should be added to the list and hen's egg should be eliminated therefrom.

§ Valá-Taila has been mentioned in the treatment of Mudha-garbha (Chapter XV, Chikitsita Sthánam) and the Traivrita-Ghrita has been described in the treatment of Mahá-Vátavyádhi (Chapter V, Chikitsita Sthánam).

patients, and those of **moderate** potency should be employed in respect of persons possessed of a middling sort of bodily strength, while weak persons should be treated with Vastis (enemas) of **mild** potency. An experienced physician should thus apply Vastis (enemas) with due regard to the nature of the season, the strength of the patient, the nature and intensity of the disease under treatment and of the Doshas involved therein and to the nature of the potency of the ingredients to be used in charging the Vasti (enema).* 34.

Loosening or disintegrating (**Utkles'ana**—lit. irritating) enemas (*i e.*, those possessed of the virtue of dislodging and disintegrating the accumulated Doshas in the system) should be employed at the outset and corrective ones (**Dosha-hara**) should then be employed, while those exerting a soothing influence on the organism (**Sams'amana**) should be employed last of all towards the close of the treatment   35.

**Different Vastis :**—An **Utklesana** (disintegrating) Vasti consists of castor seeds, *Yashti-madhu, Pippali, Saindhava, Vacha, Habushá* and *Phala* (Triphalá —Madana-phala, according to others) pasted together. A **Dosha-hara-vasti** (corrective enema) consists (of a solution) of *Yashti-madhu, Kutaja seeds and Madana-phala* with Kánjika and cow's urine. A **Samsodhana-Vasti** (soothing enema) consists of *Priyangu, Yashti-madhu, Musta and Rasánjana* with cow's milk. 36—38.

**Mádhu-Tailika Vasti :**—Now we shall describe in short the process of applying a **Mádhu-Tailika**

---

* S'ivadása, the commentator of Chakradatta, quotes two additional lines as being incorporated in Sus'ruta's text which, when translated, would be as follows :—Better use a Vasti of milder potency but never use on of strong potency than what is necessary and this is recommended especially in cases of delicate persons.—*Ed.*

Vasti (enema) which should be resorted to only in respect of kings or king-like personages as well as in respect of women, old men, infants and persons of delicate constitutions for the purposes of eliminating the Doshas (accumulated in the organism) and of improving the strength and complexion. The use of this remedy does not entail any strict observance of continence or of any particular rules, diet, conduct, or conveyance on the part of the patient, nor is it attended with any possible complication though it is quite on a par with any other kind of Vasti as regards its excellent and highly beneficial therapeutic virtues. It may thus be applied at any time by an experienced physician in the manner of a Nirudha-Vasti (enema) whenever the patient wishes to be treated therewith. Equal parts of honey, oil and the decoction of castor roots, half a Pala of *S'ata-pushpá*, a quarter Pala of *Sanidhava*, and one entire *Madana* fruit should be mixed together by stirring the whole with a ladle. The whole compound thus prepared should be injected lukewarm into the rectum of the patient. This measure is called the **Madhu-Tailika-Vasti.*** 39.

**Yukta-ratha & Dosha-hara Vastis :—** The **Yukta-ratha Vasti** consists in injecting a medicinal solution surcharged with *Vacha, Madhuka* (honey),† oil, meat-essence, *Saindhava, Pippali, Madana* fruit, and the decoction (of Eranda) into the bowels of a patient.

---

\* The quantity of the fluid should be nine Prasritas in all cases of the **Madhu-Tailika** Vasti and such-like Vastis (enemas).—*Dallana.*

† Vacha, salt, Madana-phala, Pippali, each should be one Karsha ; honey and oil four Prasritas and two Karshas each, and the decoction of Eranda roots four Prasritas and two Karshas.—*Dallana.*

In the text we find "**Madhuka**" which generally means Vashti-madhu. Here, however, it should mean "**honey**". This is evident from Dallana's commentary.

A compound of *Deva-dáru, Vará* (Triphalá), *Rásná, S'ata-pushpá, Vacha,* honey, asafœtida and *Saindhava* salt, used together as a Vasti, is called the **Dosha-hara Vasti.** 40-41.

**Siddha-Vasti :**—This Vasti should be prepared with the decoction of *Pancha-mula,* mixed with oil, honey and a paste of *S'atáhvá, Pippali* and *Saindhava* salt. Similar Vastis consisting of a decoction of *Yava, Kola* and *Kulattha,* and mixed with a paste of *Pippali, Saindhava, Yashti-madhu* and honey may also be used. This kind of Vasti is called a **Siddha-Vasti.** 42-43.

**Mustádika-Vasti :**—A Pala measure of each of the following drugs, *viz., Mustá, Páthá, Amritá* (Guduchi), *Tiktá, Valá, Rásná, Punarnavá, Manjishthá, Aragvadha, Us'ira, Tráyamáná, Gokshura* as well as of those included within the group of minor (Svalpa) *Pancha-mula,* and eight *Madana* fruits should be boiled with an Ádhaka measure of water down to its quarter part. The decoction thus prepared should again be boiled with the admixture of a Prastha measure of milk. The boiling should be continued till the watery part is completely evaporated and the milk alone is left behind. It should be then strained (through a piece of cloth). This (cooked) milk should be mixed with honey, clarified butter,* and the extract of meat of any Jángala animal, each measuring a quarter of the (above-prepared milk) and a Karsha measure each of the following drugs, *viz.,* powdered *S'atáhvá, Phalini* (Priyangu), *Yashti-madhu, Vatsaka, Rasánjana* and *Saindhava.* The application of the above in the manner of a Vasti proves curative in Váta-rakta, urinary complaints (Prameha), Edema, Hæmorrhoids, Gulma, retention

---

* According to Dallana, however, a Pala measure of each of honey and clarified butter should be added.

of urine, Hæmorrhage (Rakta-Pitta), Erysipelas, fever, and a looseness of the bowels. It acts as an aphrodisiac and vitalising tonic ; it also invigorates the eye-sight and is anti-colic in its action  It is known as the **Mustádi-Vasti** and is the best of all the Ásthápana enemas. 44.

A judicious physician may prepare, in the light of the principle laid down in connection with the preparation and application of Vastis in general, hundreds of different other kinds of Vastis (enemas) with a due consideration of the virtues of their respective ingredients (drugs) and the nature of the disease under treatment. Applications of Vastis are forbidden during the continuance of an undigested meal in the stomach. Proper rules of diet and conduct should be observed, and day-sleep should not be indulged in, after being treated with a Vasti  45-46.

The compound **Mádhu-Tailika Vasti** is so called from the facts of its being principally composed of **Madhu** (honey) and **Taila** (oil)  The term **Yukta-Ratha Vasti** owes its nomenclature to the fact of its imposing no restriction as regards riding in carriages (Rathas), or on horses and elephants after their application. The **Siddha-Vasti** derives its name from the uniform success (Siddhi) which attends its application in a large number of cases of bodily distempers and from its irresistible power in improving the strength and complexion of the body. **Mádhu-Tailika Vastis** are recommended to persons of easy and luxurious habits as well as in respect of those whose bowels can be easily moved, or who are in the habit of being daily treated with emulsive measures (Sneha-karma) and whose organisms are marked by scanty accumulations of the bodily Doshas. A **Siddha- asti** does not produce any distress or discomfort, since it is mild in potency and is applied in only three quarters of the usual dose (nine **Prasritas** only) and does not entail any strict observance of the regimen of diet and conduct (such as the previous administration of emetics and purgatives, etc.), and since it produces a satisfactory result by a single application. 47.

Thus ends the Thirty-eighth Chapter of the Chikitsita Sthánam in the Sus'ruta Samhitá which deals with Niruha-Vastis.

## CHAPTER XXXIX.

Now we shall discourse on the treatment of distressing symptoms* which are manifested in a patient **(Áturopadrava-Chikitsitam).** 1.

The digestive fire **(Káyágni)** of a person naturally grows dull† after the exhibition of emetics and purgatives, after the administration of a **Niruha-Vasti**, after the internal application of a **Sneha** and after **blood-letting**. It is further lessened by the eating of extremely heavy (difficult of digestion) articles of fare, just as a low or dull fire is extinguished by a heavy load of fuel. Light meals taken in small quantities, on the other hand, increase the digestive fire under these circumstances, just as light fuel in small quantities serves to re-kindle a low fire. 2.

The quantity of diet should be proportionate to the Dosha (morbific diathesis) eliminated from the organism. The quantity of the Dosha or Doshas eliminated consists of three measures, *viz.*, one **Prastha**,‡ half an **Ádhaka** or an **Ádhaka** (at most). The first is the lowest, the second is the intermediate and the last named measure (one **Ádhaka**) should be deemed as the highest quantity (of the Dosha that can be eliminated under the circumstances). 3.

**Yavâgu** (gruel) prepared with a small quantity of rice (Tandula) should be given once, twice or thrice respect-

---

\* By "distressing symptoms" are generally meant those complications that follow the exhibition of emetics, purgatives, Vastis, etc.

† We have been told that the digestive fire is kindled by the exhibition of emetics, purgatives, etc., but here we are told just the reverse. The solution is that the digestive fire is ultimately kindled by these measures, whereas, immediately after the exhibition, it becomes dull and sluggish.

‡ The Prastha measure here means thirteen Palas and a half.

ively in cases of the eliminated Dosha being a Prastha, half an Ádhaka or an Ádhaka in quantity. 4.

After this a quarter part of the quantity of rice or grain otherwise deemed proper and adequate for the patient, should be cooked in the form of **Vilepi**. The rice or the grain (used in the preparation) should be well boiled, without the addition of any Sneha (oil or clarified butter) or salt. 5.

It should then be (passed through a piece of cloth and) made non-slimy, and should be taken in the above-prescribed manner with a clear (pure) soup of *Mudga*-pulse. The patient should then be given a diet measuring half the quantity of his usual one. The food, in this case, should be well saturated with any oleaginous substance (Sneha). The meal of the patient in the next stage should consist of well-boiled rice measuring three parts only of his usual diet and should be made palatable to the taste and sufficient to stimulate the sense-organs. The meal in this case, should be taken with the transparent surface of clarified butter (*Ghrita-manda*). After this period the patient should be allowed to take his full meal with well-prepared soups of venison, etc. 6-7.

The above order of taking one-fourth, half and three-fourths of the usual meal applies in cases of deficient, intermediate (moderate), or satisfactory action of a purgative. 8.

Peyás, taken in an aggravated condition of the deranged Pitta, and Kapha, or by a person addicted to drinking habits or subsequent to a deficient exhibition of emetics and purgatives, may give rise to an increased (mucous) secretion (Abhishyanda) in the organism. **Tarpana** measures (demulcent food) should, therefore, be deemed beneficial in these instances. 9.

A person is likely to fast from any of the following

causes, *e. g.*, pain, unattainment of wished-for objects, penance, bereavement, and mental distraction. Rules enjoined to be observed after a course of purgatives should as well be adhered to in such cases. 10.

An Ádhaka, half an Ádhaka and a Prastha measure should similarly be the quantity of excretion in connection with a course of purgatives under the three different degrees of its action. But some are of opinion that there may be no fixed quantity of excretion in this case, since purgation should not be considered satisfactory until the S'leshmá (mucus) of the system has come out.\* A purgation should be considered satisfactory when the S'leshmá comes out and in that case no more purgative should be given. The strength (**Bala**) of a patient has been laid down to be of three degrees, consequently the rules of diet and conduct should be similarly determined. A **strong** patient should observe the regimen of diet only once, one of middling strength (**Madhya-bala**) twice, while a **weak** patient thrice. Certain authorities, however, assert that this order of diet should be observed by the patients with an impaired, intermediate and keen digestion. 11.

Lest the Doshas might become aggravated by the appetite already kindled by the observation of the rules of diet prescribed for the purpose, the patient should be made to take his meal in the following order at this stage. Sweet and bitter articles of fare should be partaken of at the outset of a meal, followed by oleaginous, acid, saline and pungent food. After this, sweet, acid and saline food should again be taken followed by

---

\* Here a line is not found in the printed edition of the Sus'ruta Sambitá, which is evident from Dallana's commentary and supported by S'rikantha Datta in his commentary on Vrinda. The line is as follows :—

"ग्रे षान्तलाद्विरेकर्थ न तामिच्छन्ति तद्विदः"।

articles of sweet and bitter tastes. Dry (Ruksha) and demulcent food should be enjoined in succession in the course of a meal. The meals of a healthy person should then be prescribed. 12.

Light diet should be given for a week after the internal use of a Sneha and after the exhibition of emetics. A patient should observe a proper regimen of recoupment of his health, after having been subjected to a course of blood-letting or treated with a course of S'odhana remedy (purgative). Intervals of three days should be allowed between two successive applications of a Vasti and the period of the third interval thus allowed, should be determined according to the requirements of each case.* 13.

A patient suffering from an ulcer (Vrana) or recently treated with emulsive measures (Sneha-karma) or cleansing (emetics or purgatives) measures, or afflicted with any affection of the eyes or with fever attended with dysentery (Jvarátisára) resembles a vessel of unbaked clay fitted with oil, *i.e.*, such a patient is greatly liable to the derangement of the Doshas. 14.

An irascible mood or fit of anger (in such a person) agitates his Pitta and produces Pitta-origined distempers;† physical labour and grief cause a distracted state of the mind; and gratification of sexual desires (in such a state) brings on such dangerous diseases as convulsions, epileptic fits, paralysis, aching pain in the limbs, swelling about the anus, cough, hiccup and

---

* Some commentators explain this verse to mean that the patient should observe the rules of diet and conduct (prescribed hereafter) for a period of three days after each application of a Vasti, but after the third application the rules of diet and conduct should be determined according to requirements.

† The Pitta-origined distempers are thirst, burning sensation, etc.

emission of blood-streaked semen and hæmorrhage from the vagina. 15-A.

Day-sleep under the circumstances. gives rise to the affections of the deranged Kapha, viz., enlargement of the spleen (Plihodara), catarrh, jaundice, edema, fever, loss of consciousness, a sense of physical langour, indigestion, an aversion to food, and causes the patient to become overwhelmed with the quality of Tamas which produces in him a desire for sleep. 15-B.

Talking in a loud voice aggravates the Váyu and is attended with such grave consequences as pain in the head, blindness, inertness, loss of the faculty of smell, dumbness, deafness, dislocation of the jaw-bones (Hanumoksha), Adhi-mantha, facial paralysis, paralysis of the eye-balls (Netra-stambha), thirst, cough, insomnia, shaking of the teeth and similar other distempers (due to an aggravation of the Váyu). 15 C.

Riding (on horse-back, etc.) under the circumstances may cause vomitings, swoons, vertigo, a sense of fatigue, stiffness of limbs, and the serious functional derangements of the sense organs. A long continuance in a sitting posture or bathing may give rise to pain in the region of the pelvis; while, on the contrary, excessive walking under the circumstances aggravates the Váyu and is attended with pain in the knee-joints, atrophy of the thighs, edematous swellings of the localities, or the form of disease known as Páda-harsha (sensitiveness in the feet). 15-D.

The use of cold water and other cold things*(such as paste of Sandal, etc.) under the circumstances tends to aggravate the bodily Váyu and brings on an aching

---

* In place of "शीतसम्भोगतोयानां" Gayadása reads] "शीतभोजनतोयानां" which means the use of cold food and drink, This reading seems to be better.—Ed,

pain in the limbs, Śula (gastralgia), stuffedness of the injested food in the stomach (Vishtambha) and inflation of the abdomen (Ádhmána) and shivering. An undue exposure to the sun and wind produces fever and discoloration of the complexion. The use of any unwholesome and incompatible diet as well as food taken before the complete digestion of the previous meal tends to produce serious distempers and may ultimately result in death. The use of incongenial fare undoubtedly leads to the deterioration of the strength and complexion of the body. A man of irregular and intemperate habits, who eats voraciously like an animal, suffers from indigestion which is the cause (source) of a number of physical distempers. 15.

In all these instances the real cause of the distress should be first ascertained, which should be then remedied with proper **antidotal** measures and remedies 16

**Articles of Diet :**—A diet consisting of cooked *Shashti* grain (Tandula) or matured *S'áli* rice, *Mudga* pulse as well as (the soup of the flesh of) an Ena, Láva, hare, peacock, Tittiri, or deer, and such other light food should be given to a patient after the exhibition of **emetics** and **purgatives.** 17.

Thus ends the Thirty-ninth Chapter of the Chikitsita Sthánam in the Sus'ruta Samhitá which deals with the treatment of distressing symptoms which are manifested in a patient.

# CHAPTER XL.

Now we shall discourse on the treatment which consists in employing the (inhalation of) medicated fumes, snuffs, (errhines) and gargles **(Dhuma-Nasya-Kavala-Graha-Chikitsita).** 1.

Dhuma (fumes) may be divided into five groups,* *viz.*, Práyogika (capable of being daily used), Snehana (soothing), Vairechana (expectorant),† Kásaghna (anti-cough) and Vámaniya (emetic). 2.

**Materials of different Dhuma-varti :** —The drugs of the *Eládi* group, excepting *Kushtha* and *Tagara*, should be pasted together. A space of eight fingers out of the entire length of a stem of *S'ara* weed twelve fingers long should be covered with a piece of silk cloth and plastered with the coat of the preceding paste. This stick should be burnt and used in the **Práyogika** Dhuma pána. The pith (pulp) of oleaginous fruits, wax and resin, *Guggulu*, etc., with the admixture of a Sneha (oil or clarified butter) should be used in the **Snehana-Dhuma.** The drugs included into Śiro-Virechana group should be used in **Vairechana Dhuma.** *Vrihati, Kanta-kárikà, Trikatu, Kása-marda, Hingu, Ingudi-bark,‡ Manah-s'ilá, Guduchi, and Karkata-s'ringi* and such other drugs which allay cough should be used in the **Kásaghna-Dhuma.** Nerves, skin, horns, hoops, shells of a crab, dried fish, dry meat or worms, etc., and

---

\* Charaka, however, divides Dhuma into three classes only—*viz.*, Práyogika, Snaihika and Vairechanaka, and includes the Kása-hara into the Práyogika, and Vámaniya into the Vairechana Dhuma.

† The term Vairechana here means S'iro-Virechana by means of fumes.

‡ Some commentators mean to explain "इङ्गदीत्वक्" as Ingudi and cardamom instead of as Ingudi-bark. This seems to be better.

such other emetic drugs should be used in the **Vâma-niya-Dhuma**. 3.

**Formation of the pipe used in Dhuma-Pána:**—The pipe to be used in respect of an inhaler should be made of one or other of the same substances\* of which the pipes of enema-syringes (Vasti-Netra) are made. The girth of such a pipe should be equal to that of the small finger at its mouth with an inner aperture or calibre as large as a *Kaláya* pulse, and its girth at the root or base should be equal to that of the thumb, while the girth of the inner apertureor near (at the root) should be sufficiently large to allow the Dhuma-Varti (made of S'ara weed) to fit in. The length of the pipe should be forty-eight fingers† in respect of a Práyogika, thirty-two fingers in respect of a Snehana, twenty-four fingers in respect of a Vairechana, sixteen fingers in respect of a Kásaghna (anti-cough) and Vámaniya (emetic) Dhuma. The girth of the aperture (channel) should be equal to that of a stone of the *Kola* fruit in respect of the tube to be used in the last two cases (Kásaghna and Vámaniya). The tube to be employed in fumigating an ulcer should be eight fingers in length and equal to a *Kaláya* pulse in outer girth, while the girth of the inner orifice should be sufficient to allow a *Kulattha* pulse to pass in. 4.

The medicinal stick (Varti) should be lubricated

---

\* See Chapter XXXV, Para. 7, Chikitsita Sthána.

† Charaka's description of the pipes, (Chapter V, S'lokasthána) corresponds closely to that of Sus'ruta, except in the case of Práyogika pipe, where Charaka's reading is somewhat ambiguous. There it may be construed to mean thirty-six as well as forty-eight fingers. Jatu-karna, however, explicitly asserts forty-eight fingers to be the length of the pipe in question. Vrinda is in a fix, and solves the difficulties by explaining that in cases of an aggravation of Kapha and an abundance of Doshas, the length of the pipe should be thirty-six fingers.

with a Sneha (clarified butter, etc). It should then be attached to one end of the pipe (Netra) and lighted. The patient should sit in an easy and comfortable posture, maintain a cheerful frame of mind and carefully inhale the medicinal fumes with his eyes cast down straight towards the ground. 5.

**Metrical Texts :**—The fumes should be first inhaled through the mouth and then through the nostrils; whether inhaled through the mouth or the nostrils they should be invariably exhaled through the mouth. Inhaled through the mouth, they should not by any means be exhaled through the nostrils, as such a course (of exhaling through the nostrils) would act wrongly and impair the eye-sight. 6.

The fumes (Dhuma) should be specially inhaled through the nostrils, in connection with a **Práyogika** inhalation, while they may be inhaled both through the mouth and the nostrils in **Snehana-Dhuma.** They should be inhaled through the nostrils alone in an act of **Vairechana** inhalation and through the mouth only in the two remaining cases (**Vámaniya** and **Kaphaghna**). 7.

**Mode of inhalation :**—In an act of **Práyogika** inhalation, the stick (Varti) should be dried in shady places protected from the wind. The stem of the *S'ara* weed inside the Varti should then be removed. The Varti should then be lighted with a live charcoal and fixed to the end of the pipe (Netra) and then the patient should be asked to inhale the fumes. The same method should be followed in respect of **Snehana** and **Vairechana** ones. In the other cases of smoking (**Kásaghna** and **Vámaniya**) the fumigating drugs (Varti) should be placed over a bed of smokeless burning charcoal contained in an earthen saucer. Another saucer furnished with an aperture at its top or middle should be fitted over the former saucer and the inhaling pipe should be fitted into this aperture, and the fumes should be inhaled (through the mouth). On the subsidence of the fumes the remaining portion of the stick should be cast into the fire and the patient should continue to inhale the fumes till the complete elimination of the aggravated Doshas from his organism. This is the rule and means of inhalation (Dhuma-pána). 8.

**Prohibitive Cases :**—Any kind of smoking (Dhuma-pána) is forbidden to a person afflicted with anger, fear, bereavement, fatigue, and in a heated state of the body and after fasting. It is also forbidden in cases of poisoning, hæmorrhage (Rakta-pitta), alcoholism, swooning, burning sensation of the body, thirst, jaundice, dryness of the palate, vomiting, head-disease, eructation, Timira, urinary complaints (Prameha), abdominal enlargement with dropsy (Udara), inflation of the abdomen and Urddha-váta, and in respect of infants, old and enfeebled persons, as well as of those treated with purgatives and Ásthápana-vasti. It is also forbidden to enciente women, those suffering from insomnia or a parched condition of the body as well as to those suffering from any kind of cachexia or from Urah kshata. An act of inhaling (smoke) is also prohibited after taking a potion of honey, clarified butter, curd, and milk, fish, wine or gruel (Yavágu) as well as during the continuance of a small quantity of Kapha in the organism. 9.

**Metrical Text :**—Medicated fumes inhaled in an improper season (*viz.*, in the above-mentioned prohibited cases) bring on vertigo, fainting fits, diseases of the head and serious injury to the eyes, ears, nose and the tongue. 10.

**Time of Smoking :**—The first three kinds of inhalations should be resorted to at the close of the following twelve physical functions and acts, *viz.* sneezing, cleansing the teeth, snuffing, bathing, eating, sleeping in the day, coition, vomiting, micturition, passing stools, fits of anger and surgical operations. A Snehana-Dhuma should be smoked after sneezing, micturition, passing stools, coition or after a fit of anger. Similarly, a **Vairechana-Dhuma** should be smoked after bathing, vomiting and sleeping in the day time, while a **Práyogika-Dhuma** should be smoked after cleansing the teeth, snuffing, bathing, eating and after a surgical operation. 11.

**The therapeutic effects of Dhuma-pána :**—Smoking the Snehana-Dhuma subdues the deranged and aggravated Váyu of the body owing to the existence of the Sneha with which it is charged, as well as to a consequent sticky coating being deposited in the organism. The **Vairechana-Dhuma** facilitates the loosening and flowing out of the mucus (Kapha) owing to its dryness, non-viscidness (Vais'adya), keenness and heat-making potency. While the **Práyogika-Dhuma** tends to loosen the accumulation of mucus (Kapha) and helps its expulsion from the system by virtue of its being possessed of common therapeutic properties with both of the two preceding kinds (of Dhuma). 12.

**Memorable Verse :**—Inhalation of (medicated) fumes removes the cloudening of the faculties of the organs of sense-perception and imparts distinctness of the speech and firmness to the teeth, hair of the head and to beard. It cleanses the mouth and fills it with an aroma. 13.

The inhalation of medicated fumes guards against an attack of cough, asthma, an aversion to food and clumsy sensation in the mouth, hoarseness, excessive salivation, nausea,* somnolence, sleep, numbness of the jaws and of the nerves (Snâyu) on the back of the neck (Manyâ), catarrh, diseases of the head, ear-ache, inflammation of the eyes, and any affection of the mouth due to an aggravation of the deranged Váyu and Kapha. 14.

It behoves a physician to be fully acquainted with the effects of satisfactory and excessive smoking (Dhuma-pána). Properly administered, it is followed by a distinct alleviation of the disease (under treatment); while its excessive use is followed by a positive aggravation or non-amelioration of the disease and is likely to produce a dryness of the palate and the throat, a burning sensation in the body, thirst, fainting fits, vertigo, delirium, alcoholism, affection of the ears, nose and eyes, impairment of vision, and weakness of the body. 15.

**Mode of Smoking :** -The Práyogika-Dhuma should be smoked thrice at a time either through the mouth or through the nostrils and may be repeated thrice or four times (according to the strength of the patient and the itensity of the Dosha). The **Snaihika-Dhuma** should be inhaled until the appearance of tears in the eyes. While the **Vairechanika-Dhuma** should be smoked till the beginning of the elimination of the Doshas from the system. The **Vámaniya-Dhuma** should be smoked by a patient after he has taken a gruel of huskless sesamum (Tila-Tandula), and the **Kásaghna-Dhuma** should be inhaled between morsels of food.† Fumigation of an ulcer should be made by means of a tube attached to (the orifice of) a covered saucer. Fumigation alle-

---

\* According to Vrinda's commentator we have here "Sneezing and a sudden obstruction of breath" as an additional text.

† Dallana quotes a different reading which would mean that the Kásaghna-Dhuma should be inhaled after taking meals,

viates the pain in an ulcer, arrests its discharge and makes it clean and non-viscid. 16.

**Metrical Text:**—The processes of inhalation and fumigation have been briefly described above. Now I shall fully describe the processes of using medicinal snuffs (Nasya). 17.

**On Snuffs and Errhines:**—The term "Nasya" (Snuff) is so called from the fact of its being composed of the powders of any drugs or of any Sneha (oleaginous substance) cooked with such drug or drugs, to be stuffed into the nostrils. It may be broadly divided into two kinds, *viz.*:—**Siro-Virechana** (errhines) and **Snehana** (contributor of oleaginous principles); and may, however, be further grouped under five specific heads, *viz.*:—**Nasya, Siro-Virechana, Pratimarsha** (a medicated Sneha poured into the nostrils to be discharged into the mouth), **Avapida** (the expressed juice of any drug put into the nostrils in drops by pressing it with the palms then and there) and **Pradhamana** (a medicinal snuff blown into the nostrils with the help of a blow pipe). Of these, the Nasya (snuff) S'iro-Virechana (errhines) are pre-eminently the most effective. Pratimarsha is a Nasya while Avapida and Pradhamana are Siro-Virechana (errhines). Thus it is that the term Nasya is employed in the above five senses. The term Nasya, in the specific sense, is particularly used with reference to the snuffing of any Sneha (oleaginous substance) with a view to make up the deficient oily matter in the brain in the case of a patient complaining of a sense of void or emptiness in the head or to impart tone to the nerves and muscles of the neck, shoulders and chest, or to invigorate the eye-sight. This should be prepared with a Sneha (oleaginous substance) cooked with the drugs possessed of the virtue of subduing the deranged Váyu and Pitta and should be snuffed in by a patient affected in the head through the overwhelming preponderance of the deranged Váyu and in cases of the falling off of the teeth and hair of the head and beard, in Karna-Kshveda, acute ear-ache, Timira (cataract), loss of voice, disease of the nose, dryness of the mouth, Ava-Váhuka, premature greyness of the hair and wrinkling of the skin and other dangerous complications due to the deranged Váyu and Pitta as well as in similar other affections of the mouth. 18.

**S'iro-Virechana :**—Powders of the S'iro-Virechana drugs* or any Sneha cooked with those drugs† should be employed in the event of there being an accumulation of Kapha (mucus) in the region of the palate, throat, or head of a patient, as well as in cases of an aversion to food, head-ache, heaviness of the head, Pinasa (coryza), Ardhávabhedaka (hemicrania), worms, Pratis'yáya (catarrh), loss of the faculty of smell, hysteric convulsion (Apasmára) and in similar other diseases of the super-clavicular regions due to the action of the deranged Kapha. 19.

These two kinds of Nasya (snuffs) should be administered before meals. To a patient affected with diseases of **Kaphaja** origin they should be administered in the morning, while one suffering from any **Pittaja** complaint should use them at noon and one

---

\* The S'iro-Virechana drugs are Pippali, Vidanga, S'igru, Siddhárthaka, Apámárga, etc. See Sutrashána, Chapter XXXIX.

† S'rikantha Datta, commentator of Vrinda, says that Gayi reads शिरोविरेचनद्रव्यसिद्धेन स्नेहेनैव etc., from which it is evident that he prescribed only the Sneha cooked with the S'iro-Virechana drugs as S'iro-Virechana Nasya.

afflicted with any distemper of the deranged **Váyu** should use them in the afternoon.* 20

Before the application of a S'iro-Virechana (errhine) the patient should be asked to cleanse his mouth with a tooth-twig and by smoking. Then the regions of the neck, cheek and forehead should be fomented and softened with the application of heated palms, the patient himself being laid on his back in a dustless chamber not exposed to the sun and the wind. His head should be kept a little hung back with his arms and legs fully stretched out and expanded and a compress should be tied over the eyes. Then the physician should lift up with the fore-finger of his left hand the tip of the nose of the patient and slowly drop with his right hand a continuous jet of (medicated) Sneha into the cleansed channels of the (patient's) nostrils. The oil to be so used should be made lukewarm (D. R. —made lukewarm in the sun) and kept in a golden, silver, copper, or earthen receptacle or in an oyster shell and poured down into the nostrils of the patient by means of an oyster shell (D. R.—pipe) or (by pressing) a cotton plug (soaked in that oil). Care should be taken that the oil does not get into the eyes (while being poured into the nostrils)† 21.

**Metrical Texts :** —The patient should refrain from shaking his head or indulging in a fit of anger or

* In respect of healthy patients, the Nasya should be administered at noon in winter, in the morning in spring and autumn, and in the afternoon in summer, while in the rainy season, they should be administered at a time when the sun would be visible in the sky.— *Vriddha-Vágbhata.*

† The commentator of Vrinda adds two more conditions—*viz.*, the patient should be made to pass stools and urine before the application of the Nasya and that the Nasya should be applied at a time when the sky would be free from clouds.

speaking, sneezing or laughing at the time of any oily snuff (Sneha-Nasya) being administered unto him, as it may otherwise badly interfere with its reaching down to the desired spot or may bring on an attack of cough or coryza (catarrh) or any affection of the head or of the eyes. 22.

**Doses of a Sneha-Nasya :**—Eight drops of oil trickling down the two upper phalanges of the forefingers should be regarded as the proper quantity for the **smallest** (lit.—first) dose. A Śukti measure (thirty-two drops) is the **intermediate** (lit.—second) dose and a Páni-Śukti measure (sixty-four drops) is the **highest** (lit.—third) dose. These are the three doses (of Sneha-Nasya) which should be dertermined in proportion to the strength of the patient and of the disease under treatment An oily snuff should never be swallowed. 23.

**Metrical Text :**—An oily snuff (Sneha-Nasya) should be hawked in so as to flow along the girths (Śringátaka) of the nostrils and immediately spit out (by the patient), without retaining it in the mouth for a moment, as it may otherwise (irritate the mucous membranes of the throat, etc., and) aggravate the local Kapha. 24.

The region of the neck and the cheeks, etc., of the patient should be fomented again after the use of the oily snuff (Sneha-Nasya) and the patient should be made to smoke, and partake of a meal not composed of any phlegmagogic articles (Anabhishyandi). He should then be advised as to regimen of conduct, etc. (to be subsequently observed). Washing the head, exposure to the sun, dust and smoke, the use of any intoxicating liquor or of any other liquid or oleaginous substance, indulgence in a fit of anger and excessive driving, etc., are strictly prohibited (after the application of Sneha-Nasya). 25.

### Effects of proper, excessive, or deficient application of a Sneha-Nasya

(**M.—T.**) :—The effects of proper and excessive applications of (oily) snuffs will now be described. Lightness of the head, sound and refreshing sleep, the state of being easily awakened, alleviation of the disease, hilarity of the mind and a gladsome activity of the sense-organs in performing their respective functions, are the symptoms which attend a **proper** and **satisfactory** application (of an oleaginous medicinal snuff) Salivation, heaviness of the head, and dulness of the sense organs are the symptoms which result from an **excessive** application of a Sneha (Nasya) and the remedy in such cases consists in employing the parching measures or medicines. A case of **deficient** application (of a Sneha-Nasya) is marked by the functional derangements of the sense-organs\* and a dryness (Rukshatá) of the system without any indication of the amelioration of the disease. The remedy, in such cases, consists in a fresh application of the (oleaginous) snuff. 26.

The proper doses of an oleaginous errhine (Śiro-Vireka) should be four, six or eight drops in accordance with the strength 'of the disease and of the patient under treatment). 27.

The fra ners of the Áyurveda have particularly classified the effects of the application (of a Sneha-Nasya) into three classes, *viz.*, proper or satisfactory, deficient and excessive. The head being satisfactorily cleared (by the **satisfactory** application (of an oleaginous errhine) is marked by a sense of lightness in the head, clearness of the channels (of the mouth, throat, nostrils, etc.),

---

\*Gayi's reading, according to Dallana, as well S'rikantha's reading is "वातवेगुख्मम्" which means the functional derangement of the local Váyu.

an amelioration of the disease under treatment, healthy and vigorous workings of the sense-organs and an exhilarating sensation of the body and of the mind. Itching, clumsiness of the mouth, heaviness, saturation of the local channels (of the mouth, throat, etc.) with mucous coatings are the symptoms which mark the **deficient** action of (an oleaginous) errhine. A discharge through the nostrils of Mastulunga (the brain matter), an aggravation of the Váyu, dulness of the sense-organs and a sense of void or emptiness in the head are the indications which mark an **excessive** application of an (oleaginous) errhine. 28

Measures and remedies possessed of the virtue of subduing the deranged Kapha and Váyu should be (respectively) employed in cases of excessive and deficient applications of (an oleaginous) errhine (Nasya), while in the case of a proper and satisfactory application the patient should be made to snuff in a quantity of clarified butter on each alternate day or at an interval of two days for one, two or three weeks in succession or for any longer period as considered proper according to the exigency of the case. In a case of an overwhelming aggravation of the Váyu, the patient may be made to use the snuff (of clarified butter) even twice a day. 29.

**Avapida-Nasya :**—The Avapida-Nasya, like the Siro-Virechana Nasya, should be administered to a person bitten by a snake, or lying in a comatose or unconscious state or suffering from a disease of the head due to its being oppressed with an accumulation of fat and mucus (Abhisyanda). An Avpida-Nasya should be administered to a patient by pasting any of the (fresh) Siro-Virechana drugs and putting a few drops therefrom into the nostrils of the patient. In cases of a distraction of the mind or of a disease of a parasitic origin or of patients suffering from the effects of poisoning the fine powder (of the Śiro-Virechana drugs) should (by means of a pipe) be blown into the nostrils of the patient. Sugar, the expressed juice of the sugar-cane, milk, clarified butter or an extract of meat should be (similarly) administered in the case of a weak patient or of one suffering from an attack of Rakta-Pitta. 30.

**Metrical Texts :**—A Sneha (oil or clarified butter) cooked with the pasted drugs (of the Śiro-Virechana group) would be as beneficial as the powder (Kalka) of those drugs for the purpose of an errhine in respect of a weak, emaciated, timid, delicate or female patient. 31.

**Forbidden Cases :** —A fasting person, or one who has just taken his meal, or one suffering from an acute catarrh or coryza of a virulent type, an enciente woman, a man found to be still under the influence of an intoxicating liquor or who has taken a Sneha (oleaginous substance), water or any other liquid, or one suffering from indigestion or who has been treated with an enema (Vasti), one in an angry and excited state of mind or afflicted with thirst or who is suffering from the effects of any slow chemical poison (Gara) or fatigued or overwhelmed with grief as well as an infant, an old man, one who has voluntarily repressed any natural urging of the body or one about to take a full bath (Sirah-Snána) should be regarded unfit for treatment with (any kind of medicinal) snuffs (Nasya). Snuffing and smoke inhalation should not be resorted to in the event of the sky being (unseasonably) overcast with clouds at a time when such phenomena do not usually or ordinarily happen. 32-A.

A deficient or an excessive application of snuffs (at one time), or its extreme heat or coldness, a sudden or delayed application of the same (into the nostrils), drooping posture of the head or its movements during the application, the fact of its being used while the patient would be taking his meals, or its application in any forbidden case may produce such distressing symptoms as thirst eructations, etc., due to the action of the aggravated or decreased Doshas of the body. 32.

**Metrical Texts :**—The evils which are usually found to attend an abuse of medicinal snuffs (Nasya) or errhines (S'iro-vireka) may be grouped into two classes —those incidental to the aggravation (**Utkleśa**) of the Doshas or to the loss or waste (**Kshaya**) of the same. The distempers due to an aggravation of the Doshas should he remedied with soothing (S'amana) and corrective (S'odhana) measures and remedies, while those resulting from the loss or waste of the Doshas should be remedied with such drugs and remedies as would make up the decreased Doshas (of the system). 33.

**Pratimarsha Nasya when to be used :** —The Pratimarsha form of snuff should be resorted to on any of the following fourteen different occasions, *viz.*:—after quitting the bed in the morning, after cleansing the teeth, on the occasion of going out of the house, after having been fatigued with physical exercise, after sexual intercourse and a journey, after defecation and urination, after the use of gargles (Kavala) and collyrium (Anjana), in an empty stomach, after vomiting, just after a day-sleep and in the evening. 34.

**Their Effects :**—A Pratimarsha snuff used by a person just after rising from his bed tends to remove the waxy mucus (Mala) accumulated in the nostrils during the night and brings on a cheerful state of the mind, when used after having cleansed the teeth, it imparts a sweet aroma to the mouth and makes the teeth steady and firm (in their sockets). When used by a man on the occasion of his going out of the house, it acts as a safeguard against the troubles of smoke and dust (assailing him on the road) owing to the consequent moist mucous secretion in the nostrils. When used after the exertion of physical exercise, coition or a journey, it serves to remove the sense of consequent fatigue, and when used after micturition or defecation it tends to remove the dulness or heaviness of vision. When applied after gargling or after an application of collyrium (along the eyelids) it serves to invigorate the eye-sight. When applied on an empty stomach, it cleanses the internal channels of the body and imparts a lightness to it. Taken after an act of emesis it tends to cleanse the mucous (S'leshmá) deposit on the beds of the internal ducts of the body and thus brings on a fresh appetite for food. When taken after a day-sleep it tends to remove the sense of drowsiness and physical heaviness and purges the filthy accumulations (in the nose, etc.) thus bringing about a concentrated state of the mind. When taken in the evening it brings on a good sleep and an easy awakening. 35.

**Metrical Texts :**—The quantity of Sneha which, being lightly snuffed in, reaches down into the cavity of the mouth, should be deemed adequate for a dose of the Pratimarsha (kind of snuff\*). The benefit of using a snuff may be perceived in a variety of ways, as it tends to cure the diseases peculiar to the super-clavicular regions of the body, removes the cloudening

---

\* One drop or two, or the quantity necessary to bring about a disruption of the Doshas, is the dose of a **Pratimarsha** Nasya according to Vriddha-Vágabhata.

The four forms of **Nasya-Karma** (medicinal) snuffs, should be prescribed for patients above seven years of age. Pratimarsha is recommended in Gulma.—*Krishnátreya.*

or dulness of the sense-organs, imparts a sweet aroma to the mouth, and strength to the teeth, jaw bones, head, neck, Trika, arms and the chest, and guards against an attack of baldness, Vyanga, premature greyness of the hair and the premature appearance of wrinkles or furrows. 36-37.

**Specific use of Sneha-Nasya :**—This snuff should consist of oil in a case marked by (the concerted actions of the deranged) Kapha and Vâyu, while it should consist of **Vasá** (lard) in a case involving the action of the Vâyu alone. Similarly **clarified butter** should be used as a snuff in a case of a Pittaja disorder, while the snuff should consist of **Majjá** (marrow) in a case marked by (the concerted actions of the deranged) Vâyu and Pitta. The four different modes of using snuff have thus been described in all of which oil may be used as not being hostile in its action as regards the seats of Kapha within the organism. 38.

**Kavala-graha :**—Now we shall describe the process of using medicinal gargles (Kavala) which may be divided into four kinds, *viz.* :—The Snehi (oleaginous), Prasâdi (soothing), Śodhi (purifying) and the Ropana (healing). The oleaginous (**Snehi**) gargle should be surcharged with any oleaginous substance and should be prescribed tepid in a case marked by the action of the deranged Vâyu, while cold and sweet articles should be employed in preparing a soothing (**Prasádi**) gargle and should be prescribed in cases of the deranged Pitta. The purifying (**Śodhana**) gargles should be composed of acid, pungent and saline drugs which are parching and heat-making* in their potency and

---

\* Vrinda does not include 'parching' while Chakradatta does not include 'heat-making' as the conditions of this kind of Kavala in their respective collections.

should be employed lukewarm (for corrective purposes) in diseases due to the action of the deranged Kapha. The healing (**Ropana**) gargles should be composed of bitter, astringent, sweet, pungent heat-making* articles and should be employed in cases of ulceration (of the mouth). The therapeutic virtues and applications of the four different kinds of gargle (Kavala) have thus been described (above). 39-40.

The neck, cheeks and the forehead of the patient to be treated with gargles should be (first) fomented and softened and he should be made to take (into his mouth) *Trikatu, Vacha,* mustard-seeds, *Haritaki* and rock-salt pasted together and dissolved in any of the following articles, *viz* :—oil, Śukta, Surá, alkali, (cow's) urine or honey, and made lukewarm (before use as a gargle). 41.

**Kavala and Gandusha—distinguished (M. T.) :**—The quantity which can be easily and conveniently rolled out in the mouth is the proper dose in respect of a **Kavala,** whereas the one which cannot be so (easily and conveniently) rolled out in the mouth is called a **Gandusha.** 42.

**Kavala—how long it should be retained :**—A gargle (Kavala) should be so long held† in the mouth by a patient till the aggravated Dosha‡ would accumulate in the regions of the cheeks§ and would secrete copiously through the nostrils and

---

\* Chakradatta does not include 'pungency' and 'heat-making potency' as conditions of this kind of Kavala.

† Vrinda here reads "सञ्चारयितव्यम्", *i.e.,* 'and should be rolled out (in the mouth)'.

‡ "Dosha" here means 'Kapha'.

§ Vrinda reads "यावद्दोषपरिपूर्णंगलकपोलत्वम्" which means till the Dosha accumulates in the regions of the throat and the cheeks.

the eyes, after which the gargle (Kavala) should be every time removed and fresh ones should be taken and kept (similarly) in the mouth. The patient should during the use of a Kavala sit in an erect posture without allowing the mind to be in the least distracted. 43.

**Metrical Texts :**—Gargles (Kavala) should be similarly prepared with Sneha, milk, honey, curd, urine, meat-juice or Amla (Kánjika) mixed with the decoction (of any drug) or hot water prescribed according to the nature and intensity of the bodily Dosha or Doshas involved in the case. An amelioration of the disease, a sense of lightness and of purity in the mouth, a cheerful frame of mind and an exhilarating vigour in the organs of sense are the features which mark an act of perfect or **satisfactory** gargling (Kavala), whereas a sense of physical lassitude, salivation and a (consequent) defect in the sense of taste are the traits which mark **deficient** gargling. Thirst, an aversion to food, dryness of the mouth, a sense of fatigue and an inflammation of the mouth are the symptoms which attend an act of **excessive** gargling. These symptoms undoubtedly arise in due proportion to the nature and intensity of the corrective drugs used. 44-45.

Sesamum, *Nilotpala,* clarified butter, sugar, milk and honey\* used as a gargle (Gandusha) alleviates the (consequent) burning sensation of a burn inside the mouth. 46.

The process of using medicinal gargles (Kavala) in general have thus been briefly described.

---

\* Commentators, on the authority of Videha, hold that gargles should be used with these articles either collectively or separately in cases of burning in the mouth by an excessive use of an alkali or such other articles,

**Pratisárana :**—A Pratisárana remedy may be of four kinds, *viz.*, that prepared with a **Kalka** (paste), **Rasa-kriyá, honey** and with **powders.** Prepared with the appropriate drugs, such a compound should be rubbed gently with the tip of a finger in a case of an affection of the mouth. An intelligent Physician may exercise his discretion in selecting the drugs to be used in the preparation of such a remedy. The symptoms of a satisfactory or unsatisfactory Pratisárana should be respectively identical with those of a Kavala. The ranges of therapeutic applications are also co-extensive in both the cases. In other words the diseases of the mouth which yield to the use of medicinal gargles, equally prove amenable to that of Pratisárana remedies. The diet in both the cases should be composed of light and non-phlegmagogic articles of food. 47.

Thus ends the Fortieth Chapter of the Chikitsita Sthánam in the Susruta Samhitá which deals with the inhalation of medicinal fumes, snuffs, and gargles.

## Here ends the Chikitsita Sthánam.

# THE SUSHRUTA SAMHITA
## KALPA-STHANAM
(Section on Toxicology).

—:o:—

## CHAPTER I.

Now we shall discourse on the mode of preserving food and drink from the effects of poison **(Anna-pána-Rakshá-Kalpa)**. 1.

Dhanvantari, the King of Kás'i, the foremost in virtue and religion and whose commands brook no disobedience or contradiction, instructed his disciples, Sus'ruta and others (in the following words). 2.

Powerful enemies and even the servants and relations of the sovereign in a fit of anger to avenge themselves on the sovereign sometimes concoct poisonous compounds and administer the same to him, powerful though he may be, by taking advantage of any defect or weak point in him. Sometimes the ladies (of the royal house-hold) are found to administer to the king various preparations (of food and drink), which often prove to be poisonous, from a foolish motive of securing his affection and good graces thereby, and sometimes it is found that by the embrace of a poisoned girl **(Visha-Kanyá)**,*

---

\* A girl slowly habituated to taking poison or poisoned food is called a **Visha-Kanyá**, such a girl presented to a king by a pretending friend of the state often managed to hug her royal victim into her fatal embrace. The poison operates through the perspiration, proving almost instantaneously fatal through the act of dalliance.

he dies almost instantaneously. Hence it is the imperative duty of a royal physician to guard the person of the king against poisoning. 3.

The minds of men are restless and uncontrollable like an unbroken horse. Faith is a rare thing in the human society and hence a crowned head should never believe any one\* in this world. 4.

**The necessary Qualifications of a Superintendent of the Royal Kitchen :**—A king should appoint a physician for the royal kitchen (to superintend the preparations of the royal fare). He should be well-paid and possess the following qualifications He should come of a respectable family, should be virtuous in conduct, fondly attached to the person of his sovereign, and always watchful of the health of the king. He should be greedless, straight-forward, god-fearing, grateful, of handsome features, and devoid of irascibility, roughness, vanity, arrogance and laziness. He should be forbearing, self-controlled, cleanly, compassionate, well-behaved, intelligent, capable of bearing fatigue, well-meaning, devoted, of good address, clever, skilful, smart, artless, energetic and marked with all the necessary qualifications (of a physician) as described before. He should be fully provided with all kinds of medicine and be highly esteemed by the members of his profession. 5.

**The necessary features of a Royal kitchen :**—The Royal kitchen should be a spacious chamber occupying an auspicious (south-east) corner of the royal mansion and built on a commendable site. The vessels and utensils (to be used in a royal kitchen) should be kept scrupulously clean. The kitchen should

---

\* A Royal Physician is an honourable exception in this respect.

be kept clean, well lighted by means of a large number of windows and guarded with nets and fret works (against the intrusion of crows, etc.) None but the trusted and proved friends and relatives should have access to the royal kitchen, or hold any appointment therein. Highly inflammable articles (such as hay, straw, etc.) should not be stacked in the royal kitchen whose ceiling should be covered with a canopy The Fire-god should be (daily) worshipped therein. The head or managar of the royal cooks should generally possess the same qualifications as those of a physician. The bearers and cooks in the royal kitchen should have their nails and hair clipped off and should bear turbans. They should be cleanly, civil, clever, obedient, good-looking, each charged with separate duties, good-tempered, composed in their behaviour, well-bathed, greedless, determined, and prompt in executing the orders of their superiors. A physician of the royal kitehen should be very cautious and circumspect in the discharge of his duties, since food is the main stay of life, and the sole contributor to the safe continuance of the body. Every one employed in a royal kitchen such as, bearers, servers, cooks, soup-makers, cake-makers (confectioners), should be placed under the direct control and supervision of the physician of the kitchen. 6.

**Characteristic features of a poisoner :**—An intelligent physician well qualified to ascertain the true state of one's feelings from the speech, conduct, demeanour and distortions of the face, would be able to discover the true culprit (**poisoner**) from the following external indications. A giver of poison does not speak nor does he answer when a question is put to him. He swoons or breaks off suddenly in the middle of his statement, and talks incoherently and indistinctly like a fool. He is found suddenly and listlessly to press the joints of his fingers or to scratch the earth, to laugh and to shiver. He will look frightened at the sight of others (indifferently), and will cut (straw or hay) with his fingernails, and his colour changes constantly. He will scratch his head in an agonised and confused state, and will look this way and that, trying to slip away by a back or side door, thus betraying his guilty conscience by his confusion. 7.

An innocent man, unjustly arraigned before the royal tribunal might from fear or precipation, become (confused and) liable to make untrue statements (and thus be unjustly convicted). Hence the king should first of all test the sincerity and fidelity of his servants ascertaining the non-poisonous character of the boiled rice, drink, tooth-twigs, unguents, combs, cosmetics, infusions, washes, anointments (with sandal pastes, etc.), garlands (of flowers, etc.), clothes, bedding, armour, ornaments, shoes, foot cushions, the backs of horses and elephants and snuffs (Nasya), Dhuma (tobacco smoking), collyrium and such other things (reserved for the use of the king). 8-9.

**Indications of poisoned food and drink, etc. :**—The indications by which the poisonous character of food, drink, etc. (to be used by a king) may be detected are described first and the medical treatment is dealt with secondly. A portion of the food prepared for the royal use should be first given to crows and flies and its poisonous character should be presumed, if they instantaneously die on partaking of the same. Poisoned food burns making loud cracks, and when cast into the fire it assumes the colour of a peacock's throat, becomes unbearable, burns in severed and disjointed flames and emits irritating fumes and it cannot be speedily extinguished. The eyes of a Chakora bird are instantaneously affected by looking at such poisoned food and a Jivajivaka dies under a similar condition. The note of the cuckoo becomes hoarse and a Krauncha (heron) becomes excited. A peacock moves about and becomes sprightly, and a Śuka and a Sáriká scream (in fear). A swan cackles violently and a Bhringarája (of the swallow class) raises its inarticutate voice. A Prishata (a species of spotted deer) sheds tears and a monkey passes stools. Hence these birds and animals should be kept in the royal palace for show and entertainment as well as for the protection of the sovereign master. 10.

The vapours arising from poisoned food when served for use give rise to a pain in the cardiac region and produce headache and restlessness of the eyes. As an antidote, a preparation of *Kushtha*, *Rámatha* (asafœtida), *Nalada* and honey mixed together should be used as an **Anjana** (along the eye-lids) and a medical compound of the same drugs should be snuffed into the nostrils. A plaster composed of *S'irisha*, turmeric, and sandal pasted together or simply a sandal paste should be used over the region of the heart in such cases 11.

A poison affecting the palms of the hands, produces a burning sensation in them and leads to the falling off of the finger-nails. The remedy in such cases consists in applying a plaster of *S'yamá*\*, *Indra*, *Gopa soma* and *Utpala* pasted together. 12.

Poisoned food partaken of through ignorance or

---

\* Some explain "S'yámá" as "S'yámá-latá"; others explain it as "Priyangu". Dallana explains "Indra" to mean "Indra-Váruni", "Gopa" to mean "Sáriva" and "Soma" to mean "Guduchi". Others, however, take "Indra-Gopa" as one word and explain it to mean a kind of insect known by that name, and they take "Soma" to mean "Soma-latá" in the ordinary sense of the word.

folly, produces a stone-like swelling and numbness of the tongue, a loss of the faculty of taste and a pricking burning pain in that organ attended with copious mucous salivation. The measures and remedies already laid down in connection with the treatment of cases of poisonous vapours as well as those to be hereinafter described in connection with the use of a poisoned tooth-twig should be adopted. 13.

Food mixed with poison, when it reaches the Ámâs'aya (stomach), gives rise to epileptic fits, vomiting, dysenteric stools (Atisâra), distention of the abdomen, a burning sensation, shivering and a derangement of the sense-organs. Under such circumstances an emetic consisting of *Madana, Alâvu, Vimbi* and *Kos'âtaki* pasted together and administered through the medium of milk, curd and *Udasvit* (Takra) or with rice-washings should be understood as the proper remedy. 14.

Food mixed with poison, if it reaches the Pakvás'aya (intestines), gives rise to a burning sensation (in the body), epileptic fits, dysenteric stools (Atisára), derangements of the organs of sense-perception, rumbling sounds in the abdomen and emaciation, and makes the complexion (of the sufferer) yellow. In such a case a purgative composed of clarified butter and *Nilini* fruits should be the first remedy. As an alternative, remedies to be described lateron (in the next chapter) in connection with the effects of **Dushi-Visha** (slow chemical poison) should be adopted and used, saturated with milk-curd (Dadhi) or honey. 15,

All liquid substances such as wine, milk, water, etc., if anywise poisoned, are found to be marked with variegated stripes on their\* surface and become covered

---

\* The colours of the different poisoned articles vary in each case and this is elaborately described by Vágbhata in his Samhitá.

over with froth and bubbles. Shadows are not reflected in such (poisoned) liquids and if they ever are, they look doubled, net-like (porous) thin and distorted. 16.

Preparations of potherbs, soups, boiled rice and cooked meat are instantaneously decomposed, and become putrid, tasteless and omit little odour when in contact with poison. All kinds of food become tasteless, smellless and colourless when in contact with poison. Ripe fruit, under such conditions, is speedily decomposed and the unripe ones are found to get prematurely ripe. 17—18.

If the tooth-twig be anyway charged with poison its brush-like end is withered and shattered and if used gives rise to a swelling of the lips and the tongue and about the gums. In such a case, the swollen part should be first rubbed (with any leaf of rough fibre) and then gently rubbed with a plaster composed of *Dhátaki* flowers, *Pathyá*, stones of *Jambuline* (black-berry) and honey pasted together. As an alternative, the part should be gently rubbed and dusted over with a plaster of powdered *Amkotha* roots or *Sapta-chchada* bark or seeds of *S'irisha*, pasted together with honey. The same remedies should be applied in the cases of affections due to the use of a poisoned tongue-cleanser or a poisoned gargle (Kavala). 12—20.

Poisoned articles for Abhyanga (oils and unguents) look thick, slimy or discoloured and produce, when used, eruptions on the skin which suppurate and exude a characteristic secretion attended with pain, perspiration, fever and bursting of the flesh. The remedy in such a case consists in sprinkling cold water over the body of the patient and in applying a plaster of sandal wood, *Tagara, Kushtha, Us'ira, Venu-patriká* (leaves of bamboo), *Soma-valli, Amritá, S'veta-padma* (lotus),

*Káliyaka* and cardamom pasted together (with cold water). A potion of the same drugs mixed with the urine of a cow and the expressed juice of *Kapittha* is equally commended in the present instance. Symptoms which mark the use of poisoned armour, garments, bedding, cosmetic, washes, infusions, anointments, etc. and the remedies for these are identical with those consequent upon the use of poisoned unguents. 21-22.

A poisoned plaster (if applied to the head) leads to the falling off of the hair and to violent headache, bleeding through the mouth and the nostrils, etc., and the appearance of glands on the head. The remedy in such a case consists in the application of a plaster made of black earth treated (Bhávita) several times with the bile of a Rishya (a species of deer), clarified butter and the expressed juice of *S'yámá*, *Pálindi* (Trivrit) and *Tanduliyaka* (in succession). The expressed juice of *Málati* (flower) or of *Mushika-parni*, fluid-secretions of fresh cow-dung and house-soot as external applications are also beneficial in such cases. 23.

In cases of poisoning through head-unguents or through a poisoned turban, cap garland of fllowers, or bathing water, measures and remedies as laid down in connection with a case of poisoned Anulepana should be adopted and applied. In a case of poisoning through cosmetics applied to the face, the local skin assumes a bluish or tawny brown colour covered with eruptions like those in cases of Padmini-kantaka and the symptoms peculiar to a case of using a poisoned unguent become manifest. The remedy in such a case consists in the application of a plaster composed of (white) sandal wood, clarified butter, *Payasyá, Yashti madhu, Phanji*, (Bhárgi), *Vandhujiva* and *Panarnavá*. A potion of honey and clarified butter is also beneficial in this case. 24-25.

A poisoned elephant usually exhibits such symptoms as restlessness, copious salivation and redness of the eyes. The buttocks, the penis, the anal region and the scrotum of its rider coming in contact with the body of such an elephant are marked by eruptions. Under such conditions both the animal and its rider should be medically treated with the remedies laid down in the treatment of poisoning through an unguent. 26.

A poisoned snuff (Nasya) or poisoned smoke (Dhuma) produces bleeding from the mouth and nose, etc., pain in the head, a discharge of mucus and a derangement of the functions of the sense-organs. The remedy in such cases consists in drinking and snuffing\* a potion of clarified butter duly cooked with the milk of a cow or such other animal together with *Ativishá*, *Vacha* and *Mallikâ* flower (as Kalka). A poisoned garland (of flowers) is characterised by the loss of odour and by the fading and discolouring of its natural colour, and when smelt produces headache and lachrymation. Remedies laid down under the heads of poisoning through vapour (Dhuma) and through cosmetics for the face (Mukha-lepa) should be used and applied. 27-28.

The act of applying poisoned oil into the cavity of the ears impairs the faculty of hearing and gives rise to swelling and pain in that locality and to the secretion (of pus) from the affected organs. The filling up of the cavity of the ears with a compound of clarified butter, honey and the expressed juice of *Vahuputrá* (Sátávari)†

---

\* Dallana explains this couplet to mean that clarified butter cooked with milk and Ativishá should be given for drink, and that cooked with Vacha and Málati flower as an errhine.

† Dallana says that some read "वहुपवायाः" and explain "वहुपचा" to mean "मयूरशिखा ।"

or with the juice of *Soma-valka* in a cold state prove curative in such cases. 29

The use of a poisoned Anjana (collyrium) to the eyes is attended with copious lachrymation, deposit of an increased quantity of waxy mucus (in the corners of the eyes), a burning sensation, pain (in the affected organs), impairment of the sight and even blindness. In such a case the patient should be made to drink a potion of fresh clarified butter (Sadyo-ghrita)* alone or with pasted *Pippali* which would act as a Tarpana (soother). Anjana prepared with the expressed juice of *Mesha s'ringi*, *Varuna*-bark, *Mushkaka* or *Ajakarna* or with *Samudra-phena* pasted with the bile (Pitta) of a cow should be applied to the eyes, or the one prepared with the (expressed juice of the) flower of *Kapittha, Mesha-s'ringi, Bhallátaka, Bandhuka* and *Amkotha* separately. 30.

The case which is incidental to the use of a paste of poisoned sandals, is marked by a swelling in the legs, secretion from the affected organs, complete anesthesia of the diseased locality and the appearance of vesciles thereon. Those due to the use of poisoned shoes or foot-stools exhibit symptoms identical with those of the above case and the medical treatment in all of these cases should be one and the same. Ornaments charged with poison lose their former lustre and give rise to swelling, suppuration and the cracking of the parts they are worn on. The treatment in these cases due to the use of poisoned sandals and ornaments should be similar to the one advised in connection

---

* Some are inclined to take "सद्यः" as an adverb meaning "instantly" and modifying "पेयम्" meaning thereby that clarified butter should be instantly taken.

with that due to the use of poisoned unguents (Abhyanga). 31-32.

**General Treatment :**—The symptoms which characterise cases of poisoning commencing with "poisoning through poisoned smoke" and ending with that due to the use of "poisoned ornaments" should be remedied with an eye to each of the specific and characteristic indications, and the medicine known as the **Mahá-sugandhi Agada** to be described hereafter should be administered as drink, unguent, snuff and Anjana. Purgatives or emetics should be exhibited and even strong venesection should be speedily resorted to in cases where bleeding would be beneficial. 33-34.

The drugs known as *Mushiká* and *Ajaruhá* should be tied round the wrists of a king as prophylactics to guard against the effects of poisoned food, since either of these two drugs (in virtue of their specific properties) tends to neutralise the operativeness of the poison. A king surrounded by his devoted friends shall cover his chest (with drugs of heart-protecting virtues) and shall drink those preparations of clarified butter, which are respectively known as the *Ajeya* and the *Amrita* Ghritas*. He should drink regularly every day such wholesome cordials as honey, clarified butter, curd, milk and cold water and use in his food the meat and soup of the flesh of a peacock, mungoose, Godhá (a species of lizard), or Prishata deer. 35—A.

**The mode of preparing the Soup :**—The flesh of a Godhá, mungoose, or deer should be cooked and spiced with pasted *Pálindi* (Trivrit), *Yashtimadhu* and sugar. The flesh of a peacock should be similarly cooked and spiced with sugar, *Ativishá*

---

* See Kalpa-Sthána, Chapter II. Para 27, and Chapter VII. para 5, respectively.

and Sunthi and that of a Prishata deer with *Pippali* and *S'unthi*. The soup of *S'imbi* taken with honey and clarified butter should, similarly, be deemed beneficial (as being possessed of similar antitoxic properties). An intelligent king should always use food and drink of poison-destroying properties. In a case of imbibed poison, the heart should be protected (with a covering of anti-poisonous drugs) and the patient should be made to vomit (the contents of his stomach) with a potion composed of sugar, *Pippali*, *Yashti-madhu*, honey and the expressed juice of sugar-cane dissolved in water. 35-36.

Thus ends the first Chapter of the Kalpa-sthána in the Sus'ruta Samhitá which deals with the mode of protecting food and drink (from the effect of poison).

# CHAPTER II.

Now we shall discourse on the chapter which treats of the indications (effects, nature and operations) of Sthávara (vegetable and mineral) poisons **(Stha´vara-Visha-Vijna´niyam)**. 1.
 **Stha´vara-poison : its Source** (M. T.)— There are two kinds of poison *viz.*, that obtained from immobile things (Sthávara) and that obtained from mobile creatures **(Jangama)**. The sources of the Sthávara (vegetable and mineral) poison are ten, while those of the Jangama (animal) poison are sixteen in number. The ten sources from which a **Stha´vara** poison may be obtained are roots, leaves, fruits, flowers, bark. milky exudations, pith (Sára', gum (Niryása), bulb and a mineral or metal (Dhátu). 2 - 3.
 **Names of the different Vegetable and Mineral poisons :**—*Klitaka, As'va-mára, Gunjá, Subandha\*, Gargaraka, Karaghátá, Vidyuch-chhikhá and Vijayá* are the eight **root-poisons** *Visha-Patriká, Lambá, Avaradáruka, Karambha* and *Mahá-Karambha* are the five **leaf-poisons** The fruits of *Kumudvati, Renuká, Karambha, Mahá-Karambha, Karkotaka, Venuka, Khadyotaka, Charmari, Ibha-gandhá, Sarpa-ghátí, Nandana* and *Sára-páka*, numbering twelve in all, are the twelve **fruit-poisons.** The flowers of *Vetra, Kadamba, Vallija (Nárácha—D. R), Karambha* and *MahaKarambha* are the five **flower-poisons.** The bark, pith and gum of *Antra-páchaka, Kartariya, Sauriyaka, Kara-ghátá, Karambha, Nandana* and *Varátaka* are

---

\* Lambá, according to Gayı—D. R.

the seven **bark-poisons, pith-poisons and gum-poisons**. The milky exudations of *Kumudaghni*, *Snuhi* and *Jála-Kshiri* are poisons and are known as the three **Kshira-Vishas**, Phenásma-bhasma (white arsenic) and Haritála (yellow orpiment) are the two **mineral poisons**. *Kála-kuta, Vatsa-nábha, Sarshapaka, Pálaka, Kardamaka, Vairátaka, Mustaka, S'ringi-visha, Prapaundarika, Mulaka, Hálahala, Mahá-visha* and *Karkataka*, numbering thirteen in all, are the **bulb-poisons**. Thus the number of poisons obtained from the vegetable and mineral world (Sthávara) amount to fifty-five in all. 4-11.

**Metrical Text:**—There are four kinds of *Vatsa-nábha* poisons, two kinds of *Mustaka* and six kinds of *Sarshapaka*. The remaining ones have no different species. 12.

**Effects of poison on the human organism :**—**Root**-poisons or poisonous roots produce a twisting pain in the limbs, delirium and loss of consciousness. A **leaf**-poison or poisonous leaf gives rise to yawning, difficult breathing and a twisting pain in the limbs. A **fruit** poison is attended with a swelling of the scrotum, a burning sensation in the body and an aversion to food. A **flower**-poison gives rise to vomiting, distensions of the abdomen and loss of conssciousness. A **bark**-poison, or **pith**-poison, or **gum**-poison is marked by a fetour in the mouth, roughness of the body, headache and a secretion of Kapha (mucus from the mouth). The effects of the poisonous **milky** exudations (of a tree, plant or creeper) are foaming from the mouth, loose stools (diarrhœa) and a curvature (drawing back) of the tongue, whereas a **mineral** poison gives rise to pain in the heart, fainting and a burning sensation in the region of the palate. All these are slow poisons proving fatal only after a considerable length of time. 13.

**Effects of Bulb-poisons:**—Now we shall describe in full the respective effects of the bulb-poisons which are very strong (Tikshna) in their actions The bulb-poison known as the **Kálakuta** produces complete anesthesia, shivering and numbness. Paralysis of the neck and yellowness of the stool, urine and of the eye-balls are the symptoms produced in a case of **Vatsanábha**-poisoning. Retention of stool and urine (Ánáha), disorders of the palate and the appearance of glands are the effects of a case of **Sarshapa** poisoning. Loss of speech and weakness of the neck are the symptoms in a case of **Pálaka** poisoning. Water-brash loose stools (diarrhœa) and a yellowness of the eyes mark a case of **Kardamaka**-poisoning. Pain in the limbs and diseases of the head are produced in a case of **Vairátaka**-poisoning. Shivering and a numbness of the limbs are the effects of a case of **Mustaka**-poisoning. Lassitude, a burning sensation in the body and an enlargement of the abdomen mark a case of **S'ringi-visha**-poisoning. An enlargement of the abdomen and redness of the eyes are the symptoms of **Pundarika**-poisoning. A discolouring of the complexion, vomiting hic-cough, swelling and a loss of cousciousness are the effects of the **Mulaka**-poison. Difficult breathing and a tawny brown colour of the skin mark a case of **Hála-hala**-poisoning. Aneurysm (Granthi) on the region of the heart and a piercing pain in the same are the symptoms in a case of **Mahá-visha**-poisoning ; while a case of **Karkataka**-poisoning is marked by laughing, gushing of the teeth and jumping up (without any cause). 14

**Specific properties of the above-named Bulb-poisons:**—These thirteen kinds of bulbous poisons should be deemed as very strong\* in their potency and they possess the following ten properties in common. They are parching (Ruksha) and heat-making (Ushna) in their potency. They are sharp (Tikshna) and subtle (Sukshma) *i.e.*, have the power of penetrating into the minutest capillaries of the body and are instantaneous (Ásu) in their effects. They first permeate the whole organism and become subsequently digested (Vyaváyi) and disintegrate the root-principles of the body (Vikási). They are non-viscid (Vis'ada), light in potency (Laghu) and indigestible (Apáki). 15.

A poison aggravates the bodily Váyu in virtue of its parching quality and vitiates the blood and the Pitta through its heat-generating property. It overwhelms the mind (produces unconsciousness) and tends to disintegrate the limbs and muscles in virtue of its sharpness and penetrates into and deranges the minutest capillaries owing to its extreme subtile essence. It proves speedily fatal owing to its speedy activity and spreads through the entire organism (which is the very nature of a drug) on account of its rapid permeating or expansive quality. It annihilates the root-principles (Dhátus) as well as the Doshas and the Malas (excreta) of the body through the power of disintregation, and does not addhere to any spot therein owing to its non-viscidness. It baffles the efficacies of other drugs and thus becomes unremediable on account of the extreme lightness (of its potency), and it cannot be easily assimilated owing to its innate indigestibility. It thus proves troublesome for a long time. 16.

---

\* The text has "Ugra-Viryáni" (strong in potency). Gayi reads "Agra-Viryáni" (of great poteney).

A poison of whatsoever sort, whether animal, vegetable, or chemical, which proves almost instantaneously fatal (within a day) should be regarded as possessed of all the ten aforesaid qualities. 17.

**Definition of Dushi-visha** (weak and slow poison):—A poison whether animal, vegetable or chemical, not fully eliminated from the system and partially inherent therein, enfeebled, of course by anti-poisonous remedies, is designated a **Dushi-visha** (weak and slow poison) which is even extended to those the keenness of potency whereof is enfeebled by the sun, the fire and the wind, as well as to those which are found to be naturally devoid of some of the ten aforesaid natural qualities of a poison. A Dushi visha, owing to its enfeebled or attenuated virtue and as a necessary consequence of its being covered over with the bodily Kapha, ceases to be fatal though retained in the system for a number of years. 18.

**Symptoms of weak and slow poisoning :**—A person afflicted with any sort of **Dushi-Visha** develops such symptoms as, looseness of stool (diarrhœa), a discoloured complexion, fetor in the body, bad taste in the mouth, thirst, epileptic fits, vomiting (D. R.—vertigo), lassitude, confused speech and all the symptoms of Dushyodara.* A Dushi-Visha lodged in the **Ámásaya** (stomach) gives rise to diseases due to the combined action of the Váyu and Kapha; seated in the **Pakvásaya** (intestines) it brings on diseases due to the deranged condition of the Váyu and Pitta and leads to the falling off of the hair. The patient becomes rapidly atrophied, and looks like a wingless bird. When it attacks the **Rasa,** etc.† of the system

---

\* See Chapter VII. para 10, Nidána-sthána.

† These are the seven fundamental principles of the body.

it produces the diseases* peculiar to the root or vital principles of the body. Its action on the body becomes aggravated on a cloudy day and by exposure to cold and wind. 19-21.

**Premonitory Symptoms of Dushi-Visha poisoning :**—Now hear me first describe the premonitory symptoms (of its aggravation). They are as follow :—Sleepiness, heaviness (of the limbs), yawning, a sense of looseness (in the joints), horripilation and aching of the limbs. These are followed by a sense of intoxication after meals, indigestion, disrelish for food, eruptions of circular patches (Mandala) on the skin, urticaria (Kotha), fainting fits, loss of the vital principles of the organism (D. R—loss of flesh), swelling of the face and the extremities (D.R.—Atrophy of the hands and legs), ascites (Dakodara), vomiting, epileptic fits, Vishama-jvara, high-fever and an unquenchchable thirst. Moreover, some of these poisons produce insanity. Some of them are characterised by an obstinate constipation of the bowels (Ánáha), others, by an involuntary emission of semen while a few others produce confused speech, Kushtha (leprosy), or some other similar disease. 22.

**Derivative Meaning of " Dushi-Visha ":**—A constant use of some particular time,† place and diet as well as constant and regular day-sleep tends (slowly) to poison the fundamental root-principles

---

\* See Chapter xxvii, Sutra Sthána.

† By " the particular **time**" is meant a cloudy and windy day as well as the rainy season. By "the particular **place**" is meant a marshy country, and by "the particular **diet**" is meant wine, sesamum, Kulaltha-pulse, etc. as well as physical exercise, sexual intercourse, fits of anger, etc.

(Dhátus) of the body and this (slow) poison is consequently known as the Dushi-Visha. 23.

**Symptoms of the different stages of Stha´vara poisoning :**—In the first stage of a case of poisoning by a Stha´vara (vegetable or mineral) poison, the tongue becomes dark brown and numbed, and epileptic fits and hard breathing follow in its wake. The second stage is marked by such symptoms as shivering, perspiration, burning sensation, itching and pain in the body; when seated in the Áma´s´aya (stomach) it causes pain in the region of the heart. The third stage is marked by a dryness of the palate and severe (colic) pain in the stomach. The eyes become discoloured, yellow-tinted aud swollen. When seated in the Pakva´s´aya (intestines) it produces hic-cough, cough, and a sort of pricking pain and rumbling sound in the Antra (intestines). The fourth stage is marked by an extreme heaviness of the head. The fifth stage is marked by salivation, discolouring of the body and a breaking pain in the joints. It is marked also by the aggravation of all the Doshas and pain in the Pakvádhána (intestines ?). The sixth stage is characterised by loss of consciousness or excessive diarrhœa; while the seventh stage is marked by a breaking pain in the back, the shoulders and the waist and a complete stoppage (of respiration)*. 24.

**Treatment :**—In the first stage the patient should be made to vomit and to drink cold water after that. Then an **Agada** (Anti-poisonous remedy) mixed with honey and clarified butter should be given him. In the second stage, the patient should be first made to vomit as in the preceding stage and then a purgative

---

\* The seven stages of the poisoning are due to the poisoning of the seven fundamantal root-principles (Dhátus) of the body in succession.

should be given him. Anti-poisonous potions, medicated snuffs (Nasya) and Anjanas possessed of similar virtues are beneficial in the third stage. An anti-poisonous potion through the vehicle of a Sneha (clarified butter) is efficacious in the fourth stage. In the fifth stage the patient should be given an antipoisonous medicine with the decoction of *Yashti-madhu* and honey. In the sixth stage the treatment should be as in a case of diarrhœa (Atisára) and the use of a medicated snuff in the form of an Avapida is recommended. The latter remedy (Avapida-Nasya) should be applied in the seventh stage as well and the scalp after being shaved in the shape of a Káka-pada* (crow's claw) should also† be incised with a small incision. The incised flesh and the (vitiated) blood should also be removed. 25.

**Koshátakyádi Yavágu :**—After adopting the respective measures enjoined in respect of the several stages of poisoning, the patient should, in the interval of any two stages be made to drink in a cold state a gruel (Yavágu) prepared with the decoctions of *Koshátaki* (Ghoshá), *Agnika* (Ajamodá), *Páthá, Suryavalli, Amritá, Abhayá, S'irisha, Kinihi, S'elu, Giryáhvá*, (white Aparájitá), the two kinds of *Rajani,* the two kinds of *Punarnavá, Harenu, Trikatu, Sárivá*, and *Balá* (D.R. Sárivá and Utpala) mixed with honey and clarified butter. This is beneficial in both the cases of (animal and vegetable) poisoning. 26.

---

\* The particular form of shaving the hair, in which the part of the scalp from and above the forehead only is shaved is technically called a **Káka-pada.**

† The particle "và" means that the measures laid down in respect of the treatment of a Jangama poison viz. beating the patient on the head, forehead, etc., should also be resorted to.

**Ajeya-Ghrita :**—Clarified butter should be duly cooked with an adequate quantity of water and the Kalka of *Yashti-madhu, Tagara, Kushtha, Bhadra-dáru, Harenu, Punnága, Elá, Ela-váluka, Nága-kes'ara, Utpala,* sugar, *Vidanga, Chandana, Patra, Priyangu, Dhyámaka,* the two kinds *Haridrá,* the two kinds of *Vrihati,* the two kinds of *Sárivá, Sthirá* (Sála-parni) and *Sahá* (Pris'ni-parni). It is called the **Ajeya-Ghrita.** It speedily destroys all kinds of poison in the system and is infallible in its efficacy. 27.

**Vishári-Agada :**—A patient afflicted with the effects of **Dushi-Visha** inherent in the system should be first fomented and cleansed by both emetics and purgatives. The following anti-poisonous Agada (medicine) should then be taken daily. The recipe of this Agada is as follows:—*Pippali, Dhyámaka, Mámsi, Sávara* (Lodhra), *Paripelava*\*, Suvarchiká,* small *Elá, Toya* (Bálaka) *and Suvarna-Gairika* should be taken with honey. It destroys, when taken, the Dushi-Visha (slow chemical poisoning) in the system. It is called the **Vishári-Agada** and its efficacy extends also to cases of all other kinds of poisoning. 28.

**Treatment of the Supervening Symptoms of poisoning :**—Cases of fever, burning sensation in the body, hic-cough, constipation of the bowels, loss of semen, swelling, diarrhoea, epileptic fits, heart-disease, ascites, insanity, shivering, and such other supervening symptoms (consequent on the effects of a Dushi-Visha inherent in the system) should be treated with remedies laid down under the respective heads of the aforesaid diseases in accompaniment with (suitable) anti-poisonous medicines. 29.

---

\* "Paripelava" means either "Dhanyáka" or "Kaivartta-Mustaka".

**Prognosis :**—A case of Dushi-Visha poisoning in a prudent and judicious person, and of recent growth is easily cured, while palliation is the only relief that can be offered in a case of more than a year's standing. In an enfeebled and intemperate patient, it should be considered as incurable. 30.

Thus ends the sceond Chapter of the Kalpa Sthána in the Sus'ruta Samhitá which treats of the Sthávara and jangama poisons.

# CHAPTER III.

Now we shall discourse on the subject of (the nature, virtue, etc. of) animal poisons **(jangama-visha-vijnániya)**. 1.

We have briefly said before that there are sixteen situations of poison in the bodies of venomous animals. Now we shall deal with them in detail. 2.

**Locations :**—An animal poison is usually situated in the following parts, *viz*; the sight, breath, teeth, nails, urine, stool, semen, saliva, menstrual blood, stings, belching*, anus, bones, bile, bristles (Śuka) and in the dead body of an animal. 3.

Of these, the venom of celestial serpents lies in their sight and breath, that of the terrestrial ones in their fangs while that of cats, dogs, monkeys, Makara (alligators?), Frogs, Páka-matsyas (a kind of insect), lizards (Godhá), mollusks (Snails), Prachalákas (a kind of insect), domestic lizards, four-legged insects and of any other species of flies such as mosquitoes, etc., lies in their teeth and nails. 4.

The venom of a Chipita, Pichchataka, Kasháya-vásika, Sarshapa-vásika, Totaka, Varchah-kita, Kaundilyaka and such-like insects lies in their urine and excreta. The poison of a mouse or rat lies in its semen, while that of a Lutá (spider) lies in its saliva, urine, excreta, fangs, nails, semen and menstrual fluid (ovum). 5—6.

The venom of a scorpion, Viśvambhara, Rájíva-fish, Uchchitinga (cricket) and a sea-scorpion lies in their

---

* Vriddha-Vágbhata reads Alaji-S'onite in place of "Visardhita."

saliva. The venom of a Chitra-śirah, Saráva, Kurdiśata, Dáruka, Arimedaka and Sáriká-mukha, lies in their fangs, belching, stool and urine. The venom of a fly, a Kanabha and leeches lies in their fangs. The poison lies in the bones of an animal killed by any poison, as well as in those of a snake, a Varati and a fish*. The poison lies in the bile of a Śakuli, a Rakta-ráji and a Cháraki fish. The poison lies in the bristles (Śuka) and the head of a Sukshma-tunda, an Uchchitinga (cricket), a wasp, a centipede (Śatapadi), a Śuka, a Vala bhika, a Śringi and a bee. The dead body of a snake or an insect is poisonous in itself. Animals not included in the above list should be deemed as belonging to the fang-venomed species *i.e.*, the poison lies in their fangs. 7—11.

**Memorable Verses :**—The enemies of a sovereign poison the pastures, water, roads, food-stuffs and smoke (Dhuma) of their country and even charge the atmosphere with poison in the event of his making incursions into their country. The poisonous nature of the foregoing things should be ascertained from the following features and should be duly purified (before use). 12-A.

**Characteristic Features and Purifications of poisoned water, etc :**—A sheet of poisoned water becomes slimy, strong-smelling, frothy and marked with (black-coloured) lines on the surface Frogs and fish living in the water die without any apparent cause. Birds and beasts that live (in the water and) on its shores roam about wildly in confusion (from the effects of poison), and a man, a horse or an elephant, by bathing in this (poisoned) water is afflicted

---

* Some read 'वरटीमत्स्य' (Varati fish) as one word—the name of a species of fish.

with vomiting, fainting, fever, a burning sensation and swelling of the limbs. These disorders (in men and animals) should be immediately attended to and remedied and no pains should be spared to purify such poisoned water. The cold ashes, of *Dhava, Aśva-karna, Asana, Páribhadra, Pátalá, Siddhaka, Mokshaka, Rája-druma* and *Somavalka* burnt together, should be cast into the poisoned pool or tank, whereby its water would be purified ; as an alternative, an Anjali-measure (half a seer) of the said ashes cast in a Ghata-measure\* (sixty-four seers) of the required water would lead to its purification. 12-B.

A poisoned ground or stone-slab, landing stage or desert country gives rise to swellings in those parts of the bodies of men, bullocks, horses, asses, camels and elephants that may chance to come in contact with them. In such cases a burning sensation is felt in the affected parts and the hair and nails (of these parts) fall off. In these cases, the poisoned surface should be purified by sprinkling it over with a solution of *Ananta* and *Sarva-gandha* (the scented drugs) dissolved in wine (Surá)†, or with (an adequate quantity of) black clay‡ dissolved in water or with the decoction of *Vidanga, Páthá,* and *Katabhi.* 12. C.

Poisoned hay or fodder or any other poisoned foodstuff produces lassitude, fainting, vomiting, diarrhœa or even death (of the animal partaking thereof). Such cases should be treated with proper anti-poisonous medicines

---

\* Jejjata explains 'Ghata' as a pitcher, *i.e.*, a pitcher-ful of water.

† Dallana holds that the use of the plural number here in " सुराभिः " means that honey, treacle, etc. should also be used with wine.

‡ Dallana says that some read ' earth of an ant-hill' in place of 'black clay for its anti-poisonous properties.

according to the indications of each case. As an alternative, drums and other musical instruments smeared with plasters of anti-poisonous compounds (Agadas)* should be beaten and sounded (round them). Equal parts of silver (*Tára*), mercury (*Sutára*) and *Indra-Gopa* insects with *Kuru-Vinda*† equal in weight to that of the entire preceding compound, pasted with the bile of a Kapila (brown) cow, should be used as a paste over the musical instruments (in such cases). The sounds of such drums, etc. (pasted with such anti-poisonous drugs) are said to destroy the effects of even the most dreadful poison. 12-D.

**Poisons of the Atmosphere and its purification :**—The dropping of birds from the skies to the earth below in a tired condition is a distinct indication of the wind and the smoke (of the atmosphere) being charged with poison. It is further attended with an attack of cough, catarrh, head ache, and of severe eye-diseases among persons inhaling the same wind and smoke. In such cases the (poisoned) atmosphere should be purified by burning quantities of *Lákshá, Haridrá, Ati-vishá, Abhayá, Abda* (Musta), *Renuka, Elá, Dala* (Teja-Patra), *Valka* (cinnamon), *Kushtha* and *Priangu* in the open ground. The fumes of these drugs would purify the **Anila** (air) and the **Dhuma** (smoke) from the poison they had been charged with. 12.

**Mythological origin of poison** (Visha): —It is stated in the Scriptures that a demon named Kaitabha obstructed in various ways, the work of the self-origined Brahmá when he was engaged in creating this world. At this the omnipotent god grew

---

\* See Chapter VII, Kalpa-Sthána.

† 'Sárivá' according to Dallana. 'Bhadra-musta' according to others.

extremely wrathful. The vehement wrath of the god gradually swollen and inflamed, at last emanated in physical forms from his mouth and reduced the mighty, death-like, roaring fiend to ashes. But the energy of that terrific wrath went on increasing even after the destruction of the demon, at the sight of which the gods were greatly depressed in spirit. The term **Visha** (poison) is so called from the fact of its filling the gods with *Vishāda* (depression of spirits). After that the god of creation, having finished his (self imposed) task of creating this world, cast that wrath both into the mobile and the immobile creations Just as the atmospheric water which is of imperceptible and undeveloped taste, acquires the specific taste of the ground or soil it falls upon, so it is the very nature of the (tasteless) Visha that it partakes of the specific taste (Rasa) of a thing or animal in which it exists. 13.

**Properties of poisons :**—All the sharp and violent qualities are present in poison. Hence poisons should be considered as aggravating and and deranging all the Doshas of the body. The Doshas aggravated and charged with poison forego their own specific functions. Hence poison can never be digested or assimilated in the system. It stops the power of inhaling. Expiration (exhalation of the breath) becomes impossible owing to the internal passages having been choked by the deranged Kapha. Consequently a poisoned person drops down in an unconscious state even when life is still present within his body. 14

**Nature and Location of Snake-poison :**—The poison of a snake like the semen in an adult male lies diffused all through its organism. As semen is gathered up, dislodged and subsequently emitted through the urethra by being agitated (by contact with woman, etc.), so the poison in a snake is gathered up and secreted through the holes of its **fangs** under the conditions of anger and agitation. The fangs being hook-shaped, a snake cannot secrete its poison without lowering its hood just after a bite. 15.

**General treatment of poisoning:**—Since a poison of whatever sort is extremely keen, sharp and heat-making in its potency, a copious sprinkling with cold water should be used in all cases of poisoning. But since the poison of an insect is mild and not too much heat-making in its potency and as it engenders a large quantity of Váyu and Kapha in the organism, measures of fomentation (Sveda) are not forbidden in a case of insect-bite. A bite by a strongly poisoned insect, however, should be treated as a snake-bite to all intents and purposes. 16.

The poison of a venomed dart or of a snakebite courses through the whole organism of the victim but it is its nature that it returns to the place of **hurt** and **bite** respectively. A man eating, from culpable gluttony, the flesh of such an animal, just dead (from the effects of poison), is afflicted with symptoms and diseases peculiar to the specific pathogenetic virtues of the poison with which the dead body is charged, and, in the long run, meets with his doom. Hence the flesh of an animal killed by a venomed dart or a snake-bite (should be considered as fatal as the poison itself and) should not be taken immediately after its death. The flesh of such an animal, however, may be eaten after a period of forty eight minutes (Muhurta) from its death after the portions of the **hurt** and the **bite** have been removed. 17.

**Symptoms of taking poison internally:**—Whoever passes a black sooty stool with loud flatus, or sheds hot tears and drops down with agony, and whose complexion becomes discoloured, and whose mouth becomes filled with foam, should be considered as afflicted with poison taken internally (**Visha-pita**). The heart of such a man (dying from the effects of internal poisoning) cannot be burnt in fire ; since the poison from its very nature lies extended in the whole viscera of the heart, the seat of cognition*. 18.

**Fatal bites :** — A man bitten by a snake in any of the vulnerable parts of the body, or near (the root of) an *As'vatthva* tree, or a temple, at the cremation ground or on an ant-hill, or at the meeting of day and night, or at the crossings of roads or under the influence of the Bharani or Maghá asterisms (astral mansions) should be given up as lost. The poison of a hooded cobra (Darvri-kara) proves instantaneously fatal. All poisons become doubly strong and operative in summer (Ushna)†. In cases of persons suffering from indigestion, urinary complaints, or from the effects of deranged Pitta or oppressed with the heat of the sun (sun-stroke) as well as infants, old men, invalids, emaciated persons, pregnant women, men of timid disposition, or of a dry temperament, or oppressed with hunger, or bitten on a cloudy day, the poisons become doubly strong and operative. 19-20.

On the other hand, a snake-bitten person, into whose body an incision is unattended with bleeding, or on whose body the strokes of lashes leave no marks, nor

---

\* In the Charaka Samhitá also we come across identical expressions of opinion as to the seat of poison in the dead body of an animal or man, dying from poison from a poisoned dart or snake-bite or from poison administered internally. See chapter xxiii, chikitsá-sthána— Charaka Samhitá.

† In place of "उर्ध्वं" some read 'अर्द्र'. This would mean "if bitten in the upper part of the body."

does horripilation appear even after a copious pouring of cold water on the body, should be likewise given up as lost. A case of snake-bite in which the tongue of the victim is found to be coated white and whose hair falls off (on the slightest pull), the bridge of whose nose becomes bent and the voice hoarse, where there is lockjaw and the appearance of a blackish-red swelling about the bite,—such a case should be given up as hopeless. 21 22.

The case in which thick, long lumps of mucus are expectorated accompanied by bleeding from both the upward and the downward orifices of the body with distinct impression of all the fangs on the bitten part, should be given up by the physician. 23.

A case of snake-bite marked by the symptoms of an insane state like that of a drunkard and accompanied by severe distressing symptoms (Upadrava), as well as loss of voice and complexion and an absence of the circulation of blood* and by other fatal symptoms should be abandoned and no action need be taken therein. 24.

Thus ends the third Chapter of the Kalpa-Sthána in the Sus'ruta Samhitá which treats of animal poisons.

* The text has "Avegi". Kártika explains it to mean "with suppression of the natural urgings, *ie.*, of stool, urine, etc.

# CHAPTER IV.

Now we shall discourse on the Chapter which treats of the specific features of the poison of a snake-bite (**Sarpa-dashta-Visha-Vijnániya**). 1.

Having laid himself prostrate at the feet of the holy and wise Dhanvantari, the master of all the S'ástras, Sus'ruta addressed him as follows :—"Enlighten and illumineus, O Lord, on the number and classification of snakes, on the nature of their poison and on the distinguishing marks of their respective bites", whereupon Dhanvantari, the foremost of all physicians replied as follows :—Innumerable are the families of serpents, of which Takshaka and Vásuki are the foremost and the most renowned. These are supposed to carry the earth\* with the oceans, mountains and the islands on their heads and are as powerful and furious as the blazing fire, fed upon the libations of clarified butter. I make obeisance to those who constantly roar, bring down rain, scorch the whole world (with the heat of their hundred-headed venom) and are capable of destroying the universe with their angry looks and poisonous breath. It is fruitless, O Sus'ruta, to enter into a discourse on the treatment of their bites as they are beyond the curative virtues of all terrestrial remedies. 2-A.

**Classification :**—I shall, however, describe in due order, the classification of the terrestrial snakes whose poison lies in their fangs wherewith they bite the human beings (and other animals). They are eighty in number, classified into five main genera, namely, the

---

\* In the Hindu mythology the earth is supposed to rest on the heads of snakes, the inmates of the infernal region.

**Darvi-kara** (hooded), **Mandali** (hoodless and painted with circular patches or rings of varied colours on their skin), **Rájimán** (hoodless and striped), **Nirvisha** (non-venomous or slightly venomous) and **Vaikaranja** (hybrid species). The last named is also, in its turn, divided into three sub-divisions only, *viz.*, the Darvi-kara (hooded), the Mandali (hoodless and ring-marked) and the Rájimán (striped ones). 2.

Of these there are twenty-six kinds of Darvi-kara snakes, twenty-two of the Mandali species, ten of the Ráji-mán class, twelve of the Nirvisha (non-venomous) species and three of the Vaikaranja (hybrid) species. Snakes born of Vaikaranja parents are of variegated colours (Chitra) and are of seven different species (three of these being Mandali (marked with rings) and (four) Rájila (marked with stripes). 3.

### Classification of snake-bites :—A

snake trampled under foot, or in a fit of anger or hunger, or anywise terrified or attacked, or out of its innate malicious nature, will bite a man or an animal. The bites of these snakes highly enraged as they are, are grouped under three heads by men conversant with their nature, *viz.*, **Sarpita** (deep-punctured), **Radita** (superficially punctured) and **Nirvisha** (non-venomous) bites. Some of the authorities on snake-bites, however, add a fourth kind *viz.*, Sarpángábhihata (coming in contact with the body of a serpent). 4·A.

### Their specific Symptoms :—The bite in

which one, two or more marks (punctures) of fangs of considerable depth are found on the affected part attended with a slight bleeding as well as those which are extremely slender and owe their origin to the turning aside and lowering of its mouth (head) immediately after the bite and are attended with swelling and the characteristic changes (in the system of the victim) should be known as the **Sarpita** bite. A (superficial) puncture (or punctures) made by the fangs of a snake and the affected part being attended with reddish, bluish, whitish or yellowish lines or stripes is called the **Radita** bite, which is characterised by the presence of a very small quantity of venom in the punctured wound. A **Nirvisha** (non-venomous) bite is marked by the presence of one or more fang-marks, an absence of swelling and the presence of slightly vitiated blood at the spot and is not attended with any change in the normal (physiological) condition of the person bitten. The contact of a snake with the body of a naturally timid person may cause the aggravation of his bodily Váyu and produce a swelling of the part. Such a man is said to be **Sarpángábhihata**\* (affected by the touch of a snake). 4.

A bite by a diseased or agitated snake or by an extremely old or young one, should be considered as considerably less venomous. The poison of a snake is inoperative in a country resorted to by the celestial Garuda (the king of birds), or by the gods, Yakshas, Siddhas and Brahmarshis, as well as in one in which there are drugs of anti-venomous virtues. 5.

**Characteristic features of the different Species of snakes :**—Those having hoods and marked with spots resembling a wheel or a plough, an umbrella or a cross (Svastika) or a goad (Amkusa) on their heads and are extremely swift, should be known as the **Darvi-kara** snakes. Those which are large and slow and marked with parti-coloured

---

\* It should be noted here that coming in contact with thorns and nails, etc., if unnoticed, may also produce in the minds of persons the fear of having been bitten by a snake and may thus produce the effects of such poisoning.

ring-like or circular spots on their skin, and have the glow of the sun or fire should be known as **Mandali** snakes, while those which are glossy and whose bodies are painted with parti coloured horizontal, perpendicular and lateral stripes, should be known as the **Rájiman** species  6.

**Features of the different Castes amongst snakes :**—The snakes whose skin is lustrous like a pearl or silver, is coloured yellow and looks like gold and emits a sweet smell, should be regarded as belonging to the **Bráhmana** species of snakes. Those which are glossy, extremely irritable in their nature and marked with spots on their skin resembling the discs of the sun and moon, or of the shape of a conchshell (Ambuja) or an umbrella, should be regarded as belonging to the **Kshatriya** species. The snakes of the **Vaiśya** caste are coloured black or red or blackish grey or ash-coloured or pigeon-coloured and are (crooked or hard in their structures) like a Vajra. The snakes which resemble a buffalo or a leopard in colour and lustre or are rough-skinned or are possessed of a colour other than the preceding ones should be considered as belonging to the **Śudra** class.  7

The poison of all hooded snakes (Phani) deranges and aggravates the bodily **Váyu**, that of the Mandali (circular spotted) species aggravates the **Pitta**, while that of the Rájimán (striped) class aggravates the bodily **Kapha**. The poison of a snake of hybrid (Vaikaranja) origin aggravates the **two** particular **Doshas** of the body which its parents would have separately aggravated—a fact which helps us to ascertain the species to which its parents belong.  8.

**Particular habits of different kinds of snakes :**—Now hear me describe the special habits of each of these families of snakes. A snake of the Rájimán species, is found abroad in the fourth or the last quarter of the night, the Mandali snakes are found to be out in the three preceding watches, while the Darvi-kara snakes are found to be abroad (in quest of prey) only in the day time. 9.

A Darvi-kara snake of tender age, a middle-aged Rájimán snake and an old Mandali snake are as fatal as personified death. A snake of extremely tender age, as well as the one roughly handled by a mungoose, or oppressed with water, as well as an extremely old and emaciated one, or one which is extremely frightened or has recently cast off its slough should be considered as mild-venomed. 10-11.

**Names of the different Species of Darvi-kara Snakes:**—Snakes known as Krishna-Sarpa, Mahá-krishna, Krishnodara, Śveta-kapota, Valá haka, Mahá-Sarpa, Śankha-pála, Lohitáksha, Gavedhuka, Parisarpa Khanda-phana, Kakuda, Padma, Mahá-Padma, Darbha-pushpa, Dadhi-mukha, Pundarika, Bhrukuti-mukha, Vishkira, Pushpábhikirna, Giri-sarpa, Riju-sarpa, Śvetodara, Mahá-śiras, Alagarda and Aśi-visha belong to the family of Darvi-kára snakes. 12

**Names of the different Species of Mandali Snakes:**—Snakes known as Ádarsha-mandala, Śveta-mandala, Rakta-mandala, Chitra-mandala, Prishata, Rodhra-pushpa, Milindaka, Gonasa, Vriddha-gonasa, Panasa, Mahá-panasa, Venu-patraka, Śiśuka, Madana, Pálimhira, Pingala, Tantuka, Pushpa-pándu, Shadga, Agnika, Vabhru, Kasháya, Kalusha, Párávata, Hastábharana, Chitraka and Enipada belong to the family of the Mandali species of snakes. 13.

**Names of the different species of Rájimán Snakes:**—Snakes known as Pundarika, Ráji-chitra, Angula-ráji, Vindu-ráji, Kardamaka, Trina-s'oshakas, Sarshapaka, S'veta-hanu, Darbha-pushpa, Chakraka, Godhumaka, Kikvisáda belong to the **Rájimán** family of snakes. 14

### Names of the different species of Nirvisha snakes :—The Galagoli, S'uka-patra, Ajagara, Divyaka, Varsháhika, Pushpa-s'akali, Jyoti-ratha, Kshirika, Pushpaka, Ahi-patáka, Andháhika, Gauráhika and the Vriks'he-s'aya belong to the **Nirvisha** (non-venomous) group of snakes. 15.

### Names and Origin of the different species of Vaikaranja snakes :—The Vaikaranja snakes are the cross-bred of the above first three species, viz., Darvi-kara, etc, and are known as Mákuli, Potagala and Snigdha-ráji. Those born of a Krishna-sarpa father and Gonasi mother or the contrary are known as Mákuli. A Rájila father and Gonasi mother or the contrary bring forth a (hybrid species known as the) Potagala, and a Krishna-sarpa father and a Rájimati mother or the contrary produce a Snigdha-ráji snake. According to several authorities, the poison of a snake of the first of these three hybrid sub families partakes of the nature of that of its father while that of the remaining two partakes of the nature of their mother. 16.

### Sub-families of the Vaikaranja Snakes :—Seven other sub-families arise out of the three aforesaid families of Vaikaranja snakes and are known as Divyelaka, Lodhra-pushpaka, Ráji-chitraka, Potagala, Pushpábhikirna, Darbha-pushpa and Vellitaka. Of these the first three species resemble the Rájila and the last four resemble the Mandali species of snakes. Thus we have finished describing the eighty different families of snakes. 17.

**Characteristic features of Male and female snakes :**—The eyes, the tongue, the mouth and the head of a male serpent are large, while those of a female snake are small. Those which partake of both these features and are mild-venomed and not (easily) irritable, should be considered as hermaphrodite (Napumsaka). 18.

Now we shall describe the general features of snake-bites :—Why does snake-poison prove instantaneously fatal like a sharp sword, thunder-bolt or fire ? Why is it that a case of snake bite, if neglected even for a very short time (Muhurta) at the outset, terminates in the death of the patient without (even) giving him an opportunity of speaking ? 19-20.

From the general characteristics of the bites, it should be presumed that they may be divided into three kinds. We shall, therefore, describe in detail the specific features of the bites of these three kinds (instead of all of them separately). It will be both beneficial to the patient and will leave no room for the confusion of the physician. From the specific features of these three kinds of snake-bites should be inferred all other snake-bites. 21.

**Specific symptoms of a bite by a Darvi-kara snake:**—A black colour of the skin, eyes, nails, tooth, urine and stool and the seat of the bite, roughness of the body and heaviness of the head, pain in the joints, weakness of the back, neck and waist, yawning, shivering, hoarseness of the voice, a rattling sound in the throat, lassitude, dry eructation, cough and difficult breathing, hiccough, upward course of the bodily Váyu, pain (S'ula) and consequent aching of the limbs, thirst, excessive salivation, foaming in the mouth, choking of the external orifices of the body (such as the mouth and the nostrils) and peculiar pains (such as the pricking, piercing pain in the body) due to the aggravation of the bodily Váyu,—these are the specific symptoms of a bite by a snake of the **Darvi-kara** species. 22.

**Specific symptoms of a bite by a Mandali snake :**—Yellowness of the skin, etc., longing for cold, a sensation as if the whole interior is being burnt with scorching vapours, extreme burning sensation in the body, thirst, a sensation of intoxication, delirium, fever, hæmorrhage through both the upper and the lower channels, sloughing of the flesh, swelling and suppuration in the affected part, a jaundiced sight, a rapid aggravation (of the Pitta) and the presence of various sorts of pain peculiar to the derangement of the of the bodily Pitta,—these are the specific symptoms of a bite by a snake of the **Mandali** species. 23.

**Specific symptoms of a bite by a Rájimán snake :**—Whiteness of the skin, etc., Sita-Jvara (catarrhal fever), horripilation, a numbness of the limbs, a swelling about the seat of the bite, flowing out of dense phlegm (from the mouth), vomiting, constant itching of the eyes, a swelling of and a rattling sound in the throat, obstruction of breath, delirium, peculiar pain and troubles characteristic of the deranged Kapha in the body,—these are the specific symptoms of a bite by a snake of the **Rájimán** species 24.

**Specific symptoms of bites by snakes of different sexes and ages, etc. :**—The sight or the pupils of the eyes of a person bitten by a male snake, is turned upward. A bite by a female serpent exhibits such smyptoms as downcast eyes and appearance of veins on the forehead, while that by a hermaphrodite (Napumsaka) snake makes the patient look sidelong. A person bitten by a pregnant snake produces yellowness of the face and tympanites. A bite by a newly delivered snake causes Śula (pain), bloody urination and an attack of tonsilites (Upa-jihvikā) in the victim. A person bitten by a hungry serpent craves for food. A bite by an old serpent is marked by a slow and mild character of the different stages of poisoning. A bite by a snake of tender age is marked by a rapid setting of the characteristic poisonous symptoms which are found to be mild in their nature. A bite by a non-venomous serpent is marked by the absence of any of the specific symptoms of poisoning. According to several authorities, a bite by a blind serpent brings on blindness in its train. An Ajagara (Boa-constructor) is found to actually swallow up the body of its prey, to which should be ascribed the death of the victim in such a case (resulting from the crushing of bones and strangulation) and not to the effects of any poison. A person bitten by a snake of instantaneously fatal poison, drops down dead at the moment of the bite as if struck by a sharp weapon or by lightning. 25.

**Symptoms of the different stages of poisoning from the bites of a Darvi-kara Snake :**—The poison of all species of snakes (snake-bites) produces **seven** distinct stages of transformation (in the organism of a person bitten by one of them). The poison of a snake of the **Darvi-kara** species affects and vitiates the blood (vascular system) in the first stage of its course or its physiological transformation in the body. The blood thereby turns black, imparting its hue to the complexion and giving rise to a sort of creeping sensation in the body, as if ants have been creeping over it. In the second stage the poison affects the principle of flesh, turns it deep black and produces swellings and Granthis all over the body. In the third stage it invades the principle of Medas (adipose tissues ?) in the body, giving rise to a sort of mucous discharge from the seat of bite, heaviness in the head, perspiration and numbness of the eyes. In the fourth stage the poison enters the Koshtha (abdomen?) and aggravates the Doshas, especially Kapha, producing somnolence, water-brash and a breaking sensation in the joints. In the fifth stage, it penetrates into the principle of bone, deranges the Prána (vital principle) and impairs the Agni (digestive fire), giving rise to hiccough, a burning sensation in the body and a breaking pain in the joints. In the sixth stage, it enters the principle of Majjan (marrow) and greatly deranges the Grahani (the large intestines ?) giving rise to a sense of heaviness of the limbs, dysentery, pain in the heart and epileptic fits. In the seventh stage it permeates the principle of semen, extremely aggravates the vital nerve-governing Váyu known as the Vyána, dislodges the Kapha even from the minutest capillaries, producing secretions of lump-like phlegm from the mouth, a breaking pain in the waist and the back, impaired functions of the mind and of the body, excessive salivation, perspiration and a suppression of breath. 26.

**Different stages of poisoning from the bites of a Mandali Snake :**—In the first stage of bite by a **Mandali** snake, the poison affects the blood (vascular system), which being thus vitiated produces shivering (lit. coldness) followed by a burning sensation in the body and pallor (yellowness) of the skin. In the second stage the poison contaminates the flesh which causes an extreme yellowness of complexion attended with a burning sensation in the body and yellowness about the seat of the bite. In the third stage, the poison affects the principle of Medas (adipose tissues) producing numbness of the eyes, thirst, slimy exudation from the wound (bite) and perspiration as in the case of a bite by a Darvi kara snake described before. In the fourth stage, it enters the Koshtha (cavity of the trunk) and produces fever. In the fifth stage, it produces a burning sensation throughout the whole organism. The sixth and the seventh stages are identical with those of the foregoing (Darvi-kara bite). 27.

**Different stages of poisoning from the bite of a Rájiman Snake :**—The poison of a Rájiman snake in the first stage of poisoning, vitiates the blood whicht is turned pale yellow producing the appearance of goose-skin of the victim who looks white. In the second stage, it contaminates the flesh, giving rise to an extreme paleness of complexion, prostration and swelling of the head. In the third stage, it affects the principle of Medas, giving rise to haziness of the eyes, deposit of filthy matter on the teeth, perspiraion and secretions from the nostrils and the eyes. In the fourth stage, it enters the Koshtha (abdominal cavity) and produces paralysis of the nerves of the neck (Manyá) and heaviness of the head. In the fifth stage, it gives rise to loss of speech and brings on S'ita-Jvara (catarrhal fever). The sixth and the seventh stages of the poisoning are identical with the preceding kind. 28.

**Memorable Verses :**—A snake-poison is found to successively attack the seven Kalás or facio described before (in Chapter IV. Śárira Sthána), and gives rise respectively to the seven stages of poisoning. The interval of time during which a deadly poison leaves a preceding Kalá and, carried forward by the bodily

Váyu, attacks the succeeding one, is called its **Vegán-tara** (the intervening stage). 29-30.

**Different Stages of poisoning in cases of lower animals:**—A lower animal bitten by a snake first becomes swelled up and looks steadfast and distresse d. In the second stage of poisoning, salivation, horripilation and pain in the heart set in. The third stage is marked by pain in the head and drooping of the neck and of the shoulder. In the fourth stage, it shivers, gnashas its teeth, drops down unconscious and expires. Some experts hold that there are only three stages of poisoning in the case of a lower animal, the fourth being included therein. 31.

**Different Stages of poisoning in cases of birds:**—A bird, bitten by a snake, looks stead-fast and becomes unconscious in the first stage of poisoning. The second stage is marked by an extreme agitated condition of the bird and the third stage ends in death. According to several authorities there is only a single stage of poisoning in the case of a bird. A snake-poison cannot penetrate far into the body of a cat, mungoose, etc. 32-33.

Thus ends the fourth Chapter of the Kalpa Sthánam in the Sus'ruta Samhitá which treats of the specific features of the poison of a snake-bite.

# CHAPTER V.

Now we shall discourse on the Chapter which deals with the medical treatment of snake-bites **(Sarpa-dashta Kaipa-Chikitsitam).**

**General treatment of Snake-bites :—** In all cases of snake-bites ligatures of cloth, skin, soft fibre or any other soft article (consecrated with the proper Mantras), should first of all be bound four fingers apart above the seat of the bite in the event of its occurring in the extremities, inasmuch as such a proceeding would arrest the further (upward) course of the poison in the body. As an alternative, the seat of the bite should be incisioned, bled and cauterized where such a ligature would be found to be impossible. Incision, cauterization, and sucking (of the poisoned blood from the seat of the bite) should be highly recommended in all cases of snake-bites. The cavity of the mouth should be filled with a linen* before sucking (the blood from the wound). It would do the man bitten by a snake an immense good if he could bite the serpent that had bitten him or failing that, bite a clod of earth without any loss of time. 2-3.

The seat of the bite by a Mandali snake should not, however, be cauterized inasmuch as the preponderant Pittaja character of the poison, aggravated by the application of the heat, might lead to its speedy expansion or coursing in the system. 4.

**Mantras :—**A physician well-versed in the Mantras of anti-venomous potency should bind a

---

\* Dallana recommends burnt earth or the earth of an ant-hill or ash for the purpose of filling up the mouth before sucking the poisoned blood.

ligature of cord consecrated with appropriate Mantras which would arrest a further spread of the poison. The Mantras full of occult energy of perfect truth and divine communion, disclosed by the Devarshis and Brahmarshis of yore, never fail to eliminate the poison from the system, and hold their own even in cases of deadliest poisons. Elimination of the poison with the help of Mantras, full of the energy of Brahmá, of truth and austerities, is more rapid than under the effects of drugs. 5.A.

A man, while learning the **Mantras**, should forego sexual intercourse, animal diet, wine, honey, etc., should be self-controlled and clean in body and spirit and (before learning the **Mantras**) shall lie on a mattress of *Kus'a-grass*. For the successful application of his newly acquired knowledge (Mantras), he shall devotedly worship the gods with offerings of perfumes, garlands of flowers, edibles, (animal) oblations, etc., and with the appropriate Mantras sacred to them as well as with burnt offerings, since a Mantra chanted by a man in an unclean spirit or body, or accented or uttered incorrectly will not take effect. The medicinal compounds of anti-venomous drugs should also be employed in such cases. 5.

**Blood-letting in Snake-bite :**—A skillful physician should open the veins round the seat of the bite and bleed the affected part. The veins of the fore-head and the extremities should be opened in the case where the poison would be found to have spread through the whole organism. The poison will be found to have been fully eliminated with the passage of the blood (from the incisioned wound). Hence bleeding should be resorted to as it is the best remedy in a case of snake-bite. 6-A.

Plasters of anti-poisonous drugs (Agada) should be applied all round the seat of the bite after scarifying it, which should be sprikled with water mixed with (red) Sandal wood and *Us'ira* or with their decoction. The appropriate Agada compounds (according to the nature of the bite) should be administered through the medium of milk, honey and clarified butter, etc. In the absence of these, the patient should be made to take (a solution of) the black earth of an ant-hill (dissolved in water). As an alternative, (a paste of) *Kovidára*, *S'irisha*, *Arka* and *Katabhi* should be prescribed for him. The patient should not be allowed to take oil, the soup of *Kulattha*-pulse, wine and *Sauviraka*. The patient should be made to vomit with the help of any other suitable liquid available, since vomiting in most cases leads to the elimination of the poison from the system. 6.

### Specific treatment of the bite by a hooded (Darvi-kara) Snake :—In the case of a bite by a hooded (**Darvi-kara**) snake, bleeding by opening the veins should be resorted to in the first stage of poisoning. In the second stage, the patient should be made to drink an Agada compound with honey and clarified butter. In the third stage, anti-poisonous snuffs (Nasya) and collyrium (Anjana) should be employed. In the fourth stage, the patient should be made to vomit, and medicated Yavágu (gruel) mentioned before (in connection with vegetable poison—see Chapter II, para. 26, Kalpasthána) should then be given him for drink. In the fifth and the sixth stages, after the administration of cooling measures, strong purgatives and emetics should be administered and the foregoing medicated Yavágu (gruel) should be administered to the patient. In the seventh stage, strong medicated Avapida-snuffs and

strong collyrium of anti-venomous efficacy should be employed for the purification (purging) of the head. Superficial incisions like the marks of crow's feet should be made on the scalp and the affected flesh and blood should be removed. 7.

**Specific treatment of bites by a Mandali Snake :**—In the first stage of a case of poisoning by the bite of a **Mandali** snake, the treatment is the same as in the corresponding stage of a Darvi-kara (cobra) bite. In the second stage, an Agada compound should be given with honey and clarified butter and after making the patient vomit the preceding medicated Yavágu (gruel) should be administerd to him. In the third stage, after the exhibition of drastic purgatives and brisk emetics, a proper and suitable medicated gruel should be administered. In the fourth and the fifth stages, the treatment would be the same as in the corresponding stages of a Darvi-kara (cobra) bite. In the sixth stage, the drugs of the Madhura (Kákolyádi) Gana taken with milk prove efficacious. In the seventh stage, anti-venomous Agada compound in the shape of Avapida (snuff) would neutralise the effects of poison. 8.

**Specific treatment of Rájiman-bites :**—In the first stage of a case of **Rájiman**-bite, bleeding should be resorted to and an Agada should be administered with milk and honey. In the second stage, emetics and an anti-venomous Agada should be given to the patient. In the third, fourth and fifth stages, the treatment should be the same as in the corresponding stages of a case of Darvi-kara-bite. In the sixth stage, the use of the strongest (anti-venomous) collyrium and in the seventh stage, that of an Avapida (snuff) of similar virtue should be prescribed. 9.

**Contra-indication to blood-letting in cases of Snake-bites:**—In the case of an infant, an old man, or an enciente woman having been bitten by a snake, all the foregoing remedies in milder doses with the exception of blood-letting should be employed according to the requirements of the case. 10.

**Dosage of Collyrium, etc., to be resorted to in cases of different beasts and birds :**—The quantity of medicated collyrium (Anjana) to be used and blood to be let out in the case of a goat or a sheep bitten by a snake should be equal to those laid down in connection with a similar human patient, while the quantity should be doubled in the case of a cow or a horse. In the case of a camel or a buffalo it should be trebled, while in the case of an elephant, it should be quadrupled Birds of whatsoever species in a similar predicament should, however, be treated only with sprays of cold water and cooling medicated plasters. 11.

**General dosage of medicines in cases of Snake-bites :**—In cases of snake-bites, collyrium to the weight of one Máshaka (Máshá) should be used at a time. The dosage of medicated snuff (Nasya), potions and emetics being respectively double, quadruple and eight times thereof. But a wise physician should treat a case of snake-bite with a full regard to the nature of the country, season, temperament, as well as to the intensity and the particular stage of poisoning the case has reached. 12-13.

We have described the anti-venomous measures and remedies applicable to the different stages of poisoning (by a snake-bite) We shall now deal with the specific treatment of poisoning of either kind according to the physical symptoms developed in the patient. Blood-letting should be speedily resorted to in the case where the poisoned limb had become discoloured, rigid, swollen and painful. Curd, Takra, honey, clarified butter and meat-soups should then be given to the patient affected with a poison marked by a preponderance of the aggravated **Váyu** and by a craving for food. A person affected with a poison marked by a predominance of the aggravated **Pitta** would have thirst, epileptic fits, perspiration and a burning sensation in the body and should be treated with shampooing with cold hands and with cold baths, and cooling medicinal plasters. A person affected with a poison marked by a predominance of the aggravated **Kapha** and bitten in the winter would have cold salivation, epileptic fits and intoxication and should be treated with strong emetics. 14

**Specific treatment of the different Supervening Symptoms :**—Purgatives should be exhibited in the event of the patient being oppressed with such symptoms as pain and burning sensation in the abdomen, Ádhmána (tympanites), retention of urine, stool and flatus, painful urination and other troubles of the deranged Pitta. **Collyrium** should be applied (along the eyelids) in the case of a swelling of the eyeballs, somnolence, discolouring of the eye, cloudiness of vision and discoloured appearance of all objects The head of the patient should be cleansed (purged) with medicinal errhines (**Nasya**) in the case of pain and a heaviness of the head, lassitude, lock-jaw, constriction of the throat (Gala-graha) and violent wryneck (Manyá-stambha). Powders of such drugs of the S'iro-virechana group as are of strong potency, in the shape of **Pradhamana** Nasya should be blown into the nostrils of the patient suffering from the effects of poisoning in the case where such symptoms as loss of consciousness, upturned eyes and drooping of the neck would set in. The veins of his forehead and of the extremities should be instantly opened. When such opening of the veins would not be attended with (the desired) bleeding superficial incisions in the shape of cow's feet (Káka-pada) should be made by an experienced surgeon on the scalp of the patient. These failing, the incisioned bits of flesh mixed with blood should be removed and the decoction or powders of a *Charma-vriksha* (Bhurja patra) should be applied to the incisions. Dundubhis (small drums) smeared with anti-venomous plasters should be sounded around the patient. The patient thus restored to consciousness should be treated with both purgatives and emetics. A complete elimination of the poison from the system is a very difficult task but it is indespensably necessary, since the least remnant of the poison may again be aggravated in course of time and cause lassitude, discolouring of the complexion, fever, cough, headache, swelling, emaciation (Sosha), cataract, blindness, catarrh (Pratiśyáya), aversion to food and nasal catarrh (Pinasa). These diseases and any other supervening symptoms of poisoning should be treated according to the injunctions laid down under their specific heads with a careful consideration of the **Dosha** or **Doshas** involved in each case. 15.

The ligature should then be removed, the seat of the bite incisioned and an Agada plaster should be applied there, so inasmuch as the poison is found to be lodged in a condensed form (in the puncture of the fangs) and is likely to be afterwards aggravated (if not fully eliminated). 16.

**Remedy for aggravated Doshas due to poison:**—If the Váyu of the body be found to be in an aggravated condition, even after a careful elimination of the poison from the system with the help of suitable Mantras, measures and medicinal remedies, it should be pacified and restored to its normal condiiton with any Vâyu-pacifying Sneha, etc., other than oil. The use of fish, *Kulattha*-soup and acid articles (fermented rice-gruel, etc.) is forbidden. The aggravated **Pitta** in such a case should be remedied with the application of a Sneha-Vasti and with the decoction of drugs prescribed in cases of Pittaja-fever, while the deranged **Kapha** should be corrected with Kapha-subduing remedies or with (the decoction of) the drugs of the *Aragvadhâdi* Gana mixed with honey, or with a diet consisting of bitter and parching (Ruksha) articles of food. 17.

A person found to be unconscious from the effects of a fall from an uneven ground or from the top of a tree or precipice as well as a drowned man rescued unconscious, or one in a state of suspended animation owing to strangulation should be treated according to the injunctions and with remedies laid down in connection with the treatment of persons who have become unconscious from the effects of poisoning (mentioned in the present chapter). 18.

If a deep seated incision (Prachchhita) in, or an extremely tight fastening (Arishta) around the seat of the bite, or an application of extremely irritant plasters or any such other application thereon gives rise to a local swelling which emits a bad smell and slimy matte it should be inferred from these that the inherent poisor in such a case has putrefied the flesh of the affecte part which can be made amenable to medicine onl with the greatest difficulty. 19-A.

**Sypmtoms of wounds from poisoned darts, etc:** The poisonous character o a **dart** or of an **arrow** with which a person has been pierced (Digdha-viddha) should be inferred from the following symptoms, *viz.,* flow of black-coloured blood from an immediately inflicted wound, suppuration, a constant burning sensation (in the incidental ulcer) and sloughing of black coloured, putrefied and morbid flesh mixed with a mucopurulent discharge from the wound, and thirst, vertigo, epileptic fits, a burning sensation in the body and fever. 19.

**Treatment of a poisoned wound :**—In a case where all the above symptoms of poisoning are present whether in a case of snake-bite or of a bite by a spider (Lutá), or in a case of being pierced with a venomed arrow, or in a case of poisoning of any kind, where putrefaction has set in, the putrid flesh of the incidental ulcer should be judiciously removed and the vitiated blood of the locality should be speedily extracted by applying leeches thereto. The system of the patient should then be cleansed with purgatives and emetics and the affected part of his body should be profusely sprayed or washed with the decoction (of the bark) of a **Kshiri-Vriksha** A poultice prepared with the anti venomous drugs of cool potency mixed with clarified butter (washed a hundred times and) placed inside the folds of linen should also be applied. In the event of its being caused by the insertion or introduction of a bone\* of any animal, the bone of which is poisonous in itself, the measures and remedies laid down above as well as those prescribed under the treatment of the "Pitta-poisoning" should be adopted and used. 20.

---

\* Dallana holds that by the word "bone" in the text should be understood all the different sources of poison, *viz.*, fæces, urine, nail, tooth, bristle, etc., of an animal.

**Recipe of different Agadas :—Mahágada :**—The powders of *Trivrit, Vis'alyá, Yashti-madhu*, the two kinds of *Haridrá, Raktá* (Manjishthá), *Narendra* (Áragvadha), the five kinds of officinal salt and *Tri-katu*, pasted with honey, should be placed inside a horn. This Agada or anti-poisonous compound used as snuff (Nasya), collyrium and anointment acts as a good neutraliser of poison. It is irresistible in its potency and is of mighty efficacy. It is called the **Mahágada.** 21.

**Ajitágada :**—A compound made of powdered *Vidanga, Páthá, Tri-phalá, Ajamoda, Hingu, Chakra* (Tagara), *Tri-katu*, the five kinds of officinal salt and *Chitraka*, pasted with honey, should be kept for a fortnight inside a cow's horn covered with a lid of the same material. This anti-venomous compound (Agada) is known as the **Ajitágada** and is efficacious in cases of both vegetable and animal poisoning. 22.

**Tárkshyágada :**—A compound made of the fine powders of *Prapaundarika, Deva-dáru, Mustá, Kálánusáryá, Katu-rohini, Sthauneyaka, Dhyámaka, Padmaka, Punnága, Tális'a, Suvarchiká, Kutannata, Elá*, white *Sindhu-vára, S'aileya, Kushtha, Tagara, Priyangu, Lodhra, Jala* (Bálaka), *Svarna-Gairika, Mágadha*, (red) *Chandana* and *Saindhava* salt, taken in equal parts and pasted with honey, should be kept inside a horn. This Agada is called the **Tárkshyágada** and is capable of neutralising the effects even of the poison of a Takshaka. 23.

**Rishabhágada :**—A compound made of the powders of *Mánsi, Tri-phalá, Murangi, Manjishthá, Yashti-madhu, Padmaka, Vidanga, Tális'a, Sugandhiká, Elá, Tvak, Kushtha, Teja-patra, Chandana, Bhárgi, Patola, Kinihi* (Apámárga), *Páthá, Mrigádani, Karkatiká, Fura* (Guggulu), *Pálindi, As'oka, Kramuka* and flowers of *Surasi* and of *Bhallátaka*, well pasted with honey and with the bile of a boar (Varáha), Godhá, Peacock, S'allaka, cat, Prishata (deer) and of mungoose, should be preserved inside a horn. This anti-venomous medicine is called the **Rishabhágada**. Snakes never visit the house of the fortunate and mighty one wherein this well prepared remedy is preserved. Venomous insects dare not come within the precincts of such a mansion and even their poison loses its quickness and fatal character. The sound of trumpets and drums, smeared with this compound and blown upon and beaten, tend immediately to destroy the effects of poison. If a poisoned patient would only look at the banner plastered with this Agada the poison from his system would be thereby eliminated. 24

**Sanjivana Agada :**—A compound made of the powders of *Láksha, Harenu, Nalada, Priyangu*, the two kinds of *S'igru, Yashti-madhu, Prithviká* (Elá) and *Haridrá*, pasted with honey and clarified butter, should be preserved inside a cow's horn and covered in the above manner. This anti venomous medicine is called the **Sanjivana Agada** and should be used as snuff, collyrium and drink. It is capable of restoring even a man apparently dead (by poisoning) to life. 25.

**Darvi-kara- Rájila -Vishahara-Agada :**—An Agada consisting of the powders of *S'leshmátaka, Katphala, Mátulunga, S'vetá, Girihvá, Kinihi*, sugar and *Tanduliya* should be regarded as the best remedy in cases of poisoning by Darvi kara or Rájila-bites. 26.

**Mandli-Vishahara Agada :**—One part each of *Dráksha, Sugandhá, Naga-vrittiká*\* and *Samangá*

---

\* Dallana says that in place of "Sugandhá Naga-vrittiká" some read "Sugandhá Naga-mrittiká" which means "the sweet-scented earth of the mountain" known to be possessed of anti-poisonous virtues.

(Varáha kránta), two parts each of the following drugs, *viz.*,—leaves of *Surasá, Vilva, Kapittha,* and of *Dádima,* and half a part each of the following, *viz.* : (leaves of) black *Sindhuvára, Amkotha* and *Gairika,* should be powdered together and mixed with honey. This anti-venomous medicine (Agada) is highly efficacious especially in the case of poisoning by a Mandali-bite. 27.

**Vamśa-tvagádi Agada:**—An Agada should be prepared with the scrapings of green bamboo (Vamśa-tvak), *Ámalaka, Kapittha, Tri-katu, Haimavati, Kushtha, Karanja*-seeds, *Tagara* and *S'irisha* flowers, pasted with cow's bile. Used as a plaster, snuff or collyrium, it destroys the poison of a spider, mouse, serpent or any other (poisonous) insect. Used as a collyrium (over the eye-lids), as a plaster over the umbilical region, or as a Varti (plug), it removes the obstruction of stool, urine and Váyu (flatus, etc.), or of a foetus in the womb. Used as a snuff or a collyrium, its curative potency is manifest even in such dangerous eye-diseases as Kácha, Arman, Kotha, Patala and Pushpa. 28.

**Pancha-Śirisha Agada:**—A potion consisting of a decoction of the roots, flowers, bark, seeds and sprouts of a *S'irisha* tree, taken with honey, the five officinal kinds of salt and a profuse quantity of powdered *Tri-kutu,* proves speedily efficacious in a case of poisoning by an insect-bite. 29.

**Sarva-Kámika Agada :**—An Agada prepared with *Kushtha, Tri-katu, Dárvi, Madhuka* (flower), the two kinds of salt (Saindhava and Sauvarchala), *Málati* (flower), *Nága-pushpa* and all the drugs of the *Madhura* (Kákolyádi) group and pasted with the juice of *Kapittha* and mixed with honey and sugar destroys all sorts of poison specially that of a mouse (Mushika). 30.

**Ekasara Agada :**—The following drugs viz., *Somarāji* seeds and *Somarāji* flowers,* *Katábhi, Sindhu-vára, Choraka, Varuna, Kushtha, Sarpa-gandhá, Saptalá, Punarnavá,* flowers of *S'irisha, Áragvada* and of *Arka, S'yámá, Ambashthá, Viḍanga, Ámra, As'mantaka,* black earth and *Kuravaka* comprise the **Ekasara Agada.** These should be applied singly† or in combination of two or three to destroy the effects of poison. 31.

Thu- ends the fifth Chapter of the Kalpa-Sáthána in the Sus'ruta Samhitá which deals with the medical treatment of snake-bites.

\* Some explain "सोमराजिफलं पुष्पं" to mean 'Somarāji, Phala (Madana) and Pushpa (Nága-kes'ara).'

† Some explain "एकश्रो द्विस्त्रिश्रो वापि" to mean that the Agada should be used "once, twice or thrice" according to the requirements in each case.

# CHAPTER VI.

Now we shall discourse on cases of rat-poisoning (**Mushika-kalpa**). 1.

**Different varieties of rats (M. Text):** —Now hear me enumerate the names of the different families of **Mushika** (rats) briefly referred to before as having their poison in their **semen,** classified according to their different names, features and the medical treatment to be employed for the neutralisation of the effects of their poison. They are eighteen in number and are named as follows :—Lálana, Putraka, Krishna, Hamsira, Chikkira, Chhuchhundara, Alasa, Kasháya-daśana, Kulinga, Ajita, Chapala, Kapila, Kokila, Aruna, Mahá-Krishna, S'veta, Mahá-Kapila and Kapotábha. 2.A

**General symptoms of rat-poisoning :**—The blood of any part of a human body coming in contact with the semen of any of these different classes of rats or scratched with their nails, teeth, etc., previously besmeared with their semen (S'ukra) is vitiated and gives rise to the appearance of Granthi (nodes), swelling, Mandala, eruptions of circular erythematous patches on the skin, Karniká (eruptions of patches resembling the calycle of a lotus flower), pimples (pustules) violent and acute erysipelas, Kitima (keloid tumours), breaking pain in the joints, extreme pain (in the body), fever, violent epileptic fits, anemia, aversion to food, difficult breathing, shivering and horripilation. 2.

**Specific symptoms and treatment of rat-poisoning :**—The general symptoms of rat-poisoning have been briefly described above. Now hear me specially describe the symptoms of the bites by the different families of rats (Mushika). A bite by a rat of the **Lálana** class is marked by a copious flow of saliva, hic-cough and vomiting. The patient in such a case should be made to use a lambative made of the roots of *Tanduliyaka* mixed with honey. A bite by a rat of the **Putraka** family is marked by a sense of physical langour, yellowness of the complexion and the appearance of nodular glands (Granthi) resembling young rats. A compound of *S'irisha* and *Ingudi* pasted together and mixed with honey should be given to the patient as a lambative in this case. A bite by a rat of the **Krishná** (black) class in foul weather and more especially on a cloudy day is characterised by the vomiting of blood. A pasted compound of *S'irisha* fruit and *Kushtha* with the washings of the ashes of *Kims'uka* (flower) should be given to the patient in such a case. 3-A.

A bite by a rat of the **Hansira** species brings on an aversion to food, yawning and horripilation. In such a case emetics should be first given to the patient who should be then made to drink a decoction of the drugs of the *Áragvadhádi* group. A bite by a rat of the **Chikkira** class is accompanied by headache, swelling, hic-cough and vomiting. In such a case an emetic consisting of the decoction of *Jálini*, *Madana* fruit and *Amkotha* should be prescribed. A bite by a venomous Mushika of the **Chhuchchhundara** (mole) species gives rise to diarrhœa (watery stool), numbness of the muscles of the neck and yawning. In this case an alkaline compound prepared of the ashes of the dry plants of barley (Yava-nála), *Rishabhi* (Átma-guptá) and *Vrihati* should be prescribed*. 3-B.

* **Different reading.**—A bite by a Mushika of the Chhuchchhundara

A bite by a rat of the **Alasa** species is characterised by a numbness of the neck, an upward coursing of the Váyu, fever and pain at the seat of the bite. In this case the patient should be made to take the **Mahágada** with honey and clarified butter as a lambative. A bite by a rat of the **Kasháya-dasana** species is marked by somnolence or excessive sleep, atrophy (Sosha) of the heart and a general emaciation of the body. In such a case a lambative made of the bark, pith and fruit (seeds) of *S'irisha* mixed with honey should be given to the patient to lick. A bite by a rat of the **Kulinga** species is marked by pain, swelling and stripe-like marks about the seat of the bite, the remedy consisting in a lambative made of the two kinds of *Sahá* (Mudga-parni and Másha-parni) and *Sindhuvára* pasted together and mixed with honey. 3-C.

A bite by a rat of the **Ajita** species is characterised by vomiting, epileptic fits (fainting), a catching pain at the heart (Hrid-graha) and blackness of the eyes. The patient in such a case should be made to lick a compound made of (the roots of) *Pálindi* (Trivrit) pasted with the milky juice of *Snuhi* and mixed with honey. A bite by a rat of the **Chapala** species is marked by vomiting, epileptic fits and thirst, and the remedy in this case should consist of a lambative made of *Tri-phalá*, *Bhadra-káshtha* (Deva-dáru) and *Jatá-mánsi* (D.R.—Yava) pasted together and mixed with honey. A bite by a rat of the **Kapila** species is followed by Kotha (putrefaction) of the bite, appearance

class produces thirst, vomiting, fever, weakness, numbness of the muscles of the neck, swelling, abscess on the back, loss of the sense of smell and Visuchiká. A compound of Chavya, Haritaki, S'unthi, Vidanga, Pippali, S'vetaka-seeds and the ashes of (the plants of) Vrihati pounded together and mixed with honey should be prescribed in this case.—Gayadása.

of nodular glands (Granthi) and fever. The remedy consists in the use of a lambative made of *Tri-phalá*, *S'vetá*\* (white Aparájitá) and *Punarnavá* pasted together and licked with honey. A bite by a rat of the **Kokila** species is attended with high fever, an intolerable burning sensation in the body and the appearance of nodular glands (Granthi). Clarified butter duly cooked with the decoction of *Varshábhu* and *Nilini* (Indigo plants) should be administered in such a case. 3-D.

A bite by a rat of the **Aruna** (vermilion coloured) species is marked by an extremely aggravated condition of the bodily Váyu and the symptoms peculiar to it. A bite by a rat of the **Mahá-krishna** (extremely black) species leads to an aggravated condition of the Pitta, while a bite by one of the **Mahá-sveta** class ushers in an aggravation of the bodily Kapha. The blood of a person is vitiated by the bite of a rat of the **Mahá-kapila** family, while the bite by one of the **Kapota** species leads to the derangement of all the four principles *viz.*, the three Doshas (Váyu, Pitta and Kapha) as well as of the blood. Their bites are accompanied by a violent swelling of the affected locality, the appearance of nodular glands (Granthi) and such other erythematous and eczematous growths as Mandala, Karniká and Pidaká (Pustules). 3-E.

Three Prastha measures† each of clarified butter, curd and milk should be duly cooked with the duly prepared decoction of *Karanja*, *Áragvadha*, *Tri-katu*,

---

\* Some explains "S'vetá Punarnavá" to mean "white Punarnavá." Gayadása reads "S'reshthá" in place of "S'vetá" in which case also the white species of Punarnavá is evidently meant.

† According to Dallana, the recipe of this Ghrita is as follows:— One Prastha each of clarified butter, curd and milk, two Palas each of Karanja, etc., and sixteen seers of water to be boiled down to four seers, the drugs of the Kalka weighing one seer in all.

*Vrihati, Ams'umati* and *Sthirā* (Kákoli), and with *Trivrit, Tila, Amritá* (Gulancha), *Chakra, Sarpa-gandhá,* (black) earth* (of an ant-hill) and the barks of *Kapittha* and *Dádima* as Kalka. The whole should be duly cooked over a gentle fire. The Ghrita thus prepared would destroy the poison of the five kinds of rats *viz.*, Aruna, etc. As an alternative, clarified butter duly cooked with the expressed juice of *Kákádani* and *Káka-máchi* should be given to the patient in such cases. A wise physician shall have recourse to bleeding or venesection in these cases and the system of the patient should be cleansed by purgatives and emetics. 3.

**General Treatment:**—The general measures to be adopted in the case of a bite by a rat of whatsoever class are as follows:—The seat of the bite should be first cauterized (with boiling clarified butter), and blood-letting should be resorted to (by opening the veins of the patient). The seat of the bite should then be marked with superficial incisions and a plaster of *S'irisha, Rajani, Kushtha, Kumkuma* and *Amrita* (Gulancha) should be applied. The patient should be made to vomit with the decoction of *Jálini* or with that of *S'ukákhyá* and *Amkotha* boiled together. The (powdered) roots of *S'ukákhya, Kos'dvati, Madana* fruits and *Devadáli* fruits should be administered with curd for the elimination by vomiting the (internal) poison (if any). The patient should be made to take (with curd) the compound consisting of *Phala* (Madana), *Vacha, Devadáli* and *Kushtha* pasted with the urine of a cow (as an emetic). This remedy neutralises the effects of the poison of all species of venomous rats. 4.-A

A compound composed of *Trivrit, Danti* and *Tri-*

---

* In place of "सपगन्धा समृत्तिका" some reads "सपंगन्धाहिमृत्तिका", while Jejjata reads "सपंगन्धागमृत्तिका।"

*phala* should (if necessary) be employed as a purgative (in such a case). A compound prepared with the pith of *S'irisha* and the pulp of its fruits should be used (if necessary) as an errhine (S'iro-virechana). The watery secretion of fresh cow-dung mixed with a profuse quantity of (powdered) *Tri-katu* should be used as collyrium. The patient should be made to lick a compound prepared with the expressed juice of the fruits of *Kapittha* and with honey and the serous secretion of (fresh) cow-dung, or a lambative made of *Rasánjana, Haridrá, Indra-yava, Katuki* and *Ati-vishá* with honey should be given to the patient in the morning. A potion of medicated clarified butter duly cooked with the roots of *Tanduliyaka* should be given to the patient for drink. As an alternative, clarified butter, duly cooked with the five parts (*viz.*, roots, bark, fruits, leaves and flowers) of a *Kapittha* tree or with the roots of *Áshphotá*, should be prescribed. 4.

The poison of a venomous Mushika (rat or mole) even though (apparently) eliminated from the system may sometimes still be aggravated in cloudy days or in foul weather. In such a case, all the above measures as well as the remedies laid down under the treatment of **Dushi-visha** should be resorted to. The round protruding edges (Karniká) of an ulcer, incidental to a rat-bite, whether benumbed or painful, should be excised (D.R.—made to suppurate) and should be treated with purifying or cleasing remedies according to the deranged Dosha or Doshas involved in each case. 5-6.

**Causes of Rabies :**—The bodily Váyu in conjunction with the (aggravated) Kapha of a jackal, dog, wolf, bear, tiger or of any other such ferocious beast affects the sensory nerves of these animals and overwhelms their instinct and consciousness. The tails, jaw-bones (D. R.— neck) and shoulders of such infurated animals naturally droop down, attended with a copious flow of saliva from their mouths. The beasts in such a state of frenzy, blinded and deafened by rage, roam about and bite each other. 7-A.

**Symptoms of Hydrophobia :**—The limb or part of the body of a person bitten by such a rabid and (consequently) poisonous animal loses its sensibility of touch, and a copious flow of dark sooty blood is emitted from the seat of the bite. The patient in such a case generally exhibits all the symptoms which mark a case of poisoning by a venomed arrow. 7-B.

**Prognosis :**—A person bitten by a rabid animal barks and howls like the animal by which he is bitten, imitates it in many other ways and, bereft of the specific functions and faculties of a human subject, ultimately dies. If a person, bitten by a rabid animal, sees its (imaginary) image reflected in water or in a mirror, he should be deemed to have reached an unfavourable stage of the disease. 7-C.

**Symptoms of Jala-trása :**—If the patient in such a case becomes exceedingly frightened at the sight or mention of the very name of **water**, he should be understood to have been afflicted with **Jala-trása** (Hydrophobia) and be deemed to have been doomed. Such a case of Jala-trása (water-scare) even in an unbitten person or in a healthy person, if frightened (by such a scare), whether waking or in sleep, should be regarded as a fatal symptom. 7.

**Treatment :**—In the case of a bite by a rabid animal, the seat of the bite should be profusely bled (by pressing it) so as to let out all the (vitiated) blood. It should then be cauterized with (boiling) clarified butter and pasted with any of the aforesaid Agada, or the patient should be made to drink a potion of matured clarified butter. Clarified butter mixed with the milky exudation of an *Arka* plant, as well as a compound of white *Punarnavá** and *Dhuttura*† should be prescribed for the patient as an errhine. 8-A.

**Treatment of bites by rabid dogs :—** A compound of pasted sesamum mixed with its oil, treacle and the (milky) juice of a *Rupiká* plant eliminates the poison of a rabid dog (Alarka) from the system as a gale of wind drives a pack of clouds before it. A quantity of rice, two Tolás (one Karsha) in weight of the roots of *S'ara-pumkha* and half a Karsha weight of *Dhuttura* (roots) should be pasted together with the washings of rice. The paste should be covered with (seven) *Dhustura* leaves and baked (on the fire) in the shape of an Apupaka (cake). The cake thus prepared should be given, at the proper time of taking a medicine, to a person bitten by a rabid dog for a complete nullification of the poison. But the use of these cakes is attended with certain other troubles at the time of their digestion and these troubles become subdued by a retiring to in a dry but cool chamber away from water. The patient (after the subsidence of the troubles) should be bathed the next day and a diet of boiled *S'áli* or *Shashtika* rice with tepid milk‡ should be prescribed for him. On the third and on the fifth day, the aforesaid anti-venomous compound should again be administered in half doses to the patient for the elimination of the poison. 8-B.

\* Some explain "S'vetá Punarnavá" to mean "white Punarnavá", but others explain it to mean "S'vetá (Katabhi) and Punarnavá".

† Some commentators prescribe the roots of Dhustura to be taken, while others hold that its fruits should be used.

‡ Dallana says that in place of "चौरेणोष्णेन" Gayadása reads "गव्येनाज्येन", that is to say, the diet should be taken with clarified butter.

The person in whom the poison (of a rabid dog or jackal, etc.) is spontaneously aggravated has no chance of recovery. Hence the poison should be artificially aggravated (and then remedied) before reaching that stage of aggravation. The patient should be bathed at the crossing of roads or on the bank of a river with pitcherfuls of water containing gems and medicinal drugs and consecrated with the appropriate Mantra. Offerings of cooked and uncooked meat, cakes and levigated pastes of sesamum as well as garlands of flowers of variegated colours should be made to the god (and the following Mantra should be recited). "O thou Yaksha, lord of Alarka, who art also the lord of all dogs, speedily makest me free from the poison of the rabid dog that has bitten me." Strong purgatives and emetics should be administered to the patient after having bathed him in the above manner, since the poison in a patient with an uncleansed organism may sometimes be aggravated, even after the healing of the incidental ulcer. 8.

The poison of a (rabid) dog, etc., lies in the teeth and tends to aggravate the Pitta and the Váyu and hence the patient bitten by such animals is found to imitate their cries and nature. A patient afflicted with such poison cannot be saved even with the greatest care. The seat of a scratch made by the nails or teeth of any of those animals should be rubbed (and the poisoned blood should be let out). It should then be sprinkled over with tepid oil, since the poison in this case aggravates only the Váyu of the system. 9-10

This reading of Gayadása seems to be the better one, as the use of clarified butter in such cases is supported by the custom of our country.

Thus ends the sixth Chapter of the Kalpa-sthána in the Su'sruta Samhitá which deals with the symptoms and treatments of rat-poison.

# CHAPTER VII.

Now we shall discourse on the Chapter which treats of the sounds of a (medicated) drum, etc., possessed of anti-venomous virtues **(Dundhubhi-Svaniya).** 1.

**Ksharágada:**—The woods of *Dhava, As'vakarna, Tinis'a, Palás'a, Pichu-marda, Pátali, Páribhadraka, Ámra, Udumbara, Karahátaka, Arjuna, Kakubha, Sarja, Kapitana, S'leshmátaka, Amkotha, Ámalaka, Pragraha, Kutaja, S'ami, Kapittha, As'vmantaka, Arka, Chira-vilva, Mahá-vriksha, Arushkara, Aralu, Madhuka, Madhu-s'igru, S'áka, Goji, Murvá, Tilvaka, Ikshuraka, Gopa-ghantá* and *Arimedá\** should be taken (in equal parts) and burnt down to ashes. The said ashes should be dissolved in the urine of a cow and filtered (through a piece of linen) in the manner of preparing an alkali. This alkaline solution should then be duly boiled (till it would assume a transparent blood-red hue and slimy character), and the powders of *Pippalimula, Tanduliyaka, Varánga, Chochaka, Manjishthá, Karanja, Hasti-Pippali, Maricha, Utpala, Sárivá, Vidanga, Griha-dhuma* (soot of a room), *Anantá, Soma, Saralá, Váhlika, Guhá, Kos'ámra,* white mustard seeds, *Varuna, Lavana, Plaksha, Nichula, Vardhamána, Vanjula, Putra-s'reni, Sapta-parna, Dandaka, Ela-váluka, Nága-danti, Ativishá, Abhayá, Bhadra-dáru Kushtha,*

---

\* The plants of these should be taken in full *i.e.* with their leaves, roots, branches, etc. The prepared ash should be dissolved in cow's urine weighing six times the combined weight of the ashes. Dallana says that, Gayadása does not read "S'irisha, Pichumarda, Kakubha, Arushkara and Madhu-S'igru" in the list.

*Haridrá* and *Vachá* together with pulverised (dead) iron (taken in equal parts)* should be added to it. Then it should be boiled again and preserved in an iron pitcher after it had been duly prepared in the manner of an alkali. 2.

**Metrical Texts :**—Dundhubhis (drums), banners and the gate ways of houses should be smeared with this alkaline preparation, hearing the sound as well as the sight and touch whereof would lead to the complete elimination of the poison from the system of the patient. This medicine is known as the **Kshárá-gada** which is equally efficacious in cases of S'arkará (gravel), stones in the bladder, Hæmorrhoids, Váta-Gulma, cough, S'ula (colic), Udara (abdominal dropsy), indigestion, Grahani, extreme aversion to food, general œdema of the body and violent asthma. The remedy is applicable in all cases of poisoning of whatsoever type and acts as a sure antidote to the poison of the serpents headed by the dreadful Takshaka. 3.

**Kalyánaka Ghrita :**—An adequate quantity of clarified better duly cooked with (the decoction and Kalka of) the drugs known as *Vidanga, Tri-phalá, Danti, Bhadra-dáru, Harenu, Tális'a-patra, Manjishthá, Kes'ara, Utpala, Padmaka, Dádima, Málati* flower, the two kinds of *Rajani*, the two kinds of *Sáriva*, the two kinds of *Sthirá, Priyangu, Tagara, Kushtha,* the two kinds of *Vrihati, Ela-váluka,* sandal wood and

---

\* The total weight of these powders to be added should be one thirtieth part of the prepared alkaline solution. Dallana says that Gayadása counts only thirty and he does not read "Maricha, Soma, Guhá, Lavana, Chakra and Ála in the text. We do not, however, find Chakra and Ála in the text. We have, on the other hand, the names of some more drugs which are believed to be mere interpolations from the marginal notes of some manuscripts.

*Gavákshi,* is known as the **Kalyánaka Ghrita.** The curative efficacy of this Ghrita extends to cases of poisoning, Grahápasmára (hysteria due to the influence of malignant stars and planets), Jaundice, Gara-dosha (slow chemical poisoning), asthma, sluggishness of appetite, fever and cough. It is commended to consumptive patients, as well as to men suffering from scantiness of semen and women afflicted with sterility. 4.

**Amrita Ghrita :**—An adequate quantity of clarified butter duly cooked with the seeds of Apámárga and of the two kinds of S'vetá, *S'irisha,* and *Kákamáchi* (previously) pasted with the urine of a cow is known as the **Amrita-Ghrita.** It embraces within the pale of its therapeutic virtues all cases of poisoning and is capable of bringing back an apparently dead man to life. 5.

**Mahá-sugandhi Agada :**—The following drugs *viz.,* (red) sandal wood, *Aguru, Kushtha, Tagara, Tila-parnika, Prapaundarika, Nalada, Sarala, Deva-dáru, Bhadra-s'ri* (white sandal wood), *Yavaphalá, Bhárgi, Nili, Sugandhiká, Káleyaka, Padmaka, Madhuka, Nágara, Jatá* (a variety of Jatá-mámsi), *Punnága, Elá, Elaválu, Gairika, Dhyámaka, Balá, Toya, Sarjarasa, Mámsi, Sita-pushpá, Harenuká, Tális'a-patra,* small *Elá, Priyangu, Kutannata, S'áila pushpa, S'aileya, Patra, Kálánu-Sárivá, Tri-katu, S'ita-s'iva,*\* *Kásmarya, Katu-rohini, Somaráji,* \Ati-visha, *Prithviká, Indra-váruni, Us'ira, Varuna, Musta, Nakha, Kustumburu,* the two kinds of *S'vetá,* † the two kinds of

---

\* Dallana explains "S'ita-s'iva" to mean "camphor". Others explain it to mean "S'ami."

† The text has "S'vetá" in the dual number meaning the two kinds of "S'vetá' *viz;* white Vacha and white Aparájitá. Dallana gives only

*Haridrá, Sthauneya, Láksha*, the five kinds of officinal salts, *Kumuda, Utpala, Padma*, flower of *Arka*, flowers and fruits of *Champaka, As'oka, Sumanas, Tilaka* (sesamum), *Pátali, Sálmali, S'elu, S'irisha, Surasi, Trina-s'uli* and of *Sindhuvára*, flowers of *Dhava, As'vakarna*, and *Tinisa, Guggula, Kumkuma, Vimbi, Sarpákshi* and *Gandha-Nákuli* should be carefully collected and pasted with honey, clarified butter and the bile of a cow and should be kept inside a horn (or a receptacle made of that material). This medicine, which is the best of all anti-venomous medicinal preparations, would rescue from the jaws of death, a patient even with drooped down shoulders and sunk and upturned eyes. It is capable of destroying in a moment the irresistible fire-like poison even of the dreadful infuriated Vásuki, the king of serpents. This Agada which consists of eighty-five ingredients is called the **Mahá-sugandhi Agada** and is the most potent of all anti-venomous remedies. It should constantly be in the possession of a king. Smeared with the present preparation he is sure to be a favourite with all his subjects and to shine with his sovereign majesty even amidst his enemies. 6.

A physician well versed in the natures of poisons, should adopt all remedial measures excepting the heat-engendering ones in all types of poisoning. But this rule would not be applicable in a case of insect-bite inasmuch as the poison of an insect is cool in its potency and hence would be aggravated by the application of any cooling measures. 7.

"Vachá" as its synonym, which shows he takes the word in the singular number and not in the dual as in the printed text. This appears to be the correct reading, for otherwise the number of the drugs in the list would be more than eighty-five.

**Rules of diet and conduct :**—Wholesome diets which have been enumerated in the chapter on Anupána-Vidhi, should be prescribed in cases of poisoning after a due consideration of the nature, habit, and temperament of the patient who should be warned against the use of unwholesome ones. The use of Phánita (liquid treacle), *S'igru, Sauvira*, the taking of meals before the digestion of the previous ones, the group of Nava-Dhánya (unmatured corn), wine, sesamum, oil and *Kulattha*-pulse, sleep in the day time, sexual intercourse, physical exercise, fits of anger and exposure to the sun are forbidden in the case of a poisoned patient. 8.

**Symptoms of elimination of poison :** —The restoration of the deranged Doshas and of the vital principles (Dhátus of the body) to their normal state, a natural craving for food and drink, the normal colour and condition of the tongue and of the urine and the normal state and functions of the mind and of the sense-organs in a poisoned patient would indicate the full and complete elimination of the poison from his system. 9.

Thus ends the Seventh Chapter of the Kalpa-Sthána in the Sus'ruta Samhitá which treats of the sounds of medicated drums, etc.

# CHAPTER VIII.

Now we shall discourse on insects, *i.e.* the measures, etc. to be adopted in cases of insect-bite, etc. **(Kita-Kalpa).** 1.

Various kinds of worms and insects (Kita) germinate from the semen, fecal matter, urine, putrid eggs and putrid carcases of serpents which are marked by Vátaja, Pittaja (Ágneya) and Kaphaja (Ambuja) temperaments. The poisons of these vermin which are nothing but insects (Kita), are apt to be most dangerous in the long run on account of their being acted upon by the Doshas and may be divided into four* groups. 2.

**Insects of Vátaja Temperament :—** The eighteen classes of insects known as the Kumbhinasa, Tundikeri, Śringi, Śata-Kuliraka, Uchchitinga, Agnináma, Chichchitinga, Mayuriká, Avartaka, Urabhra, Sáriká-mukha, Vaidala, Śaráva-kurda, Abhiráji, Parusha, Chitra-śirshaka, Śata báhu and the Rakta-ráji are possessed of a **Vátaja** temperament and their poison tends to aggravate and derange the bodily **Váyu** and produce the specific diseases due thereto. 3.

**Insects of Pittaja Temperament :—** The twenty-four families of insects known as the Kaundilyaka, Kanabhaka, Varati (asp), Patra-vriśchika, Vinásiká, Brahmaniká, Vindula (D.R.-Viluta), Bhramara,

---

* Dallana says that the four groups are to be determined according to the origin of the insects from the semen, etc. of a Darvi-kara, Mandali, Rájila, or a Vaikaranja serpent. To us it seems, however, that the groups should be Vátaja, Pittaja, Kaphaja and Sannipátaja.

Váhyaki, Pichchita, Kumbhi, Varchah-kita, Arimedaka, Padma-kita, Dundubhika, Makara, Sata-pádaka (centipede), Panchálaka, Páka-matsya, Krishna-tunda, Gardabhi, Klita, Krimi-Sarái and the Utklesaka are of a fiery *i. e.* **Pittaja** temperament and their poison tends to derange and aggravate the bodily **Pitta** and produce the specific diseases due to the derangement of that Dosha. 4.

### Insects of Kaphaja Temperament:

—The thirteen families of insects known as the Visvambhara, Pancha-s'ukla, Pancha-krishna, Kokila, Saireyaka Prachalaka, Valabha, Kitima, Suchi-mukhá, Krishna-Godhá, Káshaya-Vásika, Kita-gardabhaka and the Trotaka are possessed of Saumya *i.e.*, **Kaphaja** temperament, and their poison aggravates and deranges the Kapha and produces the specific diseases which owe their origin to the deranged condition of that Dosha. 5.

### Insects of Sánnipátika Temperament:

—The twelve kinds of insects known as the Tungi-nása, Vichilaka, Tálaka, Váhaka, Koshthágári, Krimikara, Mandala-Puchchhaka, Tunga-nábha, Sarshapika, Avalguli, Sambuka and the Angi-kita are dangerously fatal in their bite. A person or an animal bitten by any of these dangerous insects exhibits stages and symptoms similar to those of a case of a snake-bite and their poison tends to derange and aggravate the three Doshas (**Sánnipátika**) of the body and produce the specific symptoms thereof. 6-A.

### Symptoms of their bite:

—The seat of the bite seems as if on fire or being burnt with strong alkali and is characterised by a red, yellow, white or vermillion colour. The symptoms which are developed in the entire course of the poisoning (or are found to supervene) in cases of their bites are fever, breaking and aching pain (in the limbs), horripilation, vomiting, thirst, a burning sensation in the body, loss of consciousness, yawning, shaking of the limbs, difficult breathing, hic-cough, (sometimes) a burning and (at others) a cold sensation (in the seat of the bite), eruption of pustules, swelling (in the affected locality), appearance of nodular glands (Granthi), circular erythematous patches (Mandala) on the skin, ring-worm, Erysipelas, Kitima (Keloid Tumour) and Karniká (round about the seat of the bite) as well as any other symptoms peculiar to the **Dosha** aggravated by the poison of each species. 6.

The other characteristic features of the poison of these (fatal and strong-poisoned) insects should be speedily ascertained by comparing the symptoms of aggravation of the **Dushi-Visha** (consequent thereon) and by examining the effects of the application of different anti-poisonous plasters as well. 7.

These are the characteristic features of sharp-poisoned insects; now hear me describe those of the mild-poisoned ones. The symptoms which are manifest in the case of a bite by such an insect are salivation (Praseka), an aversion to food, vomiting, heaviness in the head, a slight sensation of cold and the appearance of pustules and urticaria according to the deranged Dosha aggravated by the species of the biting insect. 8.

The pulverised bodies of these insects possessing, as they do, the characteristic features of Dushi-Visha or enfeebled poison (lying inherent in a human system) is turned into a **Gara** or chemical (combinative or resultant) poison, if administered (internally) with any medicine or externally with any plaster. 9.

We shall henceforth describe the distinctive traits of one insect from another of the same species according to the classification and general characteristics and incurability of their bites. 9.

**The Kanabha class of Insects :**—The Trikantaka, Kuni, Hasti-kaksha and the Aparájita are the four kinds of insects that belong to the **Kanabha** group and are extremely painful in their bites giving rise to swelling, aching in the limbs, heaviness of the body and a black aspect at the seat of the bite. 10.

**The Gaudheyaka class of Insects :**— The five kinds of insects known as the Prati-surya, Pinga-bhása, Bahu-varna, Mahá-śiras and the Nirupama belong to the **Gaudheyaka** class. The stages and the symptoms of a bite by an insect of this group are often identical with (or mistaken for) a snake bite and are marked by all its characteristic pain and the appearance of dreadful Granthis (nodular glands) of varied colours and shapes. 11.

The six kinds of insects known as the Gala-goli, S'veta-krishná, Rakta-ráji, Rakta-mandala, Sarva-s'vetá, and the Sarshapiká belong to one and the same species. A bite by any of these insects excepting by a Sarshapiká is attended with a burning sensation and slimy exudation from and swelling in the seat of the bite, that of the Sarshapiká being accompanied by an attack of dysentery (Atisára) and pain at the heart. 12.

**Śata-padi** (centipede) :—The **S'ata-padi** (centipede) species is divided into eight kinds, *viz.*, the Parusha (rough), Krishna (black), Chitra (of variegated colours), Kapiliká (tawny brown), Pitaka (yellow), Raktá (red), S'vetá (white) and the Agni-prabhá (resembling fire in virtue). A bite by any of these insects is attended with swelling, pain and a burning sensation in the heart. A bite by one of the Śvetá or the Agni-prabhá species is marked by all the aforesaid symptoms as well as by violent epileptic fits, an intolerable burning sensation and eruptions of white pustules (Pidakà). 13.

**Manduka** (frogs):—The Mandukas (frogs) are divided in eight different species *viz*., the Krishna, Sára, Kuhaka, Harita, Rakta, Yava-varnábha, Bhrikuti and the Kotika A bite by any of these is accompanied by an itching sensation in the seat of the bite and a flow of yellow-coloured foam from the mouth. A bite by one of the Bhrikuti or Kotika species gives rise to the aforesaid symptoms as well as a burning sensation, vomiting and a severe attack of epileptic fits in addition thereto. 14.

A bite by one of the **Vis'vambhara** species of insects is followed by Sita-jvara (catarrhal fever) and an eruption of white pimples (Pidaká) in the shape of mustard seeds round about the seat of the bite. A bite by one of the **Ahinduka** species is marked by piercing pain, a burning sensation, itching and swelling (in the affected locality), as well as by delirium. A bite (contact) by one of the **Kandumaká** species is followed by a yellowness of the complexion, vomiting, dysentery and fever, etc. A bite by one of the **S'uka-vrinta** or such like species is attended with itching and Kotha (urticaria) and the bristles of the insects are found to be adhering to the affected locality. 15.

**Pipiliká** (Ants):—There are six kinds of Pipiliká (ants) *viz*., the Sthula-s'irshá, Samváhiká, Bráhmaniká, Kapiliká and the Chitra-varná. A bite by any of these is attended with imflammatory swelling and a burning sensation (in the seat of the bite) resembling those produced by contact with fire. 16.

**Makshiká** (stinging flies):—Flies (Makshiká) may be divided into six species *viz*., the Kántáriká, Krishná, Pingaliká, Madhuliká, Káshàyi and the Sthàliká. A bite by any of these is accompanied by swelling and a burning sensation. A bite by one of the Sthálika or the Káshayi species, however, is marked by the preceding symptoms as well as by the eruption of pustules (Pidaká), with supervening symptoms in addition thereto. 17.

**Maśakas** (Mosquitoes) :—Mosquitoes (Mas'akas) are divided into five species, *viz.*, the Sámudra, Parimandala, Hasti-maśaka, Krishna and the Parvatiya. A mosquito (Maśaka)-bite is characterised by a severe itching and swelling of the affected locality; while the symptoms which mark a bite by a Parvatiya one are similar to those of a bite by fatally venomous insects, and a sting of the points of their antennæ is followed by the appearance of pustules (Pidaká) attended with a burning sensation and suppuration therein, when scratched by the finger-nails. The characteristic features of a bite by **Jalaukas** (leeches) with the mode of treatment thereof have already been described 18.

**Memorable Verses :**—The poisons of the Gaudheyaka, Stháliká, Svetá, Agni-samprabhá, Bhrikuti and the Kotika belonging to their respective classes are incurable. 19.

Contact with the dead body, stool or urine of a venomous animal is accompanied by itching and a burning sensation, pricking pain, eruption of Pidaká (pustules), ulcers and Kotha as well as by a slimy and painful exudation. The local skin is found to suppurate and the treatment would be the same as in the case of a wound by an envenomed arrow. 20.

A bite which is neither depressed nor raised, but very much swollen with pain (round about), but unattended with any pain in the seat itself just after the bite, should be regarded as not easily amenable to any medical remedy. 21.

A bite by an insect of strong and acute poison should be treated as a snake-bite and the three-fold remedies to be employed in snake-bites according to the three-fold divisions of snakes should also be employed in these cases. The measures of fomenting, plastering and hot-washing would prove efficacious in these cases, except in the event of an insect-bitten patient having been found to have been fainting away on account of suppuration and sloughing in the seat of the bite, in which case all kinds of cleansing (emetic, purgative, etc.) and anti-poisonous measures should be adopted. 22-23.

Plasters of S'*irisha*, *Katuka*, *Kushtha*, *Vacha*, *Rajani*, *Saindhava*, milk, marrow, lard (Vasá), clarified butter, S'*unthi*, *Pippali* and *Deva-dáru* in the form of Utkáriká (poultice-like preparation) should be used in fomenting (the seat of the bite). As an alternative, the fomentation with the drugs of the S'*ála-parnyádi* Gana in the same (Utkáriká) form should be considered equally efficacious in the case. 24.

In the case of a **Scorpion** bite, the affected part should not be fomented. It might, however, be fumigated with vapours of the drugs to be dealt with later 'on. The medicinal remedies (Agadas) applicable in the several cases are here separately described. 25-26.

**Recipes of remedies in different cases :**—An anti-venomous compound (**Agada**) consisting of *Kushtha*, *Chakra* (Tagara), *Vachá*, *Vilva*-roots, *Páthá*, *Suvarchiká*, house-soot and the two kinds of *Haridrá* is efficacious in the case of a bite by a **Trikantaka** insect. An Agada consisting of house-soot, *Rajani*, *Chakra*, *Kushtha* and the seeds of *Palás'a* destroys the poison of a **Gala-goli** insect. An Agada composed of *Kumkuma*, *Tagara*, S'*igru*, *Padmaka* and the two kinds of *Rajani*, pasted with water, proves curative in the case of a bite by a **S'ata-padi** (centipede). An Agada consisting of *Mesha-s'ringi*, *Vachá*, *Páthá*, *Nichula*, *Rohini*, and *Bálaka* is efficacious in all kinds of **Manduka**-poisoning. An Agada consisting of *Vacha*, *As'va-gandhá*, *Ati-balá*, *Balá*, *Ati-guhá* (Sála-parni) and *Aguhá* (Pris'niparni) nullifies the poison of a **Vis'vambhara** insect. An Agada consisting of *S'irisha*, *Tagara*, *Kushtha*, the two kinds of *Haridrá*, *Ams'u-mati* and the two kinds of *Sahá* destroys the poison of an **Ahinduka** insect. Cooling measures should be adopted in the night time in the case of a **Kandumaka**-bite, since the poison which is aggravated by the sun's rays in the day does not prove amenable to any remedy, if applied at that time. An Agada consisting of *Chakra*, *Kushtha* and *Apámárga* is efficacious in a case of **Suka-vrinta**-bite. As an alternative, the earth of a black ant-hill pasted with the expressed juice of *Bhringa* would prove efficacious in such cases. A plaster prepared with the earth of a black ant-hill and the urine of a cow proves curative in cases of bites of flies, ants and mosquitoes. The treatment of a case of a bite by a **Prati-suryaka** is the same as that of a snake-bite. 27-36.

**Origin and Classification of Scorpions:**—Scorpions are divided into three classe, *viz.*, the mild-poisoned ones (Manda-visha), those whose poison is neither mild nor strong (Madhya-visha), and the strong-poisoned ones (Mahá-visha). Scorpions germinating from cow-dung* or from any other rotten substances are **Manda-visha**. Those which germinate from (decomposed) wood or (decayed) bricks are **Madhya-visha** (with poison neither mild nor strong);

---

* Dallana says that by cow-dung (Gomaya) is meant the dung, the urine etc. of not only a cow, but of a buffalo, etc. as well

while those which originate from the decmposed carcase of a snake or from any other poisonous putrid organic matter are **Tikshna-visha** (strong-poisoned). The first group of scorpions includes twelve different species, the second three and the third and last fifteen, thus making thirty* species in all. 37-38.

**Specific traits and Characteristics of mild-poisoned Scorpions :**—Scorpions which are black (Krishna) or dark-brown (S'yáva) or of variegated colours (Karbura) or yellow (Pándu) or coloured like the urine of a cow or rough or dark blue (Mechaka) or white or red or greenish (S'ádvala) or red mixed with white (Rakta-s'veta)† or provided with hair on their bodies (Romas'a) should be regarded as **Manda-visha** (mild poisoned ones). A bite by a scorpion of this species is accompained by pain (in the seat of the bite), shivering, numbness of the limbs and a flow of blackish blood (from the punctures of the bite). In the case of a bite at any of the extremities, the pain courses upward, accompained by a burning sensation, perspiration, swelling of the bitten part and fever. 39

**Madhya-visha Scorpions :**—Scorpions of the **Madhya-visha** (mild-poisoned) class are red (Rakta) or yellow (Pita), or tawny (Kapila). All of them are ash-coloured in their belly and provided with three joints or links. They germinate from the stool, excreta, eggs and putrid carcases of the three (aforesaid) groups of snakes and respectively partake of the nature of the

---

\* According to Gayadása the total number of the three classes of scorpions would be twenty-seven, of which the first (mild-poisoned) class consists of eleven, the second consists of three and the third of thirteen.

† In place of "white, red and whitish red" some read "white, red and little red" (Arakta)," while others make it "white in the abdomen (S'vetodara), red and white."

serpent whose fecal matter, etc. they originate from. A bite by a scorpion of this species is accompanied by a swelling of the tongue, an incapacity of deglutition and violent epileptic fits. 40.

**Tikshna-visha Scorpions :**—The keen-poisoned (**Tikshna-visha**) scorpions are either white or parti-coloured (Chitra) or blackish (S'yámala) or reddish white (Rakta-s'veta) or red-bellied or blue-bellied or reddish or bluish yellow or reddish blue or bluish white; others are reddish brown and are (further divided into four classes), viz., three-jointed (like those of the previous class) or one-jointed or two-jointed or jointless. The poison of this group of scorpions, varying in colour and shape, is extremely dreadful and should be regarded as the veritable robber of vitality. They germinate from the putrified dead body of a snake or any poisoned animal. A bite by a member of any of these families produces those physiological transformations in the body of its victims which mark the different stages of a snake-bite, and gives rise to pustular eruptions (Sphota) on the skin accompanied by vertigo, a burning sensation (in the body), fever and excessive discharge of black-coloured blood from the channels (mouth and nostrils, etc.). And hence their bite proves so rapidly fatal. 41.

**Treatment of Scorpion-bites :**—A bite by a scorpion of the middle-venomed or strong-venomed class should be treated as a case of snake-bite to all intents and purposes. In a case of a bite by a mild-venomed one, the affected seat should be sprinkled over with the Chakra-Taila or with a tepid oil duly cooked with the drugs of the *Vidáryádi* group. The affected locality should be (repeatedly) fomented with the application of poultices in the Utkáriká form prepared with anti-venomous drugs (S'irisha, etc.). The seat of the bite should then be marked with superficial incisions (scratches) and should be gently rubbed (Prati-sárana) with powders of *Haridrá*, *Saindhava*, *Trikatu* and the fruit and flower of *S'irisha*. The tender leaves of *Surasá* pasted with the juice of *Mátulunga* and the urine of a cow in a lukewarm state, or lukewarm (i.e., fresh) cow-dung should be employed in plastering and fomenting the affected part. Potions of clarified butter mixed with honey, milk mixed with a profuse quantity of sugar and honey, treacle mixed with cold water and perfumed with *Chatur-játaka*, or cold milk mixed with treacle should be recommended as drinks. Fumigation (Dhupana) with the compound made of the feathers of the tail of a cock or a peacock, Saindhava, oil and clarified butter pasted together and burnt is a speedy destroyer of scorpion-poison. As an alternative, the fumes (Dhuma) of a compound made up of *Kusumbha* flower, the two kinds of *Rajani* and *Kodrava* straw mixed with clarified butter applied to the region of the arms speedily destroys the poison of a venomous insect in general and of a scorpion in particular. 42.

**Spider-bites :**—Cases of **Lutá** (venomous spider)-bite (lit.—poison of a Lutá) are the most difficult to diagnose and cure. The diagnosis of such a case puzzles the head of many an experienced physician, while novices in the art of healing find it a very difficult matter. In a case of doubt or of conflicting indications pointing equally both to the venomous and non-venomous character of the bite, a physician should employ anti-poisonous remedies of such a character as would not prove hostile (to the natural temperament and vital principles of the patient's system nor to the course of food and drink he is enjoined to take or naturally takes), since the Agadas are applicable only in cases of poisoning and, applied otherwise in healthy non-poisoned persons, would produce all kinds of discomfort. Hence it is incumbent on a physician to gather conclusive evidence of the poisonous nature of the bite at the very outset. A physician, failing to ascertion the existence of poison, proves more fatal in many cases than the bite itself. 43.

**Development of Lutá-poison :**—As the first sprouting of a tree does not enable a man to correctly ascertan the species, so the poison of a venomous spider in its first stage of incubation into the body, does not develop any specific symptoms sufficiently potent to throw any light on its nature, nor does it give any hint as to its correct diagonosis. A spider (Luta)-poison latent in a human organism, is marked by a slight itching sensation in the seat of the bite, as if the poison were shifting from one place to another\* in that locality, by the presence of Kotha (urticaria), and by an indistinctness of colour on the first day of its incubation. On the second day the seat of the bite becomes swollen at the end and sunk in the middle and the characteristic marks of biting show themselves. On the third day the specific symptoms (fever, shivering, etc.) of the poison of the animal set in. On the fourth day the poison is aggravated. On the fifth day the symptoms and disorders peculiar to its aggravated condition are present. On the sixth day the poison begins to course through the organism and envolopes the Marmas (or the vulnerable parts). On the seventh day

---

\* In place of "Prachala" Gayadása reads "Prabala," *i.e.*, strong and says that the poison becomes stronger and stronger with the lapse of time.

the poison is diffused throughout the whole organism, becomes extremely aggravated and proves fatal. 44.

**Potency :**—The poison of spiders (Lutâ) which are acutely and violently venomous proves fatal in the course of a week. That of a middle-poisonous one would take a little more time in order to prove fatal, while a bite by one of the mild-poisonous brings death within a fortnight. Hence a physician should try his best with anti-venomous remedies for the complete nullification of the poison immediately after the bite. 45.

**Location :**—A spider is found to secrete seven kinds of poison through the seven different parts or principles of its body, *viz.*, saliva (Lálá), nails (claws), urine, fangs, ovum (Rajas), fecal matter and semen, and such poison is either keen or mild in its potency, or follows a middle path between the two (keen and mild). 46.

**Characteristics of poison according to its seat in the body of a spider :**—The poison which is secreted with the **saliva** (of a spider) gives rise to non-shiftting superficial Kotha (urticaria) attended with itching and slight pain. The poison from a scratch with the tips of its **claws**, is attended with swelling, itching, horripilation and a sense as if fumes had been escaping from the body. Any part of the body coming in contact with the **urine** of a spider is marked by a (slight) blackness of skin in the middle of the point of contact and redness at its edge, and the affected part is cracked. In a case of **fang**-poison (actual bite) the seat of the bite is marked by fixed circular patches and becomes indurated and discoloured. The poison in this case is strong. A part of the body touched with the **Rajas, semen,** or with **fecal matter** of a (venomous) spider is marked by eruptions of pustules which assume a yellow colour like that of a ripe Ámalaka or Pilu. 47.

Thus far we have described the effects of spider-(Lutâ)-poison according to its seat in the body of the insect and to the period of its aggravation. Now we shall describe the mythological accouut of the origin of these insects and the curable and incurable natures of their bites together with the course of medical treatment to be followed in each case. 48.

**Mythological account of the origin of Lutá :**—Once upon a time, it is said, king Visvámitra went to the hermitage of the holy Vasishtha and by his actions aroused the wrath of the holy sage. Drops of perspiration were thereupon produced on the forehead of that holy and celestially brilliant sage and trickled down on the stacks of hay culled and gathered (Luna) by the holy sages for the use of the (celestial) cow, and behold ! they (the drops of sweat) were transformed into innumerable dreadful and venomous spiders (**Lutá**) which, up to this day, are found to infest the articles of royal use for the iniquity of that royal sage (Vis'vámitra). They are called **Lutás** (spiders) from the fact of their being germinated from the drops of perspiration of the holy sage Vas'ishtha fallen on the culled (Luna) stacks of hay and they are sixteen in number. 49.

**The different names of spiders and the general symptoms of their bites :—** The poison of spiders is divided into two classes—curable with difficulty and incurable. Of the sixteen kinds of spiders, the bites or poisons of eight may be cured with the greatest difficulty, while those of the remaining eight are incurable. The Tri-mandalá, Svetá, Kapilá, Pitiká, Ála-vishá, Mutra-vishá, Raktá and the Kasaná are the **eight** species of spiders which belong to the first group. A bite by any of them is attended with an aching pain in the head, pain and itching about the seat of the bite and the symptoms and disorders peculiar to the aggravated Váyu and Kapha. The Sauvarniká, Lája-varná, Jálini, Eni-padi, Krishna-varná, Agni varná, Kákándá and the Málá-guná belong to the second group and their bites are marked by bleeding, fever, a burning sensation, dysentery and disorders due to the concerted action of all the three deranged Doshas of the body, and the bitten part putrefies. Eruptions of various sorts and pustules and large circular patches as well as large, soft and shifting swellings, red or brown in colour, appear on the skin about the affected part. These are the general features of spider (Lutá)-bites. Now we shall describe the characteristic symptoms which are developed by bites of the several classes of spiders and the course of medical treatment to be adopted in each case. 50-51.

**Specific symptoms of spider-bites and their treatment :**—A bite by a spider of the **Tri-mandalá** species is marked by a flow of black-coloured blood from the bite which is transformed into an open ulcer. It is also attended with deafness, impaired or cloudy vision and a burning sensation in the eyes. In such cases, a compound consisting of *Arka* roots, *Rajani*, *Nákuli* and *Pris'ni-parniká* should be employed as snuff as well as in drink (Pána), enemas (Vastis) and ointments etc. A bite by a spider of the **S'vetá** species is followed by the eruption of white-coloured pustules attended with itching, burning sensation, epileptic fits, fever, erysipelas and pain in and secretion from the bite. An Agada consisting of *Chandana, Rásná, Elá, Harenu, Nala, Vanjula, Kushtha,*

*Lámájjaka, Chakra* and *Nalada* is efficacious in such a case. A bite by a **Kapilá** spider is characterised by eruptions of copper-coloured pustules of an indurated nature accompanied by a sense of heaviness in the head, a burning sensation, vertigo and darkness of vision (Timira). The remedy in such a case consists of an anti-poisonous Agada composed of *Padmaka, Kushtha, Elá, Karanja, Kakubha*-bark, *S'thirá, Arkaparni, Apámárga, Durvá* and *Bráhmi*. A case of bite by a **Pitiká** spider is marked by an eruption of hard pustules, vomiting, fever, colic (Śula) and redness of the eyes, and the remedy consists in the application of an Agada, composed of *Kutaja, Us'ira, Kinihi, S'elu, Kadamba* and *Kakubha*-bark. A case of bite by an **Ála-vishá** spider is marked by the bright red colour of the seat of the bite, eruption of pustules like mustard seeds, parchedness of the palate and a burning sensation in the body. The remedy in such a case should consist of an Agada composed of *Priyangu, Hrivera, Kushtha, Lámajja, Vanjula, S'ata-pushpá* and the sprouts of the *Pippala* and the *Vata* trees. The case of bite by a spider of the **Mutra-vishá** class is attended with putrefaction (of the affected locality), erysipelas, a flow of blackish blood (from the seat of the bite), cough, difficult breathing, vomiting, epileptic fits, fever and a burning sensation. The remedy in such a case consists in *Manah-s'ilá, Ála, Yashti-madhu, Kushtha, Chandana, Padmaka* and *Lámajja* pasted together and mixed with honey. The case of bite by a spider of the **Raktá** species is marked by eruptions of yellow-coloured pustules full of blood and coloured red in the extremities (round the seat of the bite), with a burning sensation and slimy secretion. The Agada in such a case should be prepared with *Toya* (Bálaka) *Chandana, Us'ira,*

*Padmaka* and the bark of *Arjuna, S'elu* and *Amrátaka*. A bite by a spider of the **Kasaná** class is attended with a flow of slimy cold blood (from the bite), and with cough and difficult breathing, the treatment being the same as in the case of a bite by a spider of the Ratká class. 52-59.

A bite by a spider (Lutá) of the **Krishná** class smells of fecal matter and is attended with a scanty flow of blood, as well as with fever, epileptic fits, vomiting, burning sensation, cough and difficult breathing. The treatment of such a patient should be taken in hand without holding out any definite hope of recovery and the remedy in this case should consist of an Agada composed of *Elá, Chakra, sarpákshi, Gandha-nákuli, Chandana* and the drugs known as the *Mahá-sugandhi* (as described in the Dundubhi-svaniya chapter). The case of bite by an **Agni-varná** spider is marked by a burning sensation in the seat of the bite, excessive secretion (of blood), fever, a sort of sucking pain, itching, horripilation, a burning sensation in the body and eruptions of pustules. In a case of this type, the patient may be treated with the Agada prescribed for the treatment of a bite by a spider of the Krishná class but no hopes should be held out. 60-61.

**General Remedies:**—An Agada made of *Sárivá, Us'ira, Yashti-madhu, Chandana, Utpala* and *Padmaka* may be used with advantage in cases of spider-bites of all types. The bark of *S'leshmátaka* and *Kshira-pippala* should be deemed equally efficacious in all cases of spider-bites, and these may be employed in any shape, viz., as snuff, potion, unguent, etc. 62.

We have described (the symptoms and the treatment of the bites of) the eight classes of spiders which can be cured with difficulty. Those of the two classes (of the other group whose bites are generally incurable) have also been described above, as being sometimes found amenable to medicine (with the greatest difficulty). Now hear me describe (the symptoms and the treatment of the bites of) the remaining six species which are incurable. 63. A.

**Specific Symptoms of the incurable cases of Spider-bites :**—A bite by a spider of the **Sauvarniká** species is marked by swelling and a frothy secretion and a fishy smell from the seat of the bite, and is followed by cough, difficult breathing, fever, thirst and violent fainting fits. A bite by a **Lája-varná** spider is marked by a flow of flesh-smelling and fetid blood from its seat as well as by a burning sensation, dysentery, fainting fits and pain in the head. A case of bite by a spider of the **Jálini** species is very severe and is marked by a cracking of the seat of the bite which is striped with lines as well as by numbness, difficult breathing, parchedness of the palate and continued dizziness of the head. The bite by an **Eni-padi** spider resembles the seeds of black sesamum in shape and is marked by thirst, fever, fainting fits, vomiting, cough and difficult breathing. A bite by a **Kákándaká** spider is marked by an excruciating pain and a reddish-yellow colour at its seat. A bite by a **Málá-guná** spider is characterised by a cracking of the seat of the bite in several parts and is marked by a red colour, smoky smell, extreme pain, fever and epileptic fits. 63.

Treatment of the incurable cases of spider-bites should, however, be taken in hand by a wise physician with a due consideration of the aggravated Dosha or Doshas in each case with the exception of making incisions (chheda-karma). 64. A.

**Surgical Treatments :**—In all cases of the curable types of spider-bites, the affected part should at once be cut open and removed with a Vriddhi-patra instrument and the incisioned part should then be cauterised with a red-hot Jambvoshtha instrument in the absence of any fever or such like distressing symptoms and in the event of its not occurring in any of the vulnable parts of the body (Marmas). The act of cauterisation should be continued until the patient himself (through pain) prohibits the continuation of the same. If the affected part is found to be attended with a slight swelling, it should be cut open and removed. It should then be plastered with a paste of the (Mahá-sugandhi and such other) Agada mixed with *Saindhava* and honey or with the paste of *Priyengu, Haridrá, Kushtha, Samangá* and *Yashti-madhu*. A potion composed of the decoction of *Sárivá*, the two kinds of *Yashti-madhu,*\* *Drákshá, Payasyá, Kshira-morata, Vidári* and *Gokshura* mixed with honey should be administered to the patient. The affected part should be washed with a cold decoction of the bark of the *Kshiri-vrikshas*. Any other distressing symptoms should be remedied with anti-poisonous measures with an eye to the deranged Doshas involved in the case. 64.

Any of the (ten-fold) remedial measures of Nasya (snuff), medicated collyrium, unguents (Abhyanjana), potions (Pána) Dhuma (fumigation), Avapida form of snuff, gargling, emesis, purging and blood-letting by the application of leeches should be adopted in a case of spider-bite according to its requirements. 65.

---

\* Mention of Madhuka twice in the list shows that one part each of both the kinds Vashti-madhu (liquorice)—grown on lands and in water—should be taken.

All cases of bites by any insect or by any snake, and ulcers incidental to those bites should be carefully treated with measures and remedies laid down in connection with snake-bites as long as the stage of inflammation and suppuration would last. The growths (if any) of pappillæ (Karniká) around the seat of the bite should be removed after the subsidence of the swelling by the application of a plaster consisting of *Nimba* leaves,\* *Trivrit, Danti, Kusumbha* flower, *Rajini*, honey, *Guggulu, Saindhava* salt, *Kinva* and the dung of a pigeon pasted together, and such diet as would not aggravate the effects of poison should be carefully prescribed. The papillatous growths (Karniká) due to the poison of any kind should be scratched with a proper surgical instrument in the event of their being hard and painless and should then be plastered with a paste of purifying (Sodhaniya) drugs (such as Nimba leaves, etc.) mixed with honey. 66.

The specific features and treatment of the bites by the one hundred and sixty-seven types of insect are now described. The subjects mentioned but not included within these one hundred and twenty chapters (from the commencement of the book) would be dealt with in detail in the latter part of the present treatise (Uttara Tantara). 67 68

We have not heard of a holier discourse than the medical science on account of the eternal and imperishable character of the Áyurveda (the science of life) from its tested merit and its beneficial effects upon the created beings and since it is always worshipped by the whole human race for the fact of its fully explaining

\* Gayadása reads "S'ikhi" (Lángalaki) and "Vams'a" (scrapings of bamboo) in place of "Nimba-patra". He also reads "Danta" (tooth of a cow) in place of "Kinva."

the import of words (*i.e.* delineation of its specific subjects). Who ever stores up in his memory and acts up to these sacred and worshipful injunctions on the science of life propounded, as it is, by the nectar-origined sage (Dhanvantari), the preceptor of all physicians and equal to the celestial Indra in respect of majesty, enjoys happiness both in this world and in the next. 69.

Thus ends the eighth Chapter of the Kalpasthána in the Sus'ruta Samhitá which treats of the measures to be adopted in the case of an insect-bite.

## Here ends the Kalpa Sthána.

**UNIVERSITY OF CALIFORNIA LIBRARY**
Los Angeles
This book is DUE on the last date stamped below.

AUG 26 1999

DUE 2 WKS FROM DATE RECEIVED

MAY 19 2000

CPSIA information can be obtained
at www.ICGtesting.com
Printed in the USA
BVHW081701040119
537058BV00007B/98/P